Pathological Basis of Veterinary Diseases

Pathological Basis of Veterinary Diseases

Edited by Anthony Burton

MURPHY & MOORE
www.murphy-moorepublishing.com

Published by Murphy & Moore Publishing,
1 Rockefeller Plaza,
New York City, NY 10020, USA
www.murphy-moorepublishing.com

Pathological Basis of Veterinary Diseases
Edited by Anthony Burton

International Standard Book Number: 978-1-63987-422-4 (Hardback)

Cataloging-in-Publication Data

Pathological basis of veterinary diseases / edited by Anthony Burton.
p. cm.
Includes bibliographical references and index.
ISBN 978-1-63987-422-4
1. Veterinary pathology. 2. Pathology. 3. Veterinary medicine. I. Burton, Anthony.
SF769 .P38 2022
636.089 607--dc23

TABLE OF CONTENTS

PREFACE

Veterinary disease refer to an impairment that leads to a modification in the vital functions of animals. These diseases are an important area of study as they affect the economy and may transmit the causative agents to the humans. There are several reasons which have been cited for the spread of diseases, like poor sanitation, nutritional defects, pathogenic defects, improper management, etc. Pathogenic defects include certain organisms that produce toxins and harmful elements that upset the metabolic activity of animals. Viruses and bacteria are the most common disease-causing agents. They are microscopic and multiply rapidly under favorable conditions. Other pathogenic causative agents include fungi and protozoans. These pathogens live inside or outside the animal's body and alter vital functions by suppressing their immune system. This book unfolds the innovative aspects of pathological basis of veterinary disease which will be crucial for the progress of this field in the future. It will also provide interesting topics for research which interested readers can take up. Scientists and students actively engaged in this field will find this book full of crucial and unexplored concepts.

After months of intensive research and writing, this book is the end result of all who devoted their time and efforts in the initiation and progress of this book. It will surely be a source of reference in enhancing the required knowledge of the new developments in the area. During the course of developing this book, certain measures such as accuracy, authenticity and research focused analytical studies were given preference in order to produce a comprehensive book in the area of study.

This book would not have been possible without the efforts of the authors and the publisher. I extend my sincere thanks to them. Secondly, I express my gratitude to my family and well-wishers. And most importantly, I thank my students for constantly expressing their willingness and curiosity in enhancing their knowledge in the field, which encourages me to take up further research projects for the advancement of the area.

Editor

1

Inflammatory profiles in canine intervertebral disc degeneration

Nicole Willems[1], Anna R. Tellegen[1], Niklas Bergknut[1], Laura B. Creemers[2], Jeannette Wolfswinkel[1], Christian Freudigmann[3], Karin Benz[3], Guy C. M. Grinwis[4], Marianna A. Tryfonidou[1*] and Björn P. Meij[1]

Abstract

Background: Intervertebral disc (IVD) disease is a common spinal disorder in dogs and degeneration and inflammation are significant components of the pathological cascade. Only limited studies have studied the cytokine and chemokine profiles in IVD degeneration in dogs, and mainly focused on gene expression. A better understanding is needed in order to develop biological therapies that address both pain and degeneration in IVD disease. Therefore, in this study, we determined the levels of prostaglandin E2 (PGE_2), cytokines, chemokines, and matrix components in IVDs from chondrodystrophic (CD) and non-chondrodystrophic (NCD) dogs with and without clinical signs of IVD disease, and correlated these to degeneration grade (according to Pfirrmann), or herniation type (according to Hansen). In addition, we investigated cyclooxygenase 2 (COX-2) expression and signs of inflammation in histological IVD samples of CD and NCD dogs.

Results: PGE_2 levels were significantly higher in the nucleus pulposus (NP) of degenerated IVDs compared with non-degenerated IVDs, and in herniated IVDs from NCD dogs compared with non-herniated IVDs of NCD dogs. COX-2 expression in the NP and annulus fibrosus (AF), and proliferation of fibroblasts and numbers of macrophages in the AF significantly increased with increased degeneration grade. GAG content did not significantly change with degeneration grade or herniation type. Cytokines interleukin (IL)-2, IL-6, IL-7, IL-8, IL-10, IL-15, IL-18, immune protein (IP)-10, tumor necrosis factor (TNF)-α, and granulocyte macrophage colony-stimulating factor (GM-CSF) were not detectable in the samples. Chemokine (C-C) motif ligand (CCL)2 levels in the NP from extruded samples were significantly higher compared with the AF of these samples and the NP from protrusion samples.

Conclusions: PGE_2 levels and CCL2 levels in degenerated and herniated IVDs were significantly higher compared with non-degenerated and non-herniated IVDs. COX-2 expression in the NP and AF and reactive changes in the AF increased with advancing degeneration stages. Although macrophages invaded the AF as degeneration progressed, the production of inflammatory mediators seemed most pronounced in degenerated NP tissue. Future studies are needed to investigate if inhibition of PGE_2 levels in degenerated IVDs provides effective analgesia and exerts a protective role in the process of IVD degeneration and the development of IVD disease.

Keywords: Low back pain, Dog, PGE_2, Prostaglandin, Herniation, Chondrodystrophic, Non-chondrodystrophic

Background

Intervertebral disc (IVD) disease is a common spinal disorder in dogs and humans and is characterized by clinical signs ranging from back pain to neurological deficits. IVD disease is preceded by IVD degeneration with a similar etiopathogenesis in dogs and humans [1]. Chondrodystrophic (CD) dogs are predisposed to explosive extrusion of the nucleus pulposus (NP) (Hansen type I) of degenerated thoracolumbar and cervical IVDs, mainly between 3 and 7 years of age. Non-chondrodystrophic (NCD) dogs are predisposed to protrusion of the annulus fibrosus (AF) (Hansen type II) of degenerated lumbosacral and caudal cervical IVDs at 6 to 8 years of age, and NP extrusion of degenerated thoracolumbar IVDs [2–5]. Hansen type II annular protrusion does occur in CD dogs, but less commonly [6, 7].

The onset of IVD degeneration at a cellular level is characterized by a gradual replacement of notochordal

* Correspondence: m.a.tryfonidou@uu.nl
[1]Department of Clinical Sciences of Companion Animals, Faculty of Veterinary Medicine, 3584 CM Utrecht, The Netherlands
Full list of author information is available at the end of the article

cells by chondrocyte-like cells in the NP. In this respect, the NP of CD dogs contains primarily chondrocyte-like cells already by one year of age, while notochordal cells remain the predominant cell type in the NP of NCD dogs during their lifetime. In the latter, notochordal cells in some IVDs are substituted and degeneration occurs at a much later age [1, 8, 9]. In both types of dogs, a decrease in proteoglycan content, a shift in collagen type II to collagen type I in the extracellular matrix of the NP, together with a disruption of the lamellae in the annulus fibrosus (AF) is seen during IVD degeneration [10, 11]. Furthermore, in degenerated discs, nerve endings extend into the deeper layers of the AF and into the NP, in contrast to healthy discs, in which only the outer third of the AF is innervated. Stimulation of nociceptors in the AF and dorsal longitudinal ligament is related to pain [12, 13]. A nociceptive response can either be evoked by a mechanical or inflammatory stimulus. Various inflammatory mediators have also been suggested to play a role in the catabolic processes in human NP and AF tissue, including prostaglandin E_2 (PGE_2), interleukins (IL-1α, IL-1β IL-6, IL-8), and tumor necrosis factor α (TNF-α) [14–16]. In NP cells from experimental CD dogs with surgically induced IVD degeneration increased levels of TNF-α and IL-1β were shown in vitro [17]. While knowledge of the involvement of inflammatory mediators in human IVD degeneration has substantially increased over the last years [14–16, 18–34], only limited studies have focused on cytokine and chemokine profiles in IVD degeneration in dogs, and mainly focused on gene expression [17, 35, 36].

PGE_2 is the most common prostanoid and plays an important regulatory role in physiological as well as pathological processes. It is synthesized by two cyclooxygenase (COX) isoforms, COX-1 and COX-2, by conversion of arachidonic acid into prostaglandin H_2 (PGH_2) and isomerization of PGH_2 to PGE_2 by prostaglandin E synthases. COX-2 expression is highly restricted under physiological conditions, but can be rapidly induced in response to inflammatory stimuli and is therefore believed to play an important role in the PGE_2 production involved in degenerative processes [27, 37]. Current therapies of IVD disease aim at alleviating pain by administration of corticosteroids, non-steroidal anti-inflammatory drugs (NSAIDs), and/or opioids, by physical therapy, or by surgery. Among the numerous NSAIDs available, oral selective COX-2 inhibitors are primarily used for managing clinical signs, as they reduce inflammation and relieve pain, but cause less gastrointestinal side effects [38, 39]. Delivery of COX-2 inhibitors directly into the avascular IVD has been suggested as an alternative route of administration to enhance the local efficacy and to minimalize systemic side effects. A recent study in experimental CD dogs has shown the biocompatibility and safety of intradiscal injection of a hydrogel loaded with a selective COX-2 inhibitor [40]. As PGE_2 is one of the inflammatory mediators in human IVD herniation that has been shown to sensitize nerves and induce pain, the efficacy of intradiscal delivery of NSAIDs is likely to be limited to IVD disease with a clear inflammatory profile [41]. We hypothesize that PGE_2 levels are higher in degenerated and herniated (protruded or extruded) IVDs of CD and NCD dogs compared with non-degenerated or non-herniated IVDs. Therefore, we determined the levels of PGE_2, cytokines, chemokines, and matrix components in IVDs from CD and NCD dogs with and without clinical signs of IVD disease and correlated these to degeneration grade or herniation type. In addition, we investigated COX-2 expression in histological IVD samples of CD and NCD dogs.

Methods

Collection and preparation of samples for biochemical analyses

IVDs collected post-mortem

A total of 19 IVDs, with a Thompson grade I and II, were collected from 7 laboratory (3 CD, 4 NCD) dogs that were euthanized in unrelated animal experiments (experiment numbers: DEC 2007.III.08.110, DEC 2009.III.06.050),and a total of 34 samples, with a Pfirrmann grade II, were collected from 15 laboratory (CD) dogs from previous animal experiments (DEC 2012.III.05.046, DEC 2013.III.02.017). All animal experiments were approved by the Ethics Committee of Animal Experiments (DEC) of Utrecht University. None of the dogs had a history of clinical signs of IVD disease. NP and AF tissues were isolated from the spine and collected separately, snap frozen in liquid nitrogen, and stored at −80 °C until further analysis.

IVDs collected during surgical treatment

A total of 123 IVDs were collected from 76 client-owned dogs that were referred to the University Clinic for Companion Animals in Utrecht with IVD disease that required surgical intervention. The diagnosis of IVD disease was confirmed on MRI or CT. Dogs were classified as CD and NCD and divided into subgroups, based on the Pfirrmann grade on T2-weighted MR images [42, 43]. In 10 samples of 6 dogs, in which no MRI was available, grading of the IVD was performed on CT images [43]. The medical history and records of the dogs were screened for information on prior medical treatment of IVD disease and the duration of this treatment.

Diagnostic imaging

Diagnostic imaging was performed in fully anesthetized client-owned dogs, according to standard practice. MRI images were obtained with a 0.2 Tesla open MRI system (Magnetom Open Viva, Siemens AG, Erlangen, Germany) by using multipurpose flex coils until 2013, and thereafter with a 1.5 Tesla scanner (Ingenia, Philips Healthcare, Best, The Netherlands) by using a small-extremity or a posterior coil. For each examination a coil was chosen that fitted around the body of the patient as closely as possible. Sagittal T2-weighted (T2W) images were acquired using a turbo-spin echo pulse sequence with the following parameters: repetition time = 2500–3048 ms, echo time = 110–120 ms, field of view = 50 x 160/160 x 350 mm, acquisition matrix = 100 x 256/200 x 235 mm, voxel size = 0.6 x 0.8/0.8 x 1.03 mm slice thickness = 2 – 2.5 mm. CT images were obtained with a third-generation single-slice helical CT-scanner (Philips Secura). Contiguous 2 mm thick slices with 1 mm overlap were obtained with exposure settings of 120 kV and 260 mA.

Surgical treatment

Client-owned dogs were anesthetized according to standard of care. Collection of IVDs was achieved through standard surgical procedures, depending on the location of disc herniation: ventral decompression in the cervical area, dorsolateral hemilaminectomy in the thoracolumbar area, and dorsal laminectomy in the lumbosacral area. In dogs with nuclear extrusion (Hansen type I), free NP material was collected from the epidural space in the spinal canal, and AF material was collected during ventral fenestration preceding the ventral decompression for cervical disc herniations, or when an additional lateral fenestration was performed after hemilaminectomy for thoracolumbar disc herniations. In dogs with lumbosacral annular protrusion (Hansen type II), partial discectomy consisting of annulotomy and nucleotomy, allowed separate collection of NP and/or AF tissue. In 3 dogs, an adjacent IVD was fenestrated, and AF and/or NP material was collected. The treatment decision (discectomy, nucleotomy, fenestration) was taken during surgery and depended on the state of the AF and the position of the NP. Each surgeon documented the type of herniation (NP extrusion (Hansen type I) or AF protrusion (Hansen type II)) and type of collected material (NP or AF) in the surgical report.

NP and/or AF tissues were collected in separate vials during surgery, snap frozen into liquid nitrogen within minutes after collection, and subsequently stored at −80 °C until further analysis. Details of the samples are shown in Table 1 and in Additional file 1.

Biochemical analyses of IVDs collected post-mortem and intra-operatively

Prior to analyses, samples were weighed, and 400 µl and 750 µl lysis buffer (cOmplete lysis M EDTA buffer, Roche diagnostics Nederland B.V., Almere, The Netherlands) was added to NP and AF tissue, respectively. Tissues were lysed in a TissueLyser II (Qiagen, Venlo, The Netherlands) for 2x 60 s at 20 kHz. After centrifugation for 15 min at 14.000 g, the volume of the supernatant of each sample was measured and separated from its pellet. A volume of 80 µl was filtered over a 0.22 µm nylon spin-X centrifuge tube filter (8169, Costar, Corning Incorporated, NY, USA) and stored at −80 °C in aliquots for cytokine measurements.

Glycosaminoglycan and DNA assays To determine GAG and DNA, supernatants and pellets were digested in a papain buffer (250 µg/ml papain (P3125-100 mg, Sigma-Aldrich) + 1.57 mg cysteine HCL (C7880, Sigma-Aldrich)) at 60 °C overnight. The 1.9-dimethylmethylene blue (DMMB) assay was used to determine GAG content [44]. A volume of 16 mg DMMB (341088 Sigma-Aldrich) was added to 5 ml 100 % ethanol and incubated overnight on a roller bench. A solution of 2.37 g NaCl and 3.04 g glycine in 1 l distilled water with a pH set at 3.00 was sterilized by using a 0.22 µm syringe filter (SLGSV255F Millex-GS Syringe Filter Unit, Merck Millipore, Darmstadt, Germany), added to the DMMB solution, and stored at 4 °C, protected from light. Pellets were diluted 1:1000 and supernatants 1:150 in PBS-EDTA. A volume of 100 µl of the dilutions and standards was pipetted into a 96-wells microplate (655199 PS microplate, Greiner Bio-One, Alphen aan den Rijn, Netherlands), and prior to spectrophotometric analysis, 200 µl of DMMB was added to each well. The ratio of absorption at 540 to 595 nm was measured by using a microplate reader (Multimode detector DTX 880, Beckman Coulter). Chondroitin sulphate from shark cartilage (C4384, Sigma-Aldrich) was used as a standard to calculate GAG concentrations. The Quant-iT™ dsDNA Broad-Range assay kit in combination with a Qubit Fluorometer (Invitrogen, Carlsbad, USA) was used according to the manufacturer's protocol to determine the DNA content.

PGE_2, and cytokine assays PGE_2 levels were determined in the supernatants by using a colorimetric competitive enzyme immunoassay kit (PGE_2 high sensitivity EIA kit, ENZO Life Sciences BVBA, Antwerp, Belgium). A magnetic canine cytokine bead panel based on Luminex® xMAP® technology (#CCYTOMAG-90 K/CCYTOMAG-90 K-PX13); Milliplex® MAP kit, Millipore Corporation, Billerica, USA) was used to measure twelve different cytokines and chemokines in supernatants: TNF-α, granulocyte-macrophage colony-stimulating factor (GM-CSF), IL-2, IL-6, IL-7, IL-8, IL-10, IL-15, IL-18, chemokine (C-C motif) ligand 2 (CCL2), chemokine (C-X-C motif) ligand 1 (CXCL1), chemokine (C-X-C motif) ligand 10 (CXCL10). Supernatants were diluted 1:2 and were measured according to the manufacturer's instructions. All biochemical values were corrected for weight of the sample.

Table 1 Sample classification details

Samples biochemistry					Samples histopathology		
# Dogs	CD dogs		NCD dogs		# Dogs	CD dogs	NCD dogs
	58		40			15	10
Age – median	5 years		2 years		Age – median (range(yrs))	10 year	7 years
(range(mths – yrs))	(1–11)		(8–12)			(2–10)	(1–10)
Spinal location	NP	AF	NP	AF	Spinal location		
# IVDs	35	30	36	41	# IVDs	19	18
Cervical (C1 – T1)	13	21	10	16	Cervical (C1 – T1)	ND	ND
Thoracolumbar (T1 – L1)	21	12	2	ND	Thoracolumbar (T1 – L1)	5	8
Lumbar (L1 – S1)	11	7	23	25	Lumbar (L1 – S1)	14	10
Unknown	7	7	1	ND	Unknown	ND	ND
Degeneration					Degeneration		
Grade 1 (non-surgical)	ND	ND	9[a]	10[a]	Grade 1	2	8
Grade 2	32[b]	32[c]	9	9	Grade 2	4	7
Grade 3	7	6	8	8	Grade 3	3	3
Grade 4 + 5	13[d]	9[d]	10	12 + 2	Grade 4 + 5	3 + 3	3
Displacement					Displacement		
NP in situ (non-surgical)	27[b,c]	27[b,c]	9[a]	10[a]	NP in situ	ND	
Nuclear extrusion	24	18	12	7	Nuclear extrusion	ND	
Annular protrusion	1	2	15	24	Annular protrusion	ND	
Treatment					Treatment		
No treatment	9	9	14	20	No treatment	ND	
Treatment	24	21	20	20			
NSAID < 1 wk	7	8	7	4	NSAID < 1 wk	ND	
NSAID > 1 wk	6	7	8	9	NSAID > 1 wk	ND	
Steroids < 1 wk	4	2	1	ND	Steroids < 1 wk	ND	
Steroids > 1 wk	4	3	2	2	Steroids > 1 wk	ND	
Other medication	3	1	2	5	Other medication	ND	
Unknown	2	ND	2	1	Unknown	ND	

[a]Samples collected from experimental dogs
[b]9 samples collected from experimental dogs (non-surgical); 17 samples collected in a previous study [40]
[c]4 samples collected from experimental dogs (non-surgical); 17 samples collected in a previous study [40]
[d]1 sample collected via fenestration
[e]Samples collected from experimental dogs;17 samples collected in a previous study [40]

Collection of post-mortem IVDs for histology

IVDs collected post-mortem

Post-mortem, 37 IVDs were collected from vertebral columns of 16 client-owned dogs that were euthanized for diseases other than IVD disease and submitted for necropsy to the Department of Pathobiology at the Faculty of Veterinary Medicine, Utrecht University, and from 9 experimental dogs in unrelated cardiovascular experiments (DEC 2007.II.01.029, DEC 2011.07.065). Permission to collect material from the client-owned dogs was granted by the owners. None of the dogs had a reported history of back problems. Details of the dogs of which material was collected for histology are shown in Table 1.

Diagnostic imaging

Within 24 h after euthanasia or death, the vertebral column (T11 – S1) was harvested by using an electric multipurpose saw (Bosch, Stuttgart, Germany). Within 1 h after dissection, sagittal T2W MR images were obtained with a 0.2 Tesla open MRI system (Magnetom Open Viva, Siemens AG) as described earlier. All lumbar IVDs were graded on midsagittal T2W images according to the Pfirrmann score by two independent investigators (NW, AT) [42].

Histology and immunohistochemistry

After scanning, all muscles were removed and the vertebrae were transected transversely with a band saw

(EXAKT tape saw, EXAKT Advanced Technologies GmbH, Norderstedt, Germany), resulting in spinal units (endplate – IVD – endplate). These units were then transected sagittally into two halves by using a diamond band pathology saw (EXAKT 312 saw; EXAKT diamond cutting band 0.1 mm D64; EXAKT Advanced Technologies GmbH, Norderstedt, Germany). Midsagittal slices (3 – 4 mm) were cut from one half and fixed in 4 % neutral buffered formaldehyde and decalcified in EDTA. Samples were dehydrated in graded alcohol series, rinsed in xylene, and embedded in paraffin. Sections (5 μm) were cut, deparaffinized and rehydrated, and stained with both hematoxylin (109249, Merck)/eosin (115935, Merck), and with picrosirius red (saturated aqueous picric acid: 36011, Sigma-Aldrich, sirius red: 8015, Klinipath)/alcian blue (alcian blue: 05500, Sigma-Aldrich; glacial acetic acid: 100063, Merck). Histological sections were assessed for the presence of inflammatory cells, and evaluated according to a histological grading scheme described by Bergknut et al. [45].

Immunohistochemistry for COX-2 was performed on 5 μm sections mounted on KP plus glass slides (Klinipath B.V., Duiven, The Netherlands). After deparaffinization and rehydration sections were treated with Dual Endogenous Enzyme Block (S2003, Dako, California, USA) for 10 min at room temperature to block nonspecific endogenous peroxidase, followed by 2 washing steps of each 5 min with tris buffered saline containing 1 % Tween 20® (TBS-T). Sections were treated with TBS bovine serum albumin (BSA) 5 % solution to block nonspecific binding for 60 min at room temperature. Subsequently they were incubated with a primary mouse anti-human monoclonal COX-2 antibody (#160112 Clone CX229, Cayman, Ann Arbor, USA) diluted 1:800 in TBS-BSA 5 % overnight at 4 °C. The following day sections were incubated with peroxidase-labelled polymer (K4007; Envision anti-mouse, Dako) and antibody binding was visualized by using diaminobenzidine (DAB; K4007; Dako). Sections were counterstained with hematoxylin solution (Hematoxylin QS, Vector, Peterborough, UK), rehydrated and mounted in permanent mounting medium. The percentage of COX-2 positive chondrocytes in the NP, and in the dorsal AF (DAF) was determined by manual counting by a blinded independent investigator (AT).

Statistical analyses

Data were analyzed by using R statistical software, package 2.15.2 (http://www.r-project.org/). A multiple linear regression model was used to analyze the effect of multiple explanatory variables on corrected PGE_2, GAG, and DNA levels for the wet weight of the tissues. Furthermore, in order to be able to compare this study with previous reports [40], PGE_2 levels were also corrected for DNA content. Data were logarithmically transformed to achieve normality. Two separate models were employed to investigate the association of explanatory variables 'grade' (Pfirrmann grade I – IV) and 'herniation' (NP in situ, NP extrusion, AF protrusion) with inflammatory parameters. Variables incorporated into both models were 'dog' (CD, NCD), 'tissue' (NP and AF), 'treatment' (no treatment, NSAID administered less than (<) 1 wk, NSAID administered more than (>) 1 wk, corticosteroids (cort) < 1 wk, cort > 1 wk, other) and their interaction. Residual plots and quantile-quantile (QQ)-plots were used to check the critical assumptions of linearity, equal variance at all fitted values and the assumption of normally distributed residuals. The Cox proportional hazards regression model was used for analysis of the COX-2 values, that did not approximate a normal distribution after log transformation. 'Grade' (Pfirrmann grade I – IV) and 'breed' (CD, NCD) and their interaction were incorporated into this model. Calculations were performed on values distracted from 100 %. In the absence of COX-2 positive cells the sample was set at 100 % and right censored. Histological reactive changes in the IVDs were statistically evaluated by using the nonparametric Kruskal-Wallis test, followed by a Mann–Whitney U-test. The Spearman's correlation coefficient was calculated to estimate the correlation between the presence of inflammatory cells ('yes' or 'no') and COX-2 positive cells.

For all statistical models, regression coefficients were estimated by the maximum likelihood method. Model selection was based on the lowest Akaike Information Criterion (AIC). Confidence intervals were calculated and stated at the 99 % confidence level to correct for multiple comparisons. Differences between treatments were considered significant if the confidence interval did not include 0, whereas hazard ratios were considered significant if the confidence interval did not include 1. Significant differences and the corresponding confidence intervals are represented in Additional file 2.

Results

Extracellular matrix components and inflammatory profiles in relation to stage of degeneration

GAG content normalized for wet weight did not significantly change with degeneration grade according to Pfirrmann (Fig. 1a and b). In grade IV + V samples the GAG content in the NP was significantly lower than in the AF (Fig. 1a). DNA expressed as μg/mg wet weight was significantly lower in grade II samples compared with grade IV + V samples (Fig. 1b). Due to sample limitations, samples that were above the upper range of the PGE_2 assay (>1000 pg/ml) were set at 1000 pg/ml. PGE_2 levels normalized for wet weight were significantly lower in grade I NP samples compared with those in grade II, III, and IV + V NP samples (Fig. 2a). PGE_2 levels normalized for DNA were significantly lower in grade I samples

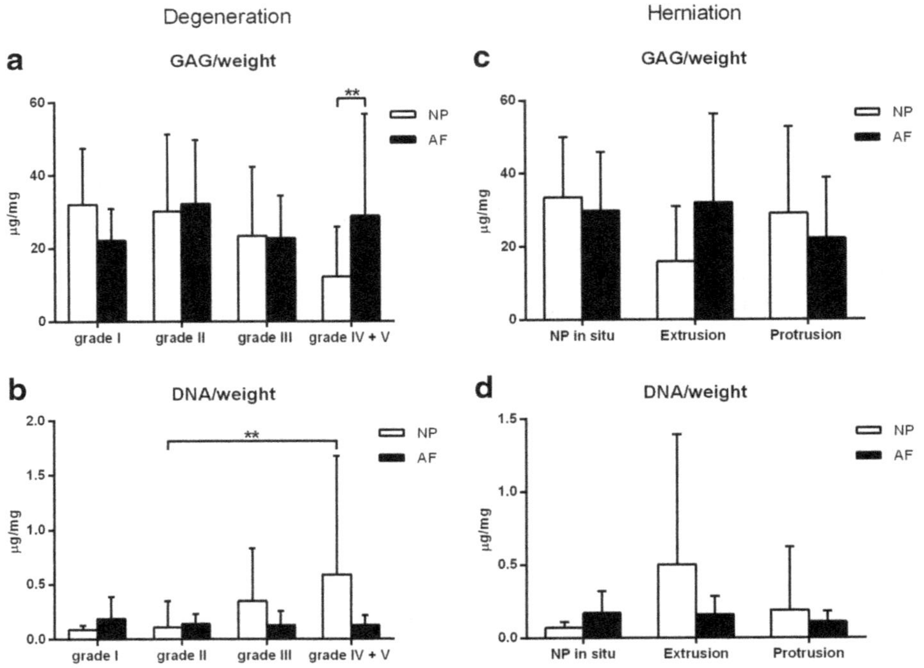

Fig. 1 Mean + standard deviation GAG and DNA content normalized for weight in the nucleus pulposus (NP) and annulus fibrosus (AF) per Pfirrmann grade (**a**, **b**) and per herniation (**c**, **d**). **a**. GAG/weight levels were significantly higher in the AF compared with the NP in grade IV + V samples. **b**. DNA/weight was significantly lower in the NP of grade II samples compared with grade IV + V. **c** and **d**. Normalized GAG and DNA levels did not significantly differ between herniation groups. No significant differences were shown between dog (CD/NCD) or treatment (no treatment, NSAID < 1 wk, NSAID > 1 wk, corticosteroids (cort) < 1 wk, cort > 1 wk, other) groups, hence these groups are not shown separately. ** Indicate significant difference at a 99 % confidence level

compared with grade II, III, and IV + V samples regardless of the tissue origin (NP/AF), dog type (CD/NCD), or treatment group (no treatment, NSAID < 1 wk, NSAID > 1 wk, cort < 1 wk, cort > 1 wk, other) (Fig. 2b). Cytokines IL-2, IL-6, IL-7, IL-8, IL-10, IL-15, IL-18, IP-10, TNF-α, and GM-CSF were not detectable in the samples. Chemokine CCL2 was measured in 66/120 samples and chemokine CXCL1 in 119/120 samples. CXCL1 and CCL2 expressed as pg/gram wet weight did not significantly change with degeneration (Fig. 2c and d). There were no significant differences between treatment groups.

Extracellular matrix components and inflammatory profiles in relation to herniation of NP and AF

GAG and DNA (Fig. 1c and d) and CXCL1 (Fig. 2d and e) expressed as pg/gram wet weight were not significantly different between herniation groups. PGE_2 levels normalized for either DNA content or wet weight, were significantly lower in non-herniated samples compared with extruded and protruded samples of NCD dogs, regardless of the tissue origin (NP/AF), or treatment group (no treatment, NSAID < 1 wk, NSAID > 1 wk, cort < 1 wk, cort > 1 wk, other). CCL2 levels in the NP from extruded samples were significantly higher compared with the AF of these samples and the NP from protrusion samples regardless of the dog breed (CD/NCD) (Fig. 2f). There were no significant differences between biochemical parameters of CD and NCD dogs or treatment groups.

Pfirrmann grade II samples from this study were compared with Pfirrmann grade II samples obtained from experimental CD dogs (Fig. 3a) [40]. As sample weights were not available in the previous study, PGE_2 was normalized for DNA. In this combined Pfirrmann grade II dataset, PGE_2/DNA in the NP was significantly higher in extruded samples compared with Pfirrmann grade II IVDs with the NP in situ. To compare this combined Pfirrmann grade II dataset to the complete dataset, we have normalized PGE_2 for DNA (Fig. 3b and c).

Histology and COX-2 expression

Histological scores according to the grading scheme by Bergknut et al. ranged from 7 – 12 (median = 8) for Pfirrmann grade1, 8 – 27 (median = 14) for Pfirrmann grade II, 14 – 20 (median =19) for Pfirrmann grade III, and 18 – 26 (median = 21) for Pfirrmann grade IV + V. In 5/37 IVDs from 3/16 dogs ventral bone formation was seen in grade I – V IVDs. Histology revealed no inflammatory cells or fibroblasts in the NP of Pfirrmann grade I – V IVDs, and in the dorsal AF of Pfirrmann grade I IVDs. However, in higher degeneration grades,

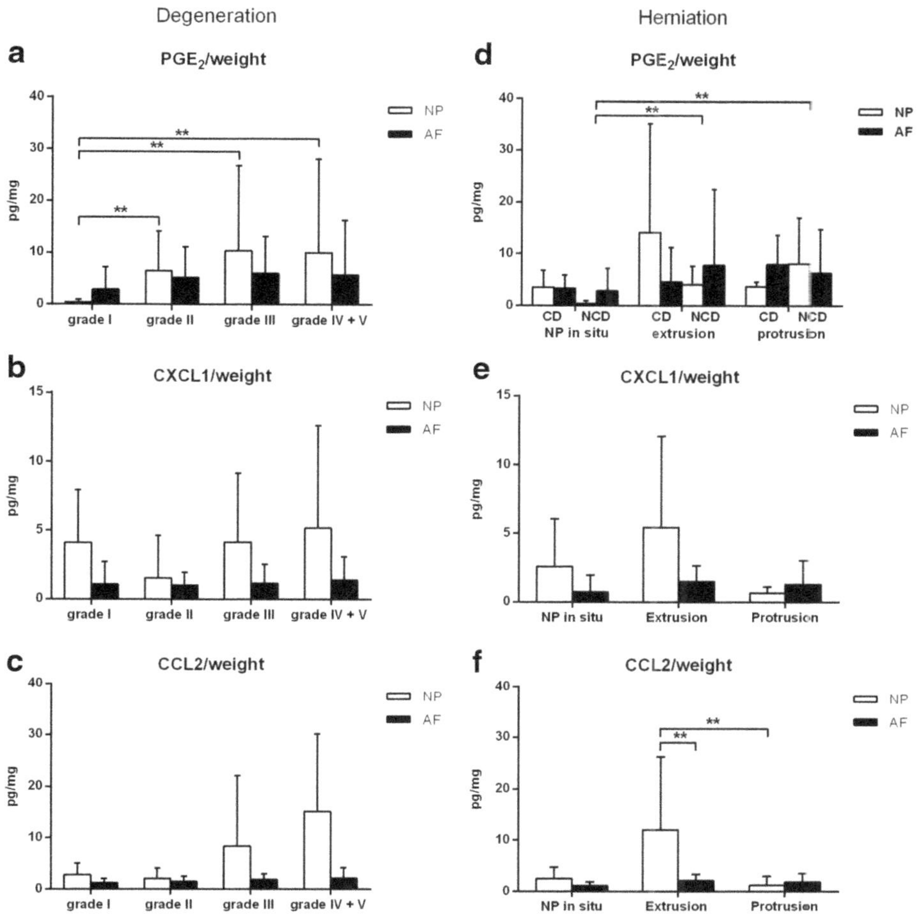

Fig. 2 Mean + standard deviation PGE_2 and chemokine (CCL2 and CXCL1) levels normalized for weight in the nucleus pulposus (NP) and annulus fibrosus (AF) per Pfirrmann grade (**a**, **b**, **c**) and per herniation (**d**, **e**, **f**). **a**. PGE_2 levels expressed as pg/mg wet weight in grade I NP samples were significantly lower compared with grade II, III, and IV + V NP samples. **c**, **b** and **c**. CCL2 and CXCL1 levels normalized for weight did not significantly change with degeneration. **d**. PGE_2 levels did not significantly differ in the NP and AF between the three herniation groups. **e**. CXCL1 levels did not significantly differ between herniation groups. **f**. CCL2 levels normalized for weight in the NP from extruded samples were significantly higher compared with the AF of these samples and the NP from protruded samples. No significant differences were shown between treatment (no treatment, NSAID < 1 wk, NSAID > 1 wk, corticosteroids (cort) < 1 wk, cort > 1 wk, other) groups, hence these groups are not shown separately. ** Indicate significant difference at a 99 % confidence level

focal infiltration of macrophages, proliferation of fibroblasts and capillaries were detected in the dorsal and/or the ventral ligament, extending into the outer layers of the dorsal and ventral AF, respectively (Fig. 3). Macrophages and proliferation of fibroblasts were present in 0 % (0/10), 10 % (1/10), 83 % (5/6) and 55 % (6/11) of the IVDs scored a Pfirrmann grade I, II, III, IV + V, respectively. Numbers of macrophages and fibroblasts in grade IV + V IVDs were significantly higher than in grade I, and in grade III significantly higher than in grade I and II. Protrusion of the AF was seen in a grade II and a grade IV + V IVD.

Percentages of COX-2-positive cells in the NP and dorsal AF of grade I and grade II tissue were significantly lower compared with the NP and dorsal AF of grade IV + V samples (Fig. 4 and Fig. 5). The presence of macrophages and fibroblasts in the dorsal AF was moderately correlated (Spearman's $\rho = 0.4$, p-value = 0.003) with COX-2 positive cells in the dorsal AF.

Discussion

To our knowledge this is the first study that describes levels of COX-2, PGE_2, cytokines, chemokines, and matrix components in IVDs from CD and NCD dogs with and without clinical signs of IVD disease and degeneration. PGE_2 levels were significantly higher in degenerated IVDs compared with non-degenerated IVDs, and they were also higher in herniated (protruded and extruded) IVDs from NCD dogs compared with non-herniated IVDs of NCD dogs. In contrast to PGE_2

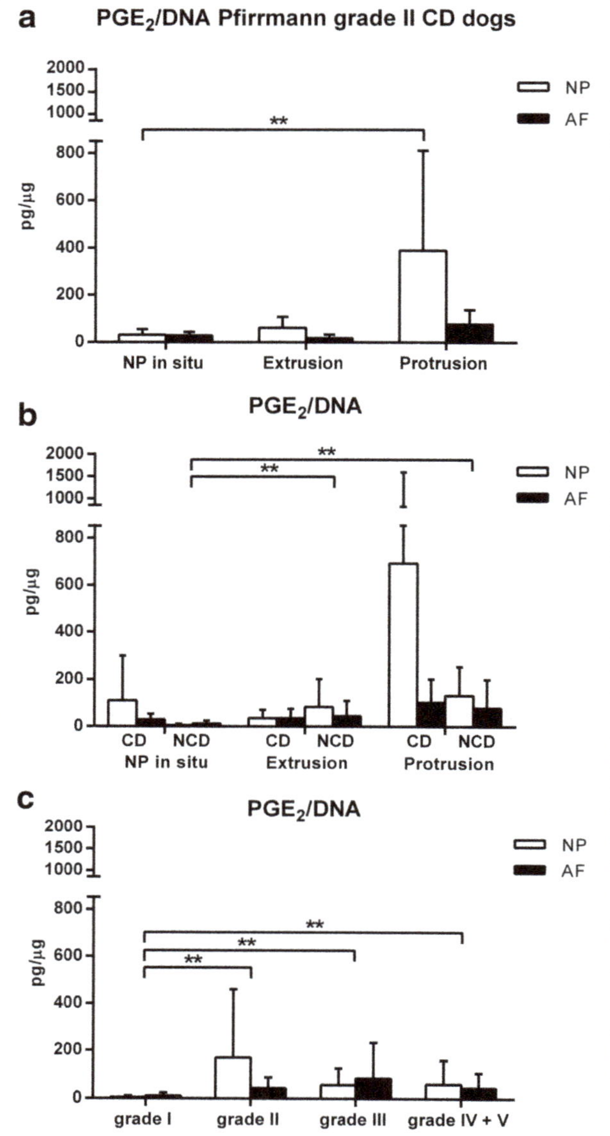

Fig. 3 Mean + standard deviation PGE_2 levels normalized for DNA content in the nucleus pulposus (NP) and annulus fibrosus (AF) in Pfirrmann grade II samples obtained from experimental chondrodystrophic (CD) dogs (**a**), and in the complete dataset (CD and nonchondrodystrophic (NCD) dogs) per Pfirrmann grade (**b**), and per herniation (**c**). **a**. PGE_2 levels expressed as pg/µg DNA in the NP of CD dogs were significantly higher in extruded grade II samples compared with NP in situ samples. **b**. PGE_2 levels normalized for DNA were significantly lower in grade I samples compared with grade II, III, and IV + V samples regardless of the tissue origin (NP/AF), dog group (CD/NCD), or treatment group (no treatment, NSAID < 1 wk, NSAID > 1 wk, corticosteroids (cort) < 1 wk, cort > 1 wk, other). **c**. PGE_2 levels expressed as pg/µg DNA were significantly lower in non-herniated samples compared with extruded and protruded samples in NCD dogs, regardless of the tissue origin (NP/AF), or treatment group (no treatment, NSAID < 1 wk, NSAID > 1 wk, corticosteroids (cort) < 1 wk, cort > 1 wk, other). ** Indicate significant difference at a 99 % confidence level

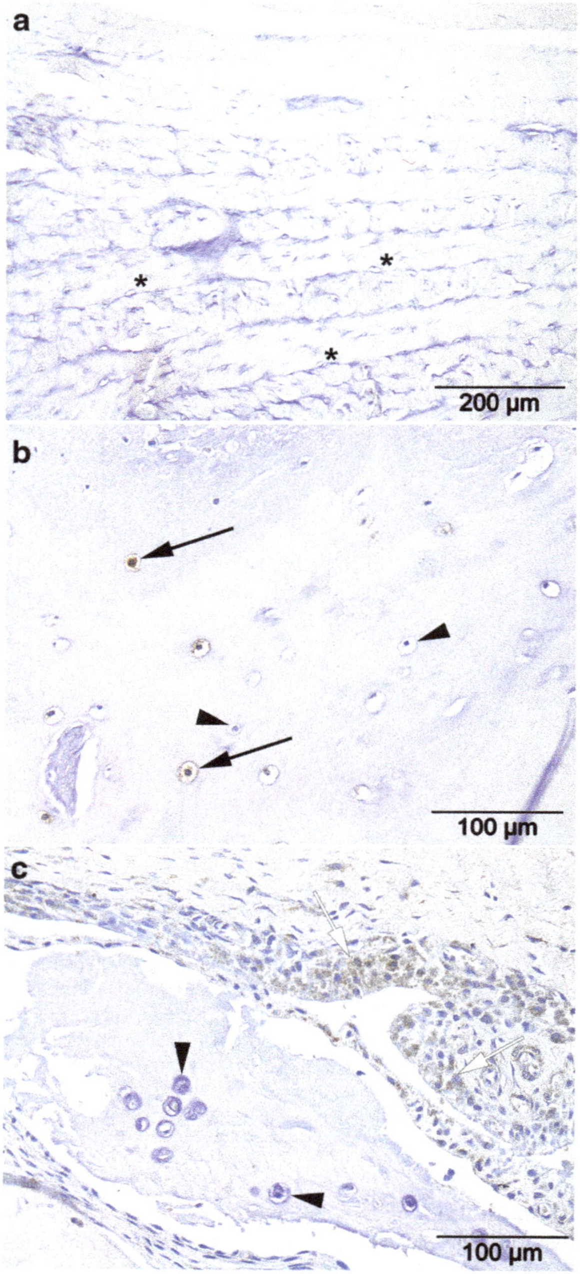

Fig. 4 Representative histological images of the annulus fibrosus (AF) of intervertebral discs (IVDs) graded according to Pfirrmann stained with a COX-2 antibody and counterstained with hematoxylin. **a**. The dorsal AF of a non-degenerated Pfirrmann grade 1 IVD consisted of well-organized lamellae with COX-2 negative spindle-shaped fibroblasts (*asterisks*). **b**. In the dorsal AF of a degenerated Pfirrmann grade IV IVD lamellar organization was lost and COX-2 negative chondrocytes (*arrowheads*) as well as COX-2 positive chondrocytes (*arrows*) were present. **c**. The dorsal AF of a Pfirrmann grade V IVD consisted of COX-2 negative chondrocytes (*arrowheads*), whereas COX-2 positive macrophages (*open arrows*) were situated in the dorsal ligament

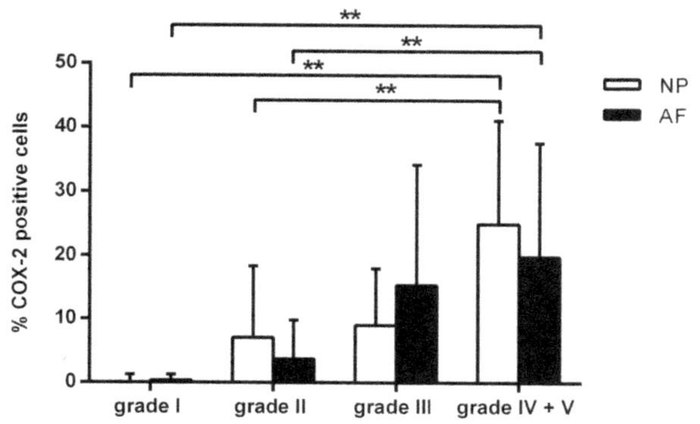

Fig. 5 Percentage of COX-2-positive cells in the nucleus pulposus (NP) and annulus fibrosus (AF) per Pfirrmann grade. The NP and AF of grade I and grade II samples were significantly lower compared with the NP and AF grade IV + V samples. ** Indicate significant difference at a 99 % confidence level

levels in Pfirrmann grade II IVDs from CD dogs with (a limited number of) protruded IVDs, PGE_2 levels in extruded IVDs were not significantly different from IVDs with the NP in situ. Furthermore, COX-2 protein expression was significantly higher in degenerated IVDs compared with non-degenerated IVDs. These results are consistent with findings in herniated human lumbar IVD cells that produced increased PGE_2 levels spontaneously in vitro compared with PGE_2 levels in control IVD cells [15].

Contrary to PGE_2 levels, COX-2 expression in the NP and AF and numbers of macrophages in the dorsal and ventral ligaments were increased in advanced stages of degeneration. Histological results of non-herniated degenerated IVDs in our study are consistent with histological findings described in studies on canine herniated IVDs. In extruded IVDs an acute inflammatory reaction has been described, characterized by neutrophils and macrophages, while in protruded IVDs a more chronic inflammatory reaction has been described, characterized by macrophages, lymphocytes and plasma cells [46, 47]. Macrophages do not only have a phagocytic function, but secret next to cytokines also a number of growth factors, e.g. fibroblast growth factor, transforming growth factor beta, that can induce neovascularization and mediate cell proliferation and differentiation [48]. The focal infiltrates of macrophages, proliferation of fibroblasts and capillaries, and the new bone formation as was seen histologically in some IVDs are reactive tissue changes that might reflect a process of tissue repair. Although a physiological inflammatory response to aseptic tissue injury primarily serves to promote tissue repair, macroscopic findings may reflect an excessive inflammatory response. This response may have detrimental effects on tissue integrity, and may contribute to the pathogenesis of IVD degeneration and/or disease.

Significantly higher PGE_2 levels in degenerated NP tissues compared with non-degenerated IVDs were observed. Although not significantly different, PGE_2 levels and COX-2 expression in grade II and IV + V IVDs were consistently higher in the NP of degenerated IVDs compared with AF, while the contrary was true for non-degenerated IVDs. In Pfirrmann grade II samples from CD dogs, PGE_2 levels in the NP were significantly higher in Pfirrmann grade II IVDs with protrusion compared with IVDs with the NP in situ. This may indicate that the production of inflammatory mediators is more pronounced at the NP level. We cannot exclude that NP and AF cells respond differently to inflammatory stimuli and mechanic stress and hence produce different levels of PGE_2, as also suggested by others based on in vitro experiments in rat IVD cells [49]. Cytokine and chemokine profiles in this study are largely consistent with limited veterinary publications. The significantly increased CCL2 levels in NP tissue of dogs with Hansen type I herniation compared with AF tissue and NP tissue in dogs with Hansen type II herniation are in line with other studies reporting upregulated gene expression levels of CCL2 in dogs with extrusion of the NP [35]. Furthermore, increased CCL2 protein expression and CCL2 production levels have been reported in human prolapsed IVDs [28]. No studies in canine tissues, and only limited studies in human tissues, have determined cytokine and/or chemokine levels by using a (multiplex) sandwich immunoassay, and have shown increased levels of IFN-γ, IL-1, TNF-α, and CCL2, in epidural lavage fluid and in cell culture media, which complicates comparison of results [51–53]. Cytokine levels of IL-2, IL-6, IL-7, IL-8, IL-10, IL-15, IL-18, IP-10, TNF-α, and GM-CSF were not detected in NP and AF tissues of this study, consistent with downregulated gene expression levels of IL-2, IL-6, IL-10, and TNF-α in herniated canine IVDs [35]. Nevertheless, our findings seem to be in contrast with increased protein and gene expression levels of TNF-α and IL-1 in human IVDs [23–25, 28, 29, 54]. Given the short half-life of TNF- α and cytokines [55, 56], and that all samples collected from degenerated IVDs were obtained during surgery and in several cases after flushing of the spinal canal, we cannot rule out degradation of cytokines/chemokines by the collection, preparation, and storage process. Although several studies have shown that IVD cells have the capacity to produce PGE_2, we cannot rule out that PGE_2 levels were influenced by infiltration from the epidural space.

Despite elevated PGE_2 levels in degenerated NP tissue in this study, GAG content was not significantly different between healthy and degenerated IVDs, while severely degenerated AFs (grade IV + V) had a higher GAG content compared with the NP. The latter may be explained by the presence of GAG-producing chondrocytes in the AF, known to be present in later stages of degeneration [45], or by the presence of unidentified GAG-rich herniated NP and/or inner AF material in AF samples. These findings are in contrast with the decrease in GAG content with increasing IVD degeneration described in literature [1, 11]. One plausible explanation for this discrepancy lies in the scoring system of degeneration prior to surgery and the matrix heterogeneity of the degenerated NP tissue, discussed in detail below. Interestingly, cell density (DNA/weight) in our study was significantly higher in the NP of severely degenerated IVDs compared with mildly degenerated IVDs. These findings touch upon findings in human IVD degeneration, in which cell density in the inner AF and NP of severely degenerated (Thompson grade V) specimens was significantly higher compared with lower grades [57, 58].

The results on the effects of PGE_2 on proteoglycan metabolism are conflicting.PGE_2 at concentrations much lower than those involved in inflammation have been demonstrated to be chondroprotective [59]. PGE_2 has been described to have anti-catabolic effects by down-regulating the expression and synthesis of IL-1, TNF- α, and matrix metalloproteinases (MMPs), and to have anabolic effects by to inducing the expression, synthesis and secretion of IGF-I, and stimulating collagen and proteoglycan synthesis, important factors in anabolic processes [16, 60–62]. In vitro, low concentrations of PGE_2 have been described to stimulate proteoglycan synthesis in rat chondrocytes, whereas higher doses have been described to decrease proteoglycan synthesis in NP cells [16, 61]. Furthermore, degradation of proteoglycans was not inhibited by a range of PGE_2 concentrations in osteoarthritic chondrocytes [60]. These possible protective effects of PGE_2 might have resulted in preservation of GAG content in the course of IVD degeneration. Nevertheless, these results should be interpreted with care, as GAG content of the studied tissues may have been affected by confounding factors explained below.

There are several confounding factors that may affect the results in the current study, including the factors that influence the scoring system of degeneration and the matrix heterogeneity of the degenerated NP tissue. Extruded NP tissue displaced into the vertebral canal results in narrowing of the disc space and a T2-hypointense area within the IVD on MRI. Hence, we cannot exclude that prior to the extrusion incident the IVD may have been assessed with a lower Pfirrmann score. Moreover, in CD dogs, calcification of the NP could have negatively influenced the signal intensity in the NP [63, 64]. In addition, in both CD and NCD dogs, IVDs may have been graded falsely higher due to hemorrhage or inflammation, that may have influenced the appearance of the IVD on MR images. Matrix heterogeneity is common in degenerating NP tissue. In human IVDs several disc-specific locations are described with a high variation in GAG and water content, suggestive of focal damage and degeneration [65]. Although this has not yet been described in dogs, we cannot rule out that tissues collected during surgery may have originated from specific GAG-rich areas in the IVD, that inherently are more prone to extrusion/protrusion compared with degenerated fibrotic tissue. Furthermore, due to sample limitations PGE_2 values higher than 1000 pg/ml could not be measured reliably, but could have resulted in an underestimation of the highest samples. Lastly, a relatively high percentage of dogs in this study was treated prior to surgery with anti-inflammatory drugs, e.g. NSAIDs and corticosteroids. Dogs that did not respond to anti-inflammatory drugs initially, were treated with other drugs, e.g. opioids, GABA-agonists. Although treatment groups were categorized, duration of treatment and dosages used showed a high variation, and might have had an influence on the results.

From a clinical perspective, decompression surgery is recommended if dogs present with clinical signs, and diagnostic work-up indicates compression of neural tissue (spinal cord and/or nerve roots) due to extruded material. With regard to an intradiscal application that provides controlled release of an anti-inflammatory drug, future studies should focus on protruded IVDs. Obviously, this would indicate development of an application in NCD dogs, as disc protrusion rarely occurs in CD dogs. IVDs ideally should be early degenerated (Pfirrmann grade II – III), without irreversible anatomical malformations due to degenerative changes.

Conclusion

In this study we have shown that PGE_2 levels, and CCL2 levels in degenerated and herniated tissues were significantly higher compared with non-degenerated and non-herniated tissues. COX-2 expression in the NP and AF and numbers of macrophages in the AF increased with advancing degeneration stages. Although macrophages invade the dorsal and ventral AF as degeneration progresses, the production of inflammatory mediators seems most pronounced in degenerated NP tissue. Future studies are needed to investigate if inhibition of PGE_2 levels in degenerated IVDs provide effective analgesia and exerts a protective role in the process of IVD degeneration and the development of IVD disease.

Abbreviations
AF: Annulus fibrosus; AIC: Akaike information criterion; BSA: bovine serum albumin; CCL2: chemokine (C-C motif) ligand 2; CD: chondrodystrophic; Cort: corticosteroids; COX: cyclooxygenase; CT: computed tomography; CXCL1: chemokine (C-X-C motif) ligand 1; DEC: Animal Experiments Committee (Dutch: Dierexperimentencommissie); DMMB: dimethylmethylene blue; EDTA: ethylenediaminetetraacetic acid; GAG: glycosaminoglycan; GM-CSF: granulocyte-macrophage colony-stimulating factor; IL: interleukin; IVD: intervertebral disc; MMP: matrix metalloproteinases; MR: magnetic resonance; NCD: non-chondrodystrophic; NP: nucleus pulposus; NSAIDs: non-steroidal anti-inflammatory drugs; PGE_2: Prostaglandin E_2; TBS: tris buffered saline; TNF-α: tumor necrosis factor α; T2W: T2-weighted.

Competing interests
The authors declare that they have no competing interests.

Author's contributions
NW drafted the manuscript, and participated in the study design, acquisition, analysis and interpretation of data. AT, NB, and JW participated in the acquisition and analysis of data. CF and KB participated in the acquisition and analysis of cytokine assays, and critically revised the manuscript. GG participated in the histological examination of the IVDs. LC participated in the study design, interpretation of data, and critically revised the manuscript. BM and MT participated in the study design, acquisition and interpretation of data, and critically revised the manuscript. All authors read and approved the final manuscript.

Acknowledgements
This research forms part of the Project P2.01 IDiDAS of the research program of the BioMedical Materials institute, co-funded by the Dutch Ministry of Economic Affairs, Agriculture and Innovation. The financial contribution of the Dutch Arthritis Foundation is gratefully acknowledged (IDiDAS, LLP22, and LLP12). We would like to acknowledge the assistance of Hans Vernooij in the statistical analysis and Saskia van Dongen in performing the biochemical assays.

Author details
[1]Department of Clinical Sciences of Companion Animals, Faculty of Veterinary Medicine, 3584 CM Utrecht, The Netherlands. [2]Department of Orthopaedics, University Medical Center, 3584 CX Utrecht, The Netherlands. [3]NMI Natural and Medical Sciences Institute at the University of Tuebingen, Regenerative Medicine II, 72770 Reutlingen, Germany. [4]Department of Pathobiology, Faculty of Veterinary Medicine, 3508 TD Utrecht, The Netherlands.

References

1. Bergknut N, Rutges JP, Kranenburg HC, Smolders LA, Hagman R, Smidt HJ, et al. The dog as an animal model for intervertebral disc degeneration? Spine (Phila Pa 1976). 2012;37(5):351–8.
2. Schmied O, Golini L, Steffen F. Effectiveness of cervical hemilaminectomy in canine Hansen Type I and Type II disc disease: a retrospective study. J Am Anim Hosp Assoc. 2011;47(5):342–50.
3. Suwankong N, Meij BP, Voorhout G, de Boer AH, Hazewinkel HA. Review and retrospective analysis of degenerative lumbosacral stenosis in 156 dogs treated by dorsal laminectomy. Vet Comp Orthop Traumatol. 2008;21(3):285–93.
4. Macias C, McKee WM, May C, Innes JF. Thoracolumbar disc disease in large dogs: a study of 99 cases. J Small Anim Pract. 2002;43(10):439–46.
5. Cudia SP, Duval JM. Thoracolumbar intervertebral disk disease in large, nonchondrodystrophic dogs: a retrospective study. J Am Anim Hosp Assoc. 1997;33(5):456–60.
6. Brisson BA. Intervertebral disc disease in dogs. Vet Clin North Am Small Anim Pract. 2010;40(5):829–58.
7. Levine JM, Levine GJ, Kerwin SC, Hettlich BF, Fosgate GT. Association between various physical factors and acute thoracolumbar intervertebral disk extrusion or protrusion in Dachshunds. J Am Vet Med Assoc. 2006;229(3):370–5.
8. Hansen HJ. A pathologic-anatomical study on disc degeneration in dog, with special reference to the so-called enchondrosis intervertebralis. Acta Orthop Scand Suppl. 1952;11:1–117.
9. Smolders LA, Bergknut N, Grinwis GC, Hagman R, Lagerstedt AS, Hazewinkel HA, et al. Intervertebral disc degeneration in the dog. Part 2: chondrodystrophic and non-chondrodystrophic breeds. Vet J. 2013;195(3):292–9.
10. Adams MA, Roughley PJ. What is intervertebral disc degeneration, and what causes it? Spine (Phila Pa 1976). 2006;31(18):2151–61.
11. Roughley PJ. Biology of intervertebral disc aging and degeneration: involvement of the extracellular matrix. Spine (Phila Pa 1976). 2004;29(23):2691–9.
12. Brisby H. Pathology and possible mechanisms of nervous system response to disc degeneration. J Bone Joint Surg Am. 2006;88 Suppl 2:68–71.
13. Freemont AJ, Peacock TE, Goupille P, Hoyland JA, O'Brien J, Jayson MI. Nerve ingrowth into diseased intervertebral disc in chronic back pain. Lancet. 1997;350(9072):178–81.
14. Ahn SH, Cho YW, Ahn MW, Jang SH, Sohn YK, Kim HS. mRNA expression of cytokines and chemokines in herniated lumbar intervertebral discs. Spine (Phila Pa 1976). 2002;27(9):911–7.
15. Kang JD, Georgescu HI, McIntyre-Larkin L, Stefanovic-Racic M, Donaldson 3rd WF, Evans CH. Herniated lumbar intervertebral discs spontaneously produce matrix metalloproteinases, nitric oxide interleukin-6, and prostaglandin E2. Spine (Phila Pa 1976). 1996;21(3):271–7.
16. Vo NV, Sowa GA, Kang JD, Seidel C, Studer RK. Prostaglandin E2 and prostaglandin F2alpha differentially modulate matrix metabolism of human nucleus pulposus cells. J Orthop Res. 2010;28(10):1259–66.
17. Li W, Liu T, Wu L, Chen C, Jia Z, Bai X, et al. Blocking the function of inflammatory cytokines and mediators by using IL-10 and TGF-beta: a potential biological immunotherapy for intervertebral disc degeneration in a beagle model. Int J Mol Sci. 2014;15(10):17270–83.
18. Burke JG, Watson RW, McCormack D, Dowling FE, Walsh MG, Fitzpatrick JM. Spontaneous production of monocyte chemoattractant protein-1 and interleukin-8 by the human lumbar intervertebral disc. Spine (Phila Pa 1976). 2002;27(13):1402–7.
19. Hoyland JA, Le Maitre C, Freemont AJ. Investigation of the role of IL-1 and TNF in matrix degradation in the intervertebral disc. Rheumatology (Oxford). 2008;47(6):809–14.
20. Hughes SP, Freemont AJ, Hukins DW, McGregor AH, Roberts S. The pathogenesis of degeneration of the intervertebral disc and emerging therapies in the management of back pain. J Bone Joint Surg Br. 2012;94(10):1298–304.
21. Kepler CK, Markova DZ, Hilibrand AS, Vaccaro AR, Risbud MV, Albert TJ, et al. Substance P stimulates production of inflammatory cytokines in human disc cells. Spine (Phila Pa 1976). 2013;38(21):E1291–9.
22. Le Maitre CL, Freemont AJ, Hoyland JA. The role of interleukin-1 in the pathogenesis of human intervertebral disc degeneration. Arthritis Res Ther. 2005;7(4):R732–45.
23. Le Maitre CL, Hoyland JA, Freemont AJ. Catabolic cytokine expression in degenerate and herniated human intervertebral discs: IL-1beta and TNFalpha expression profile. Arthritis Res Ther. 2007;9(4):R77.
24. Le Maitre CL, Hoyland JA, Freemont AJ. Interleukin-1 receptor antagonist delivered directly and by gene therapy inhibits matrix degradation in the intact degenerate human intervertebral disc: an in situ zymographic and gene therapy study. Arthritis Res Ther. 2007;9(4):R83.
25. Le Maitre CL, Pockert A, Buttle DJ, Freemont AJ, Hoyland JA. Matrix synthesis and degradation in human intervertebral disc degeneration. Biochem Soc Trans. 2007;35(Pt 4):652–5.
26. Le Maitre CL, Binch AL, Thorpe A, Hughes SP. Degeneration of the intervertebral disc with new approaches for treating low back pain. J Neurosurg Sci. 2015;59(1):47–61.
27. Park JY, Pillinger MH, Abramson SB. Prostaglandin E2 synthesis and secretion: the role of PGE2 synthases. Clin Immunol. 2006;119(3):229–40.
28. Phillips KL, Chiverton N, Michael AL, Cole AA, Breakwell LM, Haddock G, et al. The cytokine and chemokine expression profile of nucleus pulposus cells: implications for degeneration and regeneration of the intervertebral disc. Arthritis Res Ther. 2013;15(6):R213.
29. Purmessur D, Walter BA, Roughley PJ, Laudier DM, Hecht AC, Iatridis J. A role for TNFalpha in intervertebral disc degeneration: a non-recoverable catabolic shift. Biochem Biophys Res Commun. 2013;433(1):151–6.
30. Shamji MF, Setton LA, Jarvis W, So S, Chen J, Jing L, et al. Proinflammatory cytokine expression profile in degenerated and herniated human intervertebral disc tissues. Arthritis Rheum. 2010;62(7):1974–82.

31. Takahashi H, Suguro T, Okazima Y, Motegi M, Okada Y, Kakiuchi T. Inflammatory cytokines in the herniated disc of the lumbar spine. Spine (Phila Pa 1976). 1996;21(2):218–24.
32. Wang J, Markova D, Anderson DG, Zheng Z, Shapiro IM, Risbud MV. TNF-alpha and IL-1beta promote a disintegrin-like and metalloprotease with thrombospondin type I motif-5-mediated aggrecan degradation through syndecan-4 in intervertebral disc. J Biol Chem. 2011;286(46):39738–49.
33. Wang J, Tian Y, Phillips KL, Chiverton N, Haddock G, Bunning RA, et al. Tumor necrosis factor alpha- and interleukin-1beta-dependent induction of CCL3 expression by nucleus pulposus cells promotes macrophage migration through CCR1. Arthritis Rheum. 2013;65(3):832–42.
34. Weiler C, Nerlich AG, Bachmeier BE, Boos N. Expression and distribution of tumor necrosis factor alpha in human lumbar intervertebral discs: a study in surgical specimen and autopsy controls. Spine (Phila Pa 1976). 2005;30(1):44–53. discussion 54.
35. Karli P, Martle V, Bossens K, Summerfield A, Doherr MG, Turner P, et al. Dominance of chemokine ligand 2 and matrix metalloproteinase-2 and −9 and suppression of pro-inflammatory cytokines in the epidural compartment after intervertebral disc extrusion in a canine model. Spine J. 2014;14(12):2976–84.
36. Iwata M, Ochi H, Asou Y, Haro H, Aikawa T, Harada Y, et al. Variations in gene and protein expression in canine chondrodystrophic nucleus pulposus cells following long-term three-dimensional culture. PLoS One. 2013;8(5), e63120.
37. Brock TG, McNish RW, Peters-Golden M. Arachidonic acid is preferentially metabolized by cyclooxygenase-2 to prostacyclin and prostaglandin E2. J Biol Chem. 1999;274(17):11660–6.
38. Clark TP. The clinical pharmacology of cyclooxygenase-2-selective and dual inhibitors. Vet Clin North Am Small Anim Pract. 2006;36(5):1061–85. vii.
39. Nell T, Bergman J, Hoeijmakers M, Van Laar P, Horspool LJ. Comparison of vedaprofen and meloxicam in dogs with musculoskeletal pain and inflammation. J Small Anim Pract. 2002;43(5):208–12.
40. Willems N, Yang H, Langelaan M, Tellegen A, Grinwis G, Kranenburg H, et al. Biocompatibility and intradiscal application of celecoxib-loaded pNIPAAM MgFe-LDH hydrogels in a canine spontaneous intervertebral disc degeneration model. Arthritis Res Ther. 2015; 17(214). doi: 10.1186/s13075-015-0727-x.
41. Samad TA, Moore KA, Sapirstein A, Billet S, Allchorne A, Poole S, et al. Interleukin-1beta-mediated induction of Cox-2 in the CNS contributes to inflammatory pain hypersensitivity. Nature. 2001;410(6827):471–5.
42. Bergknut N, Auriemma E, Wijsman S, Voorhout G, Hagman R, Lagerstedt AS, et al. Evaluation of intervertebral disk degeneration in chondrodystrophic and nonchondrodystrophic dogs by use of Pfirrmann grading of images obtained with low-field magnetic resonance imaging. Am J Vet Res. 2011;72(7):893–8.
43. Harder L, Ludwig D, Galindo-Zamora V, Wefstaedt P, Nolte I. Classification of canine intervertebral disc degeneration using high-field magnetic resonance imaging and computed tomography. Tierarztl Prax Ausg K Kleintiere Heimtiere. 2014;42(6):374–82.
44. Farndale RW, Sayers CA, Barrett AJ. A direct spectrophotometric microassay for sulfated glycosaminoglycans in cartilage cultures. Connect Tissue Res. 1982;9(4):247–8.
45. Bergknut N, Meij BP, Hagman R, de Nies KS, Rutges JP, Smolders LA, et al. Intervertebral disc disease in dogs - part 1: a new histological grading scheme for classification of intervertebral disc degeneration in dogs. Vet J. 2013;195(2):156–63.
46. Kranenburg HC, Grinwis GC, Bergknut N, Gahrmann N, Voorhout G, Hazewinkel HA, et al. Intervertebral disc disease in dogs - part 2: comparison of clinical, magnetic resonance imaging, and histological findings in 74 surgically treated dogs. Vet J. 2013;195(2):164–71.
47. Royal AB, Chigerwe M, Coates JR, Wiedmeyer CE, Berent LM. Cytologic and histopathologic evaluation of extruded canine degenerate disks. Vet Surg. 2009;38(7):798–802.
48. Varol C, Mildner A, Jung S. Macrophages: development and tissue specialization. Annu Rev Immunol. 2015;33:643–75.
49. Miyamoto H, Doita M, Nishida K, Yamamoto T, Sumi M, Kurosaka M. Effects of cyclic mechanical stress on the production of inflammatory agents by nucleus pulposus and anulus fibrosus derived cells in vitro. Spine (Phila Pa 1976). 2006;31(1):4–9.
50. Miyamoto H, Saura R, Harada T, Doita M, Mizuno K. The role of cyclooxygenase-2 and inflammatory cytokines in pain induction of herniated lumbar intervertebral disc. Kobe J Med Sci. 2000;46(1–2):13–28.
51. Scuderi GJ, Cuellar JM, Cuellar VG, Yeomans DC, Carragee EJ, Angst MS. Epidural interferon gamma-immunoreactivity: a biomarker for lumbar nerve root irritation. Spine (Phila Pa 1976). 2009;34(21):2311–7.
52. Scuderi GJ, Brusovanik GV, Anderson DG, Dunham CJ, Vaccaro AR, Demeo RF, et al. Cytokine assay of the epidural space lavage in patients with lumbar intervertebral disk herniation and radiculopathy. J Spinal Disord Tech. 2006;19(4):266–9.
53. Schroeder M, Viezens L, Schaefer C, Friedrichs B, Algenstaedt P, Ruther W, et al. Chemokine profile of disc degeneration with acute or chronic pain. J Neurosurg Spine. 2013;18(5):496–503.
54. Risbud MV, Shapiro IM. Role of cytokines in intervertebral disc degeneration: pain and disc content. Nat Rev Rheumatol. 2014;10(1):44–56.
55. Tarrant JM. Blood cytokines as biomarkers of in vivo toxicity in preclinical safety assessment: considerations for their use. Toxicol Sci. 2010;117(1):4–16.
56. Oliver JC, Bland LA, Oettinger CW, Arduino MJ, McAllister SK, Aguero SM, et al. Cytokine kinetics in an in vitro whole blood model following an endotoxin challenge. Lymphokine Cytokine Res. 1993;12(2):115–20.
57. Hastreiter D, Ozuna RM, Spector M. Regional variations in certain cellular characteristics in human lumbar intervertebral discs, including the presence of alpha-smooth muscle actin. J Orthop Res. 2001;19(4):597–604.
58. Zhao CQ, Wang LM, Jiang LS, Dai LY. The cell biology of intervertebral disc aging and degeneration. Ageing Res Rev. 2007;6(3):247–61.
59. Tchetina EV, Di Battista JA, Zukor DJ, Antoniou J, Poole AR. Prostaglandin PGE2 at very low concentrations suppresses collagen cleavage in cultured human osteoarthritic articular cartilage: this involves a decrease in expression of proinflammatory genes, collagenases and COL10A1, a gene linked to chondrocyte hypertrophy. Arthritis Res Ther. 2007;9(4):R75.
60. Di Battista JA, Dore S, Martel-Pelletier J, Pelletier JP. Prostaglandin E2 stimulates incorporation of proline into collagenase digestible proteins in human articular chondrocytes: identification of an effector autocrine loop involving insulin-like growth factor I. Mol Cell Endocrinol. 1996;123(1):27–35.
61. Lowe GN, Fu YH, McDougall S, Polendo R, Williams A, Benya PD, et al. Effects of prostaglandins on deoxyribonucleic acid and aggrecan synthesis in the RCJ 3.1C5.18 chondrocyte cell line: role of second messengers. Endocrinology. 1996;137(6):2208–16.
62. Knudsen PJ, Dinarello CA, Strom TB. Prostaglandins posttranscriptionally inhibit monocyte expression of interleukin 1 activity by increasing intracellular cyclic adenosine monophosphate. J Immunol. 1986;137(10):3189–94.
63. Jensen VF, Arnbjerg J. Development of intervertebral disk calcification in the dachshund: a prospective longitudinal radiographic study. J Am Anim Hosp Assoc. 2001;37(3):274–82.
64. Jensen VF, Beck S, Christensen KA, Arnbjerg J. Quantification of the association between intervertebral disk calcification and disk herniation in Dachshunds. J Am Vet Med Assoc. 2008;233(7):1090–5.
65. Iatridis JC, MacLean JJ, O'Brien M, Stokes IA. Measurements of proteoglycan and water content distribution in human lumbar intervertebral discs. Spine (Phila Pa 1976). 2007;32(14):1493–7.

2

Canine REIC/Dkk-3 interacts with SGTA and restores androgen receptor signalling in androgen-independent prostate cancer cell lines

Yuiko Kato[1], Kazuhiko Ochiai[1*], Shota Kawakami[1], Nobuhiro Nakao[2], Daigo Azakami[1], Makoto Bonkobara[3], Masaki Michishita[4], Masami Morimatsu[5], Masami Watanabe[6] and Toshinori Omi[1*]

Abstract

Background: The pathological condition of canine prostate cancer resembles that of human androgen-independent prostate cancer. Both canine and human androgen receptor (AR) signalling are inhibited by overexpression of the dimerized co-chaperone small glutamine-rich tetratricopeptide repeat-containing protein α (SGTA), which is considered to cause the development of androgen-independency. Reduced expression in immortalised cells (REIC/Dkk-3) interferes with SGTA dimerization and rescues AR signalling. This study aimed to assess the effects of REIC/Dkk-3 and SGTA interactions on AR signalling in the canine androgen-independent prostate cancer cell line CHP-1.

Results: Mammalian two-hybrid and Halo-tagged pull-down assays showed that canine REIC/Dkk-3 interacted with SGTA and interfered with SGTA dimerization. Additionally, reporter assays revealed that canine REIC/Dkk-3 restored AR signalling in both human and canine androgen-independent prostate cancer cells. Therefore, we confirmed the interaction between canine SGTA and REIC/Dkk-3, as well as their role in AR signalling.

Conclusions: Our results suggest that this interaction might contribute to the development of a novel strategy for androgen-independent prostate cancer treatment. Moreover, we established the canine androgen-independent prostate cancer model as a suitable animal model for the study of this type of treatment-refractory human cancer.

Keywords: Androgen receptor (AR) signalling, Canine, Prostate cancer, Reduced expression in immortalised cells (REIC/Dkk-3), Small glutamine-rich tetratricopeptide repeat-containing protein α (SGTA)

Background

Prostate cancer is the most common human male cancer in Western society and is currently rising in Eastern Asia [1]. Prostate cancer accounts for about 25% of all cancers in the male population of the United States [2]. For its treatment, hormonal strategies [e.g., androgen ablation therapy and/or androgen receptor (AR) antagonists] are used to prevent AR signalling associated with the development and progression of prostate cancer. Although the majority of prostate tumours respond to androgen ablation, a proportion of the cases develop as androgen-independent pathological conditions [3]. Canine prostate cancer shows similar characteristics to human androgen-independent prostate cancer, which progresses without androgen stimulation and is refractory to anti-androgen therapy [4]. To study the similarities between the pathological conditions of both canine and human androgen-independent prostate cancer, we have established a canine androgen-independent prostate cancer cell line, CHP-1 [5].

Reduced expression in immortalised cells (*REIC*), initially discovered as a tumour suppressor gene, is identical to the Dickkopf-3 (*Dkk-3*) gene, which is a member of the Dickkopf gene family [6]. *REIC/Dkk-3* is ubiquitously expressed

* Correspondence: kochiai@nvlu.ac.jp; t.omi@nvlu.ac.jp
[1]School of Veterinary Nursing and Technology, Faculty of Veterinary Science, Nippon Veterinary and Life Science University, Tokyo 180-8602, Japan
Full list of author information is available at the end of the article

in normal cells, whereas its expression is significantly downregulated in various cancer cell types, including human and canine prostate cancer [7]. Downregulation of *REIC/Dkk-3* is associated with the malignancy of various cancer types [7–9]. Previous studies showed that overexpression of *REIC/Dkk-3* using adenoviral or plasmid vectors induces apoptosis in various cancer cell lines, but not in normal cells, via c-Jun-NH2-terminal kinase (JNK) and c-Jun activation, and endoplasmic reticulum (ER) stress signalling [7, 10–13].

Small glutamine-rich tetratricopeptide repeat-containing protein α (SGTA) is an Hsp70/Hsp90-associated co-chaperone that interacts with the hinge region of the human AR and interferes with its cytoplasmic maturation [3]. The dimerized form of SGTA was identified as a negative regulator of AR transport to the nucleus by hampering the interaction between the cytoplasmic AR complex and the dynein motor complex [14–18]. Our recent study revealed that the overexpression of *REIC/Dkk-3* in the human androgen-independent prostate cancer cell line PC3 upregulates AR signalling and restores the expression of prostate specific antigen (PSA) by interfering with the dimerization of SGTA [19].

We have previously cloned canine SGTA and showed that its expression levels were significantly higher in canine prostate cancer tissues compared to that in prostate hyperplasia [20]. In addition, we showed that canine SGTA played an inhibitory role in AR signalling both in canine and human androgen-independent prostate cancer cells [5, 20]. From these findings, we were able to hypothesize that canine SGTA leads to an androgen-independent condition in canine prostate cancer. Our aim was to investigate whether the interaction between canine REIC/Dkk-3 and SGTA affects AR signalling and might contribute to the development of new strategies in canine androgen-independent prostate cancer treatment. In this study, we describe the interaction between canine REIC/Dkk-3 and SGTA, and the role of canine REIC/Dkk-3 in AR signalling recovery, previously inhibited by SGTA.

Methods

Cell lines

The human 293 T and PC3 cell lines were provided by the American Type Culture Collection (ATCC, Rockville, MD). The canine prostate cancer CHP-1 cell line was established from a prostate mass collected immediately following surgery of a tumour-bearing, 10-year-old, castrated male Jack Russell Terrier breed dog in our university [5]. The 293 T and the CHP-1 cells were maintained in Dulbecco's modified Eagle's medium (DMEM) (Wako, Osaka, Japan) and PC3 cells were maintained in Ham's F12 medium (Wako) supplemented with 10% foetal bovine serum (FBS), penicillin (50 IU/mL), and streptomycin (50 μg/mL) under a humidified atmosphere with 5% CO_2 at 37 °C.

Mammalian two-hybrid (MTH) assay

For the MTH assay, the full-length open reading frame (ORF) of canine SGTA and REIC/Dkk-3 cDNA was cloned between the *Eco*RI and *Mlu*I sites of a pM GAL4 DNA-binding domain cloning plasmid (GAL4-DBD) and pVP16 transactivation domain cloning plasmid (VP16-AD) (Clontech Laboratories, Palo Alto, CA, USA), respectively. In addition, the full-length ORF of canine REIC/Dkk-3 cDNA was cloned between the *Xho*I and *Eco*RI sites of the pMACS KK HA(C) vector cloning plasmid (Miltenyi Biotec, Bergisch Gladbach, Germany). Primers were used in this study was described in Additional file 1: Table S1. Approximately 2×10^5 293 T cells per well in 24-well plates were co-transfected with 100 ng of pM, pVP16, pMACS KK HA(C), and pFR-Luc firefly luciferase reporter plasmid (Promega, Madison, WI, USA), and 0.2 ng of phRL-TK *Renilla* luciferase reporter plasmid (Promega). The cells were harvested 48 h after transfection, and the luciferase activity was measured using the dual-luciferase reporter assay system (Promega). The luciferase activity was normalized to the value of the *Renilla* luciferase activity [21].

Pull-down (PD) assay

A Halo-tagged canine SGTA was cloned into a pFN21A vector (Promega). To generate haemagglutinin (HA)-tag fusion proteins, the *Xho*I/*Eco*RI fragment of canine REIC/Dkk-3 cDNA was cloned into a pMACS KK HA(C) vector. The expression of Halo and HA-tagged constructs was induced in 293 T cells using the FuGENE® HD transfection reagent (Promega), and the transfected cells were grown for 48 h. Cells were harvested by centrifugation and washed with Phosphate-buffered Saline (PBS). The cells were lysed in Mammalian Lysis Buffer (Promega) with a Protease Inhibitor Cocktail (Promega) for 15 min, and the cellular debris was cleared by centrifugation. To the supernatant, 100 μL of HaloLink™ Resin (Promega), equilibrated with TBS including 0.05% IGEPAL CA-630 (TBS+), were added. The samples were incubated for 20 min at 25 °C with rotation. The supernatant was discarded; the resin was washed three times with TBS+ and resuspended in sodium dodecyl sulphate-polyacrylamide gel electrophoresis (SDS-PAGE) loading buffer. The samples were analysed by western blot analysis using an anti-Halo antibody (1:2000) (G9281, Promega), an anti-haemagglutinin (HA) tag antibody (1:2000) (MBL-561, Medical and Biological Laboratories (MBL), Aichi, Japan) (1:2000), and a horseradish peroxidase-conjugated anti-rabbit IgG antibody (GE Healthcare, Waukesha, WI, USA). Blots were developed using the EzWestLumi plus reagent (ATTO, Tokyo, Japan).

Immunostaining

Immunocytochemical co-staining for forced-expressed Halo-tagged canine REIC/Dkk-3 and endogenous SGTA in CHP-1 cells was performed using the mouse monoclonal anti-Halo antibody (1:100) (G9211, Promega) and rabbit polyclonal anti-SGTA antibody (1:100) (sc-292,025, Santa Cruz Biotechnology, Santa Cruz, CA, USA). Cells were plated and cultured to 30–40% confluence in Lab-Tek chambers (Nalgene, Rochester, NY, USA), and were transfected with the pFN21A vector containing Halo-tagged canine REIC/Dkk-3 by FuGENE HD (Promega). Forty-eight hours after transfection, the cells were fixed in 4% paraformaldehyde in 100 mM phosphate buffer and blocked with 5% normal goat serum in PBS. After the samples were incubated overnight at 4 °C with primary antibodies, they were incubated for 1 h at 25 °C with Alexa Fluor 488 anti-mouse and Alexa Fluor 594 anti-rabbit secondary antibodies (Invitrogen, Carlsbad, CA, USA). To stain the nuclei, the cells were incubated with Hoechst 33,342 (Dojindo Laboratories, Kumamoto, Japan) for 15 min at room temperature. Fluorescent staining was visualised and analysed under a fluorescence microscope system equipped with an analytical software program (BZ-9000, Keyence, Osaka, Japan).

Transactivation assays

For this experiment, 10% charcoal-stripped FBS was used for the cell culture. Both PC3 and CHP-1 prostate cancer cells (2×10^5/well in 24-well plates, 500 μL medium/well) were transfected with 100 ng of pEGFP C1 AR vector containing the full-length AR (Plasmid ID: 28,235, Addgene, Cambridge, MA, USA) [22], 100 ng of p159-pPr-luc vector containing a firefly luciferase reporter gene downstream of the rat probasin gene promoter (Plasmid ID: 8392, Addgene) [23], 100 ng of pFN21A-SGTA, 200 ng of pMACS KK HA(C)-REIC/Dkk-3, and 25 ng of phRL-tk *Renilla* luciferase reporter plasmid by using the Lipofectamine 2000 reagent (Thermo Fisher Scientific, Waltham, MA, USA). After 48 h of transfection, the cells were treated for 24 h with control vehicle (ethanol) or dihydrotestosterone (DHT) (Sigma, St Louis, MO, USA), and were assayed for luciferase activity using a Dual-Luciferase Reporter Assay System (Promega). All transfection mixes were balanced with the appropriate empty vectors in terms of the ratio of the expression vectors and total plasmids.

Immunoblotting

Total protein was extracted from the cells using Mammalian Lysis Buffer (Promega) with Protease Inhibitor Cocktail (Promega) for 15 min, and the cellular debris was cleared by centrifugation. Canine control fibroblasts were collected from normal breast tissue of an 8-year-old female Chihuahua undergoing contraceptive treatment. Western blot analysis was performed as previously described [24]. Approximately 10 μg of extracted protein were analysed with the specific primary antibodies as follows: rabbit polyclonal anti-EGFP (MBL-598, MBL), rabbit polyclonal anti-SGTA (sc-292,025), rabbit polyclonal anti-REIC/Dkk-3 (10365–1-AP, Proteintech, Chicago, IL, USA), and anti-β-actin (sc-69,879, Santa Cruz Biotechnology).

Statistical analysis

The data are shown as the mean ± SE. Student's *t*-test or one-way analysis of variance (ANOVA) followed by Bonferroni test were performed to assess the significance of differences between two or more groups, respectively. Differences were considered significant with $P < 0.05$.

Results

REIC/Dkk-3 expression in canine prostate cancer cell lines and its interaction with SGTA

Canine REIC/Dkk-3 proteins were not expressed in canine androgen-independent prostate cancer CHP-1 cells as confirmed by western blot analysis, compared with canine control fibroblasts (Fig. 1a). Further, we analysed the interaction between canine REIC/Dkk-3 and SGTA by an MTH assay in 293 T cells using co-transfection and expression of each protein cloned into GAL4-DBD and VP16-AD plasmids, respectively. The luciferase activity, which reflects the binding intensity of each fusion protein, was increased in comparison to the empty vectors used as negative controls (Fig. 1b). The PD assay, performed to confirm the interaction between canine SGTA and REIC/Dkk-3, showed that the canine fused HA-REIC/Dkk-3 was detected in the canine Halo-tagged SGTA co-expression condition (Fig. 1c). Therefore, the interaction between canine SGTA and REIC/Dkk-3 was demonstrated by both, the MTH and PD assays. To further verify the interaction between canine REIC/Dkk-3 and SGTA in canine cells, immunocytochemistry was performed on CHP-1 cells that forced-expressed Halo-tagged canine REID/Dkk-3 using anti-Halo and anti-SGTA antibodies. Immunostaining revealed that Halo-tagged REIC/Dkk-3 and SGTA showed cytoplasmic localization with a similar distribution pattern, suggesting that their interaction and functions occur in the same locations (Fig. 1d).

Canine REIC/Dkk-3 interference with SGTA dimerization

We evaluated the interference of canine REIC/Dkk-3 in SGTA dimerization by using a modified-MTH assay, which has been employed in our previous studies [19, 25].

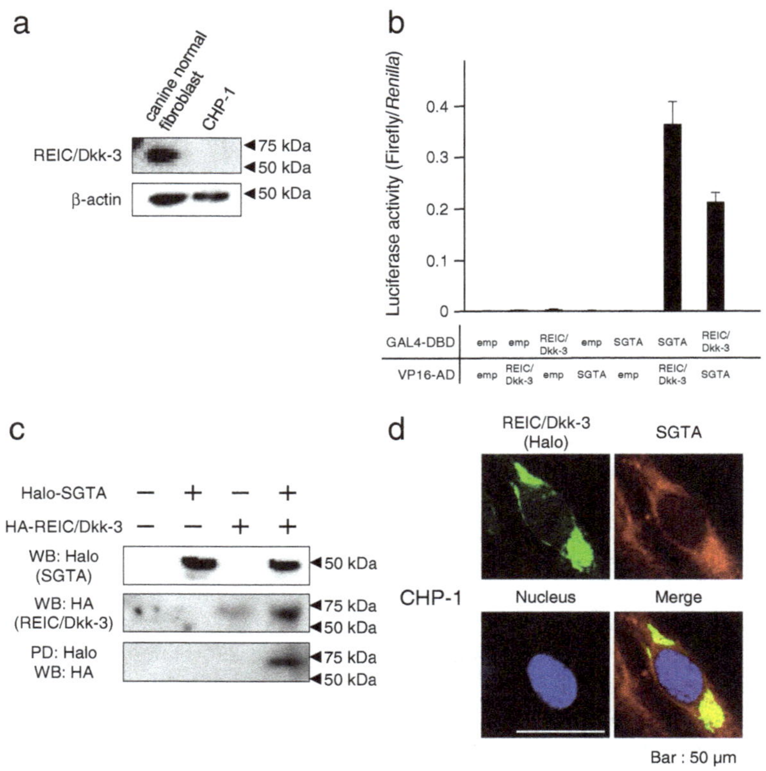

Fig. 1 Interaction between canine SGTA and REIC/Dkk-3. **a** Western blot analysis showing the expression profile of canine REIC/Dkk-3 and control β-actin in canine control fibroblasts and androgen-independent cell line CHP-1. **b** The interaction between canine SGTA and REIC/Dkk-3 was demonstrated by a mammalian two-hybrid (MTH) assay. DBD: GAL4-DNA-binding domain fusion protein. AD: VP16 transactivation domain fusion protein. The results were obtained from three independent experiments. **c** Western blot and pull-down assay results obtained from haemagglutinin (HA)-tagged REIC/Dkk-3 and Halo-tagged SGTA transfected 293 T cells lysates. **d** Co-localization of canine forced-expressed Halo-tagged REIC/Dkk-3 and endogenous SGTA was examined by double-immunofluorescence staining and observed by fluorescence microscopy. The images in green and red show the intracellular localization of Halo-tagged REIC/Dkk-3 and SGTA, respectively. The areas of overlap between REIC/Dkk-3 and SGTA are shown in yellow in the merged image

Canine REIC/Dkk-3 was co-transfected with canine SGTA, cloned in GAL4-DBD and VP16-AD plasmids, respectively. The luciferase activity was significantly decreased in the 100-ng canine REIC/Dkk-3 condition compared to the expression of canine SGTA alone (Fig. 2).

Interaction between canine REIC/Dkk-3 and SGTA regulates AR signalling activity

To evaluate the interaction between canine REIC/Dkk-3 and SGTA in the AR signal transduction pathway in canine prostate cancer, we first measured the extent of AR signalling activation by the probasin promoter-driven luciferase reporter assay [3, 19]. We expressed the AR and/or canine REIC/Dkk-3 in canine androgen-independent prostate cancer CHP-1 cells. The expression of canine REIC/Dkk-3 induced a significant increase in AR signalling with DHT stimulation (Fig. 3). This result suggests that REIC/Dkk-3 upregulates AR signalling in canine androgen-independent prostate cancer.

To investigate this mechanism, we repeated this assay in human androgen-independent prostate cancer PC3 cells. We expressed canine HA-REIC/Dkk-3 and/or Halo-SGTA together with the AR in PC3 cells (Fig. 4a). Canine REIC/Dkk-3 significantly increased, whereas canine SGTA decreased basal AR signalling and the co-expression of canine REIC/Dkk-3 recovered the signalling suppressed by SGTA in DHT-stimulated conditions (Fig. 4b). These results suggest that AR signalling is regulated by the canine REIC/Dkk-3 tumour suppressor, which interacts and interferes with SGTA functions and suppresses AR signalling in canine and human androgen-independent prostate cancer cell lines.

Discussion

Here, we demonstrated that the canine tumour suppressor REIC/Dkk-3 interacts with SGTA, which is a co-chaperone known to interact with Hsp70/Hsp90 and the cytosolic immature AR complex [3, 17, 19, 26]. Dimerized SGTA is an inhibitor of dynein motor-dependent

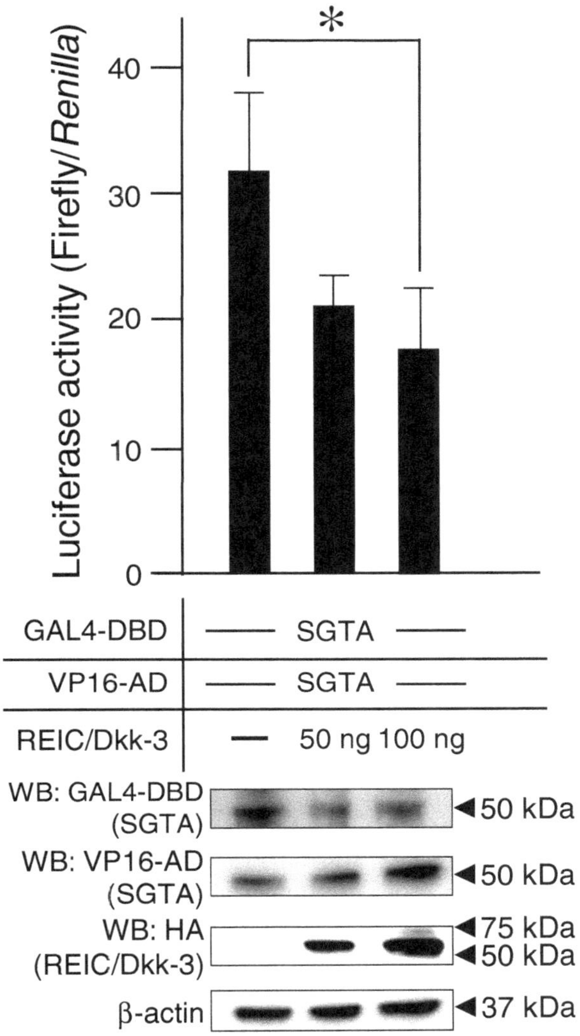

Fig. 2 Canine REIC/Dkk-3 interference in SGTA dimerization. The upper graph shows the role of canine REIC/Dkk-3, which interferes with SGTA dimerization, examined by a modified MTH assay. 293 T cells were co-transfected with DBD- or AD-fused canine SGTA plasmids and haemagglutinin (HA)-tagged REIC/Dkk-3. Luciferase activity in cell lysates was determined 48 h after transfection. The results were obtained from three independent experiments. The results show a significant difference between the SGTA alone and with the addition of 100 ng of canine REIC/Dkk-3 (*: $P < 0.05$, ANOVA). The lower panel depicts the western blot analysis showing the expression of DBD- and AD- fused canine SGTA, and haemagglutinin (HA)-tagged REIC/Dkk-3 after co-transfection in a parallel experiment with that depicted in the upper graph

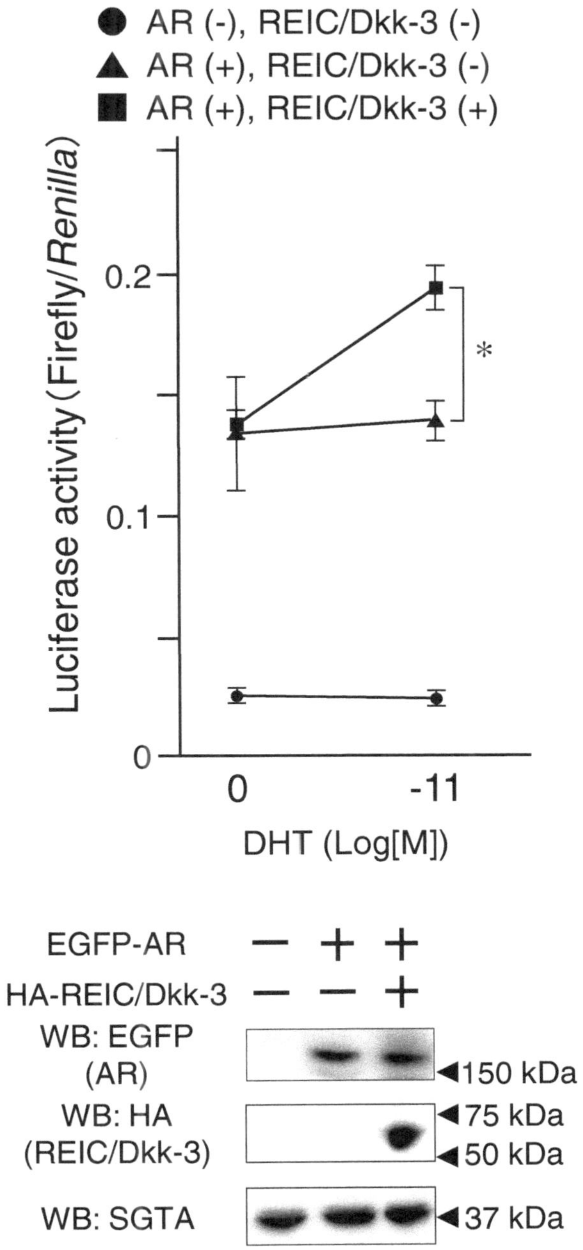

Fig. 3 Interaction between canine SGTA and REIC/Dkk-3 regulates AR signalling in canine androgen-independent prostate cancer cell line CHP-1. The upper graph shows the effects of canine REIC/Dkk-3 expression on AR signalling in the AR absent or present conditions with/without DHT stimulation in CHP-1 cells. Cells were co-transfected with the p159-pPr-Luc plasmid and treated with dihydrotestosterone (DHT). The value for the baseline was obtained using the control vehicle. The results were obtained from three independent experiments, and show a significant difference in AR activity based on REIC/Dkk-3 expression (*: $P < 0.05$, ANOVA). The lower figure shows the western blot results for the expression of EGFP-tagged AR, HA-tagged REIC/Dkk-3 and endogenous SGTA in CHP-1 cells after co-transfection in a parallel experiment with that depicted in the upper graph

AR transport and signalling, which is the cause of the androgen-independent condition in human prostate cancer [3, 17]. Canine SGTA also forms dimers and suppresses AR signal transduction [5, 20]. REIC/Dkk-3 interacts with SGTA and interferes with its dimerization

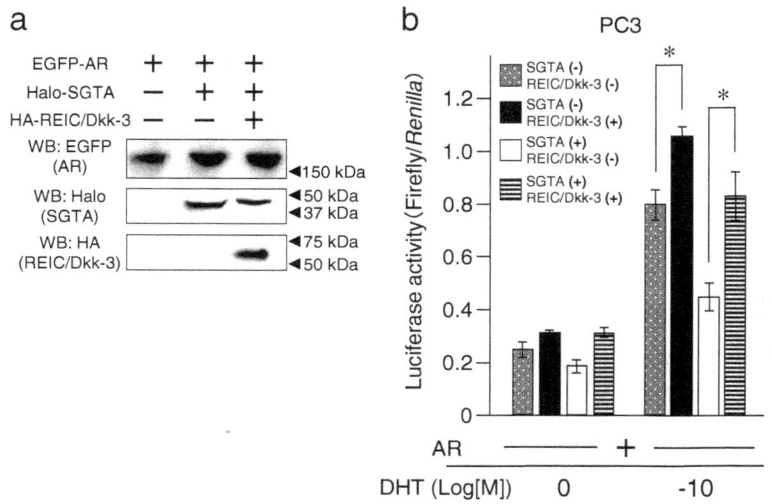

Fig. 4 Co-transfection with exogenous canine SGTA and REIC/Dkk-3 regulates AR signalling in human androgen-independent cancer cell line PC3. **a** Western blot analysis showing the expression of EGFP-tagged AR, Halo-tagged canine SGTA and HA-tagged canine REIC/Dkk-3 after co-transfection in a parallel experiment with that depicted in the graph **b**. **b** The effects of canine SGTA expression on the AR activity were examined in human prostate cancer PC3 cells under co-transfection with the AR, canine SGTA, and canine REIC/Dkk-3, with/without DHT. The results were obtained from three independent experiments, and show a significant difference in AR activity based on SGTA and/or REIC/Dkk-3 expression (*: $P < 0.05$, Student's *t*-test). All transfection mixes were balanced with the appropriate empty vectors in terms of the ratio of the expression vectors and total plasmids. The value for the baseline was obtained using the control vehicle

recovering AR translocation and signalling [19]. The interaction between REIC/Dkk-3 and SGTA shown in this study suggests that REIC/Dkk-3 may be a crucial step in the AR signalling pathway in dogs (Fig. 1b and c). Furthermore, overexpressed canine REIC/Dkk-3 interferes with SGTA dimerization and has the potential to function as an upregulator in the AR signalling pathway (Fig. 2). The underexpression of REIC/Dkk-3 in CHP-1 (Fig. 1a) suggests that the lack of this protein causes the androgen-independency in canine prostate cancer. In dogs, nearly all prostate cancers are androgen-independent, and thus, we expected that prostate cancer cell lines derived from dog e.g. DPC-1 [27], ACe-1 [28], and Leo [29] may downregulate the expression of REIC/Dkk-3.

In addition, we demonstrated that the overexpression of the canine REIC/Dkk-3 protein upregulates AR signal transduction in both canine and human androgen-independent prostate cancer cell lines. This result indicates that REIC/Dkk-3 activates AR transport by binding to SGTA and interfering with its dimerization and negative regulation (Figs. 3 and 4b). In humans, adenovirus-mediated REIC/Dkk-3 overexpression in various cancers, including prostate cancer, induces tumour specific apoptosis [7–9]. Furthermore, a canine study has shown an apoptotic function of REIC/Dkk-3 in cell lines established from a canine mammary gland tumour [30]. These results suggest that REIC/Dkk-3 has a potential role in canine androgen-independent prostate cancer as a novel anti-cancer agent.

Moreover, SGTA regulates the cell cycle, protein folding, transcription, protein transport, ubiquitin-proteasomes, and hormone receptor signalling [17, 31]. Co-chaperone proteins, including SGTA, interact with chaperones such as Hsp90 [18]. Hsp90 and other chaperone proteins are overexpressed in cancer cells with co-chaperones [18]. These events suggest that the expression of SGTA is induced by the overexpression of chaperones in various cancers types, not only prostate cancer [e.g., oesophageal squamous cell carcinoma and breast carcinoma] [31, 32]. Although upregulation of SGTA expression may not be related to hormonal signalling, overexpressed SGTA plays an important role as an inhibitor of AR signalling and confers the androgen-independent characteristics in prostate cancer [3]. In our previous study, canine SGTA was not overexpressed in prostate hyperplasia in both castrated and not castrated dogs [20]. However, castrated dogs with prostatic carcinoma highly overexpressed SGTA [20]. These results suggest that an excess of AR signalling is not a trigger for SGTA overexpression in the stage between hyperplasia and prostatic cancer in dogs, but sequentially SGTA overexpression induces the inhibition of AR signalling which leads to androgen-independency. This characteristic is remarkably similar to human androgen-independent prostate cancer. Therefore, the investigation of the relationship between AR signalling and SGTA function in canine prostate cancer allows a better understanding of the mechanisms of formation of androgen-independent prostate cancer beyond the species.

Recently, we showed that SGTA is expressed in canine prostate cancer but not in prostate hyperplasia [20]. The CHP-1 cell line, which was established from a sample of canine prostate cancer, was positive for cytokeratin AE1/AE3, an epithelial marker [5]. Although prostate cancer CHP-1 cells, which were obtained from a castrated dog, do not express the AR, the cells with AR exhibited androgen-dependent AR signalling (Fig. 3). These results suggest that CHP-1 have acquired androgen-independency followed by cancer progression. Therefore, CHP-1 may have similar characteristics to human androgen-independent prostate cancer cells, e.g. PC3 [5]. We demonstrated that REIC/Dkk-3 was not only an anti-cancer agent that induces tumour specific apoptosis but also restores AR signalling in both CHP-1 and human androgen-independent prostate cancer PC3 cells [19]. Compared to humans, castration is a very common procedure for preventing bad habits and male-specific diseases in dogs. Our results suggest that castrated dogs, and derived cells and tissues, are useful models of the study of both human and canine end-stage androgen-independent prostate cancers. The REIC/Dkk-3 and SGTA proteins are structurally and functionally well-conserved between human and dog [20, 30]; thus, our results regarding the interaction of these molecules in androgen-independent prostate cancer of human and dogs are applicable to both species. Further analysis regarding the mechanisms of the AR complex maturation via REIC/Dkk-3 and SGTA interaction in in vitro and in vivo experiments should contribute to the development of a novel strategy for the treatment of canine androgen-independent prostate cancer.

Conclusions

In conclusion, canine REIC/Dkk-3 interacts with SGTA and this interaction rescues AR signalling in both human and canine androgen-independent prostate cancers. Moreover, these results show that the role of canine REIC/Dkk-3 in AR signalling recovery can be replicated in canine prostate cancer cells. Further analyses regarding the role of REIC/Dkk-3 and SGTA interaction should contribute to breaking through refractory canine androgen-independent prostate cancer.

Abbreviations

AR: Androgen receptor; DHT: Dihydrotestosterone; ER: Endoplasmic reticulum; FBS: Foetal bovine serum; HA: Haemagglutinin; JNK: c-Jun-NH2-terminal kinase; MTH: Mammalian two-hybrid; ORF: Open reading frame; PD: Pull-down; PSA: Prostate specific antigen; REIC/Dkk-3: Reduced expression in immortalised cells; SGTA: Small glutamine-rich tetratricopeptide repeat-containing protein α

Acknowledgements

This work supported by KAKENHI scientific research grants from the Ministry of Education, Culture, Sports, Science, and Technology of Japan (No. 15 K07754).

Funding

Not applicable.

Authors' contributions

YK, SK, NN, DA and MM[1] conducted the experiments, analysed the data, and prepared the manuscript. KO, MB, MM[2], MW and TO designed this research and manuscript. All authors read and approved the final manuscript.

Competing interests

None of the authors of this paper has a financial or personal relationship with other people or organisations that could inappropriately influence or bias the content of the paper.

Consent for publication

Not applicable.

Author details

[1]School of Veterinary Nursing and Technology, Faculty of Veterinary Science, Nippon Veterinary and Life Science University, Tokyo 180-8602, Japan. [2]Laboratory of Animal Physiology, School of Animal Science, Nippon Veterinary and Life Science University, Tokyo 180-8602, Japan. [3]Department of Veterinary Clinical Pathology, Faculty of Veterinary Science, Nippon Veterinary and Life Science University, Tokyo 180-8602, Japan. [4]Department of Veterinary Pathology, Faculty of Veterinary Science, Nippon Veterinary and Life Science University, Tokyo 180-8602, Japan. [5]Laboratory of Laboratory Animal Science and Medicine, Department of Disease Control, Graduate School of Veterinary Medicine, Hokkaido University, Sapporo 060-0818, Japan. [6]Department of Urology, Graduate School of Medicine, Dentistry and Pharmaceutical Sciences, Okayama University, Okayama 700-8558, Japan.

References

1. Torre LA, Bray F, Siegel RL, Ferlay J, Lortet-Tieulent J, Jemal A. Global cancer statistics, 2012. CA Cancer J Clin. 2015;65:87–108.
2. Siegel RL, Miller KD, Jemal A. Cancer statistics, 2015. CA Cancer J Clin. 2015; 65:5–29.
3. Buchanan G, Ricciardelli C, Harris JM, Prescott J, Yu ZC, Jia L, et al. Control of androgen receptor signaling in prostate cancer by the cochaperone small glutamine rich tetratricopeptide repeat containing protein alpha. Cancer Res. 2007;67:10087–96.
4. Leroy BE, Northrup N. Prostate cancer in dogs: comparative and clinical aspects. Vet J. 2009;180:149–62.
5. Azakami D, Nakahira R, Kato Y, Michishita M, Kobayashi M, Onozawa E, et al. The canine prostate cancer cell line CHP-1 shows over-expression of the co-chaperone small glutamine-rich tetratricopeptide repeat-containing protein alpha. Vet Comp Oncol. 2017;15:557–62.
6. Tsuji T, Miyazaki M, Sakaguchi M, Inoue Y, Namba M. A REIC gene shows down-regulation in human immortalized cells and human tumor-derived cell lines. Biochem Biophys Res Commun. 2000;268:20–4.
7. Abarzua F, Sakaguchi M, Takaishi M, Nasu Y, Kurose K, Ebara S, et al. Adenovirus-mediated overexpression of REIC/Dkk-3 selectively induces apoptosis in human prostate cancer cells through activation of c-Jun-NH2-kinase. Cancer Res. 2005;65:9617–22.
8. Kawano Y, Kitaoka M, Hamada Y, Walker MM, Waxman J, Kypta RM. Regulation of prostate cell growth and morphogenesis by Dickkopf-3. Oncogene. 2006;25:6528–37.
9. Watanabe M, Nasu Y, Kumon H. Adenovirus-mediated REIC/Dkk-3 gene therapy: development of an autologous cancer vaccination therapy (review). Oncol Lett. 2014;7:595–601.

10. Hsieh SY, Hsieh PS, Chiu CT, Chen WY. Dickkopf-3/REIC functions as a suppressor gene of tumor growth. Oncogene. 2004;23:9183–9.
11. Abarzua F, Kashiwakura Y, Takaoka M, Watanabe M, Ochiai K, Sakaguchi M, et al. An N-terminal 78 amino acid truncation of REIC/Dkk-3 effectively induces apoptosis. Biochem Biophys Res Commun. 2008;375:614–8.
12. Kashiwakura Y, Ochiai K, Watanabe M, Abarzua F, Sakaguchi M, Takaoka M, et al. Down-regulation of inhibition of differentiation-1 via activation of activating transcription factor 3 and Smad regulates REIC/Dickkopf-3-induced apoptosis. Cancer Res. 2008;68:8333–41.
13. Watanabe M, Sakaguchi M, Kinoshita R, Kaku H, Ariyoshi Y, Ueki H, et al. A novel gene expression system strongly enhances the anticancer effects of a REIC/Dkk-3-encoding adenoviral vector. Oncol Rep. 2014;31:1089–95.
14. Chartron JW, VanderVelde DG, Clemons WM Jr. Structures of the Sgt2/SGTA dimerization domain with the Get5/UBL4A UBL domain reveal an interaction that forms a conserved dynamic interface. Cell Rep. 2012;2:1620–32.
15. Trotta AP, Need EF, Butler LM, Selth LA, O'Loughlin MA, Coetzee GA, et al. Subdomain structure of the co-chaperone SGTA and activity of its androgen receptor client. J Mol Endocrinol. 2012;49:57–68.
16. Hanke K, Chudak C, Kurth R, Bannert N. The Rec protein of HERV-K(HML-2) upregulates androgen receptor activity by binding to the human small glutamine-rich tetratricopeptide repeat protein (hSGT). Int J Cancer. 2013; 132:556–67.
17. Philp LK, Butler MS, Hickey TE, Butler LM, Tilley WD, Day TK. SGTA: a new player in the molecular co-chaperone game. Horm Cancer. 2013;4:343–57.
18. Trotta AP, Need EF, Selth LA, Chopra S, Pinnock CB, Leach DA, et al. Knockdown of the cochaperone SGTA results in the suppression of androgen and PI3K/Akt signaling and inhibition of prostate cancer cell proliferation. Int J Cancer. 2013;133:2812–23.
19. Ochiai K, Morimatsu M, Kato Y, Ishiguro-Oonuma T, Udagawa C, Rungsuriyawiboon O, et al. Tumor suppressor REIC/DKK-3 and co-chaperone SGTA: their interaction and roles in the androgen sensitivity. Oncotarget. 2016;7:3283–96.
20. Kato Y, Ochiai K, Michishita M, Azakami D, Nakahira R, Morimatsu M, et al. Molecular cloning of canine co-chaperone small glutamine-rich tetratricopeptide repeat-containing protein alpha (SGTA) and investigation of its ability to suppress androgen receptor signalling in androgen-independent prostate cancer. Vet J. 2015;206:143–8.
21. Ochiai K, Ishiguro-Oonuma T, Yoshikawa Y, Udagawa C, Kato Y, Watanabe M, et al. Polymorphisms of canine BRCA2 BRC repeats affecting interaction with RAD51. Biomed Res. 2015;36:155–8.
22. Stenoien DL, Cummings CJ, Adams HP, Mancini MG, Patel K, DeMartino GN, et al. Polyglutamine-expanded androgen receptors form aggregates that sequester heat shock proteins, proteasome components and SRC-1, and are suppressed by the HDJ-2 chaperone. Hum Mol Genet. 1999;8:731–41.
23. Kaczmarczyk SJ, Green JE. A single vector containing modified cre recombinase and LOX recombination sequences for inducible tissue-specific amplification of gene expression. Nucleic Acids Res. 2001;29:E56-6.
24. Watanabe M, Yang G, Cao G, Tahir SA, Naruishi K, Tabata K, et al. Functional analysis of secreted caveolin-1 in mouse models of prostate cancer progression. Mol Cancer Res. 2009;7:1446–55.
25. Ochiai K, Yoshikawa Y, Yoshimatsu K, Oonuma T, Tomioka Y, Takeda E, et al. Valine 1532 of human BRC repeat 4 plays an important role in the interaction between BRCA2 and RAD51. FEBS Lett. 2011;585:1771–7.
26. Liu FH, Wu SJ, Hu SM, Hsiao CD, Wang C. Specific interaction of the 70-kDa heat shock cognate protein with the tetratricopeptide repeats. J Biol Chem. 1999;274:34425–32.
27. Anidjar M, Villette JM, Devauchelle P, Delisle F, Cotard JP, Billotey C, et al. In vivo model mimicking natural history of dog prostate cancer using DPC-1, a new canine prostate carcinoma cell line. Prostate. 2001;46:2–10.
28. LeRoy BE, Thudi NK, Nadella MV, Toribio RE, Tannehill-Gregg SH, van Bokhoven A, et al. New bone formation and osteolysis by a metastatic, highly invasive canine prostate carcinoma xenograft. Prostate. 2006;66:1213–22.
29. Thudi NK, Shu ST, Martin CK, Lanigan LG, Nadella MV, Van Bokhoven A, et al. Development of a brain metastatic canine prostate cancer cell line. Prostate. 2011;71:1251–63.
30. Ochiai K, Watanabe M, Azakami D, Michishita M, Yoshikawa Y, Udagawa C, et al. Molecular cloning and tumour suppressor function analysis of canine REIC/Dkk-3 in mammary gland tumours. Vet J. 2013;197:769–75.
31. Yang X, Cheng L, Li M, Shi H, Ren H, Ding Z, et al. High expression of SGTA in esophageal squamous cell carcinoma correlates with proliferation and poor prognosis. J Cell Biochem. 2014;115:141–50.
32. Zhu T, Ji Z, Xu C, Peng Z, Gu L, Zhang R, et al. Expression and prognostic role of SGTA in human breast carcinoma correlates with tumor cell proliferation. J Mol Histol. 2014;45:665–77.

3

Epidemiological and pathological study of feline morbillivirus infection in domestic cats in Japan

Eun-Sil Park[1], Michio Suzuki[1], Masanobu Kimura[1], Hiroshi Mizutani[2], Ryuichi Saito[2], Nami Kubota[2], Youko Hasuike[2], Jungo Okajima[2], Hidemi Kasai[2], Yuko Sato[3], Noriko Nakajima[3], Keiji Maruyama[2], Koichi Imaoka[1] and Shigeru Morikawa[1*]

Abstract

Background: Feline morbillivirus (FmoPV) is a novel paramyxovirus found to infect domestic cats. FmoPV has been isolated in several countries in Asia and Europe and is considered to have genetic diversity. Also, it is suspected to be associated with feline renal diseases including tubulointerstitial nephritis (TIN), which affects domestic cats with a high incidence rate.

Results: To clarify the state of FmoPV infection among domestic cats in Japan, an epidemiological survey was conducted. Twenty-one out of 100 cats were found to have serum antibodies (Ab) against FmoPV-N protein by indirect immunofluorescence assay (IF) using FmoPV-N protein-expressing HeLa cells. Twenty-two of the cats were positive for FmoPV RNA in the urine and/or renal tissues. In total, 29 cats were positive for Ab and/or viral RNA. These FmoPV-infected cats were classified into three different phases of infection: RNA+/Ab + (14 cats), RNA+/Ab- (8 cats) and RNA-/Ab + (7 cats). In immunohistochemistry (IHC), 19 out of 29 cats were positive for FmoPV-N protein in kidney tissues; however, the FmoPV-N protein was located in the inflammatory lesions with severe grade in only four out of the 19 cats. Since 15 out of 29 infected cats were positive for viral RNA and Ab, approximately half of the infected cats were persistently infected with FmoPV.

Conclusions: A statistically significant difference was observed between infection of FmoPV and the presence of inflammatory changes in renal lesions, indicating a relationship between FmoPV infection and feline renal diseases. However, we could not obtain histopathological evidence of a relationship between FmoPV infection and TIN.

Keywords: Feline morbillivirus, Cat, Kidney disease, Epidemiology, Inflammation

Background

A novel paramyxovirus, feline morbillivirus (FmoPV), has recently been detected in domestic cats [1–8]. FmoPV is genetically most closely related to viruses such as canine distemper virus (CDV), measles virus (MV), rinderpest virus (RPV), peste-des-petits-ruminants virus (PPRV), phocine distemper virus (PDV) and cetacean morbillivirus (CMV), belonging to the genus morbillivirus in the family *Paramyxoviridae* [1–5]. FmoPV showed genetic diversity among isolates [3–5], and a natural recombination in the envelope protein region between viruses in different clades was also found [4]. In Germany, three groups of feline paramyxoviruses (FPaV) have been detected, and these were associated with feline chronic kidney diseases (CKD) including lower urinary tract diseases (LUTD) [5]. Phylogenetically, the first group of these viruses belongs to the same cluster of FmoPV with 99 % homology, whereas the second group represents a new cluster between FmoPV and other morbilliviruses. The third group represents a group that is distinct from FmoPV and other morbilliviruses. A seroepidemiological survey of CDV infection in Asian countries showed that domestic cats were susceptible to CDV infection, but CDV was not virulent in domestic

* Correspondence: morikawa@nih.go.jp
[1]Department of Veterinary Science, National Institute of Infectious Diseases, Tokyo 162-8640, Japan
Full list of author information is available at the end of the article

cats [9]. At the moment, it is not yet confirmed that FmoPV is classified in the genus morbillivirus or in a novel genus separate from the genus morbillivirus.

Kidney failure is one of the most important and common diseases in domestic cats. It can be divided into acute kidney disease (AKD) and chronic kidney disease (CKD), or inherent kidney disease and acquired kidney disease [10–13]. AKD, which could be caused by toxins, trauma, infection, shock, blockage of the blood flow and heart failure [11], is reversible and can affect cats of all ages. CKD affects domestic cats, especially middle-aged or older cats [14], and its prevalence increases according to age, affecting up to half of cats older than 15 years [14]. CKD could result from infection, blockages, dental disease, high blood pressure and cancer. In particular, idiopathic CKD such as pyelonephritis, glomerulonephritis and chronic tubulointerstitial nephritis (TIN) due to unknown causes has been reported extensively [10, 11, 15–17]. It is suspected that FmoPV is one of the causative agents of CKD [1, 5], such as chronic TIN. Therefore, it is important to clarify the characteristics or the pathogenicity of FmoPV and the pathogenesis in domestic cats as the natural host. In this respect, large-scale epidemiological investigation is considered to be indispensable.

In this study, epidemiological and pathological studies were performed to demonstrate the seroprevalence of FmoPV and the relationship between FmoPV and CKD in Japan. These studies revealed that the infection rate of FmoPV was considerable and FmoPV might be related to urinary tract diseases.

Results

Detection of FmoPV by RT-PCR and phylogenetic analysis

Cat urine and renal tissues were examined for the presence of FmoPV RNA by nested RT-PCR [2]. Seventeen cats (17 %) were positive for FmoPV RNA in urine, and 18 cats (18 %) were positive in renal tissues (Table 1). Among these cats, 13 cats (13 %) were both positive in urine and tissues. Four cats (4 %) were positive in the urine but negative in the tissues, whereas five cats (5 %) were negative in the urine but positive in the tissues.

Nucleotide sequences of all the PCR-positive samples were analyzed phylogenetically with those of FmoPVs in Hong Kong and Japan (Kyoto), and CDV and Nipah virus as outgroups. They were divided into three groups (Fig. 1). To determine the groups of FmoPV strains in

Table 1 Detection of FmoPV RNA by RT-PCR

		In urine ($n = 100$)	
		-	+
In kidney tissues ($n = 100$)	-	78	4
	+	5	13

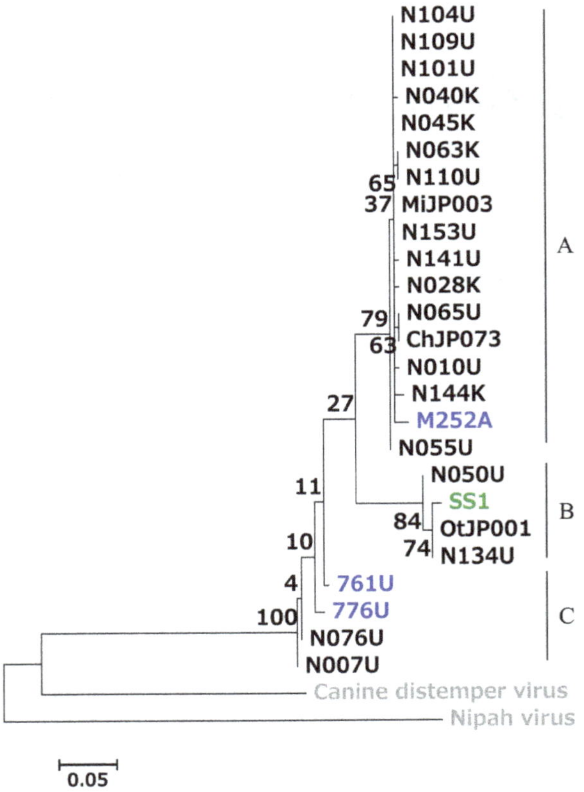

Fig. 1 Phylogenetic analysis based on partial L protein sequences of FmoPV in infected cats in Tokyo. Phylogenic tree was inferred using the maximum likelihood method in the MEGA6 package. The percentage of replicate tree in which the associated taxa clustered together in the bootstrap test (1000 replicates) is shown next to the branches. The tree is drawn to scale, and the scale bar indicates the branch length corresponding to 0.05 substitutions per site. The strains from Hong Kong and Japan (Kyoto) are represented by *blue* and *green*, respectively. Nucleotide sequences of CDV and Nipah virus are used as outgroups and represented in *gray*. Information about the strain names and accession numbers is listed in Table 2. Statistically significant differences ($P < 0.01$) were obtained in the distribution of the pairwise distances of clusters A, B and C

the phylogenetic tree are stable, pairwise distances were compared by histogram by the method described previously [18]. Statistically significant differences ($P < 0.01$) were obtained in the distribution of the pairwise distances of clusters A, B and C (data not shown). FmoPV strains from Hong Kong and some strains of Japan were grouped into the same clusters, cluster A and C, thus a phylogenetic relationship with geographic distribution of FmoPV in two countries was not observed (Fig. 1).

Detection of antibodies against FmoPV-N protein by Immunofluorescence (IF) test

To detect FmoPV-N antibodies by IF test, FmoPV-N expressing HeLa cells were prepared. The specificity of the IF test was confirmed by serum from rabbit immunized with the purified FmoPV-N and its pre-immune negative control rabbit serum. As shown in Fig. 2, FmoPV-N immunized rabbit serum reacted to FmoPV-N expressing HeLa, but not to mock-HeLa cells nor empty plasmid, pKS336, transfected HeLa cells. Negative control rabbit serum did not react to any of the HeLa cells. Specificity of the IF test was also confirmed using FmoPV antibody positive cat serum (N045) (Fig. 2). Thus, all the cat sera were tested by the IF test to detect antibodies against FmoPV-N.

Twenty-one percent of cats had Ab against FmoPV-N protein (Table 2 and Fig. 2). Ab titers ranged between 1:160 to 1:20,480 or above. The Ab titers appeared to be high in middle-aged cats (from 4 to 8 years old, Fig. 3), although not significantly. All the FmoPV antibody positive cat sera were tested negative by IF test using CDV-N expressing HeLa cells (data not shown), indicating there is no serological cross reactivity between CDV-N and FmoPV-N at least by IF test. There were four patterns: RNA+/Ab + (14 cats), RNA+/Ab- (eight cats) and RNA-/Ab + (seven cats) (Table 2) and RNA-/Ab- (71 cats, data not shown). In total, 29 out of 100 cats (29 %) were positive for Ab and/or viral RNA, thus they were considered to be FmoPV-infected. Fourteen out of 29 cats were positive for viral RNA and Ab, indicating that approximately half of the infected cats were persistently infected with FmoPV.

Histopathological examination of FmoPV infection in cat renal tissues

Histopathological examination was performed to detect FmoPV in cat renal tissues and to confirm the relationship between virus infection and tubulointerstitial nephritis by hematoxylin and eosin (HE) staining and immunohistochemistry (IHC) (Fig. 4). Among 29 cases that showed FmoPV RNA+ and/or Ab+, moderate to severe chronic interstitial nephritis was observed in 16 cases (Table 2 and Fig. 4). Mild infiltration of inflammatory cells into the renal tissues was observed in 10 cases. Three cases had no lesions. Other lesions including interstitial fibrosis, glomerulosclerosis, tubular microcystic change, proteinaceous casts and calcification were observed in some cases (data not shown). Among 71 FmoPV non-infected cats, moderate to severe chronic interstitial nephritis was observed in 29 cases. No lesions or mild infiltration of inflammatory cells into the renal tissues were observed in 25 and 15 cases, respectively. No statistically significant relationship could be confirmed between tubulointerstitial nephritis and the infection of FmoPV (Table 3, $P > 0.05$). However, a significant relationship was found between the presence of inflammatory lesions and the infection of FmoPV (Table 4, $P < 0.01$).

To prepare rabbit antibody against FmoPV-N protein for the detection of FmoPV antigens, a recombinant FmoPV-N protein with his-tag at C terminal was expressed in Sf9 insect cells using a recombinant baculovirus. The recombinant FmoPV-N was purified by Ni-NTA agarose chromatography and was confirmed by SDS-PAGE (Fig. 5). Two major bands with a molecular weight of 59 and 40 kDa were observed by SDS-PAGE. A large band was consistent with the predicted size of the FmoPV-N, while a small one is thought to be N-terminal truncated FmoPV-N, since both of them were purified by Ni-NTA agarose chromatography. Since FmoPV-positive cat serum reacted to both two bands in immunoblot, N-terminal truncated FmoPV-N was considered to be immunogenic. The purified FmoPV-N protein was subcutaneously injected into three rabbits five times. When the serum antibody titers by IF test reached

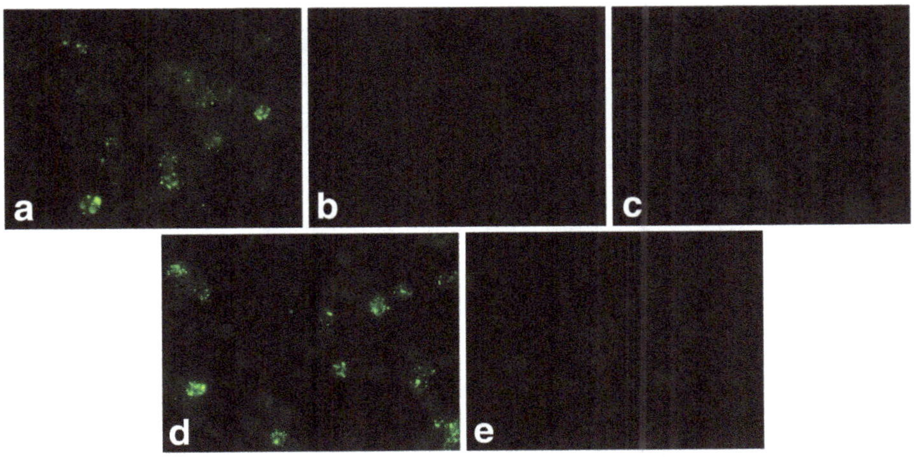

Fig. 2 IF staining. **a** FmoPV-N immunized rabbit serum strongly reacted to FmoPV-N expressing HeLa cells, but did not react to empty vector, pKS336, transfected HeLa cells (**b**), nor to mock HeLa cells (**c**). FmoPV antibody positive cat (N045, 1:40) reacted to FmoPV-N expressing HeLa cells (**d**), but did not react to mock HeLa cells (**e**). Granular *apple green* signal was observed in the cytoplasm, represented by FITC

Table 2 Detection of viral RNA, IgG and antigen

No. of cases	ID of cat	Degree of lesions	FmoPV RNA		Antibody titer in IF	IHC	Accession no.	Strain
			urine	tissue				
1[a]	N010	++	P[1]	P	>20,480	***	LC080842	N010U
2[a]	N101	++	P	P	5120	***	LC080851	N101U
3[a]	N153	+++	P	P	640	***	LC080858	N153U
4	N007	+	P	P	10,240	**	LC080841	N007U
5	N110	+	P	P	1280	**	LC080854	N110U
6	N134	++	P	P	160	**	LC080855	N134U
7	N141	+	P	P	2560	*	LC080856	N141U
8	N020	+	P	N[2]	5120	*		
9	N050	+++	P	N	640	**	LC080846	N050U
10	N104	none	P	N	1280	**	LC080852	N104U
11	N028	+++	N	P	5120	**	LC080843	N028K
12	N040	++	N	P	1280	**	LC080844	N040K
13†	N055	++	P	P	<40	***	LC080847	N055U
14	N001	++	P	P	<40	**	AB924120	OtJP001
15	N003	+	P	P	<40	**	AB924121	MiJP003
16	N073	+++	P	P	<40	*	AB924122	ChJP073
17	N076	none	P	P	<40	**	LC080850	N076U
18	N109	++	P	P	<40	*	LC080853	N109U
19	N140	+	N	N	640	*		
20	N045	++	N	P	2560	none	LC080845	N045K
21	N144	+++	N	P	640	none	LC080857	N144K
22	N063	+	N	P	<40	none	LC080848	N063K
23	N065	+	P	N	<40	none	LC080849	N065U
24	N024	+	N	N	2560	none		
25	N064	+++	N	N	2560	none		
26	N131	+	N	N	320	none		
27	N136	++	N	N	640	none		
28	N138	none	N	N	320	none		
29	N148	++	N	N	2560	none		

[a] IHC-positive in inflammatory lesions
1 positive
2 negative
+ mild
++ moderate
+++ severe
* mild
** moderate
*** extensive

above 1:10,000, the rabbits were euthanized and the sera were collected. The rabbit antibodies reacted to the recombinant FmoPV-N protein in immunoblot (data not shown).

Immunohistochemistry (IHC) was performed using the rabbit FmoPV-N antibody to detect viral antigens in tissues. Among 29 FmoPV-infected cats, 19 cats showed FmoPV-N proteins in renal tissues by IHC (Table 2). However, only four cases out of the 19 cats were positive for FmoPV-N proteins in,the tubular cells of the renal cortex and the renal medulla (Fig. 4). Extensive inflammatory cells were infiltrated around the FmoPV-N positive renal tubular cells, indicating the cats were suffered from chronic tubulointerstitial nephritis (Fig. 4a and b). Although other cases also showed mild to severe infiltration of mononuclear cells in the interstitial tissues, the distribution of FmoPV-N proteins was limited in renal tubular cells or transitional cells of the renal medulla or pelvis,

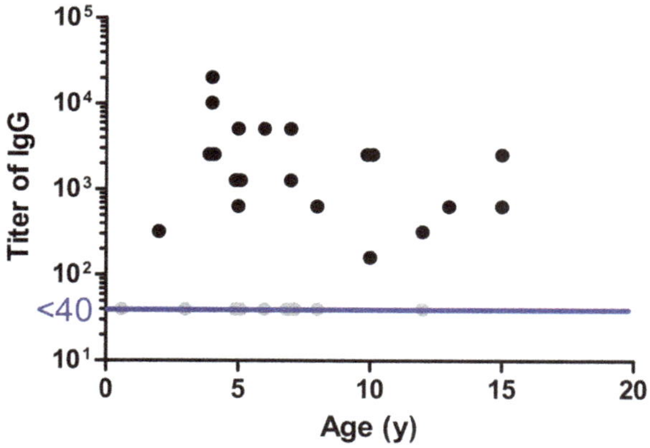

Fig. 3 The relationship between age of FmoPV-infected cats and Ab titer. Ab titers in IF test are represented by *black dots*. Sera showing Ab titers of less than 1:40 are considered negative (*gray dots*)

Table 3 The relationship between the grade of lesions and the infection of FmoPV

Infection of FmoPV	Grade of lesions				Total
	1[a] (*n*)	2[b]	3[c]	4[d]	
FmoPV-positive	3	10	16	0	29
FmoPV-negative	25	15	29	2	71

[a] No lesions
[b] Mild infiltration of inflammatory cells
[c] Moderate to severe TIN
[d] et al

but not in the inflammatory lesions (Fig. 4e and f). In all of the cases, cytoplasms of renal tubular cells were positive for FmoPV-N proteins and there were no specific intracytoplasmic or intranuclear inclusion bodies (Fig. 4). Overall, it seemed likely that FmoPV infection might be associated with feline urinary tract diseases including CKD or LUTD, although it remained inconclusive whether FmoPV causes these diseases per se or acts as a helper or bystander.

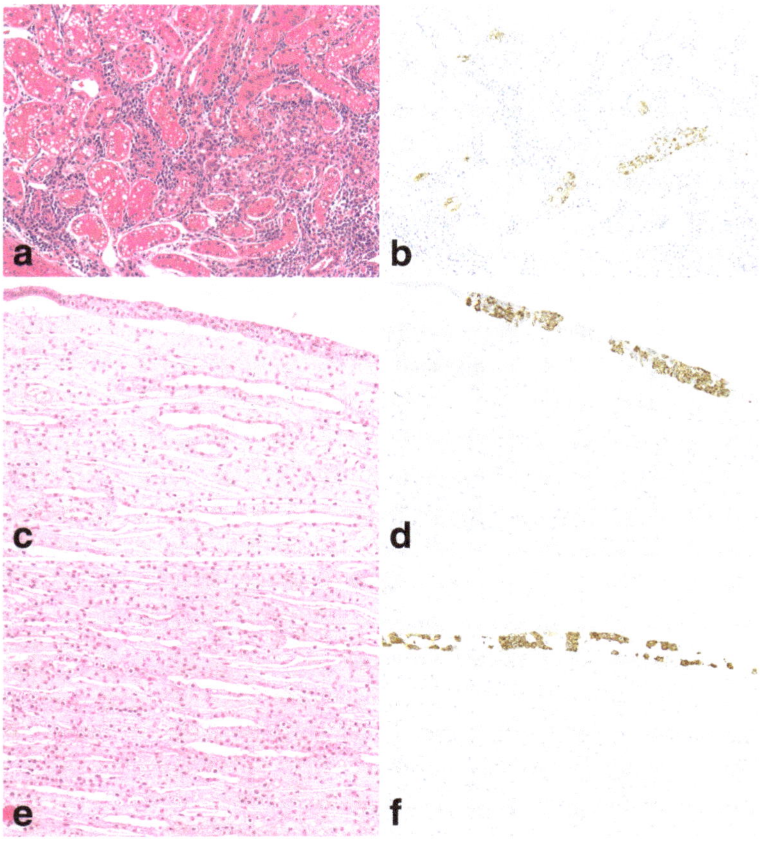

Fig. 4 IHC examination of FmoPV-infected cases. **a** FmoPV RNA+ and Ab + positive case (ID of cat: N101). Severe infiltration of inflammatory cells into the interstitial tissue or renal tubules is observed (HE staining). **b** FmoPV RNA+ and Ab + positive case (ID of cat: N110). FmoPV antigens were demonstrated in the cytoplasm of renal tubular cells (IHC). **c** FmoPV RNA+ and Ab- case (ID of cat: N055). **d** FmoPV RNA+ and Ab- case (ID of cat: N055). Transitional cells in the renal pelvis are positive (IHC). **e** FmoPV RNA+ and Ab- case (ID of cat: N076). There are no pathologic lesions in this case (data not shown, Table 2). **f** FmoPV RNA+ and Ab- case (ID of cat: N076). Renal tubular cells are positive (IHC)

Table 4 The relationship between the presence of inflammatory lesions and the infection of FmoPV

Infection of FmoPV	The presence of inflammatory lesions		Total
	Existed (*n*)	Not existed (*n*)	
FmoPV-positive	26	3	29
FmoPV-negative	44	27	71

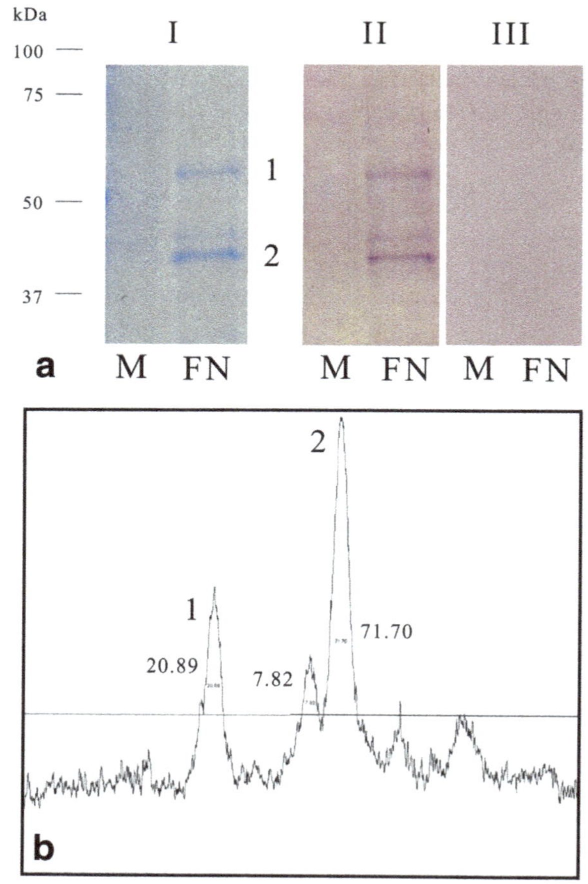

Fig. 5 Analysis of recombinant FmoPV-N protein. **a** Coomassie Brilliant Blue (CBB) staining and Immunoblot. Two major bands were stained with CBB (M; mock, FN; FmoPV-N) (I). A large band corresponded to the entire FmoPV-N with a molecular weight of 59 kDa (1), while other smaller band may correspond to a truncated FmoPV-N with a molecular weight of 40 kDa (2). FmoPV antibody positive cat serum (N028) reacted to both two bands (II). FmoPV antibody negative cat serum (N004) did not react to mock and FmoPV-N protein (III). **b** Purity of the recombinant FmoPV-Ab. An image of the stained gel was analyzed using ImageJ 1.50i and it was shown that amount of the entire FmoPV-N and the truncated protein were approximately 21 and 72 %, respectively. The purity was estimated to be 93 %

Discussion

In the present study, 22 out of 100 cats in Japan were shown to be FmoPV RNA positive in urine and/or kidney. Phylogenetic analysis of the FmoPV detected in Japan showed FmoPV was clustered in three groups. However, a phylogenetic relationship with geographic distribution of FmoPV in Japan and Hong Kong was not observed. Further, a significant relationship between FmoPV cluster and renal disease in the cat was not observed (data not shown). It is, however, necessary to compare the FmoPV sequences in cats from other regions in future to confirm this hypothesis. Recently, several partial sequences of FmoPV detected in cats in Germany were reported [5], however, we could not compare our data with them because the region of the sequences were not overlapped.

RNAs and proteins of FmoPV were detected in cat urine, sera and/or renal tissues. Anti-FmoPV Abs were also demonstrated in cat sera. FmoPV-infected cats in the present study were divided into three groups: RNA +/Ab+, RNA+/Ab- and RNA-/Ab+. Cats in the RNA +/Ab- group were considered to be in an acute phase of FmoPV infection. Cats in the RNA+/Ab + group were considered to be in either a subacute or a chronic phase of the infection. Since it is not confirmed that the nested R-PCR used in the present study detected all the FmoPV strains because of the genetic diversity of the viruses, thus it is possible that there are some false negative results in the RT-PCR. Since humoral immune response in addition to cellular immune response to the virus are thought to eliminate the virus from animals, cats in the RNA-/Ab + group were considered to be in a convalescent phase. Consequently, it appears that FmoPV could establish as an acute, subacute or chronic infection, and could be eliminated. Additionally, there were cases in which RNA of FmoPV was negative in urine but positive in renal tissues. Since approximately half of the infected cats (14 out of the 29 infected cats) were positive for viral RNA and Ab, it seems likely that cats are easily chronically or persistently infected with the virus. However, further long-term follow-up studies in FmoPV-infected cats are necessary to confirm this hypothesis.

Cat samples were collected randomly from healthy cats and sick or wounded cats, including stray cats in Tokyo. No relationships among the clinical data, except age and sex, with the infection by FmoPV could be found. The infection rate of FmoPV was significantly high in unneutered male cats ($P < 0.005$) in this study (Fig. 6). These tendencies could be due to differences of behavior patterns, such as more aggressive or active behavior in unneutered male cats than neutered male cats and female cats, and such behavior might result in an increase in opportunity of infection with FmoPV from other infected cats. The transmission of FmoPV between cats could occur in veterinary hospitals, boarding

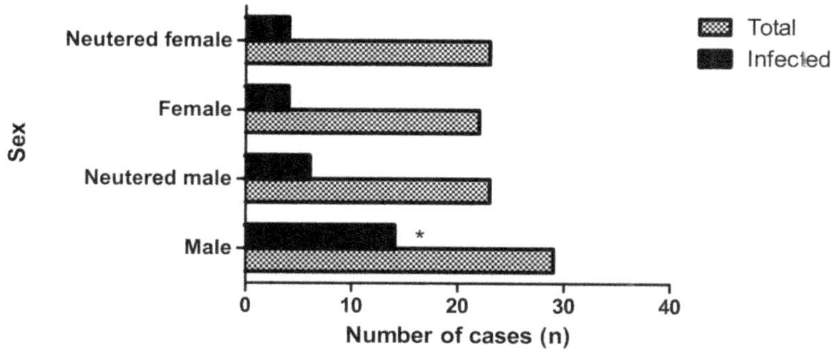

Fig. 6 FmoPV-infected cats according to sex. The infection rate of FmoPV was significantly high in unneutered male cats ($P < 0.005$)

kennels, breeding facilities, outdoors or at home. Given the high positive rate, it seemed that FmoPV might be maintained between their transmissible cats for a long time.

In a pathological examination, 25 out of 29 infected cats had renal lesions, from mild mononuclear cell infiltration to chronic tubulointerstitial nephritis. Half of them were mediate to severe cases. As a result of IHC, 19 out of 29 cats showed FmoPV-N protein in their kidney tissues. Four of the 19 cats showed severe lesions with FmoPV-N protein in the inflammatory lesions. The FmoPV-N protein-positive cells were identified to be renal tubular epithelial cells in the renal cortex, medulla and pelvis. FmoPV-N protein-positive mononuclear cells could not be found in this study, different from a report in Hong Kong [1]. These cases had RNA of FmoPV both in urine and renal tissues and relatively high IgG titer of 1: 640 to 20,480, except one case, representing the chronic phase. However, the IHC-positive sites were focally located, not distributed widely in the lesions.

In the other 15 cases, normal renal tubular cells or transitional cells of the renal medulla or pelvis were IHC-positive. No statistically significant correlations were found between the grades of lesions and the infection of FmoPV. However, a statistically significant relationship with the presence of inflammatory lesions and the infection of FmoPV was found, regardless of TIN. Consequently, no meaningful direct relationship between infection by FmoPV and chronic TIN was confirmed in this study. It might be plausible that FmoPV antigens in the lesions were already eliminated by host immune responses in the case of severe chronic TIN. A similar phenomenon was reported in other virus infectious diseases such as hemorrhagic fever with renal syndrome (HFRS) caused by hantavirus and severe acute respiratory syndrome (SARS) caused by SARS coronavirus (SARS-CoV) [19, 20]. In these cases, uncontrolled responses in cytokines and chemokines are considered to be responsible for the pathogenesis. In this regard, it would be necessary to analyze innate immune responses in cats with FmoPV.

It is well known that many viruses such as feline immunodeficiency virus, feline foamy virus, feline infectious peritonitis virus and feline leukemia virus can affect the kidneys of domestic cats, resulting in severe CKD including glomerulosclerosis, TIN, amyloidosis and pyrogranulomatous nephritis [21–27]. FmoPV is a recently identified virus, but it could affect the kidneys in infected cats. Thus, the existence or pathogenicity of FmoPV could have been underestimated.

In addition, a correlation between lower urinary tract disease (LUTD) and infection of FmoPV has been reported recently [5]. LUTD including urethral obstruction (UO) and interstitial cystitic (IC) is also an important and common disease in domestic cats [10, 11, 15–17, 28–30]. Feline calicivirus, feline herpesvirus type II and feline foamy virus have been detected in some cats with LUTD [21, 28–32]. In this study, lower urinary tract tissues or related clinical symptoms were not examined. However, it could not be excluded that FmoPV may also be related to LUTD, for two reasons: 1) only four cases had FmoPV antigens in inflammatory lesions of the renal cortex, even focal, 2) normal tubular cells of the renal medulla and transitional cells of the renal pelvis in proximity to the lower urinary tract were FmoPV antigen-positive.

Genetic diversity of FmoPV has been described extensively [3–5]. In Hong Kong, FmoPV seemed to be related to chronic TIN [1]. In Germany, it was detected in a LUTD case [5]. In addition, they detected FmoPV in a LUTD case showing 86 ~ 99 % homology compared to reported FmoPV [5]. At the moment, we could not detect FmoPV belonging to genetically diverged group found in Germany [5] among cats in Japan. We can not rule out the possibility that our RT-PCR and IHC could not detected these FmoPV RNA and N protein and their antibodies could not be detected using N proteins of FmoPV belonging to cluster C. However, it is unlikely since N proteins of paramyxoviruses in the same species are highly conserved and cross-reactive.

In our study, no clear relationship between FmoPV and chronic TIN or LUTD could be clarified although many types of FmoPV-infected cases are described.

It was suggested that FmoPV infection has a significant relationship with inflammatory reactions in the feline kidney and may be associated with urinary tract diseases. This was the first epidemiological report including seroprevalence and pathological examination of FmoPV among domestic cats in Japan. Considering the high infection rate and the genetic diversity of FmoPV, it seemed likely that FmoPV has evolved in Japan over a long period. Further retrospective and larger scale studies, including pathological studies, in other organs of cats are needed to elucidate the pathogenicity of FmoPV in cats.

Conclusions

In this study, a high prevalence of FmoPV infection in domestic cats in Japan was revealed, and a significant relationship between FmoPV infection and inflammatory lesions in the kidneys was found. Further studies are necessary to elucidate the etiology of FmoPV in domestic cats. The serological and pathological examination established in this study might be useful for further surveillance.

Methods

Cat samples

Post-mortem urine ($n = 100$), sera ($n = 100$) and renal tissue samples ($n = 100$) were obtained from cats housed in the Tokyo Metropolitan Animal Care and Consultation Center. Cats in the center were carried by owners or captured in outdoors in Tokyo. Physical state and clinical symptoms were examined and recorded at the center. Cats randomly selected in the present study were healthy, sick or wounded, varying in age from new-born to 20 years old. The sex ratio of cats used in this study was similar.

Detection of FmoPV

Total RNAs were extracted from cat urine (100 μL) and renal tissue samples (randomly selected three sites) using ISOGEN (Wako, Osaka, Japan) and a precipitation carrier (Ethachinmate, Wako), according to the manufacturer's instructions. In the reverse transcription reaction, cDNA was synthesized by random primers (SuperScript R III First-strand synthesis supermix, Invitrogen, CA, USA) from the extracted RNA. Then, a part of L-gene sequence of FmoPV with 401 bp was amplified by nested polymerase chain reaction (PCR, 94 °C 5 min/94 °C 15 s, 55 °C 30 s, 68 °C 1 min/68 °C 5 min, first PCR : 40 cycles, second PCR : 20 cycles) using puRe Taq ready-to-go PCR beads (GE Healthcare, Buckinghamshire, UK) according to the previous reports [2, 4]. The primer sets used in the nested RT-PCR were previously reported [2]. A PCR product amplified from a FmoPV positive cat was purified and cloned into the pCR™ 4-TOPO® vector (Invitrogen) and used as a positive control of the nested RT-PCR. The sensitivity of the nested RT-PCR was approximately 10 copies /reaction (data not shown).

Phylogenetic analysis

RT-PCR amplicons were separated by agarose gel electrophoresis and purified from the agarose gel using illustra™ GFX™ PCR DNA and Gel Band Purification Kit (GE Healthcare), according to the manufacturer's instruction. The purified RT-PCR amplicons were used as templates for sequencing on an ABI 3130 Genetic Analyzer (Applied Biosystems) using a BigDye Terminator v3.1 cycle sequencing kit (Applied Biosystems, CA, USA) with the first and second PCR primers. Phylogenetic analysis was performed according to previous reports [4, 33, 34]. Briefly, phylograms were constructed using with the maximum likelihood method with the Kimura two-parameter model included in the MEGA6 package. The robustness of the resulting branching patterns was tested using the bootstrap method with 1000 replicates. In the analysis, the sequences of FmoPV (Hong Kong : M252A, 761U and 776U, Japan : SS1, OtJP001, MiJP003 and ChJP073, outgroups : CDV-Acc.No. AB476401.1 and Nipah virus-Acc.No. JN808863.1) deposited in the GenBank were included in the analysis. To support the result of phylogenetic tree, pairwise distances were analyzed by MEGA6 package and a distribution of pairwise distances was represented by histogram [18]. Statistically significant differences were calculated by Welch's *t* test.

FmoPV-N protein-expressing HeLa cells

Since the nucleocapsid (N) protein of morbilliviruses is highly conserved among isolates and has immunogenic epitopes [35–37], a full-length N protein of FmoPV (761U strain, JQ411014) was expressed in HeLa cells. A plasmid pMK-RQ containing FmoPV-N cDNA was chemically synthesized (Life Technologies, Tokyo, Japan). FmoPV-N cDNA with a *Bam*HI restriction site sequence at each extremity was amplified by polymerase chain reaction (PCR) from pMK-RQ containing FmoPV-N cDNA using an N-BamHI-F primer 5'-AGG ATC CAC AAT GTC TAG TCT ATT GAG G-3' and N-BamHI-R 5'-TGG ATC CAG TTA TTT TAG AAG GTC AGT-3' and cloned into a BamHI site of pKS336 expression vector [38]. The resultant vector, pKS336-FmoPV/N, was transfected into HeLa cells, and selected by DMEM medium containing 5 % fetal calf serum (FCS) and Blasticidin S Hydrochloride (2 μg/ml, Kaken Pharmaceutical. Co, Tokyo, Japan). The generated FmoPV-N-expressing HeLa cells were mixed with mock HeLa cells at 1:1, spotted on 14-well HT-coated slide glasses (AR Brown, Tokyo, Japan), air dried and fixed with acetone at room temperature for 5 min and stored at -80 °C until use. The antigen slides were used for the immunofluorescence test described below.

Preparation of rabbit antibody against FmoPV-N protein

Recombinant FmoPV-N protein with a histidine (His)-tag at C-terminal was prepared by a baculovirus expression vector system to obtain rabbit antibody against FmoPV-N protein. First, to construct the expression plasmid, cDNA of FmoPV-N protein (761U strain, Accession No. JQ411014) was amplified by PCR using N-BamHI-F and N-BamHI-R primers and cloned into a transfer vector, pAcYM1-His-C. To construct the recombinant baculovirus containing FmoPV-N cDNA, the resulting transfer vector, pAcYM1-His-C-FmoPV/N, was co-transfected with a linearized baculovirus DNA, BaculoGold™ DNA (BD Biosciences, San Jose, CA) using X-treme 9 GENE Transfection solution (Roche, Mannheim, Germany) into Sf9 insect cells. The cells were cultured in Sf-900 TM II SFM Complete × 1 (Gibco, NY, USA) with 10 % FCS and kanamycin for 7 days at 27 °C. The medium and cells were harvested and centrifuged at 3000 rpm for 10 min at room temperature. The supernatants containing recombinant baculovirus-FmoPV/N were collected and saved at 4 °C. The cell pellets were used in SDS-PAGE to confirm the expression of his-tagged FmoPV-N protein. Baculovirus-FmoPV/N was infected to Tn5 cells to express his-tagged FmoPV-N protein. Infected Tn5 cells were harvested at 3 days post-infection and his-tagged FmoPV-N protein was purified by Ni-NTA agarose (QIAGEN, Hilden, Germany) and His-Bind® buffer kit (Novagen, San Diego, CA, USA). Purity of the purified FmoPV-N protein was analyzed by SDS-polyacrylamide gel electrophoresis (SDS-PAGE) followed by Coomassie Brilliant Blue staining (Bio-Safe TM Coomassie G-250 stain, Bio-Rad, CA, USA). Stained bands were quantified using ImageJ 1.50i [39, 40]. The purified FmoPV-N protein was subcutaneously injected into three rabbits five times. When the serum antibody titer checked by IF reached above 1:10,000, the rabbits were euthanized and sera were collected.

They reacted with FmoPV-positive renal tissues by IF, IHC and immunoblot, but did not react with FmoPV-negative renal tissues.

Immunoblot

The purified recombinant FmoPV-N protein with His-tag was separated by SDS-PAGE and electrophoretically transferred to Immu-Blot PVDF membranes (Bio Rad, CA, USA). The membranes were blocked with Blocking One (Nacalai tesque, Inc. Kyoto, Japan) at 4 °C overnight and were incubated with cat sera (FmoPV-N Ab-positive; N028, FmoPV-N Ab-negative; N004) at a dilution of 1:500 at room temperature for 2 h. Then, the membranes were incubated with horse radish peroxidase-conjugated recombinant protein A/G (Purified Recomb ® Protein A/G, peroxidase-conjugated, Thermo Scientific, MA, USA) at a dilution of 1:1000 at room temperature for 1 h. The reaction of the antibodies were visualized with EzWest-Blue (ATTO Corporation, Tokyo, Japan).

Immunofluorescence (IF) test

IF was performed to detect antibodies (Ab) to FmoPV-N protein in cat sera. Cat sera were serially diluted in phosphate-buffered saline (PBS (-)) at a dilution of 1;40 to 1;20,480. They were applied to the wells of the antigen slides described above, and reacted for 1 h at 37 °C in a humidified chamber. After washing in PBS(-), goat anti-cat-IgG (H + L) conjugated with fluorescein (FITC) (1:1000, ROCKLAND, Gilbertsville, PA) was applied and incubated for 40 min at 37 °C. IF test was performed three times for each cat serum. Rabbit antibodies against FmoPV-N protein and goat anti-rabbit-IgG (H + L) conjugated with FITC were used as the positive control. Pre-sera from the same rabbits were used as negative controls. After washing in PBS(-), the slides were examined for staining patterns under a fluorescent microscope (Olympus BX51 and Olympus DP Controller 1. 1. 1.65 (Olympus, Tokyo, Japan). The Ab titers of tested cat sera were recorded as the reciprocals of the highest dilutions producing positive staining.

Histopathological examination

Three sites including the renal cortex, medulla and pelvis were collected randomly and fixed in 10 % neutral formalin solution. Fixed tissues were embedded in paraffin, sectioned, and stained with hematoxylin and eosin (HE). For immunohistochemistry (IHC), deparaffinized sections were autoclaved at 121 °C for 10 min for antigen retrieval. Endogenous peroxidase activity was blocked by incubating sections with 3 % hydrogen peroxide in methanol at room temperature for 5 min. For the tissue blocking, sections were treated with 10 % skimmed milk in PBS(-) at 37 °C for 40 min. Then, rabbit antibodies against FmoPV-N protein (1:500 to 1:1000) were applied as primary antibodies at 4 °C overnight. Thereafter, sections were incubated with Envision System HRP-labeled polymer anti-rabbit (DAKO Japan, Kyoto, Japan) at room temperature for 40 min. Finally, the sections were visualized with 3,3'-diaminobenzidine tetrahydrochloride (Wako, Japan), and counterstained with Mayer's hematoxylin solution (Wako). Degree of lesions was scored by severity of the lesions based on degree and extensiveness of tubulointerstitial nephritis or infiltration of inflammatory cells and other associated findings including interstitial fibrosis, necrotic changes, glomerulosclerosis and calcification. Scoring criterion + was defined as mild lesion with focal infiltration of small inflammatory cells. Scoring criterion ++ was defined as moderate lesion with infiltration of moderate inflammatory cells. Scoring criterion +++ was defined as severe lesions with severe infiltration of inflammatory cells. Distribution of FmoPV-N antigens in the renal tissues by IHC were also scored. Scoring criterion * was defined as FmoPV-N antigen positive cells focally in normal renal tissues, and criterion ** was defined as FmoPV antigens in several sites, while criterion *** was defined as extensive FmoPV antigen positive cells around lesions.

Statistical analysis

Results are expressed as the number of cases. Statistical analyses were performed using StatFlex software (ver. 6, Artech Co., Ltd., Osaka, Japan). Significant differences between groups were determined by the Mann-Whitney U-test and χ^2 test.

Acknowledgement

We thank all staffs who got involved in this study at Tokyo Metropolitan Animal Care and Consultation Center.

Funding

This work was partly supported by a grant-in-aid from the Ministry of Health, Labor and Welfare of Japan (grants H25-shinkou-ippan-008) and the Research Program on Emerging and Re-emerging Infectious Diseases from Japan Agency for Medical Research and development, AMED.

Authors' contributions

EP participated in the study design, the experimental work, the analysis interpretation of the data and drafted the manuscript. MS, MK and KI participated in the study design, the experimental work, the analysis interpretation of the data and helped draft the manuscript. KM, HM, RS, NK, YH, JO and HK participated in collecting cat samples. NN and YS participated in the pathological examination. SM conceived and designed the study and participated in the analysis and interpretation of the data and writing of the manuscript. All authors read and approved the final manuscript.

Authors' information

EP, MS, MK, KI and SM are staff at the Department of Veterinary science, National Institute of Infectious Diseases. KM, HM, RS, NK, YH, JO and HK are staff at the Tokyo Metropolitan Animal Care and Consultation Center. NN and YS are staff at the Department of Pathology, National Institute of Infectious Diseases.

Competing interests

The authors declare that they have no competing interests.

Consent for publication

Not applicable.

Ethics approval and consent to participate

Post-mortem cat samples were obtained from cats housed in the Tokyo Metropolitan Animal Care and Consultation Center. Cats in the center were carried by owners or captured in outdoors in Tokyo. Cat samples were used under the approval of the Bureau of Social Welfare and Public Health of Tokyo Metropolitan Government in Japan (24-DouSou-4557). The maintenance and handling of cats were performed at the Tokyo Metropolitan Animal Care and Consultation Center (Jonanjima Branch Office) in accordance with the Act on the Welfare and Management of Animals (Article 40) of Japan.

Author details

[1]Department of Veterinary Science, National Institute of Infectious Diseases, Tokyo 162-8640, Japan. [2]Tokyo Metropolitan Animal Care and Consultation Center, Jounanjima Branch Office, Tokyo 143-0002, Japan. [3]Department of Pathology, National Institute of Infectious Diseases, Tokyo 162-8640, Japan.

References

1. Woo PC, Lau SK, Wong BH, Fan RY, Wong AY, Zhang AJ, Wu Y, Choi GK, Li KS, Hui J, et al. Feline morbillivirus, a previously undescribed paramyxovirus associated with tubulointerstitial nephritis in domestic cats. Proc Natl Acad Sci U S A. 2012;109(14):5435–40.
2. Furuya T, Sassa Y, Omatsu T, Nagai M, Fukushima R, Shibutani M, Yamaguchi T, Uematsu Y, Shirota K, Mizutani T. Existence of feline morbillivirus infection in Japanese cat populations. Arch Virol. 2014;159(2):371–3.
3. Sakaguchi S, Nakagawa S, Yoshikawa R, Kuwahara C, Hagiwara H, Asai K, Kawakami K, Yamamoto Y, Ogawa M, Miyazawa T. Genetic diversity of feline morbilliviruses isolated in Japan. J Gen Virol. 2014;95(Pt 7):1464–8.
4. Park ES, Suzuki M, Kimura M, Maruyama K, Mizutani H, Saito R, Kubota N, Furuya T, Mizutani T, Imaoka K, et al. Identification of a natural recombination in the F and H genes of feline morbillivirus. Virology. 2014;468–470:524–31.
5. Sieg M, Heenemann K, Rückner A, Burgener I, Oechtering G, Vahlenkamp TW. Discovery of new feline paramyxoviruses in domestic cats with chronic kidney disease. Virus Genes. 2015;51(2):294–7.
6. Lorusso A, Di Tommaso M, Di Felice E, Zaccaria G, Luciani A, Marcacci M, Aste G, Boari A, Savini G. First report of feline morbillivirus in Europe. Vet Ital. 2015, doi:10.12834/VetIt.833.4136.2
7. Sharp CR, Nambulli S, Acciardo AS, Rennick LJ, Felix Drexler J, Rima BK, Williams T, Paul Duprex W. Chronic infection of domestic cats with feline morbillivirus, United States. Emerg Infect Dis. 2016;22(4):760–2.
8. Marcacci M, De Luca E, Zaccaria G, Di Tommaso M, Mangone I, Aste G, Savini G, Boari A, Lorusso A. Genome characterization of feline morbillivirus from Italy. J Virol Methods. 2016;234:160–3.
9. Ikeda Y, Nakamura K, Miyazawa T, Chen MC, Kuo TF, Lin JA, Mikami T, Kai C, Takahashi E. Seroprevalence of canine distemper virus in cats. Clin Diagn Lab Immunol. 2001;8(3):641–4.
10. DiBartola SP, Rutgers HC, Zack PM, Tarr MJ. Clinicopathologic findings associated with chronic renal disease in cats: 74 cases (1973-1984). J Am Vet Med Assoc. 1987;190(9):1196–202.
11. Jeraj K, Osborne CA, Stevens JB. Evaluation of renal biopsy in 197 dogs and cats. J Am Vet Med Assoc. 1982;181(4):367–9.
12. Worwag S, Langston CE. Acute intrinsic renal failure in cats: 32 cases (1997-2004). J Am Vet Med Assoc. 2008;232(5):728–32.
13. Eaton KA, Biller DS, DiBartola SP, Radin MJ, Wellman ML. Autosomal dominant polycystic kidney disease in Persian and Persian-cross cats. Vet Pathol. 1997;34(2):117–26.
14. Boyd LM, Langston C, Thompson K, Zivin K, Imanishi M. Survival in cats with naturally occurring chronic kidney disease (2000-2002). J Vet Intern Med. 2008;22(5):1111–7.
15. Mayer-Roenne B, Goldstein RE, Erb HN. Urinary tract infections in cats with hyperthyroidism, diabetes mellitus and chronic kidney disease. J Feline Med Surg. 2007;9(2):124–32.
16. Elliott J, Barber PJ. Feline chronic renal failure: clinical findings in 80 cases diagnosed between 1992 and 1995. J Small Anim Pract. 1998;39(2):78–85.
17. Chakrabarti S, Syme HM, Brown CA, Elliott J. Histomorphometry of feline chronic kidney disease and correlation with markers of renal dysfunction. Vet Pathol. 2013;50(1):147–55.
18. Katayama K, Shirato-Horikoshi H, Kojima S, Kageyama T, Oka T, Hoshino F, Fukushi S, Shinohara M, Uchida K, Suzuki Y, Gojobori T, Takeda N. Phylogenetic analysis of the complete genome of 18 Norwalk-like viruses. Virology. 2002;299(2):225–39.
19. Tomashefski JF, Farver CF, Fraire AE. Dail and Hammar's Pulmonary Pathology. 3rd ed. New York: Springer; 2008. p. 432–4. Volume I.
20. Gu J, Korteweq C. Pathology and pathogenesis of severe acute respiratory syndrome. Am J Pathol. 2007;170(4):1136–47.
21. Greene CE. In: Greene CE, editor. Infectious Disease of the dog and cat. 3rd ed. St. Louis, Missouri: SAUNDERS; 2011. p. 92–149. 162-264.

22. Poli A, Tozon N, Guidi G, Pistello M. Renal alterations in feline immunodeficiency virus (FIV)-infected cats: a natural model of lentivirus-induced renal disease changes. Viruses. 2012;4(9):1372–89.
23. Poli A, Abramo F, Taccini E, Guidi G, Barsotti P, Bendinelli M, Malvaldi G. Renal involvement in feline immunodeficiency virus infection: a clinicopathological study. Nephron. 1993;64(2):282–8.
24. German AC, Harbour DA, Helps CR, Gruffydd-Jones TJ. Is feline foamy virus really apathogenic? Vet Immunol Immunopathol. 2008;123(1-2):114–8.
25. Reinacher M. Diseases associated with spontaneous feline leukemia virus (FeLV) infection in cats. Vet Immunol Immunopathol. 1989;21(1):85–95.
26. Fujii Y, Tochitani T, Kouchi M, Matsumoto I, Yamada T, Funabashi H. Glomerulonephritis in a ferret with feline coronavirus infection. J Vet Diagn Invest. 2015;27(5):637–40.
27. Francis DP, Essex M, Jakowski RM, Cotter SM, Lerer TJ, Hardy Jr WD. Increased risk for lymphoma and glomerulonephritis in a closed population of cats exposed to feline leukemia virus. Am J Epidemiol. 1980;111(3):337–46.
28. Buffington CA. Idiopathic cystitis in domestic cats–beyond the lower urinary tract. J Vet Intern Med. 2011;25(4):784–96.
29. Kruger JM, Osborne CA. The role of uropathogens in feline lower urinary tract disease. Clinical implications. Vet Clin North Am Small Anim Pract. 1993;23(1):101–23.
30. Lund HS, Rimstad E, Eggertsdóttir AV. Prevalence of viral infections in Norwegian cats with and without feline lower urinary tract disease. J Feline Med Surg. 2012;14(12):895–9.
31. Rice CC, Kruger JM, Venta PJ, Vilnis A, Maas KA, Dulin JA, Maes RK. Genetic characterization of 2 novel feline caliciviruses isolated from cats with idiopathic lower urinary tract disease. J Vet Intern Med. 2002;16(3):293–302.
32. Kruger JM, Osborne CA, Lulich JP. Changing paradigms of feline idiopathic cystitis. Vet Clin North Am Small Anim Pract. 2009;39(1):15–40.
33. Tamura K, Nei M. Estimation of the number of nucleotide substitutions in the control region of mitochondrial DNA in humans and chimpanzees. Mol Biol Evol. 1993;10:512–26.
34. Tamura K, Stecher G, Peterson D, Filipski A, Kumar S. MEGA6: Molecular evolutionary genetics analysis version 6.0. Mol Biol Evol. 2013;30:2725–9.
35. Ohishi K, Inui K, Yamanouchi K, Barrett T. Cell-mediated immune responses in cattle vaccinated with a vaccinia virus recombinant expressing the nucleocapsid protein of rinderpest virus. J Gen Virol. 1999;80(Pt 7):1627–34.
36. Mitra-Kaushik S, Nayak R, Shaila MS. Identification of a cytotoxic T-cell epitope on the recombinant nucleocapsid proteins of Rinderpest and Peste des petits ruminants viruses presented as assembled nucleocapsids. Virology. 2001;279(1):210–20.
37. Sheshberadaran H, Norrby E, McCullough KC, Carpenter WC, Orvell C. The antigenic relationship between measles, canine distemper and rinderpest viruses studied with monoclonal antibodies. J Gen Virol. 1986;67(Pt 7):1381–92.
38. Saijo M, Qing T, Niikura M, Maeda A, Ikegami T, Sakai K, Prehaud C, Kurane I, Morikawa S. Immunofluorescence technique using HeLa cells expressing recombinant nucleoprotein for detection of immunoglobulin G antibodies to Crimean-Congo hemorrhagic fever virus. J Clin Microbiol. 2002;40(2):372–5.
39. Rasband WS. ImageJ, U. S. National Institutes of Health, Bethesda, Maryland, USA, http://imagej.nih.gov/ij/, 1997-2012
40. Schneider CA, Rasband WS, Eliceiri KW. NIH Image to ImageJ: 25 years of image analysis. Nat Methods. 2012;9:671–5.

4

Homologous prime-boost immunization with live attenuated *Salmonella enterica* serovar Senftenberg and its preventive efficacy against experimental challenge with various strains of *S.* Senftenberg

Nitin M. Kamble and John Hwa Lee*

Abstract

Background: The heterogeneity observed regarding persistence, and subsequent fecal shedding pattern of the *Salmonella* Senftenberg (*S.* Senftenberg) serovar in chicken's calls for development of the optimized immunization strategy which can provide protection against various *S.* Senftenberg isolated. Optimization of an immunization strategy with a live attenuated *S.* Senftenberg *(Δlon and ΔcpxR)* vaccine candidate (JOL1587) was undertaken in this study to evaluate the ability of a homologous prime-boost immunization strategy (using JOL1587) to confer protection against four different *S.* Senftenberg isolates in chickens.

Results: After oral immunization with JOL1587, the humoral, mucosal and cell-mediated immune responses were significantly higher in double immunized chickens than in single immunized and control group chickens. A significant increase in the multifunctional cytokine IL-6 and in helper and cytotoxic T cell populations after a booster immunization also indicated the advantage of double over single immunization. The four different *S.* Senftenberg field isolates were characterized by their persistence levels in chickens, and were subsequently used for challenge experiments to evaluate the differences in protective efficacy conferred by single and double immunization. Chickens from the doubleimmunized group exhibited significant reduction in the shedding of all four wild-type *S.* Senftenberg challenge strains below the detection limit in the fecal samples. Single immunized chickens showed a decrease in fecal shedding, but failed to exhibit complete protection against all the challenge strains.

Conclusion: Although single immunization with JOL1587 showed a reduction in the fecal shedding of challenge strains, only the homologous prime-boost immunization strategy provided an adequate immune response for increased protection against all four challenge strains of *S.* Senftenberg from the feces of chickens.

Keywords: *Salmonella* Senftenberg, Mucosal immunity, Persistence, Fecal shedding

* Correspondence: johnhlee@jbnu.ac.kr
College of Veterinary Medicine and Bio-Safety Research Institute, Chonbuk National University, Iksan Campus 570-752, Republic of Korea

Background

The nontyphoidal serovars of the gram-negative pathogen *Salmonella* enterica are a leading cause of invasive bacterial gastroenteritis in humans [1]. According to the Centers for Disease Control and Prevention (CDC), there are 94 million cases of nontyphoidal gastroenteritis and 115,000 deaths reported annually in the worldwide human population. The *Salmonella* enterica subsp. Enterica serovar Senftenberg (*S.* Senftenberg) is one of the nontyphoidal serotypes (NTS) that was isolated from several outbreaks of gastroenteritis in humans [2–4]. *S.* Senftenberg is a gram-negative, facultative, intracellular pathogen affecting both poultry and humans [5, 6]). The *Salmonella* pathogen is transmitted to humans either through direct contact with an infected animal or by consumption of contaminated food and water. The serovar *S.* Senftenberg is primarily associated with hatcheries, but recent reports have suggested its emergence and persistence in poultry environments throughout the rearing season. This could pose a potential risk of contamination of poultry products [7, 8]. Moreover, *S.* Senftenberg cells are reported to tolerate desiccation and survive routine cleaning and disinfection procedures, enabling them to persist longer and transmit more easily to other poultry and humans [8]. The hallmark of *S.* Senftenberg infection in chickens is its high colonization of the cecum, which in turn leads to an asymptomatic carrier state in chickens [7]. Various strains of *S.* Senftenberg isolated from different poultry outbreaks were analyzed for their persistence and fecal shedding patterns in the cecum [9]. As previously reported, a coordinated immune response from the systemic and the mucosal arms of the immune system is needed for clearance of *Salmonella* infection [10]. Therefore, generation of both a systemic and a mucosal immune response locally in the intestine is essential for the control of *S.* Senftenberg colonization and fecal shedding.

Homologous immunization with a *S.* Senftenberg vaccine can be an approach for managing persistent infection of *S.* Senftenberg in hatcheries as well as poultry farms. Recently, we developed a live attenuated *(Δlon and ΔcpxR) S.* Senftenberg vaccine candidate strain (JOL1587) to provide protection against *S.* Senftenberg [11]. The fact that different *S.* Senftenberg strains exhibit variation in the fecal shedding pattern and extent of colonization in the cecum underscores the need for optimization of the immunization strategy with JOL1587. The principle objective of this study was to generate a robust systemic and mucosal immune response to prevent fecal shedding of the persistent and the non-persistent *S.* Senftenberg strains. We evaluated the mucosal and systemic immune response generated in chickens following single or double immunization with a live attenuated mutant of *S.* Senftenberg (*Δlon* and *ΔcpxR*). The ability to confer a protective immune response by mucosal immunization was evaluated by assessing the rate of fecal shedding and persistence of four different wild-type strains of *S.* Senftenberg in challenged chickens.

Methods

Preparation of the mutant and challenge strain

The attenuated mutant of *S.* Senftenberg JOL1587 was constructed by deleting the *lon* and *cpxR* genes from wild-type S. Senftenberg JOL1556 by the allelic exchange method described previously [11, 12]. Four strains of *S.* Senftenberg (JOL1557, JOL1815, JOL1816 and JOL1817) isolated from different field outbreaks in chickens and characterized for persistence in the caecum were used for the challenge study. The wild-type strains were characterized for presence of the specific pathogenicity island (SPI) related genes by PCR (Table 1). All bacterial strains were cryopreserved as frozen glycerol cultures in Luria-Bertani (LB) broth at−80 °C. The glycerol stocks were revived by streaking the thawed cultures on LB agar and incubating at 37 °C for 24 h. A single colony was picked from overnight grown culture, inoculated in LB broth at 1:20 dilution, and grown in shaker culture until the optical density at 600 nm (OD_{600}) reached 0.6. The culture was adjusted to a suitable concentration before inoculation into chickens.

Table 1 Fecal shedding of wild-type *S.* Senftenberg from challenged chickens

Challenge Strain	Group	Subgroup	Days post inoculation						
			1	3	7	9	14	21	28
JOL1557	A	A1	100[a]	100	100	100	100	100	100
	B	B1	100	60	40	40	40	40	40
	C	C1	100	60	40	40	0	0	0
JOL1815	A	A2	100	100	100	100	100	80	80
	B	B2	100	40	60	40	60	60	40
	C	C2	100	60	40	10	0	0	0
JOL1816	A	A3	100	100	100	100	100	100	100
	B	B3	100	40	0	40	40	60	60
	C	C3	100	60	40	40	0	10	0
JOL1817	A	A4	100	100	100	100	100	80	80
	B	B4	100	40	60	40	60	40	0
	C	C4	100	60	40	10	0	0	0

A: PBS inoculated group; B: Prime immunized group and C: Prime-boost immunized group

Each major group A, B and C are further sub-divided into four subgroups and challenged with JOL1557, JOl1815, JOL1816 and JOL1817, respectively

[a]Percentage population tested positive for recovery of the *S.* Senftenberg in fecal samples

Chicken immunization and challenge experiments
For chicken experimentation, female day-old layer chickens (Brown Nick, $n = 75$) were procured from JOINBIO hatchery located in the yongin-si, South Korea. The chickens were divided into three groups ($n = 25$). The strategy for the immunization and challenge study is explained in Table 2. All animals were provided with ad libitum antibiotic-free feed and water. At the fourth week of age, group A was inoculated orally with PBS to serve as a non-immunized control and groups B and C were inoculated orally with a JOL1587 suspension containing 1×10^8 colony forming units (CFUs). Further, group C was given a booster dose orally at the 8 week of age with a JOL1587 suspension containing 1×10^8 CFUs. Post-immunization and booster, the serum and intestinal lavage samples were collected from six randomly selected chickens from the pool of 25 chickens in each group.

Collection of the intestinal wash for sIgA
The intestinal lavage samples were collected for measurement of the secretory IgA levels according to a protocol described elsewhere [13]. Briefly, chickens were taken off feed for 16 h. The off-feed chickens were orally administered 5 mL of lavage solution (0.2 M Na_2SO_4, 0.2 M $NaHCO_3$, 0.1 M KCl, 0.25 M NaCl, and 16.25% polyethylene glycol in distilled water) and kept in clean, disinfected buckets. Thirty minutes post-administration, the chickens were injected intramuscularly with 200 µl of a 5% pilocarpine solution. The chickens were observed for mucinous droppings over a period of thirty minutes. The mucinous droppings were collected in microcentrifuge tubes containing 1× soybean trypsin protease inhibitor and 50 mM EDTA solution. Samples were preserved by adding 10 µL each of 5% bovine serum albumin, 10% sodium azide and 1% PMSF (phenylmethylsulfonyl fluoride). Samples were stored at −20 °C until analysis.

Table 2 Immunization and challenge strategy

Group	N	Immunization		Subgroups	Animal No.	Challenge strain
		Primary	Booster			
A	25	PBS	PBS	AI	6	JOL1557
				AII	6	JOL1815
				AIII	6	JOL1816
				AIV	6	JOL1817
B	25	JOL1587	PBS	BI	6	JOL1557
				BII	6	JOL1815
				BIII	6	JOL1816
				BIV	6	JOL1817
C	25	JOL1587	JOL1585	CI	6	JOL1557
				CII	6	JOL1815
				CIII	6	JOL1816
				CIV	6	JOL1817

Enzyme-linked immunosorbent assay (ELISA)
The development of *S.* Senftenberg-specific humoral and mucosal immunity in response to JOL1587 immunization in chickens was evaluated by estimating the variation in plasma IgG and intestinal sIgA levels by *S.* Senftenberg antigen-specific indirect ELISA. The outer membrane protein fraction (OMP) was extracted from wild-type *S.* Senftenberg as described elsewhere (Osborn and Munson, 1974). The levels of OMP specific IgG antibodies in the plasma of the immunized chickens were determined using an indirect ELISA. Briefly, 96-well Microlon® ELISA plates (Greiner Bio-One GmbH, Fricken hausen, Germany) were coated with OMP (50 µg/mL) and blocked with 5% skim milk powder in PBS. For total IgG and sIgA detection, the ELISA plates were incubated with an intestinal wash (1:5 dilution) and plasma (1:100 dilution) and then incubated with horseradish peroxidase (HRP)-conjugated goat anti-chicken IgG and IgA at a 1:100,000 dilution for 1 h. The plates were developed with o-phenylenediamine dihydrochloride substrate (Sigma-Aldrich, St. Louis, MO, USA) and read at 492 nm.

Lymphocyte proliferation assay (LPA)
The LPA stimulation indices were calculated 3 weeks post-prime- and –booster immunization to estimate the cellular immune response generated after JOL1587 immunization in chickens. From each group (A, B and C) heparinized blood samples were collected from six randomly selected chickens from the pool of 25 chickens. Cells were stimulated with soluble antigen prepared from the *S.* Senftenberg wild-type strain, as described elsewhere [14]. Soluble antigen was prepared from the wild-type *S.* Senftenberg strain JOL1556. Briefly, the overnight grown bacterial cell culture were pelleted and resuspended in PBS. The bacterial suspension was sonicated for 5 min, and pelleted by centrifugation at 5000 × *g* for 60 min at 4 °C. The supernatant containing the sonicated bacterial cell protein suspension (sbcp) was collected and used as the soluble antigen. Post-inoculation, the peripheral blood mononuclear cells (PBMCs) were separated from the heparinized blood collected from the jugular veins of five randomly selected chickens per group. Blood was carefully loaded on Histopaque-1083 (Sigma-Aldrich, St. Louis, MO, USA) and centrifuged at 400 × g for 40 min at room temperature. The buffy coat at the interface was suspended in RPMI-1640 medium (HyClone Laboratories, South Logan, UT, USA). The PBMCs were adjusted to a 1×10^6 cells/mL final concentration in the RPMI-1640 medium and distributed in triplicate to 96-well tissue culture plates. The plates were incubated with medium alone

or medium containing 4 μg/mL of the soluble antigen of *S.* Senftenberg at 40 °C with 5% CO_2 for 72 h. Cell proliferation was measured by using thiazolyl blue tetrazolium bromide (MTT) dye (Sigma-Aldrich, St. Louis, MO, USA) as per the manufacturer's protocol. The blastogenic response was expressed as mean stimulation index (SI), which was calculated as the ratio of the average OD of the stimulated/unstimulated wells.

Flow cytometry

Post-booster immunization, variations in the JOL1587-specific helper (CD3 + CD4+) and cytotoxic (CD3 + CD8 +) T cell populations were analyzed following ex vivo stimulation of peripheral blood mononuclear cells (PBMCs) with soluble antigen extracted from wild-type *S.* Senftenberg. PBMCs were separated from blood samples of five chickens from each group (A, B and C) at 1 week post-prime and booster immunization. The isolated PBMCs were stimulated ex vivo with soluble antigen extracted from wild-type *S.* Senftenberg. The stimulated PBMCs were stained with anti-CD3, anti-CD4 and anti-CD8 antibodies, as described elsewhere [15]. Briefly, a total of 1×10^6 PBMCs were stained with appropriately diluted mouse anti-chicken CD3-FITC, CD4-APC and CD8-RPE (Southern Biotech, USA). After incubation, all stained samples were washed three times with PBS and analyzed with a flow cytometer (Miltenyi Biotech, Germany). A total of 10,000 events were recorded and analyzed using the FlowJo single cell analysis software.

Relative quantification of cytokines by real-time quantitative reverse transcriptase PCR (qRT-PCR)

The cytokine response was evaluated after prime and booster immunization in PBMCs following ex vivo stimulation with the soluble antigen of *S.* Senftenberg. The qRT-PCR method was employed for relative quantification of IL-6, IFN-γ, and IL-2 cytokine mRNA levels. The RNA was isolated from PBMCs separated at ten days post prime and booster vaccination. The housekeeping gene β-actin was used as an endogenous control for normalization of the sample Ct values. The comparative $2^{-\Delta\Delta Ct}$ method was used for the relative quantification of the fold change in the cytokine mRNA levels [16].

Fecal shedding of the different strains of S. Senftenberg

At the twelve week of age, chickens from each group were further separated into four sub-groups containing six chickens each, and orally challenged individually with virulent wild-type (WT) *S.* Senftenberg strain, JOL1557, JOL1815, JOL1816, and JOL1817 (5×10^8 CFUs), respectively. For fecal shedding, the fecal samples were collected from six chickens in each sub-group using sterile, buffered peptone water (BPW, Becton Dickinson, USA). A ten-fold dilution of BPW was plated onto brilliant green agar (BGA, Becton Dickinson) and incubated at 37 °C for 24 h. Samples showing colonies on BGA were counted as positive. Negative samples were further incubated in Rappaport-Vassiliadis R10 enrichment broth (RV, Becton Dickinson) for 48 h at 42 °C. The enriched culture was picked with a sterile loop and then plated onto BGA. Samples that were positive after direct plating or after enrichment were taken as positive for harboring *S.* Senftenberg. The challenge strain was confirmed by PCR using *S.* Senftenberg serotype-specific primers. The challenge strain was distinguished from inoculated JOL1587 (*Δlon/ΔcpxR)* by using primer sets specific to *lon* and *cpxR* genes. The enumeration of the cfu per gram of tissue was performed as described elsewhere [17].

Statistical analysis

The results of this study are expressed as means ± SEM unless otherwise specified. A one-way ANOVA with Bonferroni corrections was employed to analyze statistical significance for expression levels of CD3 + CD4+ T cells, CD3 + CD8+ T cells, cytokines, plasma IgG and intestinal sIgA. The values for the individual groups were considered statistically significant if the *P*-values were ≤ 0.05 or ≤ 0.01. The fecal shedding data was converted into percentage value for comparison. All analysis was performed using the SPSS 16.0 (SPSS Inc., USA).

Results

Characterization of wild type S. Senftenberg strain

Four wild-type *S.* Senftenberg strains, JOL1557 (WT), JOL1815 (WT), JOL1816 (WT) and JOL1817 (WT) were characterized by PCR for presence of various SPI specific genes (Table 3). The PCR data indicated the size-specific amplification and presence of the SPI1, 2, 3, 4 and 5 specific analyzed genes in all four wild-type *S.* Senftenberg strain (Data not shown). The four groups of the non-immunized chickens were inoculated separately with JOL1557 (WT), JOL1815 (WT), JOL1816 (WT) and JOL1817 (WT) for evaluation of the persistence in the cecum. The bacterial recovery experiment showed that all the four wild-type strains were recovered from cecum swabs on BGA plates until week four post-inoculation.

Estimation of S. Senftenberg-specific humoral and mucosal immune responses

Indirect ELISA estimated differences in humoral and mucosal immune responses generated after single and double immunization. Immunization of the chickens with JOL1587 led to a significant rise ($P \leq 0.05$) in the IgG and sIgA levels in both the single and double immunized groups relative to the control group chickens

Table 3 List of primers used for detection of genes specificto different SPI

SPI	Primers	Sequence 5'–3'	Amplicon Size (bp)
SPI1	invAE F	CAGCGATATCCAAATGTTGC	2168
	invAE R	AAATGGCAGAACAGCGTCGTA	
	hilA F	CTGCCGCAGTGTTAAGGATA	497
	hilA R	CTGTCGCCTTAATCGCATGT	
	avr F	AGACTTATATTCAGCTATCC	1115
	avr R	ACATAACCCTGCTGTACCTG	
SPI2	aa permease F	ACCATTCAAGAGACAATTGG	1737
	aa permease R	GTCCTGTTCTGGTATTACGC	
SPI3	mgtC F	ATGAATCCCCAAAATTAAGG	1153
	mgtC R	AATCATCTGGCAAGTTAACG	
SPI4	ABC Trans F	CAGTCTATCACAGCAAGGCA	1409
	ABC Trans R	TTATCCGGAGAACAATCACG	
SPI5	pipB F	AATATTGGATGGGGGAAAAG	230
	pipB R	AACCTGACTCACGCAGACCT	

(Fig. 1). The effect of booster immunization was apparent for both the plasma IgG and intestinal sIgA responses in that levels of each increased significantly ($P \leq 0.05$) only in the double immunized group. The chickens from the single immunized group (coinciding with the timing for booster immunization) started exhibiting sharp and significant declines ($P \leq 0.05$) in both IgG and sIgA levels compared to the double immunized group. The levels of IgG and sIgA in the single immunized group became insignificant and similar to control group chickens by eleven weeks of age ($P \leq 0.05$, Fig. 1). The non-immunized control group chickens showed insignificant rise in *S.* Senftenberg-specific IgG and sIgA levels throughout the observation period (Fig. 1).

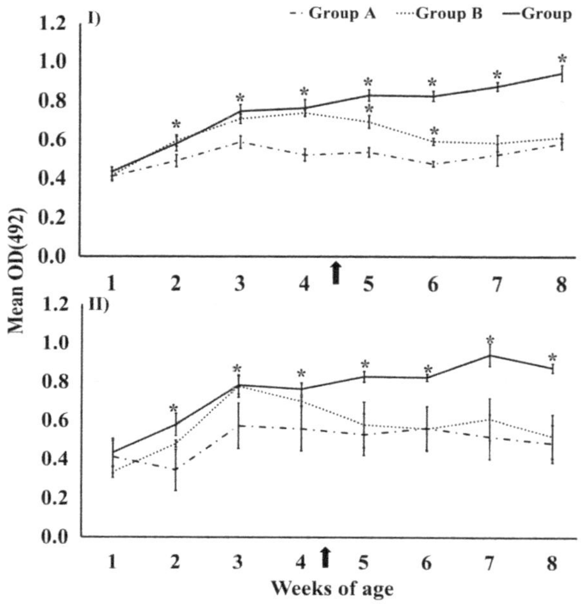

Fig. 1 Graphical representation of the OD values for evaluation of the plasma IgG and intestinal lavage sIgA responses to JOL1587 immunization in chickens. **I**) Plasma IgG levels, **II**) Intestinal lavage sIgA levels. a: PBS-inoculatec group; b: single immunized group and c: double immunized group. The arrow denotes the time of booster immunization in group C ch ckens. Values shown for each group are the mean ± SEM of antibody levels ($n = 6$). The * symbol indicates a significant increase in the antibody levels in the JOL1587 immunized chickens compared to the control group chickens ($P \leq 0.05$)

Evaluation of S. Senftenberg-specific cellular immune responses

As shown by the LPA results, the immunization of chickens with JOL1587 successfully induced an *S.* Senftenberg-specific cellular immune response in both single and double immunized groups (Fig. 2). For calculation of significant differences in the cellular immune response, the SI value for an immunized group was compared with control group chickens. The LPA results showed that the cellular immune response in the double immunized group was significantly elevated ($P \leq 0.05$) after prime (1.6-fold) as well as booster 2.0-fold) immunization (Fig. 2). The single immunized chickens, which showed a significant rise (1.7-fold, $P \leq 0.05$) in SI value after prime immunization, contrastingly showed an insignificant decline in the SI value (1.5-fold, $P \leq 0.05$) at eleven week of age.

Analyses of helper and cytotoxic T cell populations

For estimation of the differences in the helper and cytotoxic T cell populations, the CD3 + CD4+ and CD3 + CD8 + T cell populations for the immunized groups were compared with control group chickens. Both the single and double immunized chickens showed a significant increase ($P \leq 0.05$) in cytotoxic T cell populations after prime-

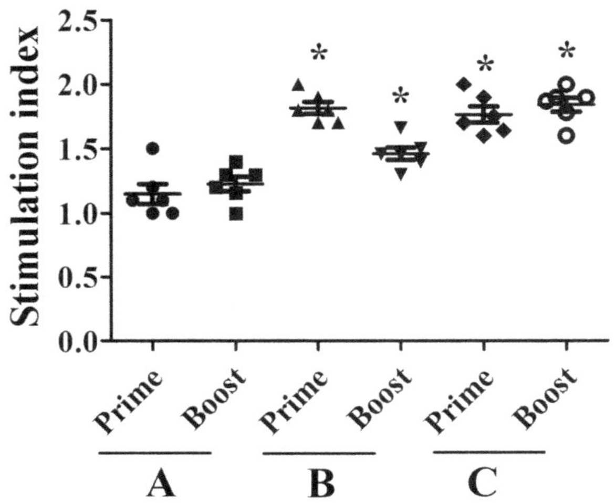

Fig. 2 Stimulation indices for measurement of a lymphocyte proliferation response in the JOL1587-immunized and control group chickens. **a** PBS-inoculated group; **b** Single immunized group and **c**: Double immunized group. The LPA assay was performed at 7 and 11 weeks of age after the prime and booster immunizations, respectively. The * symbol indicates a significant increase in the lymphocyte proliferation response in the JOL1587 immunized chickens compared to the control group chickens ($P \leq 0.05$). Total six samples were analyzed which were collected from six randomly selected chickens from group a, b and c

immunization. However, this failed to generate a significant increase in the peripherally circulating helper T cell populations as compared to the control group chickens (Fig. 3I). Our experimental data showed that the significant increase ($P \leq 0.05$) in both the helper and cytotoxic T cell populations was observed in the double immunized group only after the booster immunization (Fig. 3I). The quantitative estimation of the CD3+ CD4+ and CD3+ CD8+ T cell populations in the double immunized chickens showed these were approximately 2.5- and 1.5- fold higher than in the control group chickens, respectively ($P \leq 0.05$, Fig. 3II). After booster immunization, the levels of the CD3 + CD4+ and CD3+ CD8+ T cell populations for the single immunized and control group chickens were similar, with no fold change differences observed (Fig. 3).

Cytokine mRNA expression levels

The fold changes observed in the mRNA copy number of the IL-6, IFN-γ and IL-2 cytokines in the PBMCs from control and immunized group chickens are shown in Fig. 4. Both the single and double immunized groups showed significant upregulation ($P \leq 0.05$, Fig. 4) of the IL-6, IFN-γ and IL-2 cytokines relative to control group chickens. After quantitative estimation, IFN-γ and IL-2 cytokine mRNA expression levels were upregulated 10- and 16-fold in the single and double immunized groups, respectively ($P \leq 0.05$, Fig. 4). IL-6 showed a 16- and 24-fold increase in the single immunized group and a 16- and 46-fold increase in the double immunized group ($P \leq 0.05$, Fig. 4).

Protective efficacy against different wild-type strains of S. Senftenberg

The fecal colonization of the JOL1557, JOL1815, JOL1816, and JOL1817 from the challenged chickens was evaluated to determine the protective efficacy offered by JOL1587 immunization. The fecal samples obtained from the immunized and control group chickens showed direct and post-enrichment recovery of all the challenge strains on BGA plates. The colonization and persistence of different S. Senftenberg was studied by challenging immunized as well as control group chickens. We divided each major group A, B and C post immunogenicity study into 4 sub-groups with six birds each. Each sub-group was challenged with different wild type *S.* Senftenberg (Table 2). Post-challenge bacterial recovery from fecal samples was performed to assess the protective efficacy. The bacterial recovery data was expressed as mean CFU/gm of each *S.* Senftenberg strain recovered from each sub-group (Fig. 5). Individual variation in the CFU recovery data was observed, hence mean value was calculated for each sub-group. The control group chickens showed significantly higher recovery of *S.* Senftenberg JOL1557, JOL1815, JOL1816 and JOL1817 strain until day 9, 28, 28 and 21 than prime-boost group, respectively (GI. 5, $p < 0.05$). Within immunized group, only the prime-boost immunized group showed significantly lower and below detection limit recovery for JOL1557, JOL1815, JOL1816 and JOL1817 from day 14 post-challenge (Fig. 5; $p < 0.05$).

Some chickens showed bacterial recovery only after enrichment culture; therefore, we interpreted the enrichments and direct recovery data as positive after for infected and shedding chickens and negative for non-shedding chickens. The percent population of positive (infected and shedding) and negative (non-shedding) chickens for *S.* Senftenberg infection are shown in Table 1. Total 80 to 100% chickens from the non-immunized control group showed fecal recovery of the JOL1557, JOL1815, JOL1816, and JOL1817 challenge strains consistently up to 4 weeks post-challenge, whereas the immunized chickens showed a significant decrease in the percentage population of the chickens positive for fecal shedding of the challenge strains (Table 2). Among the JOL1587 immunized chickens, the double immunized group showed significantly higher protection against *S.* Senftenberg than the single immunized and control group chickens (Table 2). Chickens from the double immunized group showed reduction in the challenge strain shedding below the detection level in the feces from day 9 post-challenge onward (Table 2). Although the single immunized group showed a significant reduction in the

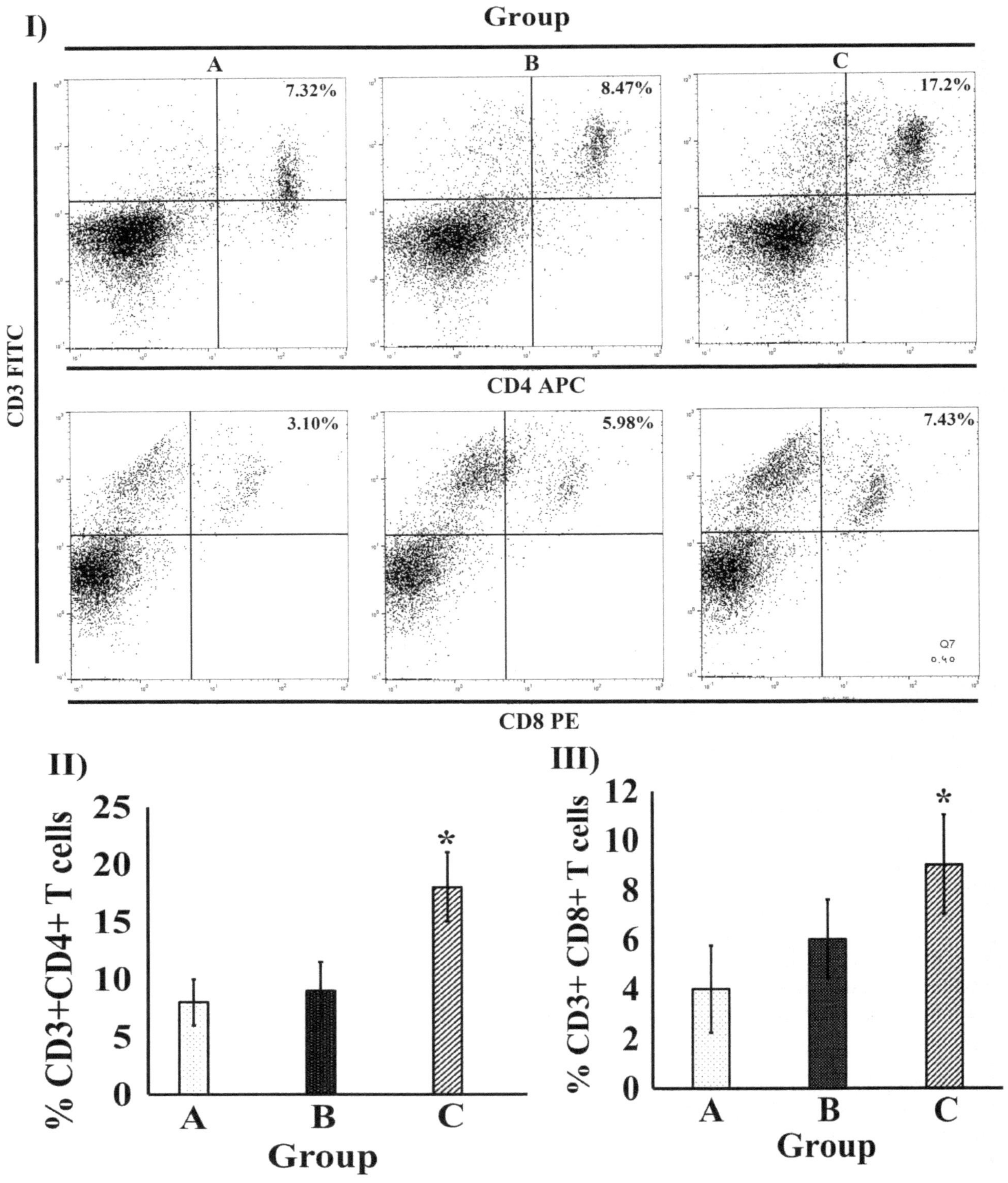

Fig. 3 (See legend on next page.)

(See figure on previous page.)
Fig. 3 FACS analysis for peripheral CD3 + CD4+ and CD3 + CD8+ T cell populations in the JOL1587-immunized and control group chickens. The isolated PBMCs were stained with appropriately diluted fluorescein-isothiocyanate (FITC)-labeled anti-CD3, allophycocyanin (APC)-labeled anti-CD4, and phycoerythrin (PE)-labeled anti-CD8 monoclonal antibodies. *a*: PBS-inoculated group; *b*: single immunized group and *c*: double immunized group. (**I**) Representative dot plots for CD3 + CD4+ and CD3 + CD8+ T cell populations. The population is represented as a percentage of gated cells; (**II**) The percentage of peripheral CD3 + CD4+ T cells; (**III**) The percentage of peripheral CD3 + CD8+ T cells. The values are shown as the mean ± SEM of five chickens per group. The * symbol indicates a significant increase in the percentage of peripheral T lymphocytes in the JOL1587-immunized chickens compared to the control group chickens ($P \leq 0.05$)

number of chickens positive for fecal shedding of the challenge strains, this group failed to show complete reduction in the shedding of wild–type *S.* Senftenberg below the detection limit from all the chickens (Table 2).

Discussion

Contrary to other *Salmonella* serovars, the pattern of *S.* Senftenberg infection in chickens is characterized by colonization of the intestinal epithelium with very little induction of the systemic immune response [18]. Information regarding the quality and magnitude of the immune response needed for optimal protection against *S.* Senftenberg infection is sparse, and many factors still need to be investigated. Previously we developed a *S.* Senftenberg mutant strainJOL1587 *(Δlon and ΔcpxR)* for immunization of the chickens against wild-type S. Senftenberg infection [11]. In this study, we evaluated the magnitude and quality of immune response generated by JOL1587 immunization in chickens. Further, the generated immune response was evaluated for its ability to protect chickens against four different wild-type isolates of *S.* Senftenberg.

Generation of *Salmonella*-specific IgG and sIgA antibodies is essential for the development of acquired immune protection against NTS [19]. Because *S.* Senftenberg colonizes and persists in the cecum of chickens, the induction of a sIgA antibody response might be beneficial for the mucosal clearance of *S.* Senftenberg. *Salmonella*-specific sIgAs in the intestinal mucosa constitute a first line of defense by preventing bacterial penetration of the intestinal barrier through the mechanism of immune exclusion [20, 21]. In this study, we evaluated the potential of single and double immunization to induce a plasma IgG and intestinal sIgA response in chickens. From the ELISA results, it was evident that double immunization induced significantly higher IgG and sIgA levels than single immunization. It is possible that the booster immunization activates memory B cells, producing an increase in antibody titer by their rapid proliferation and differentiation into plasma cells [22]. The observed decline in the magnitude of IgG and sIgA levels in the single immunized group contrary to the double-immunized group may have been due to poor systemic invasion and lower levels of colonization in the spleen. This has been observed previously after experimental parenteral inoculation with *S.* Senftenberg in chickens [7]. The ELISA results highlight the necessity of a booster immunization in this case with JOL1857 to induce better humoral and mucosal immune responses against *S.* Senftenberg infection in chickens.

Along with humoral immunity, the generation of a *Salmonella*-specific cellular immune response (CMI) is a prerequisite for the establishment of immune protection against *Salmonella* spp. in chickens [23]. The production of CD4 and CD8 T cells as part of an adaptive cellular immune response is crucial for the clearance of *Salmonella* infection in mice [24]. Activated *Salmonella*-specific CD4 and CD8 T cells migrate to infected non-lymphoid tissues and exert their effector functions to enable *Salmonella* clearance [25]. In the present study, the single and double immunized chickens showed a significant increase in their LPA and CD8 T cell responses relative to control group chickens, but failed to induce a CD4 T cell response after primary immunization with JOL1857. Following oral inoculation of attenuated *Salmonella*, the antigen-specific CD4 T cell response is initially generated in the gut-associated lymphoid tissue (GALT), a primary site for processing intestinal immunogens in mice [26]. Because *S.* Senftenberg serovars have been shown to colonize intestinal epithelial cells following oral inoculation in chickens [18], the *Salmonella*-specific CD4 and CD8 T cell responses observed in this study after primary immunization with JOL1857 may be induced in the GALT of the chickens. The fact that intestinal lymphoid tissue possesses very few naïve CD3 + CD4+ T cells could explain the low T helper cell response after primary immunization with JOL1587 [27]. Only after the booster immunization was a significant increase in the CD4 T-cell level observed in the double immunized chickens. This significant increase in the CD4 T cell levels observed following booster immunization correlates with the increased antibody titers in the double immunized chickens. *Salmonella*-specific antibodies have been shown to upregulate the cellular immune response by amplifying the processing and presentation of antigens from *Salmonella* to T helper cells in mice [28, 29]. Overall, the prime-boost chickens immunized with JOL1857 displayed a significant increase in the *S.* Senftenberg-specific CMI response compared to the single immunized chickens.

To further elucidate the role of the CMI response in *S.* Senftenberg clearance from chickens, we investigated

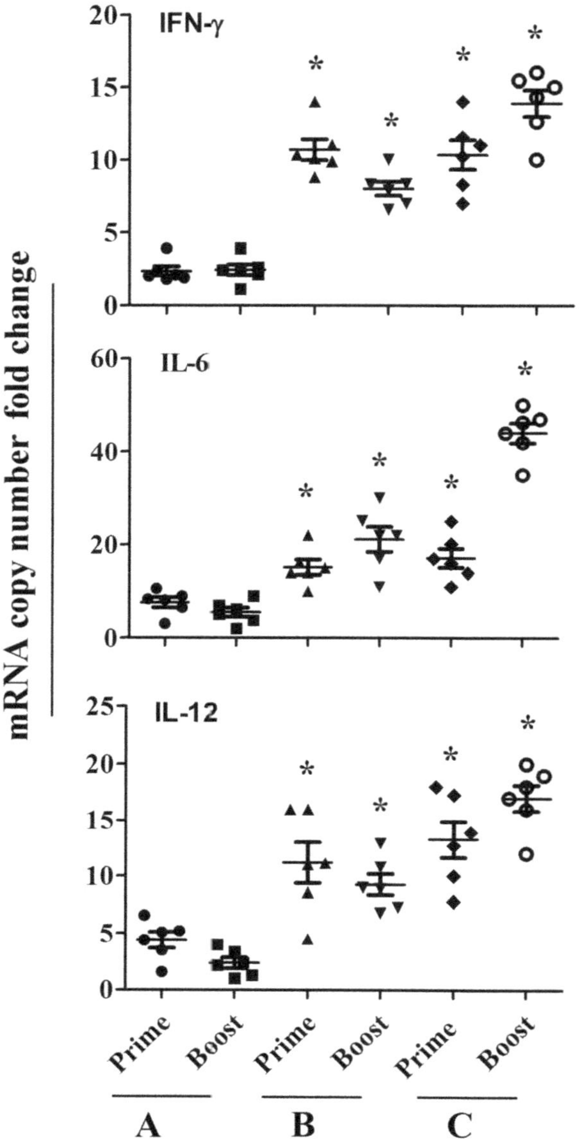

Fig. 4 The IFN-γ, IL-2 and IL-6 cytokine profiles of in vitro-stimulated PBMCs from the JOL1587-immunized and control group chickens. The relative mRNA copy numbers were determined by qRT-PCR using the comparative Ct method. I) Prime inoculation with JOL1587 at the fourth week of age and II) Prime-boost inoculation with JOL1587 at the 8 week of age. **a** PBS-inoculated group; **b** Prime immunized group and **c** Prime-boost immunized group. The * symbol indicates a significant increase in the cytokine levels for the JOL1587-immunized group compared to the control group chickens ($P \leq 0.05$).Total six splenocytes samples were analyzed which were collected from six randomly selected chickens from group a, b and c

differences in the expression patterns of the cytokines IL-2, IFN-γ and IL-6 for immunized and control groups. The chickens immunized with JOL1587 showed significant upregulation of IFN-γ, IL-2 and IL-6 after receiving the primary and booster immunizations. As studied in mice infection model, the mechanisms employed by IFN-γ, IL-2 and IL-6 for establishing protection against *Salmonella* infection are diverse in nature [30–32]. The cytokines IL-2 and IFN-γ are known to mediate immune protection against *Salmonella* by up-regulating the generation of *Salmonella*-specific cell-mediated and mucosal immunity, respectively [33, 34]. The production of IFN-γ in the intestinal mucosa is essential for the generation of mucosal immunity against *Salmonella* infection [34]. In the absence of IFN-γ in the mucosa, infection with *Salmonella* Typhimurium has been shown to produce increased invasion and disseminated infection with septicemia in mice [34]. The multifunctional cytokine IL-6 has also been shown to confer a protective effect at the mucosal level against invasive *Salmonella* infection [32, 35]. Upregulation in IL-6 levels can trigger the rapid development of a cytotoxic T cell response against *Salmonella* infection in mice [36, 37]. Our results showed a correlation between an increase in IL-6 and the production of *S.* Senftenberg-specific CD8 T cells after booster immunization in the double immunized group. Collectively, the results from the immunogenicity study for JOL1587 in chickens suggest that the prime-boost immunization protocol can induce significant humoral, mucosal, and cellular immune responses against the *S.* Senftenberg serovar in chickens.

Current evidence suggests that optimal protection against *Salmonella* infection is conferred by vaccines that produce a pattern of immune response homologous to that induced by natural infection [38]. Hence, the ability of the immune response generated in response to JOL1587 immunization to establish immune protection was evaluated by challenging the chickens orally with four different wild-type strains of *S.* Senftenberg. Systemic infection with wild-type *S.* Senftenberg in chickens was reported to be self-limiting in nature [9]. Heterogeneity regarding caecal persistence and fecal shedding for various *S.* Senftenberg strains in chickens represents a potential challenge for this serovar's suitability as a vaccine candidate [7]. The wild-type S. Senftenberg strains used in this study were tested positive for presence of SPI1, 2, 3, 4, and 5 specific gene with persistence in cecum of chicken. Evaluation of fecal shedding for the different challenge strains of wild-type *S.* Senftenberg can provide a useful means of estimating the protective efficacy conferred by JOL1587. The fecal shedding data from the protective efficacy experiments showed that, compared to the single immunization protocol, the prime-boost immunization with JOL1587 was sufficient for reduction of the wild-type *S.* Senftenberg recovery below the detection level in the feces of the chickens. Overall, the immunity generated in chickens by prime-boost immunization with JOL1587 was sufficient to protect chickens against infection with various wild-type *S.* Senftenberg strains.

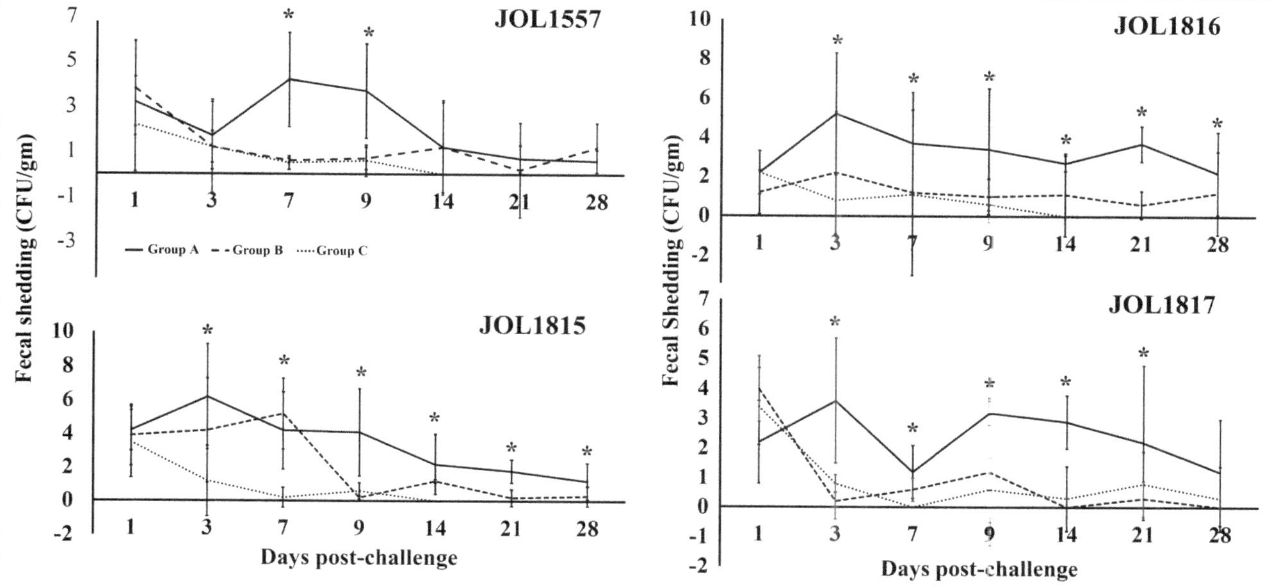

Fig. 5 Faecal shedding level of different *S.* Senftenberg isolates from immunized and control group chickens. Number of CFU of *S.* Senftenberg strains, JOL1557, JOL1815, JOL1816 and JOL1817 per gram of faecal samples from chickens orally challenged with 5×10^8 CFUs. Bacterial recovery was performed from day 1 to 28 post-challenge by direct plating and enrichment culture. Total 6 faecal samples were collected from six birds from each sub-group within major group A, B and C and processed for bacterial recovery. The data represented is mean CFU/gm ± SEM. * symbol indicates a significant amount of bacterial recovery from control group chickens compared to single and double immunized chickens

Conclusion

Our results indicate that chickens double immunized with JOL1587 can generate significant *S.* Senftenberg-specific mucosal, humoral and cell-mediated immune responses in chickens. Fecal shedding of the various *S.* Senftenberg wild-type isolates was significantly reduced below detection limit only in the double immunized chickens. In conclusion, the prime-boost immunization strategy of chickens with JOL1587 can provide a valuable method to prevent *S.* Senftenberg infection and fecal shedding in chickens.

Abbreviations

APC: Allophycocyanin; CDC: Centers for disease control and prevention; CFU: Colony forming units; ELISA: Enzyme linked immunosorbent assay; FITC: Fluorescein-isothiocyanate; NTS: Non-typhoidal serotypes; OMP: Outer membrane protein; PBMC: Peripheral blood mononuclear cell; PE: Phycoerythrin; *S.* Senftenberg: *Salmonella* Senftenberg; sbcp: Sonicated bacterial cell protein

Acknowledgments

This work was supported by a National Research Foundation of Korea (NRF) grant funded by the Korea government (MISP) [No. 2015R1A2A1A14001011].

Authors' contributions

NMK and JHL have designed and conceptualized the research topic. NMK carried out construction and animal work experimentation. JHL analysed the data. NMK and JHL have formulated the manuscript and tables. All authors read and approved the final manuscript.

Competing interests

The authors declare that there is no financial and non-financial conflict of interests.

Consent for publication

Not applicable.

References

1. L'Ecuyer PB, Diego J, Murphy D, Trovil ion E, Jones M, Sahm DF, et al. Nosocomial outbreak of gastroenteritis due to Salmonella senftenberg. Clin Infect Dis. 1996;23:734–42.
2. Mohle-Boetani JC, Farrar JA, Werner S3, Minassian D, Bryant R, Abbott S, et al. Escherichia coli O157 and Salmonella infections associated with sprouts in California, 1996–1998. Ann Intern Med. 2001;135:239–47.
3. Pezzoli L, Elson R, Little CL, Yip H, Fisher I, Yishai R, et al. Packed with Salmonella–investigation of an international outbreak of Salmonella Senftenberg infection linked to contamination of prepacked basil in 2007. Foodborne Pathog Dis. 2008;5:661–8.
4. Rushdy AA, Stuart JM, Ward LR, Bruce J, Threlfall EJ, Punia P, et al. National outbreak of Salmonella senftenberg associated with infant food. Epidemiol Infect. 1998;120:125–8.
5. Hamada S, Hashimato H, Tasaka T, Tsuchiya Y. Studieson chick salmonellosis: II. Salmonella Senftenberginfections in chicks. Jpn. J. Vet. Res. Hokkaido University. 1959;6:181–95.
6. Hu Q, Coburn B, Deng W, Li Y, Shi X, Lan Q, et al. Salmonella enterica serovar Senftenberg human clinical isolates lacking SPI-1. J Clin Microbiol. 2008;46:1330–6.
7. Boumart Z, Roche SM, Lalande F, Virlogeux-Payant I, Hennequet-Antier C, Menanteau P, et al. Heterogeneity of Persistence of Salmonella enterica Serotype Senftenberg Strains Could Explain the Emergence of this Serotype in Poultry Flocks. Roop RM, editor. PLoS ONE. 2012;7:e35782.
8. Pedersen TB, Olsen JE, Bisgaard M. Persistence of Salmonella Senftenberg in poultry production environments and investigation of its resistance to desiccation. Avian Pathol Taylor & Francis Group. 2008;37:421–7.
9. Kallapura G, Kogut MH, Morgan MJ, Pumford NR, Bielke LR, Wolfenden AD, et al. Fate of Salmonella Senftenberg in broiler chickens evaluated by challenge experiments. Avian Pathol. 2014;43:305–9.
10. Griffin AJ, McSorley SJ. Development of protective immunity to Salmonella, a mucosal pathogen with a systemic agenda. Mucosal Immunol Society for Mucosal Immunology. 2011;4:371–82.

11. Kamble NM, Lee JH. Characterization and evaluation of *Salmonella enterica s* erotype Senftenberg mutant created by deletion of virulence-related genes for use as a live attenuated vaccine. Clin Vaccine Immunol. 2016;23:802–12.
12. Kim SW, Moon KH, Baik HS, Kang HY, Kim SK, Bahk JD, et al. Changes of physiological and biochemical properties of Salmonella enterica serovar Typhimurium by deletion of cpxR and lon genes using allelic exchange method. J Microbiol Methods. 2009;79:314–20.
13. Porter RE, Holt PS. Use of a pilocarpine-based lavage procedure to study secretory immunoglobulin concentration in the alimentary tract of White Leghorn chickens. Avian Dis. 1992;36:529–36.
14. Rana N, Kulshreshtha RC. Cell-mediated and humoral immune responses to a virulent plasmid-cured mutant strain of Salmonella enterica serotype gallinarum in broiler chickens. Vet Microbiol. 2006;115:156–62.
15. Chaudhari AA, Jawale CV, Kim SW, Lee JH. Construction of a Salmonella Gallinarum ghost as a novel inactivated vaccine candidate and its protective efficacy against fowl typhoid in chickens. Vet Res BioMed Central. 2012;43:44.
16. Livak KJ, Schmittgen TD. Analysis of relative gene expression data using real-time quantitative PCR and the 2(–Delta Delta C(T)) Method. Methods. 2001;25:402–8.
17. Nandre RM, Matsuda K, Chaudhari AA, Kim B, Lee JH. A genetically engineered derivative of Salmonella Enteritidis as a novel live vaccine candidate for salmonellosis in chickens. Res Vet Sci. 2012;93:596–603.
18. Boumart Z, Roche SM, Lalande F, Virlogeux-Payant I, Hennequet-Antier C, Menanteau P, et al. Heterogeneity of persistence of Salmonella enterica serotype Senftenberg strains could explain the emergence of this serotype in poultry flocks. PLoS ONE. 2012;7, e35782.
19. MacLennan CA, Gondwe EN, Msefula CL, Kingsley RA, Thomson NR, White SA, et al. The neglected role of antibody in protection against bacteremia caused by nontyphoidal strains of Salmonella in African children. J Clin Invest. 2008;118:1553–62.
20. Holmgren J, Czerkinsky C. Mucosal immunity and vaccines. 2005.
21. Wijburg OLC, Uren TK, Simpfendorfer K, Johansen F-E, Brandtzaeg P, Strugnell RA. Innate secretory antibodies protect against natural Salmonella typhimurium infection. J Exp Med. 2006;203:21–6.
22. Galen JE, Chinchilla M, Pasetti MF, Wang JY, Zhao L, Arciniega-Martinez I, et al. Mucosal immunization with attenuated Salmonella enterica serovar Typhi expressing protective antigen of anthrax toxin (PA83) primes monkeys for accelerated serum antibody responses to parenteral PA83 vaccine. J Infect Dis. 2009;199:326–35.
23. Penha Filho RAC, Moura BS, De Almeida AM, Montassier HJ, Barrow PA, Berchieri JA. Humoral and cellular immune response generated by different vaccine programs before and after Salmonella Enteritidis challenge in chickens. Vaccine. 2012;30:7637–43.
24. Hess J, Ladel C, Miko D, Kaufmann SH. Salmonella typhimurium aroA- infection in gene-targeted immunodeficient mice: major role of CD4+ TCR-alpha beta cells and IFN-gamma in bacterial clearance independent of intracellular location. J Immunol. 1996;156:3321–6.
25. Kirby AC, Sundquist M, Wick MJ. In vivo compartmentalization of functionally distinct, rapidly responsive antigen-specific T-cell populations in DNA-immunized or Salmonella enterica serovar Typhimurium-infected mice. Infect Immun. 2004;72:6390–400.
26. McSorley SJ, Asch S, Costalonga M, Reinhardt RL, Jenkins MK. Tracking salmonella-specific CD4 T cells in vivo reveals a local mucosal response to a disseminated infection. Immunity. 2002;16:365–77.
27. Moon JJ, Chu HH, Pepper M, McSorley SJ, Jameson SC, Kedl RM, et al. Naive CD4(+) T cell frequency varies for different epitopes and predicts repertoire diversity and response magnitude. Immunity. 2007;27:203–13.
28. Barr TA, Brown S, Mastroeni P, Gray D. TLR and B cell receptor signals to B cells differentially program primary and memory Th1 responses to Salmonella enterica. J Immunol. 2010;185:2783–9.
29. Ugrinovic S, Ménager N, Goh N, Mastroeni P. Characterization and development of T-Cell immune responses in B-cell-deficient (Igh-6(–/–)) mice with Salmonella enterica serovar Typhimurium infection. Infect Immun. 2003;71:6808–19.
30. Matsui K. Role of interleukin-2 receptor expression on macrophages from Salmonella-infected mice. FEMS Immunol Med Microbiol. 1999;24:97–103.
31. Muotiala A, Mäkelä PH. The role of IFN-gamma in murine Salmonella typhimurium infection. Microb Pathog. 1990;8:135–41.
32. Weinstein D, O'Neill B, Metcalf E. Salmonella typhi stimulation of human intestinal epithelial cells induces secretion of epithelial cell-derived interleukin-6. Infect Immun. 1997;65:395–404.
33. Paetkau V, Shaw J, Caplan B, Mills GB, Lee KC. Interleukin 2 in cell-mediated immune responses. J Supramol Struct. 1980;13:271–80.
34. Bao S, Beagley KW, France MP, Shen J, Husband AJ. Interferon-gamma plays a critical role in intestinal immunity against Salmonella typhimurium infection. Immunology. 2000;99:464–72.
35. Huang F-C. Upregulation of Salmonella-induced IL-6 production in Caco-2 cells by PJ-34, PARP-1 inhibitor: involvement of PI3K, p38 MAPK, ERK, JNK, and NF-kappaB. Mediators Inflamm. 2009;2009:103890.
36. Salazar-Gonzalez R-M, Srinivasan A, Griffin A, Muralimohan G, Ertelt JM, Ravindran R, et al. Salmonella flagellin induces bystander activation of splenic dendritic cells and hinders bacterial replication in vivo. J Immunol. 2007;179:6169–75.
37. Salerno-Goncalves R, Sztein MB. Priming of Salmonella enterica serovar typhi-specific CD8(+) T cells by suicide dendritic cell cross-presentation in humans. PLoS ONE. 2009;4, e5879.
38. Viret JF, Favre D, Wegmüller B, Herzog C, Que JU, Cryz SJ, et al. Mucosal and systemic immune responses in humans after primary and booster immunizations with orally administered invasive and noninvasive live attenuated bacteria. Infect Immun. 1999;67:3680–5.

5

Report of the first clinical case of intestinal trichomoniasis caused by *Tritrichomonas foetus* in a cat with chronic diarrhoea in Brazil

Aline S. Hora[1*], Samantha I. Miyashiro[2], Fabiana C. Cassiano[3], Paulo E. Brandão[1], Archivaldo Reche-Junior[2] and Hilda F. J. Pena[1]

Abstract

Background: *Tritrichomonas foetus* is an emergent and important enteric pathogen of cats, which causes prolonged diarrhoea in cats.

Case presentation: This study describes a *T. foetus* infection in a seven-month-old, entire male domestic shorthair kitten with a six-month history of persistent large intestinal diarrhoea, faecal incontinence, prostration, apathy and weight loss. Parasites were microscopically observed and confirmed by PCR and DNA sequencing. Molecular analyses were carried out comparing the sequence obtained in this study with *T. foetus* and *T. suis*. Retrieved from GenBank. After treatment with ronidazole, the cat showed resolution of clinical signs.

Conclusions: This is the first clinical case of *T. foetus* infection in a chronic diarrheic cat in Brazil and South America, confirming the presence of this pathogen in this part of the world and highlighting the importance of this protozoa being considered in the differential diagnosis of cats presenting diarrhoea of the large intestine. Our case report enriches our knowledge on the geographical distribution of *T. foetus* in cats in Brazil and provides further understanding of the clinical significance of feline intestinal trichomoniasis in this country.

Keywords: Feline Tritrichomonosis, Large bowel diarrhea, Enteric pathogen

Background

Tritrichomonas foetus is a protozoal parasite in the order *Trichomonadida*, and family *Trichomonadidae* (Phylum Parabasalia) which also includes the genera *Trichomonas*, *Ditrichomonas* and *Pentatrichomonas* [1]. Originally described as a parasite restricted to the urogenital tract of cattle, *T. foetus* has more recently been shown to infect the gastrointestinal tract of domestic cats [2]. *T. foetus* has been reported to be a naturally occurring pathogen of the large intestine of domestic cats that colonizes the ileum, cecum, and colon, and resides in close contact with the epithelium, causing chronic large bowel diarrhoea [3, 4].

* Correspondence: alineshora@gmail.com
[1]Department of Preventive Veterinary Medicine and Animal Health, College of Veterinary Medicine, University of São Paulo, São Paulo, SP, Brazil
Full list of author information is available at the end of the article

T. foetus has been diagnosed in the domestic cat in many geographic regions including Europe (Austria, Finland, France, Germany, Greece, Italy, the Netherlands, Norway, Poland, Spain, Sweden, Switzerland, and the UK), North America (Canada and the USA), Australia/Oceania (Australia and New Zealand), and Asia (Japan and South Korea) [5]. In Brazil, to date, infection with *T. foetus* has been reported only in asymptomatic cats [6]. This case report describes a case of naturally occurring *T. foetus* infection in a kitten inhabiting in Brazil, São Paulo state and the molecular analysis of this strain.

Case presentation

A seven-month-old, entire male domestic shorthair kitten was presented to the Veterinary Hospital of the School of Veterinary Medicine – University of São Paulo, Brazil, in October 2013. This cat had a six-month history of persistent large intestinal diarrhoea, faecal incontinence, prostration, apathy and weight loss. Previously to the cat presentation at the Veterinary Hospital of the School of Veterinary Medicine, the cat was presented to veterinary practitioners and several different anthelminthics, metronidazole and sulfadimetoxin (dosage not available) were blindly administrated without success. The cat had been confined indoor, and had contact with three asymptomatic cats and a dog. Unfortunately, it was not possible to evaluate the contacting animals due to low compliance of the owner.

At physical examination, the cat showed sensibility to abdominal palpation in the mesogastric region, thickened bowel loops with faecal content, inflammation at the anal region and a body temperature of 39.2 °C. Screening tests for feline leukaemia virus - FeLV and feline immunodeficiency virus - FIV (SNAP FIV/FeLV Combo Test, Idexx Laboratories) were performed and the results were negative.

Faecal flotation was negative for the presence of nematode eggs, *Giardia* species cysts and coccidian oocysts using sugar centrifugation flotation as previously described [7].

The fresh faecal sample obtained via colon flush was suspended in an equal volume of normal saline and microscopically examined under a cover slip using 200X and 400X magnification. *Tritrichomonas* sp. was identified by direct examination, which revealed very large numbers of motile trophozoites featuring a pyriform body, which measured approximately 10 to 20 μm in length, with three free anterior flagella, an undulating membrane running the length of the body and one posterior flagellum (Fig. 1a and b). The trophozoites exhibited jerky, progressive forward motion (Additional file 1: Movie S1). The motile characteristics of *T. foetus* differ from *Giardia* sp. in that a falling leaf motility has been observed [5].

Both *T. foetus* and *Pentatrichomonas hominis* can occur in the intestinal tract of cats [6]. *P. hominis* lives as a mere commensal in the colon of cats [8] and a number of other mammalian hosts including humans, pigs, dogs, water buffalos, cows, and goats [9]. *Tritrichomonas* sp. and *Pentatrichomonas* sp. are not easily differentiated from one another by examining living material or organisms stained with routinely used histological stains [10]. Thus, molecular methods to detect *T. foetus* and *Pentatrichomonas* sp. were performed.

DNA was extracted directly from the fresh faecal sample using a commercial DNA extraction kit (DNeasy® Blood & Tissue, Qiagen), according to the manufacturer's protocol. *T. foetus* and *P. hominis* were tested using the primers and conditions previously described by Felleisen et al. [11] and Crucitti et al. [12], respectively.

Coinfection with *T. foetus* and *P. hominis* was not observed herein, unlike the prior study conducted in Brazil, in which three of the four *T. foetus*-positive cats were infected with *P. hominis*, although both studies using the same set of primers for the molecular diagnosis of both infections [6]. The amplicon corresponding to *T. foetus* (347 bp) was purified using ExoSAP-IT PCR Product Cleanup (USB Products Affymetrix, Cleveland, OH) and submitted to bidirectional DNA sequencing with BigDye 3.1 (Applied Biosystems, Carlsbad, CA), according to the manufacturer's protocols. The products were resolved using a 3500 Genetic Analyser (Applied Biosystems, Foster, CA), and the electropherograms were analysed with Phred at http://asparagin.cenargen.embrapa.br/phph/. Positions with a quality score of >20 were used to generate contiguous sequences with Cap-Contig implemented in the software Bioedit 7.0.9.0 [13]. The sequence was then submitted to BLAST/n at http://www.ncbi.nlm.nih.gov/BLAST to confirm the amplicon identities. Each sequence was aligned with homologous sequences from *T. foetus* retrieved from GenBank with CLUSTAL/W in Bioedit 7.0.9.0, and a phylogenetic tree

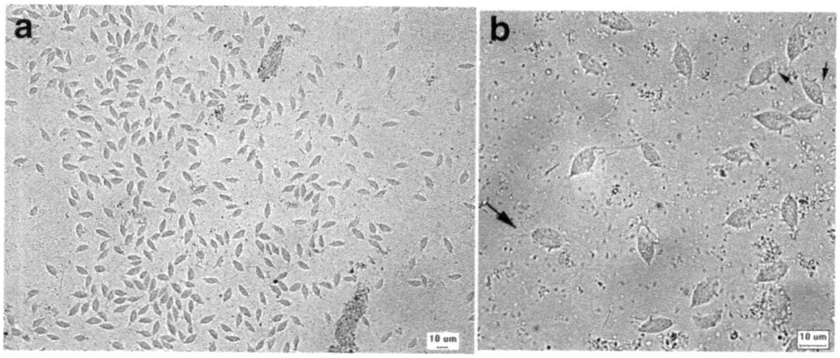

Fig. 1 *Tritrichomonas foetus* in cat faeces. **a** Numerous pyriform trophozoites. **b** The three free anterior flagella (large arrow) and the undulating membrane (*small arrows*) can be visualised in some trophozoites. Fresh preparation in saline 0.85%

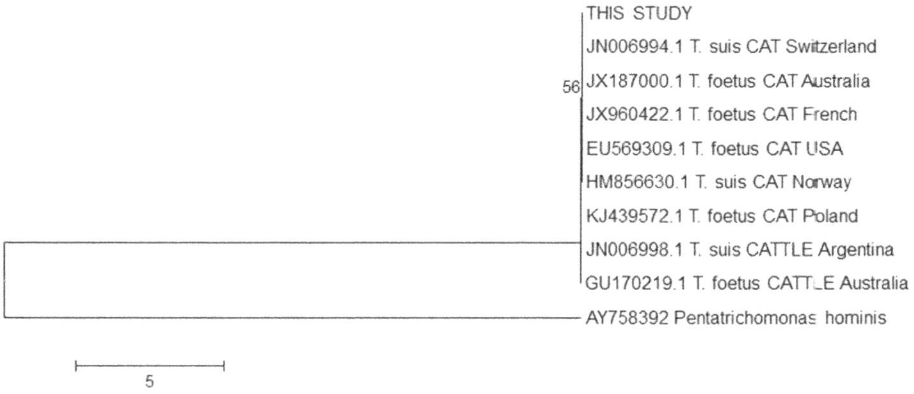

Fig. 2 Neighbor-joining maximum composite likelihood phylogenetic tree of partial sequences of *Tritrichomonas foetus* and *T. suis* internal transcribed spacer 1 (partial), 5.8S ribosomal RNA gene (complete), and internal transcribed spacer 2 (partial). *Pentatrichomonas hominis* was used as an outgroup. The numbers on the nodes indicate the bootstrap support from 1000 replications. Only bootstrap values of >50 are shown. The scale bar represents the number of substitutions per nucleotide

for the nucleotide sequences was generated using the neighbor-joining distance algorithm and the maximum composite likelihood model with 1000 bootstrap replicates using MEGA 5.0 [14]. A sequence identity matrix was performed with Bioedit 7.0.9.0. The nucleotide sequence determined in this work was submitted to GenBank under accession number KU680816.

Feline isolates and bovine isolates are morphologically indistinguishable [15]. Current evidence suggests that *T. foetus* and *T. suis* appear to correspond to the same species [15–18], as observed herein (Fig. 2). This finding is also sustained by a minor difference (0.04%) in identity in the sequences from *T. foetus* (KJ439572, GU170219) and *T. suis* (JN006998) retrieved from GenBank compared to the sequence from this study.

The kitten was treated with 30 mg/kg of ronidazole, administered orally once a day for 14 days, which resulted in improvement in faecal consistency and frequency without adverse effects. However, adverse effects, such as reversible neurological signs, including lethargy, trembling of extremities, ataxia, agitation, facial tremors and hyperesthesia, have already been observed in cats treated with this drug [19].

Discussion and Conclusions

In recent years, *T. foetus* has become increasingly recognized as an important enteric pathogen of cats. A wide geographical distribution of this pathogen has been observed [5], in South America, *T. foetus* has previously been detected in asymptomatic cats in Brazil [6]. This is the first clinical case of intestinal trichomoniasis caused by *T. foetus* in Brazil and South America, confirming the presence of this pathogen in this part of the world and highlighting the importance of this protozoa being considered in the differential diagnosis of cats presenting diarrhoea of the large intestine. Our case report enriches our knowledge on the geographical distribution of *T. foetus* in cats in Brazil and provides further understanding of the clinical significance of feline intestinal trichomoniasis in this country.

Abbreviations

FeLV: Feline leukaemia virus; FIV: Feline immunodeficiency virus; T. foetus: *Tritrichomonas foetus*; T. suis: *Tritrichomonas suis*

Funding

We are very grateful to the Fundação de Amparo à Pesquisa do Estado de São Paulo, Brazil (Grants no. FAPESP 2014/01919-0) and the Coordenação de Aperfeiçoamento de Pessoal de Nível Superior (Grant no. CAPES/PROEX 1841/2016) for funding this research.

Authors' contributions

ASH performed biomolecular tests and sequencing analysis. SIM performed clinical pathology tests. FCC handled the case when first presented to the Veterinary Hospital of the School of Veterinary Medicine – University of São Paulo, Brazil. PEB supervised the activities and contributed to the draft. ARJ supervised the clinical activities. HFJP performed parasitological testes, DNA extraction and contributed to the draft. All authors read and approved the final manuscript.

Competing interests

The authors declare that they have no competing interests.

Consent for publication

Consent was obtained from the owner of the cat for publication of this case report and any accompanying images and video.

Author details

[1]Department of Preventive Veterinary Medicine and Animal Health, College of Veterinary Medicine, University of São Paulo, São Paulo, SP, Brazil. [2]Department of Veterinary Medicine, College of Veterinary Medicine, University of São Paulo, São Paulo, SP, Brazil. [3]Veterinary Hospital, College of Veterinary Medicine, University of São Paulo, São Paulo, SP, Brazil.

References

1. Frey CF, Müller N. Tritrichomonas-systematics of an enigmatic genus. Mol Cell Probes. 2012;26:132–6.
2. Slapeta J, Müller N, Stack CM, Walker G, Lew-Tabor A, Tachezy J, et al. Comparative analysis of Tritrichomonas foetus (Riedmüller, 1928) cat genotype, T. foetus (Riedmüller, 1928) cattle genotype and Tritrichomonas suis (Davaine, 1875) at 10 DNA loci. Int J Parasitol. 2012;42:1143–9.

3. Gookin JL, Levy MG, Law JM, Papich MG, Poore MF, Breitschwerdt EB. Experimental infection of cats with Tritrichomonas foetus. Am J Vet Res. 2001;62:1690–7.
4. Xenoulis PG, Lopinski DJ, Read SA, Suchodolski JS, Steiner JM. Intestinal Tritrichomonas foetus infection in cats: a retrospective study of 104 cases. J Feline Med Surg. 2013;15:1098–103.
5. Yao C, Köster LS. Tritrichomonas foetus infection, a cause of chronic diarrhea in the domestic cat. Vet Res BioMed Central Ltd. 2015;46:35.
6. Santos CS, Jesus VLT, McIntosh D, Berto BP, Lopes CWG. Co-infection by Tritrichomonas foetus and Pentatrichomonas hominis in asymptomatic cats. Pesq Vet Bras. 2015;35:980–8.
7. Ogassawara S, Benassi S. Infecção experimental de gatos com coração de bovino parasitado por Sarcocystis sp. Arq Inst Biol (São Paulo). 1980;47:27–32.
8. Gookin JL, Stauffer SH, Levy MG. Identification of Pentatrichomonas hominis in feline fecal samples by polymerase chain reaction assay. Vet Parasitol. 2007;145:11–5.
9. Kamaruddin M, Tokoro M, Rahman M, Moshiur A, APNH S, Syafruddin D, PBS A, et al. Molecular Characterization of Various Trichomonad Species Isolated from Humans and Related Mammals in Indonesia. Korean J Parasitol. 2014;52:471–8.
10. Levy MG, Gookin JL, Poore M, Birkenheuer AJ, Dykstra MJ, Litaker RW. Tritrichomonas foetus and not Pentatrichomonas hominis is the etiologic agent of feline trichomonal diarrhea. J Parasitol. 2003;89:99–104.
11. Felleisen RSJ, Lambelet N, Bachmann P, Nicolet J, Muller N, Gottstein B. Detection of Tritrichomonas foetus by PCR and DNA Enzyme Immunoassay Based on rRNA Gene Unit Sequences. J Clin Microbiol. 1998;36:513–9.
12. Crucitti T, Abdellati S, Ross DA, Changalucha J, Dyck E, Buve A. Detection of Pentatrichomonas hominis DNA in biological specimens by PCR. Lett Appl Microbiol. 2004;38:510–6.
13. Hall TA. Bioedit: a user-friendly biological sequence alignment editor and analysis program for Windows 95/98/NT. Nucleic Acids Symp Ser. 1999;41:95–8.
14. Tamura K, Peterson D, Peterson N, Stecher G, Nei M, Kumar S. MEGA5: molecular evolutionary genetics analysis using maximum likelihood, evolutionary distance, and maximum parsimony methods. Mol Biol Evol. 2011;28:2731–9.
15. Reinmann K, Müller N, Kuhnert P, Campero CM, Leitsch D, Hess M, et al. Tritrichomonas foetus isolates from cats and cattle show minor genetic differences in unrelated loci ITS-2 and EF-1α. Vet Parasitol. 2012;185:138–44.
16. Slapeta J, Craig S, McDonell D, Emery D. Tritrichomonas foetus from domestic cats and cattle are genetically distinct. Exp Parasitol. 2010; 126:209–13.
17. Sun Z, Stack C, Šlapeta J. Sequence differences in the diagnostic region of the cysteine protease 8 gene of Tritrichomonas foetus parasites of cats and cattle. Vet Parasitol. 2012;186:445–9.
18. Kleina P, Bettim-Bandinelli J, Bonatto SL, Benchimol M, Bogo MR. Molecular phylogeny of Trichomonadidae family inferred from ITS-1, 5.8S rRNA and ITS-2 sequences. Int J Parasitol. 2004;34:963–70.
19. LeVine DN, Papich MG, Gookin JL, Davidson GS, Davis JL, Hayes RB. Ronidazole pharmacokinetics after intravenous and oral immediate-release capsule administration in healthy cats. J Feline Med Surg. 2011;13:244–50.

6

Assessment of pathogenicity and tissue distribution of infectious bronchitis virus strains (Italy 02 genotype) isolated from moroccan broiler chickens

Khadija Khataby[1,2], Faouzi Kichou[3], Chafiqa Loutfi[2†] and My Mustapha Ennaji[1*†]

Abstract

Background: Avian infectious bronchitis (IB) is one of the most important viral diseases of poultry, affecting chickens of all ages and causing major economic losses in poultry flocks. Mass vaccination is conducted in Morocco using a vaccine against Massachusetts, which is the most dominant serotype; however no information about the pathogenesis and tissue distribution of the Moroccan Italy 02 genotype was reported.
40 one-day-old specific pathogen free chickens were divided randomly into four groups. Group1, 2 and 3 were inoculated intra oculo-nasally with 103.5 EID50 of Italy02 viruses, and group 4 was kept as control. Chickens in each group were monitored for 14 days post-infection (pi).

Results: Chickens in all infected groups showed severe respiratory signs, which most of them have been reproduced on 2dpi, with varying times of appearance and disappearance. The infected birds appeared lethargic, reluctant to move, with specific respiratory clinical signs and macroscopic lesions. However no nephritis lesions or mortality were recorded in all groups. The specific histological lesions finding in all infected birds, exhibited tracheal lesions with mucosal thickening, hyperplasia of the surface epithelium, mononuclear inflammatory cell infiltrate of lamina propria. Primary and secondary bronchi, epithelial hyperplasia and mononuclear inflammatory cell infiltrate of the lamina propria were also observed. Tracheal lesions developed in all infected birds, confirm the ability of the three tested strains to induce respiratory disease. The results at 14 dpi also revealed that all strains were able to induce serological response. Virus re-isolation from infected organs and amplification of the viral RNA by real-time PCR proved the presence of the virus in lung and trachea of infected chicks. Neither re-isolation nor significant viral RNA detection were detected in the kidney.

Conclusion: The results demonstrated that the three strains Italy02 genotype emerging in Moroccan poultry farms have a wide distribution for respiratory system, without kidney damage and without causing mortality.

Keywords: Infectious bronchitis virus (IBV), Italy 02, Clinical scoring, Pathogenecity

* Correspondence: m.ennaji@yahoo.fr
†Equal contributors
[1]Laboratory of Virology, Microbiology, Quality and Biotechnologies/ Ecotoxicology & Biodiversity, Faculty of Sciences and Techniques, University Hassan II of Casablanca, Mohammedia, Morocco
Full list of author information is available at the end of the article

Background

Avian infectious bronchitis (IB) is an acute, highly contagious respiratory disease of chickens, causes major economic losses in poultry industry worldwide [1]. The IB virus (IBV) is a member of *Gammacoronavirus* genus, previously Group 3, within the Coronaviridae and it is the type species of the avian *Coronavirus* of the domestic chicken (*Gallus Gallus*)) [2].

It is generally accepted that chickens are the most important natural host of IBV and epithelial cells of the upper respiratory tract are the primary target, and intensive virus replication, predominantly in the trachea, results in respiratory signs, which are the most frequent clinical manifestation of this disease [1].

Chickens of all ages are susceptible, but the severity is great in younger ages [3], and the clinical signs include depression, coughing, dyspnea, sneezing, nasal discharge, and death [4]. However, some strains of IBV can also replicates in the ciliated epithelial cells of organs, such as the kidney, reproductive and enteric tracts, producing severe nephritis, reproductive disorders in males and females, a drop in egg production and quality in laying flocks and deep pectoral myopathy in broiler breeder may occure [5].

The transmission of IBV is mainly horizontal by direct contact via the respiratory tract from infected chickens. Infection takes place via inhalation of droplets containing the air born virus. Or indirect by contaminated feed and drinking water, including human beings, probably contribute to more local spread [6]. In addition, it has been demonstrate that certain strains of IBV may persist in small amounts in the cecal tonsils of the intestinal tract by asymptomatic way during long time [7].

IBV is an enveloped, non segmented, positive sense, single stranded RNA virus. Its genome consists of about 27.6 kb and codes for four structural proteins: the membrane (M), small membrane (E), nucleoprotein (N) and spike (S) [8]. The multimeric coiled-coil S protein is post-translationally cleaved into smaller proteins namely S1 and S2 [8]. The S1 gene contains the hypervariable regions that are responsible for the induction of neutralizing, serotype specific antibodies and protective immunity [9]. Many IBV genotypes and serotypes have been identified and have complicated efforts at control through vaccination, due to the frequent point mutations in S1 gene that can be partially or poorly neutralised by existing vaccine serotypes [10]. For this reason, the sequencing of this gene is the most useful strategy for the molecular characterization of virus isolates existing in the field and the selection of appropriate vaccines [11].

In Morocco, IBV was identified for the first time in 1983 by El Houadfi & Jones [12]. Subsequently, several reports confirmed the IBV strains related to the Massachusetts and to 4/91 genotypes [13, 14].

Recently, between 2010-2014, an epidemiological survey showed the emergence of a novel strain of Italy02 serotype with a prevalence of 32 %, co-circulating with two serotypes; Massachusetts and 4/91, with a prevalence of 66 % and 2 % respectively, that are isolated from vaccinated and unvaccinated chicken flocks [15].

Mass vaccination in Morocco is conducted using a vaccine against Massachusetts, which is the most dominant serotype, however no information about pathogenesis and tissue distribution of Italy 02 serotype, hence the objective of this present study which is reported for the first time in Morocco, aims to evaluate the pathogenicity and the tissue distribution of the three isolated Moroccan strains of IBV Italy 02 genotype in one day old experimentally infected SPF chickens. The clinical signs, tracheal ciliary activity, gross and microscopic lesions were evaluated. Serological response by the detection of IBV antibodies of the affected chicks was also checked. Re-isolation of the virus from the affected organs and RT-PCR test was used to detect virus in several tissues of infected birds.

Results

Clinical signs and gross pathological findings

Clinical monitoring of infected chicks reveals at first, apparent respiratory symptoms beginning at day 2 post-inoculation (dpi). Respiratory clinical signs were predominant in all of the inoculated groups and were intense and more severe until 7 dpi, with no clear differences in the pathogenicity of the three strains. The most prominent clinical signs were characterized by gasping, depression, sneezing, difficulty in breathing, cough, pulmonary and tracheal rales, with high scores were reported for all the tested strains with clinical score of 108, 126 and 140 for IBV/RA, IBV/MN and IBV/TU strain respectively, (Tables 1, 2 and 3).

Nasal discharge and watery eyes were also observed but were transient in some of infected by IBV/RA and IBV/MN chicks. These clinical symptoms were persisted in all groups until 12dpi. The birds infected by IBV/MN and IBV/TU appeared lethargic, reluctant to move (Fig. 1), whereas, chicks infected with by IBV/RA were not as apathetic. At autopsy, all infected chicks that were killed at 5 dpi to prevent their suffering were examined for the macroscopic lesions in the trachea, lung and kidney. These gross lesions consisted in hemorrhagic tracheitis, mucosal congestion and catarrhal exudates that mainly progressed. For the three strains used, the signs were observed in the most infected chicks with dominance in the lungs that were hemorrhagic and sometimes cyanotic at one lobe. Therefore, samples were taken at 14 dpi just for a macroscopic examination of organs to confirm whether the absence of clinical signs is correlative with the gross lesions. Whereas, gross lesions of kidney, were not observed in all inoculated chicks. During the experiment, the

Table 1 Clinical Signs scores of SPF chickens inoculated with IBV strains IBV/MN*IBV* infectious bronchitis virus

IBV/MN Strain						
Days Post inoculation	Clinical Score (0 to 3)					
	No Signs (0)	Sneezing (1)	Tracheal Rale (2)	Pulmonary Rale (2)	Sick (3)	Day Score
1	5/10	3/10	1/10	0/10	1/10	8
2	3/10	4/10	2/10	0/10	1/10	11
3	1/10	3/10	3/10	0/10	3/10	18
4	0/10	4/10	4/10	0/10	2/10	18
5	0/10	3/10	3/10	2/10	2/10	19
6	0/7	4/7	2/7	0/7	1/7	11
7	1/7	4/7	1/7	0/7	1/7	9
8	2/7	3/7	1/7	0/7	1/7	8
9	2/7	3/7	1/7	0/7	1/7	8
10	2/7	2/7	1/7	0/7	1/7	7
11	3/7	3/7	1/7	0/7	0/7	5
12	4/7	2/7	1/7	0/7	0/7	4
Total score	126					

IBV infectious bronchitis virus
SPF Specific pathogen free
IBV/MN infectious bronchitis virus sampled from Meknes Tafilalet region

non-infected control group stayed normally without clinical signs or gross lesions. The statistical analysis was not performed as the three tested strains are phylogentically related to each other and the difference in clinical and tissues scores is not very significant.

Histopathological examination

The microscopic tissues analysis was performed in the euthanized chicks at 5 dpi. This period correlates with the maximum intensity of clinical signs (which begins between 2 and 7dpi). These signs fade from the 7dpi

Table 2 Clinical Signs scores of SPF chickens inoculated with IBV strains IBV/RA*IBV* infectious bronchitis virus

IBV/RA Strain						
Days Post inoculation	Clinical Score (0 to 3)					
	No sing (0)	Sneezing (1)	Tracheal Râle (2)	Pulmonary Rale (2)	Sick (3)	Day Score
1	9/10	1/10	0/10	0/10	0/10	1
2	3/10	4/10	2/10	1/10	0/10	10
3	2/10	3/10	2/10	2/10	1/10	12
4	1/10	2/10	4/10	2/10	1/10	18
5	0/10	3/10	6/10	1/10	1/10	14
6	0/7	3/7	2/7	2/7	0/7	11
7	1/7	4/7	2/7	0/7	0/7	8
8	1/7	4/7	2/7	0/7	0/7	8
9	2/7	3/7	2/7	0/7	0/7	7
10	2/7	2/7	3/7	0/7	0/7	8
11	3/7	1/7	2/7	0/7	0/7	5
12	3/7	2/7	2/7	0/7	0/7	6
Total score	108					

IBV infectious bronchitis virus
SPF Specific pathogen free
IBV/RA infectious bronchitis virus sampled from Rabat-Sale-Azzemour Zaire region

Table 3 Clinical Signs scores of SPF chickens inoculated with IBV strains IBV/TU*IBV* infectious bronchitis virus

IBV/TU Strain						
Days Post inoculation	Clinical Score (0 to 3)					
	No sing (0)	Sneezing (1)	Tracheal Râle (2)	Pulmonary Rale (2)	Sick (3)	Day Score
1	7/10	2/10	1/10	0/10	0/10	4
2	5/10	2/10	3/10	0/10	0/10	8
3	4/10	2/10	2/10	1/10	1/10	11
4	2/10	1/10	2/10	2/10	3/10	18
5	1/10	1/10	3/10	2/10	3/10	20
6	0/7	1/7	2/7	1/7	3/7	16
7	0/7	1/7	1/7	2/7	3/7	17
8	0/7	2/7	1/7	2/7	2/7	13
9	0/7	3/7	1/7	1/7	2/7	13
10	2/7	2/7	2/7	1/7	0/7	8
11	2/7	2/7	2/7	1/7	0/7	7
12	2/7	3/7	1/7	0/7	0/7	5
Total score	140					

IBV infectious bronchitis virus
SPF Specific pathogen free
IBV/TU infectious bronchitis virus sampled from Abda-Doukkala region

with a total restoration at 12 dpi, that why we only conducted the macroscopic examination at this time. Histopathological lesions developed at 5dpi in the three groups of experimentally infected chickens, were compatible of those previously described for infectious bronchitis virus [16]. And their scoring was mainly correlating with the ranking and scoring described in previous experiments [17].

In the trachea, most detected lesions in all infected groups were characterized by mucosal thickening, hyperplasia of the surface epithelium, loss of cilia, and mononuclear inflammatory cell infiltrate (lymphocytes, plasmocytes, and macrophage) of lamina propria (Figs. 2a and b). Mean total score of severity was 3,7; 4,7 and 6,7 in birds infected by IBV/MN; IBV/RA and IBV/14/TU strains respectively. This indicates that IBV/TU strain seems to have a higher degree of pathogenicity than the other tested strains (Table 4).

In the lungs, lesions in all infected groups were mainly confined to the primary and secondary bronchi and included epithelial hyperplasia, loss of cilia, and heterophils and mononuclear inflammatory cell infiltrate (lymphocytes, plasmocytes and macrophages) of the lamina propria and peribronchial space (Fig. 3a and b). Other changes were located in the atria and parabronchi and consisted of hypertrophy and/or hyperplasia of pneumocytes. The score of these changes were from mild to moderate degree of severity and there was no big differences in the mean total score of severity among tissues infected with the 3 tested IBV strains (7,3; 8,3 and 6), thus indicating no differences in the pathogenicity of the three strains for the lung (Table 5). However, no kidney lesions were observed in chicks

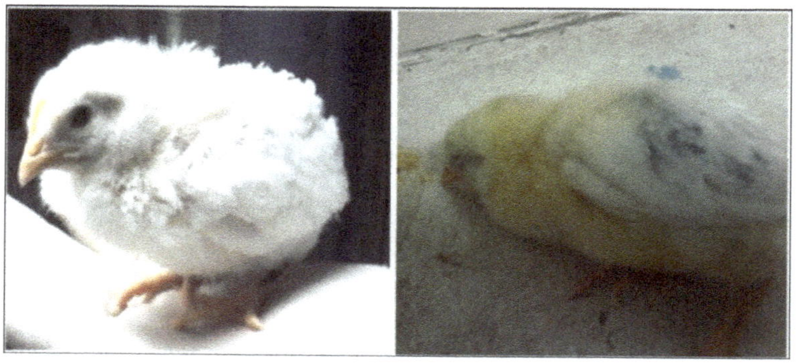

Fig. 1 Birds lethargic and reluctant to move after infection with IBV/MN strain (in the left) and with IBV/TU strain (in the right)

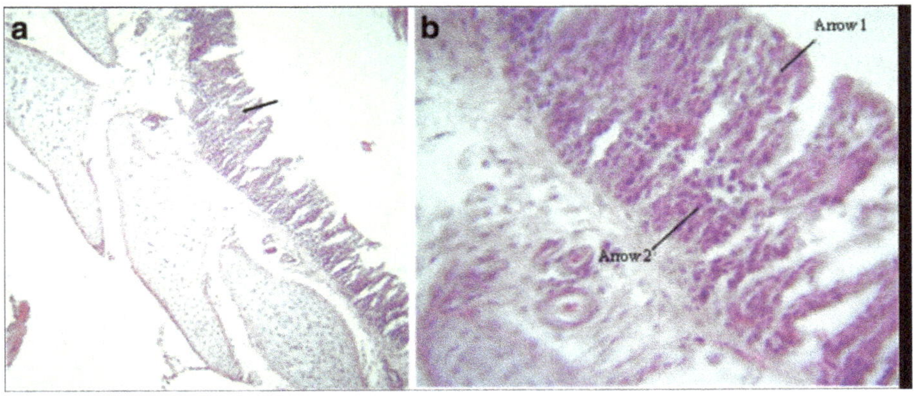

Fig. 2 a Trachea of IBV/TU inoculated chick – Severe thickening of mucosa (*Arrow*) H&E, X 62,50. **b** Trachea of IBV/TU inoculated chick – moderate hyerplasia of surface epithelium and loss of cilia (*Arrow1*) and moderate lympho- plasmocytic infiltration of lamina propria (*Arrow2*), H&E, X250

infected with the three tested strains. Tracheas and lungs of control chicks samples throughout the experiment, showed normal histological features.

Ciliostasis: tracheal ciliary activity

Ciliary activity was observed in all tracheas of infected birds at 5dpi. But the severity differed between the three strains tested; the ciliostasi caused by IBV/MN and IBV/RA strains was 25 % and 50 % for IBV/TU strain, compared to the control group (100 %). However, a partial recovery of ciliary activity in infected birds was observed at 12dpi.

Viral re- isolation

Results related to IBV distribution was checked in all tissues samples collected at 5dpi of all infected chicks. The virus was found in the trachea, lung of all strains, but in the kidney of one strain (IBV/MN) with low viral load. The effect of the virus after one passage in SPF 10 old embryonated eggs showed dwarfism and hemorrhagic spots in all over the body of the embryo, which are considered pathognomonic signs of IBV (Fig. 4).

The virus was re-isolated from all the sampled tissues with a high viral load in the trachea and lungs. No IB virus was re-isolated from the control group. Real time RT-PCR results obtained from the tissues of infected chicks at 5 dpi was closely correlating with those obtains from allantoic liquid of inoculated eggs (Table 6).

Serological response

Antibody titers against Infectious Bronchitis (Anti-IBV) in the serum collected from chickens of different groups on days 5 and 14 dpi was measured by ELISA test. In the all infected group, serum samples were negative at day 0

Table 4 Microscopic lesion scores in trachea of 5 day-old SPF chickens inoculated with field IBV strains IBV/MN, IBV/RA and IBV/TU*IBV* infectious bronchitis virus

	Lesions		Mean lesion scores in IBV infected groups of birds		
			IBV/MN	IBV/RA	IBV/TU
Trachea	Epithelium	Thickening	1	1,3	2
		Hyperplasia (1-4 +)	1	1,3	2,6
		Loss of cilia	0	0	0,6
		Degenerescence and necrosis of epithelial cells	0	0	0
		Inflammatory exudate (degenerate epithelial cells, Lc, heterophyles) on the surface	0	0,3	0,6
	Lamina propria	Oedema,	0	0,6	1
		Diffuse infiltration by mononuclear inflammatory cells (Lc, Plc, Mph)	1,3	1,3	1,3
		Mean total Score of severity	3.666	4.666	7,666

IBV infectious bronchitis virus
SPF Specific pathogen free
IBV/TU infectious bronchitis virus sampled from Abda-Doukkala region
IBV/RA infectious bronchitis virus sampled from Rabat-Sale-Azzemour Zaire region
IBV/MN infectious bronchitis virus sampled from Meknes Tafilalet region

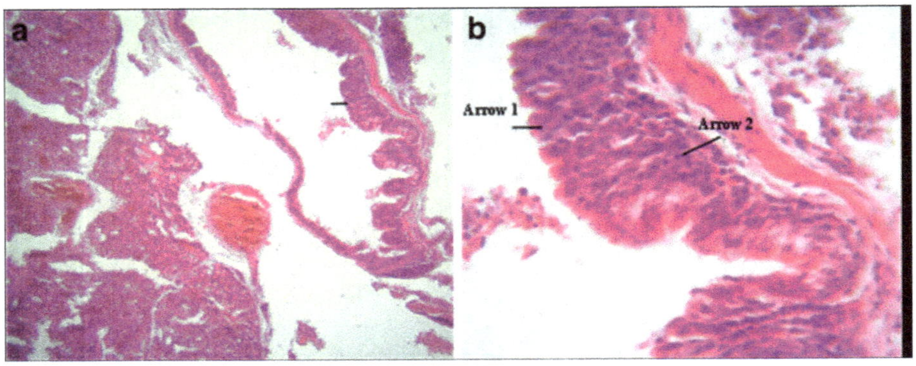

Fig. 3 a Lung of IBV/MN inoculated chick – thickening of the surface mucosa (*Arrow*) of a secondary bronchus, H&E, X 62,50. **b** Lung of IBV/MN inoculated chick – mild hyerplasia of surface epithelium (*Arrow 1*) and severe heterophilic and lympho-plasmocytic infiltration of Lamina propria (*Arrow 2*) and paeribronchial space of a secondary bronchus, H&E, X250

and 5 dpi but antibodies titers was increased at 14dpi. Serum of the control chicks was free from specific antibodies against IBV on the entire dpi.

Discussion

In the present work, we have studied the pathogenesis of IBV Italy 02 genotype which was recently detected for the first time in Morocco and also in Africa [15]. No studies on the Italy02 genotype were reported in neighboring Maghreb or other African countries. The previous study in Morocco focused the mapping serotypes circulating in poultry flocks [15], but no information is available about the pathogenicity and the tissue tropism of this new genotype (Italy02) and protective efficacy of implemented vaccines. To do that, experimental infection in one day-old SPF chickens was used to evaluate pathogenicity and tissue tropism of three Moroccan Italy02 strains (coded, IBV/MN, IBV/TU and IBV/RA).

Results showed that all the three tested strains of IBV, were capable to induce respiratory signs at 48 h pi. Infected chicken showed the various signs of depression, sneezing, difficulty in breathing, nasal discharge, cough, pulmonary and tracheal rales. Developed symptoms became severe at 5 to 7 dpi, and persisted in some chicks until 12dpi. The birds infected by IBV/MN and IBV/TU appeared lethargic, reluctant to move compared to those infected by IBV/RA. No clinical nephritis or mortalities were recorded during the course of experiment in all groups. The clinical signs and gross lesions of this genotype are in accordance with the findings that have been described previously for other serotype of IBV [18], and were in agreement with the clinical signs mentioned by Purcell and McFerran [19]. Regarding to histopathological examination of 3 sacrificed infected birds at 5dpi. The three IBV strains studied have the same severity of lesions in lung with no differences in the pathogenicity. But the

Table 5 Microscopic lesion scores in lungs of 5 day-old SPF chickens inoculated with field IBV strains IBV/MN, IBV/RA and IBV/TUIBV: infectious bronchitis virus

	Lésions		Mean lesion scores in IBV infected groups of birds		
			IBV/MN	IBV/RA	IBV/TU
Lung	Primary & secondary Bronchi	Epithelial hyperplasia	2	1,7	1
		Loss of cilia	1	1	0,7
		peribronchial infiltration by mononuclear inflammatory cells	2	1,3	0,3
		Infiltration of lamina propria by heterophils & mononuclear inflammatory cells	2	1,3	0,3
	Atria & parabronchi	Hypertrophy of pneumocytes	0	0,7	1,3
		Epithelial hyperplasia	0	0,7	1,3
	Inter-capillarysepta	hyperemia	1	1	1
		Mean of total Score of severity	7.333	7.666	6

IBV infectious bronchitis virus
SPF Specific pathogen free
IBV/TU infectious bronchitis virus sampled from Abda-Doukkala region
IBV/RA infectious bronchitis virus sampled from Rabat-Sale-Azzemour Zaire region
IBV/MN infectious bronchitis virus sampled from Meknes Tafilalet region

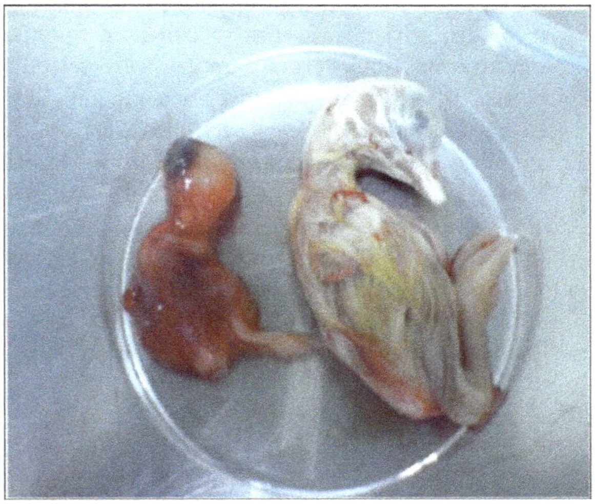

Fig. 4 Dwarfism and hemorrhage of embryos after re-isolation of the virus from experimentally infected chicks (in the left) in comparison with the control (in the right)

IBV/TU strain seems to have a higher degree of pathogenicity in the trachea than others tow tested strains. Clinical signs score and tracheal lesions developed in all infected birds confirm the ability of this new Moroccan genotype, to induce respiratory disease and is therefore regarded as having respiratory tropism. Whereas, Dolz et al, demonstrated that the Spanish Italy02 serotype capable to cause severe respiratory and renal damage [20]. The pathogenicity and clinical sing score obtained with the three strains Italy02 genotype were in accordance and common with those reported for most other serotype of IBV in different countries [21–24].

Results of virus re-isolation confirm IBV distribution in all tissues examined at 5dpi, with the three tested strains. Histopathological and gross lesions showed that the trachea is the primary site of lesions associated with IBV replication as generally reported for the IBV virus [25].

In this report, ELISA test used to evaluate levels of the Ab to IBV in all infected groups at 5 and 14dpi. ELISA method detected moderate levels of the Ab at 14dpi. This result confirms that infected chickens seroconverted against IB, after manifestation of specific clinical sings. Indeed, Ghadakchi et al. showed that ELISA could be reliable, repeatable, and sensitive for detecting IB antibodies [26].

Results obtained with Moroccan Italy02 genotype demonstrated that the three strains emerging in Moroccan poultry farms have a wide distribution for respiratory system, without kidney damage and without causing mortality.

Conclusion

The present study has revealed that the chickens infected with the three tested strains showed the specific respiratory signs with high clinical signs. These infected chicks were sero-converted at 14 dpi and confirmed the spread of the inoculated virus. In addition, the macroscopic lesions and histopathological examination revealed specific lesions of trachea and lung, without renal manifestations. The histopathology of respiratory organs demonstrated a high lesional score of IBV/TU strain which correlate with the clinical score of 140. Moreover, virus re-isolation was performed successfully for all the three tested strains. Results obtained with real time PCR in organs sampled from infected birds (trachea, lung and kidney) and from fluid allantoic in the first passage in SPF eggs, showed a significant abundance of the virus in the respiratory tract. In other words, the findings of molecular analysis of virus re-isolation are strongly correlated with the histopathological tests.

Finally, this current report justify that Italy 02 genotype isolated from different regions of Morocco is capable to induce a severe respiratory disease with a wide distribution of respiratory system. However, this genotype do not cause any kidney damage and without causing mortality.

Table 6 Viral replication detected 5 days post infection in the respiratory and nephritic tract of experimentally infected chicks*SPF* Specific pathogen free

Real time RT-PCR (Ct) for Viral strains	Organs samples			Fluid SPF eggs		
	Trachea	Lung	Kidney	Trachea	Lung	Kidney
IBV/TU	27.05	32.49	0	13.13	20.30	0
IBV RA	28.73	25.43	0	14.79	14	0
IBV/MN	30.21	27.3	30.74	13	21.41	30.74
Control	0	0	0	0	0	0

SPF Specific pathogen free
rRT- PCR real time reverse transcriptase polymerase chain reaction
Ct Cycle threshold
IBV infectious bronchitis virus
IBV/TU infectious bronchitis virus sampled from Abda-Doukkala region
IBV/RA infectious bronchitis virus sampled from Rabat-Sale-Azzemour Zaire region
IBV/MN infectious bronchitis virus sampled from Meknes Tafilalet region

Methods

Viral strains

Three IBV field strains (coded, IBV/MN, IBV/RA and IBV/TU), were isolated from trachea, lungs and kidney of broiler chickens suffering from the specific clinical signs of IB, and were previously characterized to belong to Italy02 serotype at laboratory of Biopharma between 2010- 2014 [15]. Phylogenetically, the three strains of Italy02 genotype branched and clustered with Spanish genotypes, are very closely related to Italy 497/02-1 (98.9 %); Spain/05/866 (98.9 %); and Spain/04/221 (97.4 %). The sequences of the three strains have a S1 gene nucleotide identity ranged between 96.9 % and 98.7 % when compared to each other.

These IBV strains were propagated by inoculation in 9- to 11-day-old SPF egg as described by Owen et *al* [27]. For virus titration 6-fold dilutions were inoculated into the allantoic cavity of six SPF chickens embryos, and incubation during six days at temperature of 37 °C +/- 2 °C and relative humidity of 75 % +/- 10 %. The titer is calculated following the Reed and Muench method [28].

Chickens

A total of 40 one day old SPF chickens, used for experimental infection were provided from the SPF chickens flock unit of Biopharma Laboratory, Rabat, Morocco.

Experimental infections

In order to evaluate the pathogenesis of three Moroccan viral strains, an experimental infection study was performed in SPF chickens obtained from SPF chicken flock Unit of Biopharma, Rabat, Morocco. For this purpose, 40 one-day-old SPF chickens were housed in separate isolators with negative-pressure, the bright and thermal program was the same for all birds, and water and food were provided at will. Chickens were randomly divided into four groups of 10 birds (30 chicks in the experimental and ten chicks in the control group). The infection trials were approved by the local ethics committee of Biopharma (Biopharma Ethics and Scientific Committee) directed by its veterinarian in charge, with requirement of formal ethics approval referenced as **N° 412/SB/2015**, and were carried out following strict animal welfare guidelines.

Using a micropipette, chickens in the three groups were oculo-nasally administrated with 50 µl of inoculum containing $10^{3.5}$ (EID50/ml) of virus strain, and control group was inoculated with phosphate-buffered saline (1XPBS). The specific clinical signs of IB were recorded at a rate of 2 times daily by the same observer during 14 days. Specific clinical signs of IB recorded by the same observer have included gasping, coughing, sneezing, depression, rales, and ruffled feather. Three chickens from each group were killed at 5dpi; one control animals and their tissues of trachea, lung and kidney were examined for gross lesions, and were collected for histopathology examination. Serum samples were tested for the presence of antibodies against IB using the ELISA test. Also the tracheal rings from each bird were obtained and placed in cell culture medium (D-MEM supplemented with 10 % of foetal calf serum) to evaluate tracheal ciliary activity at 5 and 12 dpi. Treatment organs of lung, trachea and kidney by the antibiotics and frozen at -80 °C were used for virus re-isolation and real time RT-PCR detection. At 14 dpi, all the birds were euthanized and necropsied for gross lesions examination before their elimination.

Histopathological examination

Sacrificed birds at 5 days of age were necropsied and gross lesions were recorded. Tissue samples from the trachea and lungs were collected and fixed in 10 % neutral-buffered formalin. They were processed for histopathological examination according to standard methods. They were dehydrated and embedded in paraffin wax. Five µm thick sections were stained with hematoxylin and eosin and examined under light microscope. Microscopic lesions in respiratory tissues were recorded and scored as described previously [17], from 0, 1, 2 and 3 (no, mild, moderate and severe, respectively). A mean of total severity index was then attributed to each IBV strains based on scores from 3 birds.

Ciliostasis: tracheal ciliary activity

Several parts of tracheal rings were prepared from each infected bird at 5dpi that coincides with the pic of the clinical signs. At 12 dpi, the ciliary activity was also evaluated from all the infected birds that have recovered. The prepared tracheal rings were immersed immediately in cell culture medium (D-MEM supplemented with 10 % of foetal calf serum), were microscopically analyzed for estimating the ciliary movement in tracheal infected and in tracheal control, and were scored on a scale from 0 (100 % activity) to 4 (no activity) [29]. The mean score of each strain was then compared to evaluate the respiratory pathogenicity.

Viral re-isolation

All individual samples of trachea, lung and kidney collected at 5 dpi from IBV-infected chickens, were immediately suspended in phosphate-buffered saline (1XPBS), treated by Gentamycin antibiotics (50 µg/g) and clarified by centrifugation at 2500 × g at 4 °C for 25 min. The homogenates samples were used and processed for IBV reisolation as previously described [30]. It's was performed by inoculation in allontoic sac route of 9–11 day old eggs, with 100 µl of homogenates and incubation during 6 days (using five eggs by sample) at temperature of 37 °C +/- 2 °C and relative humidity of 75 % +/- 10 %.

The embryos were examined for the presence of dwarfism and hemorrhagic traces (on the whole body of the embryo). The RT-PCR detection of viral RNA was performed in parallel with the homogenates tissues and the clarified allontoic fluid.

Extraction of viral RNA

Viral RNA was extracted from 200 µl of both organs samples and allantoic fluid (AF) using the Kits Macherey-Nagel according to the manufacturer's instructions. Each RNA fraction was eluted in 50 µl of RNase-free water, and subjected to reverse transcriptase RT-PCR amplification.

Real time RT-PCR

A one step Real time RT-PCR was carried out using Invitrogen kit (SuperScript® III Platinum, Life Technologies, USA). The synthesis of the cDNA first strand was performed using 5 µl total viral RNA primed with a universal pair of primers a) downstream primer, AIBV-fr, targeting N gene nucleotide positions 811–832 (5′-ATGC TCAACCTTGTCCCTAGCA-3′); and b) upstream primer, AIBV-as, targeting N gene nucleotide positions 921–941 (5′-TCAA-ACTGCGGATCA-TCACGT-3′), and the probe TaqMan targeting N gene nucleotide positions 848-875 (5′FAM-TTGGAAGTAGAGTGACGCCCAAAC TTCA-3′Tamra) [31].

The amplifications reactions (PCRs) were performed on a Smart Cycler. The following mix of each reaction was contained: 12.5 µl 2 × RT- PCR buffer mix, 0.5 µl MgSO4 (50 mM), 0.5 µl Rox (25 mM), 4.75 µl nuclease free water, 0.5 µl M-MULV reverse transcriptase enzyme (200U), 0.5 µl primers to a final concentration of 10 µM, 0.25 µl probe to a final concentration of 10 µM and 5 µl RNA template. The reaction was carried out in StepOneTM Plus real-time PCR system (Smart cycler Cepheid, USA) at 50 °C for 15 min, 95 °C for 5 min, and 40 cycles of 95 °C for 15 s and 60 °C for 45 s. All reactions amplifications were recorded, analyzed, and the threshold cycle (Ct) determined with the StepOne software (Smart Cycler).

Serological response

An enzyme-linked immunosorbent assay (ELISA) commercial kit (FlockChek (IDEXX Laboratories, Inc., Westbrook, ME, USA), was carried out on serum samples collected from experimentally infected birds for antibodies detection at 5 and 14dpi. The test was performed according to the manufacturer's instructions. Moreover, serology on SPF chicks of one day from the same rearing was also performed to ensure the negative status anti-IBV chicks antibodies used.

Abbreviations

Ct, cycle threshold; dpi, day post-infection; IB, infectious bronchitis; IBV/MN, infectious bronchitis virus sampled from Meknes Tafilalet region; IBV/RA, infectious bronchitis virus sampled from Rabat-Sale-Azzemour Zaire region; IBV/TU, infectious bronchitis virus sampled from Abda-Doukkala region; IBV, infectious bronchitis virus; M, membrane; N, nucleocapsid; Pi, post-infection; rRT- PCR, real time reverse transcriptase polymerase chain reaction; S, spike; SPF, specific pathogen free.

Acknowledgments

This work was done by Biopharma Society, Rabat, Morocco and University Hassan II of Casablanca-Ministry of Higher Education of Morocco.

Funding

This study was supported by University Hassan II of Casablanca- Ministry of Higher Education of Morocco and the Biopharma Society, Rabat, Morocco.

Authors' contributions

KK participated in the design of the study, performed the experimental infection, virological, molecular and serological studies, and drafted the manuscript. FK performed the histopathological examination and helped to draft the manuscript. CL developed the protocol of the experiment, provides technical assistance in laboratory tests and helped to draft and improves the manuscript. MME conceived of the study, participated in the design, helped to draft the manuscript, and assumes coordination. All authors read and approved the final manuscript.

Competing interests

The authors declare that they have no competing interests.

Consent for publication

Not applicable.

Ethics approval and consent to participate

The experimental protocols for this study performed in this paper were approved on the 17th December 2014 by the local ethical committee of Biopharma (Biopharma Ethics and Scientific Committee) directed by its veterinarian in charge; with requirement of formal ethics approval referenced as **N° 412/SB/2015**. All experimentations of the infected chicks were followed by a Veterinary Doctor during the period of experimentation with respect of the welfare guidelines of the Manual of Diagnostic Tests and Vaccines for Terrestrial Animals /OIE (chapter 7.8. Use of Animals in Research and Teaching), and the Guide of good manufacturing practices (GMP) for veterinary use (Specific guidelines: LPD 4 Section 28, 29 and 30).

Author details

[1]Laboratory of Virology, Microbiology, Quality and Biotechnologies/ Ecotoxicology & Biodiversity, Faculty of Sciences and Techniques, University Hassan II of Casablanca, Mohammedia, Morocco. [2]Society Biopharma, Km 2, Route de Casa, B.P. 4569, Rabat, Morocco. [3]Department of Veterinary Pathology and Public Health, Hassan 2nd Institute of Agronomy and Veterinary Medicine, B.P. 6202, Madinat Al Irfane, Rabat, Morocco.

References

1. Cavanagh D. Nidovirales: a new order comprising Coronaviridae and Arteriviridae. Arch Virol. 1997;142:629–33.
2. Cook JKA, Jackwood M, Jones RC. The long view: 40 years of infectious bronchitis research. Avian Pathol. 2012;41:239–50.

3. Glahn RP, Wideman RF, Cowen BS. Order of exposure to high dietary calcium and Gray strain infectious bronchitis virus alters renal function and the incidence of urolithiasis. Poult Sc. 1989;68:1193–204.
4. Raj GD, Jones RC. Infectious bronchitis virus: immunopathogenesis of infection in the chickens. Avian Pathol. 1997;26:677–706.
5. Balestrin E, Fraga AP, Ikuta N, Canal CW, Fonseca AS, Lunge VR. Infectious bronchitis virus in different avian physiological systems-a field study Brazilian poultry flocks. Poult Sc. 2014;93:1922–9.
6. Cavanagh D, Mawditt K, Welchman DB, Britton P, Gough RE. Coronaviruses from pheasants (Phasianus colchicus) are genetically closely related to coronaviruses of domestic fowl (infectious bronchitis virus) and turkeys. Avian Pathol. 2002;31:81–93.
7. Alexander DJ, Gough RE. A long-term study of the pathogenesis of infection of fowls with three strains of avian infectious bronchitis virus. Res Vet Sci. 1978;24:228–33.
8. Lai MM, Cavanagh D. The molecular biology of coronaviruses. Adv Virus Res. 1997;48:1–100.
9. Casais R, Dove B, Cavanagh D, Britton P. Recombinant avian infectious bronchitis virus expressing a heterologous spike gene demonstrates that the spike protein is a determinant of cell tropism. J Virol. 2003;77:9084–9.
10. Liu HJ, Lee LH, Shih WL, Lin MY, Liao MH. Detection of infectious bronchitis virus by multiplex polymerase chain reaction and sequence analysis. J Virol Methods. 2003;109:31–7.
11. Worthington KJ, Currie RJW, Jones RC. A reverse transcriptase-polymerase chain reaction survey of infectious bronchitis virus genotypes in Western Europe from 2002 to 2006. Avian Pathol. 2008;37:247–57.
12. El Houadfi M, Jones RC. Isolation of avian infectious bronchitis viruses in Morocco including an enterotropic variant. Vet Res. 1985;116:445.
13. Alarabi MAH. A field study of kidney disease among the broiler flocks in Morocco and its relationship to infectious bronchitis virus. Ph.D thesis. Rabat, Morocco: Agronomic and Veterinary Institute Hassan II; 2004.
14. El Bouqdaoui M, Mhand R, Bouayoune H, Ennaji MM. Genetic grouping of nephropathogenic avian infectious bronchitis virus isolated in Morocco. Int J Poult Sci. 2005;4:721–7.
15. Fellahi S, Ducatez M, El Harrak M, Guerin JL, Touil N, Sebbar G, Bouaiti E, Khataby K, Ennaji MM, Elhouadfi M. Prevalence and molecular characterization of avian infection bronchitis virus in poultry flocks in Morocco from 2010-2014 and the first report of Italy02 genotype in Africa. Avian Pathol. 2015;44:287-95.
16. Ficken MD. The respiratoy system. In: Riddell C, editor. Avian Histopathology. 2nd ed. Pennsylvania: American Association of Avian Pathologists; 1996. p. 89–109.
17. Nakamura K, Cook JKA, Otsuki K, Huggins MB, Frazier JA. Comparative study of respiratory lesions in two chicken lines of different susceptibility infected with infectious bronchitis virus: histology, ultrastructure and immunohistochemistry. Avian Pathol. 1991;20:241–57.
18. Seifi S, Asasi K, Mohammadi A, Shirzad MR, Pourfallah M. Serological and gross findings in broilers with AIV and IBV. Online J Vet Res. 2010;14:87–94.
19. Purcell DA, McFerran JB. The histopathology of infectious bronchitis in the domestic fowl. Res Vet Sci. 1972;13:116–22.
20. Dolz R, Vergara-Alert J, Pérez M, Pujols J, Majo´ N. New insights on infectious bronchitis virus pathogenesis: characterization of Italy 02 serotype in chicks and adult hens. Vet Mic. 2012;156:256–64.
21. Benyeda Z, Szeredi L, Mato´ T, Süveges T, Balka G, Abonyi-Tóth Z, Rusvai M, Palya V. Comparative histopathology and immunohistochemistry of QX-like, Massachusetts and 793/B serotypes of infectious bronchitis virus infections in chickens. J Comp Pathol. 2010;143:276–83.
22. Chousalkar KK, Roberts JR, Reece R. Comparative histopathology of two Serotypes of infectious bronchitis virus (T and N1/88) in laying hens and cockerels. Poult Sc. 2007;86:50–8.
23. Boroomand Z, Razeghian I, Asasi K, Mohammadi A, Hoseini A. Isolation and identification of a new isolate of avian infectious bronchitis virus IRFIBV32 and a study of its pathogenicity. Online J Vet Res. 2011;15:366–80.
24. Chacóna JL, Assayag Jra MS, Revolledoa L, Astolfi-Ferreiraa CS, Vejaranoa MP, Jones RC, Piantino Ferreiraa AJ. Pathogenicity and molecular characteristics of infectious bronchitis virus (IBV) strains isolated from broilers showing diarrhoea and respiratory disease. Br Poult Sci. 2014;55:271–83.
25. Cavanagh D, Gelb J. Infectious bronchitis. In: Saif YM, Barnes HJ, Glisson JR, Fadly AM, Mcdougald LR, Swayne DE, editors. Diseases of Poultry. Ames: Iowa State University Press; 2008. p. 117–35.
26. Ghadakchi H, Dadras H, Pourbakhsh SA, Hosseini SMH. Standardization of an Enzyme-Linked Immunosorbent Assay for Detection of Infectious Bronchitis Virus Antibody. Arch Razi Inst. 2005;59:75–83.
27. Owen RL, Cowen BS, Hattel AL, Naqi SA, Wilson RA. Detection of viral antigen following exposure of one-day-old chickens to the Holland 52 strain of infectious bronchitis virus. Avian Pathol. 1991;20:663–73.
28. Reed LJ, Muench H. A simple method of estimating fifty percent endpoints. Am J Hyg. 1983;27:493–7.
29. Cook JKA, Orbell SJ, Woods MA, Huggins MB. Breadth of protection of the respiratory tract provided by different live-attenuated infectious bronchitis vaccines against challenge with infectious bronchitis viruses of heterologous serotypes. Avian Pathol. 1999;28:477–85.
30. Ignjatovic J, Ashton F. Detection and histodifferentiation of avian infectious bronchitis viruses using amonoclonal antibody-based ELISA. Avian Pathol. 1996;25:721–36.
31. Meir R, Maharat O, Farnushi Y, Simanov L. Development of a real-time TaqMan RT-PCR assay for the detection of infectious bronchitis virus in chickens, and comparison of RT-PCR and virus isolation. J Virol Methods. 2010;163:190–4.

7

Integrated pharmacokinetic–Pharmacodynamic (PK/PD) model to evaluate the in vivo antimicrobial activity of Marbofloxacin against *Pasteurella multocida* in piglets

Qing Lin Zeng[1], Xian Mei[1], Jia Su[1], Xiao Hong Li[1], Wen Guang Xiong, Yan Lu and Zhen Ling Zeng[1,2*]

Abstract

Background: Marbofloxacin is a veterinary fluoroquinolone with high activity against *Pasteurella multocida*. We evaluated it's in vivo activity against *P. multocida* based on in vivo time-kill data in sw ne using a tissue-cage model. A series of dosages ranging from 0.15 to 2.5 mg/kg were administered intramuscularly after challenge with *P. multocida* type B, serotype 2.

Results: The ratio of the 24 h area under the concentration-time curve divided by the m nimum inhibitory concentration ($AUC_{24}TCF/MIC$) was the best PK/PD index correlated with the in vivo antibacterial effectiveness of marbofloxacin (*R2* = 0.9279). The $AUC_{24}TCF/MIC$ necessary to achieve a 1-$\log_{10}$ CFU/ml reduction and a 3-$\log_{10}$ CFU/ml (90% of the maximum response) reduction as calculated by an inhibitory sigmoid E_{max} model were 13.48 h and 57.70 h, respectively.

Conclusions: Marbofloxacin is adequate for the treatment of swine infected with P. *multocida*. The tissue-cage model played a significant role in achieving these PK/PD results.

Keywords: Marbofloxacin, PK/PD, *P. Multocida*, Tissue-cage model, Piglets

Background

The increase in drug-resistance coupled with the lack of new and effective antimicrobials indicates that modified drug-dosage regimens may be useful clinical alternatives. In the clinic, pharmacokinetic (PK) and pharmacodynamic (PD) outcomes are interrelated [1]. PK/PD modeling in veterinary medicine can be used to define the relationship between the effects of different drug concentrations and therapeutic outcomes. In short, PK/PD modeling provides a chance for dosage optimization [2]. We used the tissue cage (TC) infection model to evaluate PK and PD profiles in interstitial fluids in the presence of an active immune response [3–5].

P. multocida is a widespread pathogen that inhabits mucosal surfaces and upper respiratory tracts of clinically healthy animals [6]. It is the causative agent of fowl cholera in poultry, atrophic rhinitis in swine and hemorrhagic septicemia in buffalo and cattle [7–10]. It also plays a major role in pneumonia in swine and ruminants as an opportunistic pathogen [11].

Marbofloxacin is a synthetic third-generation fluoroquinolone that is used solely in veterinary medicine [12, 13]. It is active against Gram-negative and some Gram-positive bacteria as well as mycoplasmas and other intracellular pathogens [14, 15]. It is widely used against most of the swine respiratory pathogens including *Actinobacillus pleuropneumoniae, Haemophilus parasuis and P. multocida* [16–19].

* Correspondence: zlzeng@scau.edu.cn
[1]National Laboratory of Safety Evaluation of veterinary Drugs, College of Veterinary Medicine, South China Agricultural University, Guangzhou, China
[2]National Laboratory of Safety Evaluation (Environmental Assessment) of Veterinary Drugs, College of Veterinary Medicine, South China Agricultural University, Guangzhou, China

Marbofloxacin acts as a bactericidal concentration-dependent antibiotic similar to other fluoroquinolones. The AUC_{24}/MIC or C_{max}/MIC (peak concentration divided by the MIC) are the PK/PD surrogates that most closely reflect clinical outcomes. [20, 21]. We used an integrated PK/PD model to evaluate the in vivo antimicrobial activity of marbofloxacin against *P. multocida* in swine. This approach gives an approximation of the most effective treatment for achieving a bacteriological cure and minimizing the emergence of bacterial resistance.

Methods

Animals and tissue-cages

Twenty clinically healthy castrated crossbred piglets (~1-month Duroc ×Landrace × Yorkshire),purchased from Guangdong pig breeding farm, with body weights of 14 to 18 kg were included in the study. These animals were housed in individual pens for a week prior to experiments with a controlled temperature of 26 °C. The animals were fed antimicrobial-free feed twice a day with water available ad libitum. Tissue-cages were fabricated according to a previously published method [5]. Two tissue-cages were implanted subcutaneously in the neck of each piglet after sedation and local anesthesia. About 3–4 weeks later and after wound healing, 0.5 mL tissue-cage fluid (TCF) was sampled by percutaneous puncture. TCF samples were cultured for aerobic and anaerobic contaminants to ensure sterility before commencing the experiments.

Bacterial strain and inoculant preparation

P. multocida strain CVCC434 (type B, serotype 2) was purchased from the China Veterinary Culture Collection Centre (Beijing, China). The original bacterial culture was isolated from a piglet that died of plague in Jiang Su, China. *P. multocida* was grown on tryptic soy agar (Guangdong Huaikai Microbial, Guangzhou, China) supplemented with 5% defibrinated sheep blood (BTSA). Bacteria were cultured in Mueller–Hinton broth (Becton Dickinson, Sparks, MD, USA), with shaking at 37 °C and grown to 10^9 CFU/mL. The cells were then concentrated by centrifugation at 3000×g for 10 min and suspended in sterile 0.9% NaCl to 10^8 CFU/mL.

Drugs

Marbofloxacin was obtained as a 10% injectable aqueous solution from Yuan Zhen (Hebei, China). Marbofloxacin standard was purchased from Dr. Ehrenstorfer (GmbH) and ofloxacin was acquired from the National Institute for Food and Drug Control (Beijing, China). Pentobarbital sodium was from Jian Yang Biotechnology and procainamide hydrochloride was purchased from Xin Zheng (Tianjin).

MIC determinations

MIC values were determined by an agar dilution method as a preliminary screening according to Clinical and Laboratory Standards Institute (CLSI) reference methods. In this study, we measured the MIC of marbofloxacin against the *P. multocida* in the tissue-cage fluid by a micro dilution assay in triplicate using the tissue-cage fluid as matrix.

PK studies

Tissue cage fluid (0.5 ml) was sampled 1 h after the injection of drug and thereafter at 3, 6, 9, 12, 24, 30, 36, 48, 72 and 96 h. All the samples were centrifuged at 6000×g at 4 °C for 10 min. The supernatants were stored at −20 °C. The concentrations of marbofloxacin in tissue cage fluid were determined using a Waters 2695 series high performance liquid chromatography (HPLC) system with fluorescence detection [13, 22]. The chromatographic separation was achieved on an Agilent BDS C18 column (250 mm × 4.6 mm; internal diameter, 5 μm) at 28 °C with a thermostat column oven (Agilent 1200 series). All TCF samples were thawed at room temperature before analysis and 3 mL of trichloromethane was added to a 10 mL centrifuge tube with 200 μL tissue-cage fluids spiked with 10 μL ofloxacin internal standard, and vortexed for 1 min. The aqueous layer was discarded after centrifugation at 6000 g for 10 min and the organic layer was dried under a stream of nitrogen. The residue was suspended with 0.2 mL mobile phase and a 10 μL aliquot was taken and injected into HPLC for analysis after filtered through a 0.22 μm nylon syringe filter (JinTeng Experiment Equipment, Tianjing). The determination of marbofloxacin in the tissue cage fluid was linear within a range of 0.01–2 μg/mL and the correlation coefficient was >0.99. The lower limit of quantitation was 0.01 μg/mL. The recoveries of marbofloxacin in tissue-cage fluid were >85%. The standard deviations (SD) and the coefficients of variability (CV %) for both interday and intraday were <8% in TCF.

Tissue-cage infection and in vivo kill curve of marbofloxacin

Twenty piglets were divided into ten groups randomly, with 4 tissue-cages for each group. 24 h after 0.5 mL of *P. multocida* saline suspension (~2.0 × 10^8 CFU/mL) were injected into the sterile tissue cage; nine groups were treated with a series of marbofloxacin intramuscular injections (10%) at 0.15, 0.3, 0.5, 0.8, 1.0, 1.3, 1.6, 2.0, 2.5 mg/kg. The control group was given sterile physiological saline only. TCF samples were aspirated from the tissue-cages by percutaneous puncture at 0, 3, 6, 9, 12 and 24 h after dosing. 100 μL of tissue cage fluid was serially diluted 10-fold in saline within 1 h of sampling for CFU determinations. From each dilution, 20 μL was

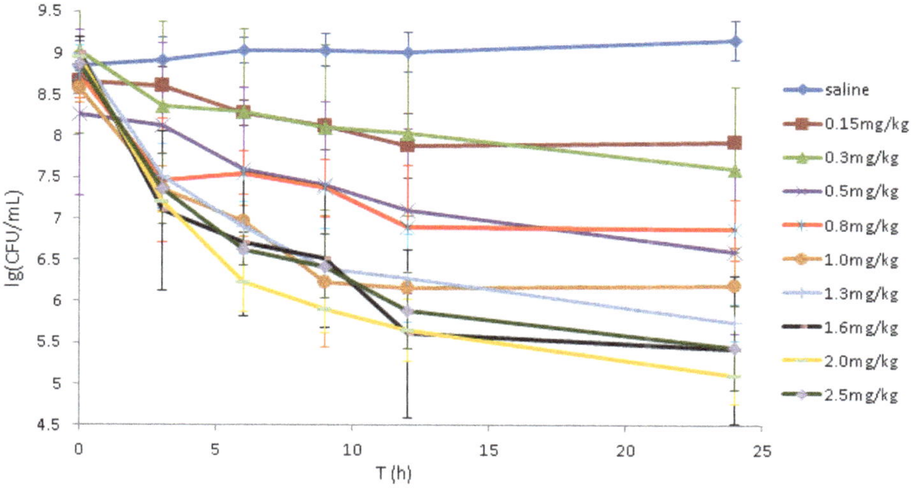

Fig. 1 In vivo time killing curve of marbofloxacin against *P. multocida* in TCF. Kb-1 means the group treated by saline. Mean log_{10}CFU/mL values only (*n* = 4 experimentations). (Excel, Microsoft Office)

spread on BTSA plated in triplicate and incubated for 16 h at 37 °C.The limit of detection was 500 CFU/mL.

Protein binding

To determination the protein binding of marbofloxacin in TCF, marbofloxacin at 0.05, 0.1, 0.5, 1 and 2 mg/L was spiked into pooled uninfected TCF in triplicate. An Amicon Centrifree Micropartition device with a 10 KDa cutoff (Millipore, Bedford, MA, USA) was used to remove the protein-bound drug as previously described [23, 24]. The marbofloxacin concentration before and after ultrafiltration and centrifugation was determined as described in the PK studies. The percent of drug bound to protein was calculated as the following equation: Bound % = (1-Cu/Ci) × 100%, where Cu is the filtrate concentration and Ci is the initial concentration.

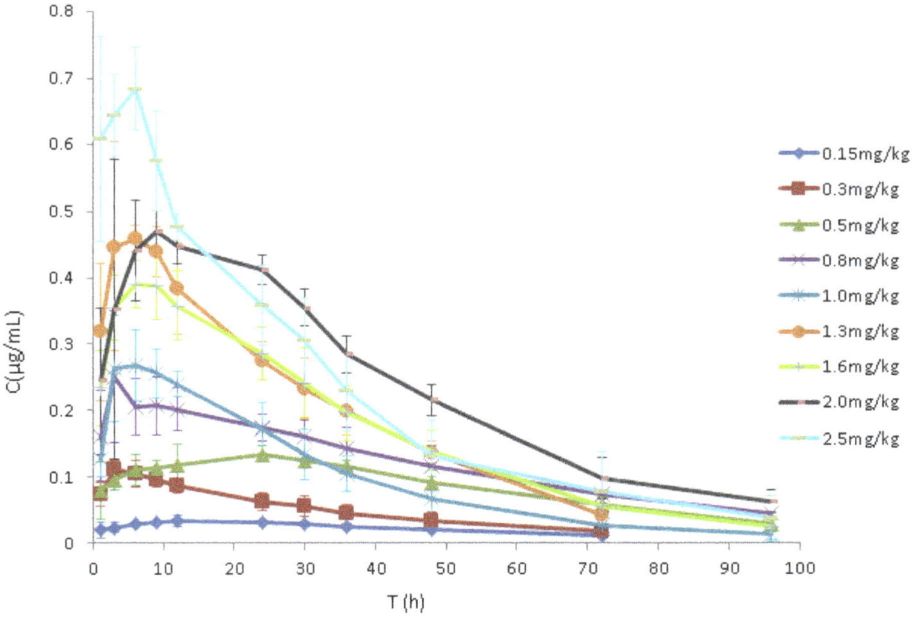

Fig. 2 Pharmacokinetic profiles of marbofloxacin in TCF. The tissue-cages were infected with *P. multocida* as described above, 24 h later administered with single intramuscularly doses of 0.15, 0.3,0.5,0.8,1.0,1.3,1.6,2.0 and 2.5 mg/kg marbofloxacin as BW. All TCF were sampled by puncture at 1, 3, 6, 9, 12, 24, 30, 36, 48, 72and 96 h after dosing. Marbofloxacin concentrations were determined using a HPLC method with fluorescence detection. But a small number of samples sampled on 96 h were undetected. Each symbol represents the mean ± standard deviation of the levels in the four tissue-cages. (Excel, Microsoft Office)

Table 1 AUC_{24} and Cmax of marbofloxacin following multiple dosages in the *P. multocida* infected tissue cage fluid

Doses(mg/kg)	AUC_{24}(h·μg/mL) (X^a ± SD)	C_{max}(μg/mL) (X^a ± SD)
0.15	0.72 ± 0.09	0.04 ± 0.01
0.3	2.04 ± 0.23	0.11 ± 0.01
0.5	2.70 ± 0.20	0.14 ± 0.01
0.8	4.65 ± 0.68	0.27 ± 0.07
1.0	5.25 ± 0.40	0.31 ± 0.07
1.3	7.89 ± 1.49	0.51 ± 0.06
1.6	8.53 ± 0.70	0.53 ± 0.06
2.0	9.70 ± 0.82	0.54 ± 0.12
2.5	12.03 ± 0.56	0.74 ± 0.10

X^a is the mean value.

Pharmacokinetic-Pharmacodynamic analysis

The MIC value was included in the calculation of the PK/PD index. According to standard methodology, an inhibitory sigmoid E_{max} model was used to assess the PK/PD index with the highest predictive value to the different indices for each dosing regimen (Eq. 1). The R^2 value was computed for the correlation between antimicrobial effectiveness and each of the PK/PD parameters.

$$E = E_{max} - (E_{max} - E_0) \times C_e^N / \left(EC_{50}^N + C_e^N\right) \quad (1)$$

E is the antibacterial effect; E_0 represents maximum drug effect 24 h after *i.m* administration. E_{max} is the change of bacterial load (Log_{10} CFU/mL) in the infected tissue-cage with no drug present. C_e is the PK/PD index magnitude. EC_{50} is the magnitude required for achieve 50% of E_{max} and *N* is the Hill coefficient that describes the sigmoid shape. PK and PD indices were calculated using a non-compartment model in WinNonlin 6.2 software (Pharsight Corporation, Mountain View, CA, USA),

Results

MIC of marbofloxacin for *P. multocida*

Tissue cage fluid was sterile as assessed by aerobic and anaerobic culture. We then determined that the MIC of marbofloxacin for *P. multocida* in tissue cage fluid was 0.12 μg/mL ex vivo. This did not change after exposure to marbofloxacin for 24 h and this number was used for PK/PD calculations.

TC infection and in vivo kill curve of marbofloxacin

We determined the in vivo antibacterial activity of marbofloxacin against P. *multocida* CVCC434. *P. multocida* inoculated into tissue cages in the absence of antibiotic was 8.79 ± 0.22 log_{10} CFU/mL averaged over all tissue cages. When marbofloxacin was administered intramuscularly, the bacterial counts for marbofloxacin-treated groups decreased by 0.72 to 3.85log_{10} CFU/mL. By this time, the control saline-treated cages had increased to 9.17log_{10} CFU/mL. Marbofloxacin exerted bactericidal activity when the dosage via intramuscular injection exceeded 1.3 mg/kg (Fig. 1).

PK study

The concentration-time profile of marbofloxacin in the infected cages were calculated as AUC_{24h} and C_{max} of

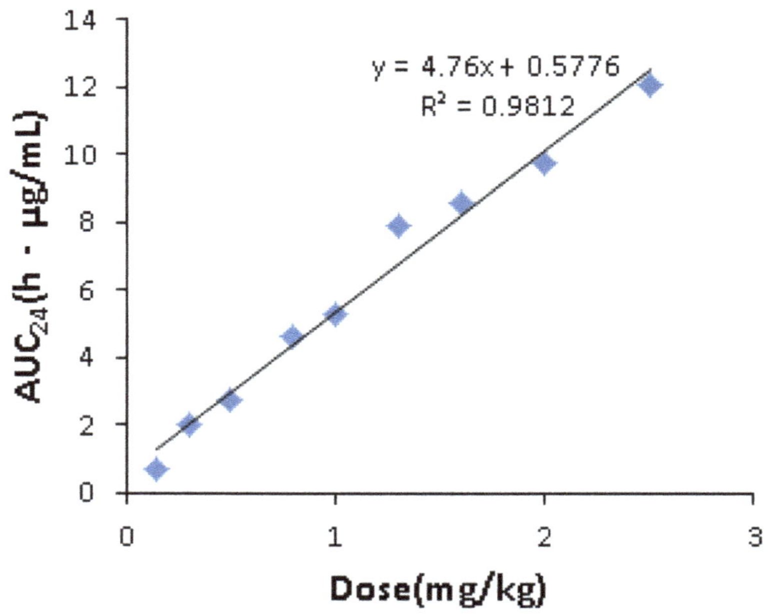

Fig. 3 Linear regression plots between administered doses and AUC_{24} values. (Excel, Microsoft Office)

Table 2 Protein binding of marbofloxacin in serum and tissue cage fluid

Spiked concentration (μg/mL)	Protein binding (X^a ± SD)	
	Serum	TCF
0.05	52.17 ± 3.36	45.71±1.30
0.1	53.84 ± 2.13	48.68±1.39
0.5	48.92 ± 2.68	46.99±0.73
1	55.58 ± 0.35	48.20±1.66
2	53.98 ± 1.42	49.90±0.40
total	52.90 ± 3.30	47.89±1.86

marbofloxacin in the tissue cage fluid following multiple dosages obtained from the measured marbofloxacin concentration data from each cage (Fig. 2 and Table 1). The mean values of AUC_{24} for marbofloxacin increased with dose escalation in the tissue cage fluid. A significant correlation (R_2 = 0.9812) was observed between AUC_{24} TCF and dosages (Fig. 3).

PB

The protein binding of marbofloxacin in tissue cage fluid was 47.89 ± 1.86% and 52.90 ± 3.30% in serum within the range of 0.05 ~ 2 mg/L for marbofloxacin (Table 2).

Magnitude of the PK/PD parameter required for efficacy

The PK parameters best predicting the in vivo of the drug were the AUC_{24}/MIC (R^2 = 0.9279), %T > MIC (R^2 = 0.8257) and C_{max}/MIC (R^2 ⁼0.9022) (Fig. 4). The magnitudes of AUC_{24}/MIC predicted for a 1-log reduction and a 3-log reduction (bactericidal) were 13.48 h and 57.70 h, respectively, and the slope of both parameters for antibacterial effectiveness was 1.41 (Table 3).

Discussion

Respiratory diseases greatly affect the production and health of swine and result in high economic losses [25]. In Europe, *P. multocida* is one of the most common bacterial species among porcine respiratory diseases and leads to atrophic rhinitis in young pigs [26]. Marbofloxacin shows excellent effectiveness for treating *P. multocida* infection through in vitro tests [16]. The protein binding of marbofloxacin was low in previous studies and was 52% for serum, 40% for tissue cage fluid in cattle and 49.4% for pig serum [3, 16]. Only free drug in the interstitial fluid is microbiologically active against extracellular bacteria [3, 27].

In the present study, the protein binding of marbofloxacin in pig serum and TCF were 52.90% and 47.89% respectively and these values were independent of concentration in the range of 0.05 ~ 2 μg/mL. The AUC_{24}TCF of marbofloxacin following single intramuscular administration (2.5 mg/kg) was estimated to be 12.03 h·μg/mL, which was lower than that in plasma (25.8 h·μg/mL) [28]. The C_{max} for tissue cage fluid was lower than previously reported in plasma (2.57 μg/mL) and tissue cage fluid (1.57 μg/mL) in pigs [28, 29].

The PK/PD model integrating the PK parameter, the in vitro MIC and PD outcome are all valuable in designing rational dosage regimens and in the measurement of susceptibility breakpoints [20, 30]. Our data indicated that AUC_{24}TCF/MIC was the best parameter that correlated with the in vivo antibacterial effects of marbofloxacin against *P. multocida*. This agrees with previous studies of marbofloxacin activity against *P. multocida* [3, 31]. We found an AUC_{24}TCF/MIC value of 100.25 h (2.5 mg/kg) that was lower than the reported value in plasma in piglets (264.10 h) [28].

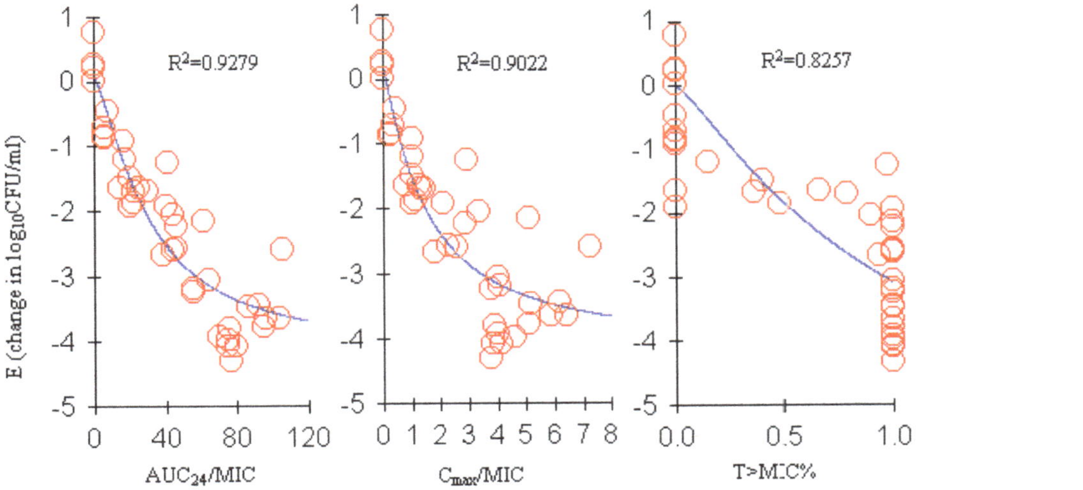

Fig. 4 Relationships between PK/PD parameters (AUC/MIC, Cmax/MIC, T > MIC %) and antibacterial effect (E) after 24 h of therapy. *R2* is the correlation coefficient. (Winnonlin software)

Table 3 PK/PD analysis of marbofloxacin in TCF infection model

Parameter(unit)	Value
E_{max} (log_{10}(CFU/mL))	0.05
E_0(log_{10}(CFU/mL))	−4.20
AUC_{24}/MIC for 1log reduction(h)	13.48
AUC_{24}/MIC EC_{50}(h)	29.78
AUC_{24}/MIC for bactericidal action(h)	57.70
Slope(N)	1.41

The AUC_{24h}TCF/MIC ratios that produced a 1-log reduction, and 50% and 90% of the maximum effect were 13.48 h, 29.78 h and 57.70 h, respectively. The AUC_{24}TCF/MIC ratio for bactericidal effects in this study was different from previous study values of 31.29, 278.08 and 50.65 h for 3-log reductions [3, 22, 31]. These differences may by accounted for by examining the ex vivo PK/PD model. This model holds the antibiotic concentration constant but this concentration would vary with time in the animal infection model [32]. In addition, the ex vivo and neutropenic murine lung infection models do not take the host immune responses into consideration. Finally, the magnitude of PK/PD indices were influenced by the bacterial load and this may influence characteristics of the PK parameters. A higher antimicrobial concentration would be required for higher pathogen loads [31, 33].

An AUC_{24}/MIC ratio exceeding a value of 125 h was reported as useful for the treatment of infections caused by Gram-negative organisms while reducing the risk of resistance induction [34–36]. In combination with the MIC_{90} (0.06 µg/mL) from two previous studies, and the PK characteristics in this study, we can infer that a dosage regimen of marbofloxacin 2.0 mg/kg (AUC_{24}TCF/MIC, 161.67 h > 125 h) was effective for the treatment of *P. multocida* infections [37, 38]. However, considering that we found an AUC_{24}TCF/MIC ratio of 57.70 h that produced a 3-log reduction in this investigation, a marbofloxacin dose of 1.34 mg/kg every 24 h is recommended for treatment of *P. multocida* infections with MIC values lower than 0.12 µg/mL. The dosage 1.34 mg/kg was calculated by the equation $AUC_{24} = 4.76 \quad \text{Dose} + 0.5776$ (Fig. 3). However, we did not assess the diffusion of marbofloxacin in lungs and the immune responses in lungs may be different from that in tissue cage fluid.

Conclusions

The present study characterized the in vivo effectiveness of marbofloxacin against *P. multocida* in a tissue cage model in pigs. The AUC_{24}TCF/MIC proved to be the PK/PD index that predicted the antimicrobial activity of marbofloxacin against *P. multocida.* Marbofloxacin presented excellent antibacterial activity with an AUC24TCF/MIC ratio of 57.70 h for a 3-log reduction in bacteria. Although this study needs to be validated by clinical treatment under practical conditions, the results indicated that it may be a critical step closer to clinical trials for optimization of dosage regimens.

Abbreviations

AUC: area under the curve; AUC_{24h}/MIC: the ratio of area under the concentration-time curve over 24 h to MIC; BW: body weight; CFU: Colony forming unit; CLSI: clinical and laboratory standards institute; C_{max}/MIC: the ratio of peak concentration to MIC; Cmax: peak concentration; CVCC: China veterinary culture collection; HPLC: high performance liquid chromatography; MIC: minimum inhibitory concentration; *P. multocida*: Pasteurella multocida;; PD: Pharmacodynamics; PK: Pharmacokinetics; T% > MIC: The percent time that marbofloxacin concentrations were above the MIC; TC: tissue cage; TCF: tissue cage fluid

Acknowledgments

Not applicable.

Funding

This work is supported financially by the National Natural Science Foundation of China (grant 31,372,480) and the National Key Basic Research Program of China (grant 2013CB127200). The funders had no role in study design, data collection and analysis, decision to publish, or preparation of the manuscript.

Authors' contributions

ZZ conceived of the study helped to draft the manuscript. QZ designed the experiment and drafted the manuscript. QZ and JS conducted the experiment and acquired the data. XM and XL analyzed the data. WX and YL participated in the revision of the manuscript. All authors read and approved the final manuscript.

Competing interests

The authors declare that they have no competing interests.

Consent for publication

Not applicable.

References

1. Frimodt-Moller N. How predictive is PK/PD for antibacterial agents? Int J Antimicrob Ag. 2002;19(4):333–9.
2. Ahmad I, Huang LL, Hao HH, Sanders P, Yuan ZH. Application of PK/PD modeling in veterinary field: dose optimization and drug resistance prediction. Biomed Res Int. 2016;
3. Cao C, Qu Y, Sun M, Qiu Z, Huang X, Huai B, et al. In vivo antimicrobial activity of marbofloxacin against Pasteurella multocida in a tissue cage model in calves. Front Microbiol. 2015;6:759.
4. Sidhu PK, Landoni MF, Aliabadi FS, Lees P. PK-PD integration and modeling of marbofloxacin in sheep. Res Vet Sci. 2010;88(1):134–41.
5. Zhang BX, Gu XY, Li YF, Li XH, Gu MX, Zhang N, et al. In vivo evaluation of mutant selection window of cefquinome against *Escherichia coli* in piglet tissue-cage model. BMC Vet Res. 2014;10
6. Holst E, Rollof J, Larsson L, Nielsen JP. Characterization and distribution of Pasteurella species recovered from infected humans. J Clin Microbiol. 1992;30(11):2984–7.
7. Blackall PJ, Pahoff JL, Marks D, Fegan N, Morrow CJ. Characterisation of Pasteurella multocida isolated from fowl cholera outbreaks on turkey farms. Aust Vet J. 1995;72(4):135–8.
8. Magyar T, King VL, Kovacs F. Evaluation of vaccines for atrophic rhinitis–a comparison of three challenge models. Vaccine. 2002;20(13–14):1797–802.
9. Kalorey DR, Yuvaraj S, Vanjanri SS, Gunjal PS, Dhanawade NB, Barbuddhe SB, et al. PCR analysis of Pasteurella multocida isolates from an outbreak of pasteurellosis in Indian pigs. Comp Immunol Microb. 2008;31(6):459–65.
10. Aalbaek B, Eriksen L, Rimler RB, Leifsson PS, Basse A, Christiansen T, et al. Typing of Pasteurella multocida from haemorrhagic septicaemia in Danish fallow deer (*Dama dama*). APMIS. 1999;107(10):913–20.

11. Boyce JD, Seemann T, Adler B, Harper M. Pathogenomics of Pasteurella multocida. Curr Top Microbiol Immunol. 2012;361:23–38.
12. Schneider M, Thomas V, Boisrame B, Deleforge J. Pharmacokinetics of marbofloxacin in dogs after oral and parenteral administration. J Vet Pharmacol Ther. 1996;19(1):56–61.
13. Aliabadi FS, Lees P. Pharmacokinetics and pharmacokinetic/pharmacodynamic integration of marbofloxacin in calf serum, exudate and transudate. J Vet Pharmacol Ther. 2002;25(3):161–74.
14. Meunier D, Acar JF, Martel JL, Kroemer S, Valle M. Seven years survey of susceptibility to marbofloxacin of bovine pathogenic strains from eight European countries. Int J Antimicrob Agents. 2004;24(3):268–78.
15. Thomas A, Nicolas C, Dizier I, Mainil J, Linden A. Antibiotic susceptibilities of recent isolates of mycoplasma bovis in Belgium. Vet Rec. 2003;153(14):428–31.
16. Dorey L, Hobson S, Lees P. Potency of marbofloxacin for pig pneumonia pathogens Actinobacillus pleuropneumoniae and Pasteurella multocida: comparison of growth media. Res Vet Sci. 2016;111:43–8.
17. Appelbaum PC, Hunter PA. The fluoroquinolone antibacterials: past, present and future perspectives. Int J Antimicrob Agents. 2000;16(1):5–15.
18. Spreng M, Deleforge J, Thomas V, Boisrame B, Drugeon H. Antibacterial activity of marbofloxacin. A new fluoroquinolone for veterinary use against canine and feline isolates. J Vet Pharmacol Ther. 1995;18(4):284–9.
19. Vilalta C, Giboin H, Schneider M, El Garch F, Fraile L. Pharmacokinetic/pharmacodynamic evaluation of marbofloxacin in the treatment of Haemophilus parasuis and Actinobacillus pleuropneumoniae infections in nursery and fattener pigs using Monte Carlo simulations. J Vet Pharmacol Ther. 2014;37(6):542–9.
20. Craig WA. Pharmacokinetic/pharmacodynamic parameters: rationale for antibacterial dosing of mice and men. Clin Infect Dis. 1998;26(1):1–10. quiz 11-12
21. MacGowan A, Bowker K. Developments in PK/PD: optimising efficacy and prevention of resistance. A critical review of PK/PD in in vitro models. Int J Antimicrob Agents. 2002;19(4):291–8.
22. Shan Q, Wang J, Yang F, Ding H, Liang C, Lv Z, et al. Pharmacokinetic/pharmacodynamic relationship of marbofloxacin against Pasteurella multocida in a tissue-cage model in yellow cattle. J Vet Pharmacol Ther. 2014;37(3):222–30.
23. Zeitlinger M, Sauermann R, Fille M, Hausdorfer J, Leitner I, Muller M. Plasma protein binding of fluoroquinolones affects antimicrobial activity. J Antimicrob Chemoth. 2008;61(3):561–7.
24. Greko C, Finn M, Franklin A, Bengtsson B. Pharmacokinetic/pharmacodynamic relationship of danofloxacin against Mannheimia haemolytica in a tissue-cage model in calves. J Antimicrob Chemoth. 2003;52(2):253–7.
25. Dayao DA, Gibson JS, Blackall PJ, Turni C. Antimicrobial resistance in bacteria associated with porcine respiratory disease in Australia. Vet Microbiol. 2014;171(1–2):232–5.
26. Pors SE, Hansen MS, Bisgaard M, Jensen HE. Occurrence and associated lesions of Pasteurella multocida in porcine bronchopneumonia. Vet Microbiol. 2011;150(1–2):160–6.
27. Zeitlinger M, Sauermann R, Fille M, Hausdorfer J, Leitner I, Muller M. Plasma protein binding of fluoroquinolones affects antimicrobial activity. J Antimicrob Chemother. 2008;61(3):561–7.
28. Hossain MA, Hc P, Jeong K, Yh J, Kim DG, Kang J, et al. Pharmacokinetic and Pharmacodynamic Evaluation of Marbofloxacin in Pig against Korean Local Isolates of Actinobacillus pleuropneumoniae. *Biomed Res Int*. 2017;2017:1–11.
29. Ding H, Li Y, Chen Z, Rizwan-ul-Haq M, Zeng Z. Plasma and tissue cage fluid pharmacokinetics of marbofloxacin after intravenous, intramuscular, and oral single-dose application in pigs. J Vet Pharmacol Ther. 2010;33(5):507–10.
30. Andes D, Craig WA. In vivo activities of amoxicillin and amoxicillin-clavulanate against Streptococcus Pneumoniae: application to breakpoint determinations. Antimicrob Agents Chemother. 1998;42(9):2375–9.
31. Qu Y, Qiu Z, Cao C, Lu Y, Sun M, Liang C, et al. Pharmacokinetics/pharmacodynamics of marbofloxacin in a Pasteurella multocida serious murine lung infection model. BMC Vet Res. 2015;11:294.
32. Xiao X, Sun J, Yang T, Fang X, Wu D, Xiong YQ, et al. In vivo pharmacokinetic/pharmacodynamic profiles of valnemulin in an experimental intratracheal mycoplasma gallisepticum infection model. Antimicrob Agents Chemother. 2015;59(7):3754–60.
33. Illambas J, Potter T, Cheng Z, Rycroft A, Fishwick J, Lees P. Pharmacodynamics of marbofloxacin for calf pneumonia pathogens. Res Vet Sci. 2013;94(3):675 81.
34. Hyatt JM, Nix DE, Schentag JJ. Pharmacokinetic and pharmacodynamic activities of ciprofloxacin against strains of Streptococcus Pneumoniae, *Staphylococcus aureus*, and Pseudomonas Aeruginosa for which MICs are similar. Antimicrob Agents Chemother. 1994;38(12):2730–7.
35. Gunderson BW, Ross GH, Ibrahim KH, Rotschafer JC. What do we really know about antibiotic pharmacodynamics? Pharmacotherapy. 2001;21(11 Pt 2):302S–18S.
36. Thomas JK, Forrest A, Bhavnani SM, Hyatt JM, Cheng A, Ballow CH, et al. Pharmacodynamic evaluation of factors associated with the development of bacterial resistance in acutely ill patients during therapy. Antimicrob Agents Chemother. 1998;42(3):521–7.
37. El Garch F, de Jong A, Simjee S, Moyaert H, Klein U, Ludwig C, et al. Monitoring of antimicrobial susceptibility of respiratory tract pathogens isolated from diseased cattle and pigs across Europe, 2009-2012. VetPath results. Vet Microbiol. 2016;194:11–22.
38. de Jong A, Thomas V, Simjee S, Moyaert H, El Garch F, Maher K, et al. Antimicrobial susceptibility monitoring of respiratory tract pathogens isolated from diseased cattle and pigs across Europe: the VetPath study. Vet Microbiol. 2014;172(1–2):202–15.

8

Host-pathogen interplay at primary infection sites in pigs challenged with *Actinobacillus pleuropneumoniae*

Elena L. Sassu[1†], Janna Frömbling[2†], J. Catharina Duvigneau[3], Ingrid Miller[3], Andrea Müllebner[3], Ana M. Gutiérrez[4], Tom Grunert[2], Martina Patzl[5], Armin Saalmüller[5], Alexandra von Altrock[6], Anne Menzel[6], Martin Ganter[6], Joachim Spergser[2], Marion Hewicker-Trautwein[7], Jutta Verspohl[8], Monika Ehling-Schulz[2†] and Isabel Hennig-Pauka[1*†]

Abstract

Background: *Actinobacillus (A.) pleuropneumoniae* is the causative agent of porcine pleuropneumonia and causes significant losses in the pig industry worldwide. Early host immune response is crucial for further progression of the disease. *A. pleuropneumoniae* is either rapidly eliminated by the immune system or switches to a long-term persistent form. To gain insight into the host-pathogen interaction during the early stages of infection, pigs were inoculated intratracheally with *A. pleuropneumoniae* serotype 2 and humanely euthanized eight hours after infection. Gene expression studies of inflammatory cytokines and the acute phase proteins haptoglobin, serum amyloid A and C-reactive protein were carried out by RT-qPCR from the lung, liver, tonsils and salivary gland. In addition, the concentration of cytokines and acute phase proteins were measured by quantitative immunoassays in bronchoalveolar lavage fluid, serum and saliva. In parallel to the analyses of host response, the impact of the host on the bacterial pathogen was assessed on a metabolic level. For the latter, Fourier-Transform Infrared (FTIR-) spectroscopy was employed.

Results: Significant cytokine and acute phase protein gene expression was detected in the lung and the salivary gland however this was not observed in the tonsils. In parallel to the analyses of host response, the impact of the host on the bacterial pathogen was assessed on a metabolic level. For the latter investigations, Fourier-Transform Infrared (FTIR-) spectroscopy was employed. The bacteria isolated from the upper and lower respiratory tract showed distinct IR spectral patterns reflecting the organ-specific acute phase response of the host.

Conclusions: In summary, this study implies a metabolic adaptation of *A. pleuropneumoniae* to the porcine upper respiratory tract already during early infection, which might indicate a first step towards the persistence of *A. pleuropneumoniae*. Not only in lung, but also in the salivary gland an increased inflammatory gene expression was detectable during the acute stage of infection.

Keywords: FTIR, Salivary gland, Acute phase proteins, Early immune response, Gene expression

* Correspondence: isabel.hennig-pauka@vetmeduni.ac.at
†Equal contributors
[1]University Clinic for Swine, Department of Farm Animals and Veterinary Public Health, University of Veterinary Medicine Vienna, Vienna, Austria
Full list of author information is available at the end of the article

Background

Actinobacillus (A.) pleuropneumoniae is the etiological agent of porcine contagious pleuropneumonia, which results in increased mortality throughout swine production worldwide [1]. The outcome of infection ranges from colonisation of the upper respiratory tract without any clinical signs to severe lung infection with peracute death. The severity has been ascribed to variation in serotype-related virulence, influenced by biotic and abiotic factors in the pig environment [1]. If the pig overcomes the acute phase of the disease, it can harbour the bacterium in chronic lung lesions, tonsillar crypts and nasal cavities. Thus, infected pigs become persistent carriers of the infectious agent [2]. The Waldeyer's ring is the first immunological and mechanical barrier faced by inhaled pathogens [3, 4]. Its failure allows persistence of *A. pleuropneumoniae* at this site or may lead to reoccurrence of acute outbreaks. Early innate immune response to respiratory disease is not restricted to the lung as the primary site of infection, but additionally involves peripheral lymphoid tissues, the liver [5] and the salivary gland [6]. The acute immune response is characterised by the self-sustaining production of acute phase proteins and inflammatory cytokines. Particularly for *A. pleuropneumoniae* the synergic action of endotoxins and the pore forming exotoxins Apx I to IV, in enhancing the production of inflammatory cytokines, such as IL-6, TNF-α and IL-1 is well known [5, 7–9]. Thus, these bacterial virulence factors can cause tissue damage, directly by Apx cytotoxic effect and indirectly by mounting an exacerbated inflammatory response.

To gain insight into the early stages of host-pathogen interaction, we experimentally challenged pigs with *A. pleuropneumoniae* using the endotracheal infection route and studied in parallel the host and the pathogen during the first few hours of infection. We investigated the mRNA expression of inflammatory cytokines and acute phase proteins in the lung, liver, salivary gland and tonsils as well as the protein levels of these markers in bronchoalveolar lavage fluid (BALF), serum and saliva samples. For studying the influence of the host milieu on the bacterial pathogen, Fourier-Transform Infrared (FTIR) spectroscopy, was employed. FTIR spectroscopy is a well-established vibrational spectroscopic technique that can be used for the generation of spectral fingerprints from a broad range of biological materials [10, 11]. Recently, chemometric assisted FTIR spectroscopy was shown to be a valuable tool for studying metabolic adaptation of bacterial pathogens to host environments. For instance, FTIR spectroscopy was successfully applied for the examination of host genotype-specific imprints on the metabolism of *Listeria monocytogenes* re-isolated from mice with different genotypes [12]. In another study, FTIR spectroscopic analysis of *Streptococcus uberis* re-isolated during the progression of the uterine clearance process of post-partum cows revealed specific *S. uberis* biotypes, which could be linked to the uterine health status [13]. This renders FTIR spectroscopy a suitable technique to investigate bacterial host adaptation on a macromolecular and metabolic level not only for human but also for animal pathogens. In our current study, we showed that already in the early stages of porcine infection *A. pleuropneumoniae* undergoes organ specific metabolic changes that mirror those detected in the host.

Methods

Animals

Ten 6–8 week-old healthy pigs (German Landrace) were used in this study. Animals were derived from a closed breeding herd of a high health status that is routinely tested negative for *A. pleuropneumoniae*, Porcine Reproductive and Respiratory Syndrome Virus (PRRSV), toxigenic *Pasteurella multocida*, endo- and ectoparasites. After arrival, all pigs tested negative for *A. pleuropneumoniae* using an Apx-II Enzyme-linked immunosorbent assay (ELISA) [14]. At arrival, animals were individually marked with ear tags and randomly assigned to a control ($n = 4$) or infection ($n = 6$) group. Within a one-week adaptation period pigs became familiar to the housing conditions. Twice a day commercial feed was supplied. Pigs were housed under specific pathogen-free conditions according to FELASA guidelines and were continuously observed during the whole experiment. A humane intervention point (HIP) checklist, which has been developed and approved previously for infection experiments with *A. pleuroneumoniae*, was used during monitoring the animals continuously for clinical signs by trained staff (participants of FELASA B training course) [15, 16]. HIP was conducted by injection of 60 mg pentobarbital/kg body weight intravenously in deep anaesthesia of the animals as soon as behavioural changes or a significant increase in body temperature reflected the development of early respiratory disease.

Experimental infection protocol

The experiment was part of a comprehensive study to characterise the early stages of inflammatory lung alterations by imaging techniques such as infrared thermography (data not published).

Pigs were not fed on the day of infection to decrease the risk of pulmonary aspiration of stomach content under anaesthesia. An acute infection trial lasting 8–10 h was carried out and included anaesthesia, surgical implantation of the central catheter into the *Vena cava cranialis*, intratracheal infection, clinical examination and collection of blood and saliva samples till scheduled euthanasia. Pigs were anaesthetized intramuscularly with

15 mg ketamine (Ursotamin®, Serumwerk-Bernburg AG, Bernburg, Germany) per kg body weight (bw) and 2 mg azaperon (Stresnil®, Janssen-Cilag GmbH, Baar, Switzerland) per kg bw. Intratracheal infection was performed under visible control using a flexible fiberoptic bronchoscope (IT3; Olympus, Hamburg, Germany) as previously described [15]. Briefly, the tip of the bronchoscope was placed cranial the *Bifurcatio tracheae* and 5 ml of inoculum was instilled gently into the main bronchi. *A. pleuropneumoniae* biotype 1-serotype 2 strain (no. C3656/0271/11, isolated from a fattening pig with respiratory symptoms during an acute outbreak of porcine pleuropneumonia in northern Germany and stored at the Institute of Microbiology, University of Veterinary Medicine, Hannover, Germany [17]) was cultivated in fresh pleuropneumonia-like organism (PPLO) liquid medium to reach an optical density of approximately 0.45 at 600 nm for infection as described elsewhere [18]. This culture was subsequently diluted 1:1000 with 154 mM sterile NaCl solution, resulting in a challenge dose of approximately 1.6×10^6 CFU per pig determined retrospectively by serial dilution and overnight culture. Control pigs were treated with 154 mM sterile NaCl (sham control). Blood and saliva samples were taken at 2 h prior to and 2, 5 and 8 h post infection and clinical scores were recorded simultaneously.

Blood samples were collected by means of the central catheter into vacutainer tubes with either EDTA for haematological examination or sodium heparin for biochemical examination as anticoagulants.

Saliva samples were obtained by allowing pigs to chew a cotton wool swab (Salivette®, Numbrecht, Germany). The cotton wool swabs were replaced in the original tube, centrifuged at 3000 × g for 10 min and the supernatants stored at−20 °C. Rectal body temperature was measured every hour. At the end of the experiment all pigs were euthanized by intravenous application of 60 mg pentobarbital (Euthadorm®, CP-Pharma, Burgdorf, Germany)/kg bw at eight to ten hours after infection and necropsy was performed immediately.

Clinical evaluation

Clinical examinations were carried out before infection and at 2, 5 and 8 h post infection (hpi) and a total clinical score was calculated for each animal at each time point. This total clinical score was obtained by summing up the single scores for six clinical parameters, as dyspnoea (heavy breathing = 1; open-mouth breathing = 2), coughing (=1), posture (sitting = 1; lying = 2), body temperature (38.0–39.5 °C = 0; >39.5 °C = 1; <38.0 °C = 2), vomiting (=1) and sudden death (=2 extra), so that an individual maximal clinical score of 10 was possible. Scores recorded at 8 hpi were statistically compared between the groups.

Post-mortem examinations

After euthanasia lungs were removed immediately from the carcasses. The severity of lung alterations was assessed using the lung lesion score (LLS) proposed by Hannan et al. [19] and as recommended by the European Pharmacopoeia for the control of vaccine efficacy (3rd edition, EDQM, Council of Europe, Strasbourg, France). Briefly, using a schematic map of the porcine lung as a guide, the organ was virtually subdivided into 74 triangles (7 triangles for cranial and middle lobes, 19 triangles for caudal lobes and 8 triangles for the accessory lobe). Then, the number of triangles with pathological lung alterations were expressed as a fraction and multiplied by five for each lobe, so that each lobe could reach a maximum score of 5, resulting in a maximum LLS of 35 when the entire lung was affected.

One main bronchus was separated from the lung by a surgical clamp. Lung tissue samples were taken from the clamped lung lobe, while the other lung lobe was lavaged with 100 ml of 154 mM sterile NaCl solution. Lung lavage fluid was collected by gently pouring in a glass container moistened inside with concentrated heparin solution. Tissue samples from the clamped main lung lobes were fixed in 10% formalin containing 2% calcium acetate for the preparation of paraffin sections. Routine histology sections were stained with hematoxylin-eosin (HE, hemalaun after Delafield). For mRNA extraction, approximately 500 mg tissue samples from liver, tonsils, salivary gland and lung were snap frozen in liquid nitrogen and then stored at −80 °C.

Blood and lung lavage fluid analyses

Leucocyte cell counts and differential blood counts were determined (Haemotology analyser, Celltag alpha, Nihon Kohden, Kleinmachnow, Germany) immediately after blood collection. Serum haptoglobin (Hp) concentrations were analysed with a colorimetric method (Tridelta Phase Haptoglobin Assay, Tridelta Development Limited, Maynooth, Ireland), while serum C-reactive protein (CRP) was determined by ELISA (Phase Porcine CRP Assay, Tridelta Development Limited).

Total leukocyte counts were determined in the undiluted lavage fluid in a Neubauer-counting chamber prior to centrifugation of the fluid (10 min, 200 × g, 4 °C). The sediment was used for further cytological examination. Cytospots were prepared for differential cell determination of the bronchoalveolar lavage fluid (BALF) by centrifugation of small amounts of resuspended sediments in a cytocentrifuge (Multifuge KR®, Heraeus, Thermo, Osterode, Germany) at 200 × g for 10 min. Cells were stained with a Pappenheim staining solution (Merck, Darmstadt, Germany) and 400 cells were differentiated at 1000 × magnification. The cell-free supernatant of lung lavage fluid was stored at −80 °C.

Analysis of gene expression in tissues

RNA was extracted and reverse transcribed as described previously [20]. The primer sequences and hybridization probes used for the detection of porcine cytokine mRNAs (IL-2, IL-4, IL-10, IL-6, INF-γ and IL-1) as well as the internal references (GAPDH, cyclophilin A and β-actin) were reported by Duvigneau et al. (2005) [21]. The primer sequences and hybridization probes for the detection of porcine stress gene mRNAs (iNOS/HO1/TNF-α) were detailed in a previous work [20]. The primer sequences used for the specific amplification of porcine CRP and Hp were described by Skovgaard et al. (2009) [5], and the primer sequence for amplification of porcine SAA was characterised by Soler et al. (2011a, b) [22, 23]. Primers used for the detection of IL-8 expression were designed for this study as follows: forward: AACAGCCCGTGTCAACATGA and reverse: TGCACT GGCATCGAAGTTCT. The suitability of the newly designed primers was verified in separate experiments by performing a dilution series using the PCR products as well as a dilution series of the cDNA pool, generated by collecting equal aliquots of all investigated cDNA samples. The dilution series, in conjunction with the melting characteristics of the PCR product, were used to optimise the assays regarding the primer concentration as well as the annealing and extension times for the PCR. Further details about the validation of the qPCR assays are provided (see Additional file 1). All primers (Invitrogen, Carlsbad, CA, USA) and probes (Eurofins MWG Operon, Ebersberg, Germany) were synthesised commercially. Specificity of the generated PCR products was verified using melt curve analysis and by randomly verifying correct fragment sizes using gel electrophoresis.

PCR assays were performed as described in [21, 24]. All samples were measured in duplicate. Each plate contained corresponding randomly assigned RT-minus controls of about 15% of all samples, the non-template controls (NTC) as well as the internal standard (IS), which was generated by pooling aliquots of all samples investigated in this study. Data were analysed as described previously [23] and normalised against cyclophilin A and β-actin. The obtained ΔΔCq values of the replicates were averaged and expressed as fold change relative to the IS.

Quantitative ELISA of serum and BALF

Serum and BALF samples were analysed for IL-6, TNF-α and IL-1 expression by means of commercially available sandwich ELISA assay (Duoset DY686, DY690B, DY681, R&D Systems, Biomedical medical products GmbH and Co KG, Vienna, Austria) according to the manufacturer's instructions with minor modifications. For the preparation of standard curves, the recombinant cytokines were diluted in the same body fluid as the samples. Therefore, serum samples from four or BALF from two healthy age-matched pigs were pooled to decrease the risk of individual variation in the matrix. For serum samples, in order to increase signal intensity, the working concentrations of capture and detection antibodies and of the streptavidin-HRP conjugate were doubled. The respective recombinant protein was diluted serially (1:2) in the serum pool. Sera were analysed undiluted and all samples, controls and standard concentrations were run in duplicate. For BALF samples, the working concentrations of antibodies and HPR-conjugates were used as recommended. The BALF pool to create the standard curves was used in the same dilution as the samples. BALF was used undiluted for TNF-α and diluted 1:4 for IL-1 and IL-6 detection. The detection limits of the assays were 150 pg/ml for IL-6, 200 pg/ml for TNF-α and 70 pg/ml for IL-1, respectively. Tetramethylbenzidine (TMB) was used for colour development and 1 M sulphuric acid as stopping solution according to the manufacturer's instructions. Optical density was measured at 450 nm and at 690 nm as the reference with an ELISA reader (Tecan, Sunrise, Grödig, Austria) and concentrations were calculated with Magellan software (Tecan) using the standard curves as allocation base.

Time-resolved fluorometry immunoassay of saliva and BALF

The concentrations of Hp and CRP in saliva and BALF samples were quantified using previously developed and validated one-step non-competitive sandwich type immunoassays based on time-resolved fluorometry technology [25, 26]. The assays used for Hp and CRP measurements comprise calibration curves with seven standards with concentrations between 10 and 1500 ng/ml approximately. This wide dynamic range allows the quantification of samples with highly varying protein concentrations. For saliva, the optimal sample dilution was 1:10 and 1:2 for Hp and CRP measurements respectively, as reported previously. However, described assays had not been evaluated for BALF samples so far, so that the procedures were modified by using optimised dilutions of 1:100 and 1:10 for Hp and CRP quantifications respectively.

Bacterial isolation and cultivation

Lung and tonsillar tissue samples, as well as nasal swabs of four control (C1-4) and six infected (I1-6) animals were examined for the presence of *A. pleuropneumoniae*. For bacterial isolation swabs from organ tissue and nostrils were streaked on Columbia sheep blood agar (Oxoid, Wien, Austria). *Staphylococcus aureus* was used as nurse to facilitate the isolation of *A. pleuropneumoniae* from organs carrying a high bacterial background microbiota, such as tonsils and nostrils [1]. Subsequent cultivation of bacteria was performed in PPLO broth (Difco™, Becton, Dickinson and Company, Franklin Lakes, USA) supplemented with 10 mg/l NAD (AppliChem GmbH, Darmstadt, Germany) for molecular analyses or grown as solid cultures supplemented with 14 g/l bacteriological agar (Oxoid) for FTIR spectroscopy (see below). All bacterial cultivations were carried out at 37 °C and 5% CO_2.

Serotype 2 specific PCR

Serotype 2 specific PCR using primers for the capsular biosynthesis genes *cps2AB* was performed to confirm the identity of *A. pleuropneumoniae* re-isolated from infected host tissue [27]. Briefly, pelleted bacteria from 2–4 ml liquid culture were re-suspended in 100 µl ddH_2O and lysed at 100 °C for 10 min. Cell debris was removed by 3 min centrifugation at 13.000 × g. 2 µl supernatant containing 50 ng/µl genomic DNA served as a template for a 25 µl PCR reaction mixture containing 5 µl 5× Green GoTaq® Flexi buffer (Promega, Madison, USA), 2.5 µl 25 mM $MgCl_2$, 0.5 µl 20 mM dNTP, 0.25 µl APPcps2F and APPcpsR Primer each (50 pmol), 0.125 µl GoTaq® Flexi DNA Polymerase (5 U/µl; Promega, Madison, USA) and 14.38 µl ddH_2O. DNA was amplified for 35 cycles with the following parameters: 30 s denaturation at 94 °C, 30 s annealing at 58 °C and 30 s elongation at 72 °C. PCR products were analysed on a 1.5% agarose gel.

DNA fingerprinting of bacteria

Genetic stability of bacteria was confirmed by M13 - PCR typing of re-isolated *A. pleuropneumoniae* and the original challenge strain grown *in vitro* as previously described by Henderson et al. [28]. Genomic DNA was isolated with the MasterPure™ DNA Purification Kit (Epicentre, Madison, USA) following the manufacturer's instructions. 2 µl genomic DNA (50 ng/µl) was used as a template for a 25 µl PCR reaction mixture containing 5 µl 5 × Green GoTaq® Flexi buffer (Promega, Madison, USA), 2.5 µl 25 mM $MgCl_2$, 0.5 µl 20 mM dNTP, 0.5 µl Primer M13 (50 pmol/µl; 5'-GAGGGTGGCGGCTCT-3'), 0.15 µl GoTaq® Flexi DNA Polymerase (5 U/µl; Promega, Madison, USA) and 14.35 µl ddH_2O. The amplification was performed using the following parameters: 35 cycles of 35 s of denaturation at 95 °C, 1 min annealing at 40 °C and 2 min of extension at 72 °C. PCR products were analysed on a 2% agarose gel.

Preparation of crude capsular extract

Crude capsule extracts (CEs) were prepared from *A. pleuropneumoniae* isolates derived from lung and tonsils of the infected pigs by mild water-phenol extraction. In brief, fresh 50 ml liquid cultures of *A. pleuropneumoniae* isolates were grown to an OD_{600} of 0.2 and bacteria were harvested by centrifugation at 6530 × g for 5 min. Per gram of bacterial mass 18 ml 1% phenol were added and capsules were extracted by shaking for 5 min at 37 °C followed by an incubation step at 4 °C for 30 min. Bacterial debris was pelleted by centrifugation at 27000 × g for 30 min at 4 °C. Supernatant was sterile filtrated with a syringe sterile filter (pore size 22 µm) to remove remaining cellular debris. The phenol solution was removed by vacuum centrifugation and CE was re-suspended in ddH_2O and immediately analysed by FTIR spectroscopy.

FTIR spectroscopy and spectral data analyses

FTIR spectroscopy was employed to investigate the impact of the host on the metabolism of *A. pleuropneumoniae* re-isolated from organs and tissues of infected pigs. Infrared spectra reflect the biochemical composition of living cells by mirroring the stretching and bending vibrations of proteins, nucleic acids, polysaccharides and fatty acids within different frequency areas [11], which makes FTIR spectroscopy a powerful and highly discriminatory tool for the generation of bacterial metabolic fingerprints and to study host-pathogen interactions [12]. For the generation of a metabolic fingerprint, a loop full of a bacterial mass of the different isolates was cultivated as a lawn on PPLO agar at 37 °C for 24 h and samples were prepared for FTIR spectroscopy as described previously [29, 30]. In brief, one loop-full of bacteria was suspended in 100 µl sterile distilled water. Subsequently, an aliquot of 30 µl cell suspension was transferred to a zinc selenide (ZnSe) optical plate (BrukerOptics GmbH, Ettlingen, Germany) and dried for 40 min at 40 °C. Infrared absorption spectra were recorded in transmission mode in the range of 4000 to 500 cm^{-1}, with a resolution of 6 cm^{-1}, zero-filling factor 4 and Blackmann-Harris 3-term apodization by the aid of a HTS-XT microplate adapter coupled to a Tensor 27 FTIR spectrometer (BrukerOptics GmbH). An average spectrum of 32 scanned interferograms was calculated with background subtraction for each spectrum. Spectral data were processed and analysed and subsequent chemometric analysis was performed using OPUS software (Version 7.2; BrukerOptics GmbH). The frequency range 1150–1100 cm^{-1} in the polysaccharide region (1200–900 cm^{-1}) provided the maximum discriminatory information to assess the tissue-related bacterial metabolic fingerprints by hierarchical cluster analysis (HCA). Most characteristic frequency areas to assess differences specifically related to the bacterial capsule were the polysaccharide region (1200–900 cm^{-1}) and the protein region (1800–1500 cm^{-1}) [11]. Dendrograms of 2nd-derivative spectra (9-point Savitzky-Golay filter) were generated using the Ward's algorithm with normalisation to repro level 30. Measurements of CE were performed with minor alterations as previously described [31].

Statistical analysis

Statistical data analysis was performed for protein and mRNA level and for the clinical score by using the SPSS software (2011, IBM, SPSS Statistics for Windows, Version 20.0, Armonk, NY, IBM Corp.). Since data were not normally distributed, non-parametrical tests were performed. For statistical evaluation of group differences between infected and sham control pigs the Wilcoxon rank sum test was used. Parameters in paired samples prior to and after infection within one group were compared by the Wilcoxon Signed-Rank test.

Results

Clinical and post-mortem findings

Four hours after infection all pigs experimentally infected with *A. pleuropneumoniae* showed signs of respiratory disease such as dyspnoea, open mouth breathing and coughing. Rare episodes of vomiting were observed in both, infected and control animals, most likely due to a side effect of anaesthesia. Control animals did not display any sign of respiratory disease (Table 1). Successful experimental infection was additionally confirmed by macroscopic and microscopic pathological lung alterations. In the lungs of all infected animals red foci of consolidation and multifocal haemorrhagic lesions associated with interlobular oedema were found (Fig. 1a). In one animal scattered layers of fibrin on the *Pleura visceralis* indicated an incipient pleurisy. Lung lesion scores of infected animals were significantly higher than those of controls as shown in Table 1 ($p \leq 0.01$). Microscopic lung tissue alterations in infected pigs were dominated by a severe neutrophilic infiltration as well as fibrin exudation into the alveolar spaces and interalveolar septa leading to an obstruction of bronchioli (Fig. 1b). The histological diagnosis was a fibrinopurulent, necrotizing and haemorrhagic pleuropneumonia (Table 1). Control pigs showed no histological signs of pleuropneumonia.

Cytological findings in blood

At no time point after infection did the total number of neutrophils in the blood differ between the two groups. Nevertheless, differences were detectable when considering singularly granulocyte fractions. As shown in Fig. 2, eight hours after infection segmented neutrophils in infected animals decreased to a significantly lower level than in control pigs, while a significant increase in immature granulocytes, both band cells and metamyelocytes, was observed in infected pigs in comparison to the sampling prior to infection. Already five hours after infection band neutrophils rose in infected pigs (Fig. 2).

BALF was harvested eight to ten hours after infection from the isolated lungs. Significantly ($p \leq 0.01$) higher total leukocyte cell counts, as well as a trend ($p = 0.057$) in lymphocytes and alveolar macrophages, were observed in infected pigs (Table 2).

Gene expression in host tissue

Gene expression of inflammatory cytokines (IL-6, IL-1 and TNF-α), chemokine IL-8, and the anti-inflammatory cytokine IL-10 was evaluated in liver, lung, salivary gland and tonsils (Fig. 3). Gene expression of iNOS, HO1, IL-2, IL-4 and IFN-γ was below the detection limit and for this reason is not mentioned further in this study (data not shown). In infected animals, IL-6 expression was significantly up-regulated in the liver ($p \leq 0.05$), lung and salivary gland (both $p \leq 0.01$) in comparison to control pigs, but in the tonsils, only a tendency was detected ($p = 0.06$). In the lung tissue of infected animals, all pro-inflammatory cytokines and IL-8 were significantly ($p \leq 0.05$) up-regulated. In addition, IL-1 expression was significantly increased ($p \leq 0.05$) in the salivary gland of infected pigs. No significant differences were found for IL-10 expression in any tissue. In the tonsils none of the investigated parameters were changed (Fig. 3A). The mRNA expression of acute phase proteins (CRP, Hp and SAA) was also assessed in the same tissues (Fig. 3B). Serum amyloid A (SAA) expression was found to be significantly up-regulated ($p \leq 0.01$) in all tissues apart from tonsils. In the salivary gland, the expression of all acute phase proteins was significantly up-regulated ($p \leq 0.01$), while in the tonsils no difference in gene expression in comparison to the control group was found.

Protein expression in serum, BALF and saliva

Concentrations of pro-inflammatory cytokines (IL-6, IL-1, TNF-α) were determined in serum and BALF and acute phase proteins (CRP and Hp) were quantified in serum, BALF and saliva. In sera of infected animals, no significant changes in inflammatory cytokines were detected (data not shown).

Interestingly, TNF-α was not detected in BALF after infection. In contrast, the median concentrations of IL-6 and IL-1 were increased in infected animals while remaining below the detection limit in control pigs. Acute phase proteins behaved similarly in serum and BALF. While Hp concentrations remained unchanged throughout the study, CRP increased significantly at eight hours after infection (Table 2.).

Table 1 Clinical score (CS), lung lesion score (LLS) and histological evaluation of lung lesions in control and infected animals

Group	Clinical score	Lung lesion score	Histological evaluation
Control ($n = 4$)	0 (0–0.75)	0 (0–0.6)	Moderate infiltrates of neutrophils and macrophages in interalveolar septa
Infected ($n = 6$)	**4** (2.75–5.5)**	**7.39** (3.1–16.56)**	Fibrinopurulent, necrotizing, hemorrhagic pleuropneumonia

**$p \leq 0.01$; Wilcoxon rank sum test
CS prior to death (8 hpi) and LLS at the time of the necropsy are expressed as median (interquartile range). Significant values are marked in bold

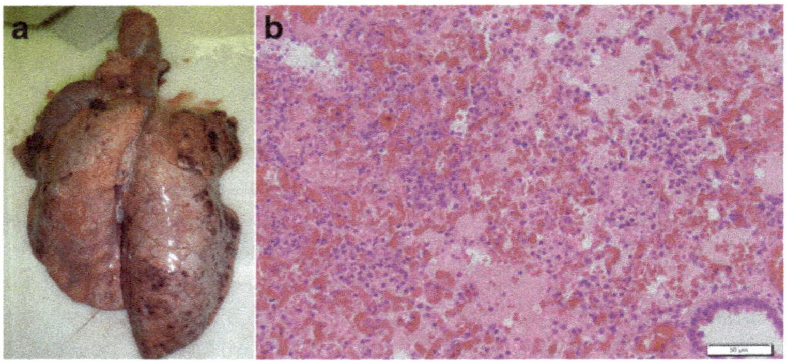

Fig. 1 Pathological lung tissue alterations in a pig 8 hpi with *A. pleuropneumoniae* serotype 2. **a** Macroscopic lung alterations are characterised by multifocal and disseminated haemorrhagic lung tissue consolidations; **b** Histopathological findings are dominated by fibrinous exudates in alveolar spaces and interlobular septa (H&E stain; bar = 50 μm)

The concentrations of CRP and Hp analysed in saliva showed increased levels in the infected animals. Specifically, at the last time point, Hp increased significantly ($p \leq 0.05$) whereas CRP showed only a trend ($p = 0.07$). In control animals no changes were detected.

Metabolic fingerprinting of *A. pleuropneumoniae* re-isolated from host tissues

A. pleuropneumoniae was isolated from the lung of all six, the tonsils of two and the nostrils of three infected animals (Table 3). Serotype 2 specific PCR (APPcps2 PCR) was used to confirm that the isolated *A. pleuropneumoniae* colonies are indeed derived from the *A. pleuropneumoniae* serotype 2 strain used for infection, [27]. The clonality and genetic stability of the isolates were checked by DNA fingerprinting via M13-PCR [28]. All isolates showed the same band pattern via M13-PCR indicating that all isolates are indeed progenitors of the strain used for infection (data not shown). FTIR spectra of all *A. pleuropneumoniae* isolates from the host tissues were recorded and subjected to chemometric analysis. Hierarchical cluster analysis (HCA) of the normalised and pre-processed spectral data revealed a distinct organ-specific clustering of the isolates, indicating organ-specific impacts on the metabolism of host passaged *A. pleuropneumoniae*. From the recorded IR spectra, the spectral window of 1150 to 1100 cm^{-1}, representing a part of the polysaccharide region, showed the highest discriminatory power, resulting in 4 major clusters (Fig. 4). While cluster A covers all isolates from the lung and the inoculation strain, isolates of the upper respiratory tract (tonsillar and nostril isolates) cluster apart from cluster A in the three clusters B-D (Fig. 4). Further passaging showed that the bacterial metabolic adaptation remained stable for the first passages. Consecutive cultivation under laboratory conditions revealed that these metabolic changes are reversible. HCA of FTIR spectral data from bacteria passed 5 times under laboratory conditions showed that isolates from the upper and lower respiratory tract are clustering together (see Additional file 2). The latter results indicate that the observed adaptation is indeed a metabolic adaptation triggered by the organ-specific environment, which is lost over time due to consecutive cultivation under laboratory conditions.

Analysis of *A. pleuropneumoniae* CEs

The metabolic fingerprints of the *A. pleuropneumoniae* lung and upper respiratory tract (nostrils and tonsils) isolates obtained by FTIR spectroscopy showed remarkable differences in the polysaccharide and the protein region. Since the capsule, which is an important virulence factor of *A. pleuropneumoniae* [32], mainly consists of polysaccharides, CE from the re-isolated bacteria were prepared. In order to retain CE associated proteins, a mild aqueous phenol capsule extraction method without further purification was used for the latter. The extracted CE was subjected to FTIR spectroscopy and subsequent chemometric analysis. HCA of the FTIR spectral date of the CEs, using the frequency areas 1800–1500 cm^{-1} (protein region) and 1200–900 cm^{-1} (polysaccharide region), revealed two major clusters: one cluster comprising of the CE spectra from the strain used for infection and its isolates derived from the lung of the infected pigs I1-4 and I6, and one cluster comprising the CE spectra from the tonsil isolates of the infected pig I4 (Fig. 5). Differential FTIR spectral analysis was carried out to search for host site-specific imprints in the CE from the re-isolated bacteria. Therefore, subtraction of a second derivate, vector-normalised, average FTIR spectrum of the CE from *A. pleuropneumoniae* lung isolates from the average spectrum of tonsillar isolates was performed (Fig. 6). The comparison between the CE of isolates revealed significant alterations within the protein (1800–1500 cm^{-1}) and carbohydrate (1200–900 cm^{-1}) regions. Higher amounts of substances absorbing at 1637 cm^{-1} were recorded in CE of lung isolates. This band can be assigned to amide I of β-pleated

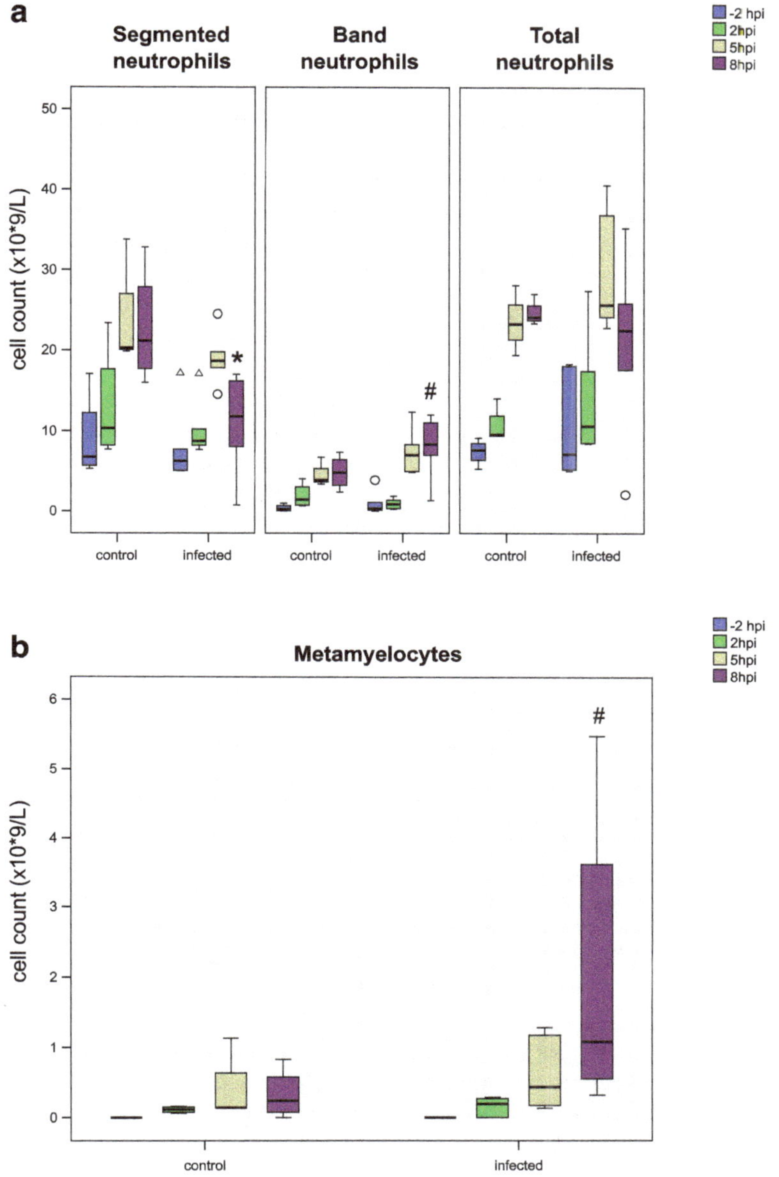

Fig. 2 Cytological findings in the blood during the course of infection. The absolute numbers of mature and immature neutrophils (**a**: total, segmented, band neutrophils, **b**: metamyelocytes) prior to and at 2, 5 and 8 hpi of control ($n = 4$) and infected ($n = 6$) animals are shown. Box-plots show median (line within the box), 25th and the 75th percentiles (box), 1.5 times the interquartile range (whiskers) and outliers (circles and triangles). *$p \leq 0.05$ Wilcoxon rank sum test in comparison to control, # $p \leq 0.05$ Wilcoxon signed-rank test in comparison to sampling prior to infection within the same group

sheet structures [33]. Another significant difference could be detected in the tonsillar CE at 984 cm^{-1} compared to the CE of the lung. Being part of the carbohydrate region this band falls into the spectral range in which O–C, C–O structures dominated by ring vibrations of carbohydrates C–O–P and P–O–P absorb [34].

Discussion

Early induced immune response is the first line of defence against many common microorganisms, including *A. pleuropneumoniae.* Its failure in eliminating the pathogen can result in the development of a chronic and persistent infection status [2, 35]; for this reason, the acute stage of porcine pleuropneumonia, where early immune response usually takes place, was investigated in this study. To induce an acute stage of infection an intratracheal infection route was applied. The experimental model used in this study resulted in diffuse bilateral pneumonia in all infected pigs and the LLS mirrored clinical signs, thus confirming the reproducibility of infection.

Table 2 Concentrations of cytokines (IL-6, IL-1 and TNF-α), acute phase proteins (CRP, Haptoglobin) and cells in different bodily fluids from control and infected animals

	Control ($n = 4$)[a]	Infected ($n = 6$, [c]$n = 3$)
BALF Cytokines:		
IL-6 (pg/ml)	ND	434.2 (ND-2491.5)
IL-1β (pg/ml)	ND	1166.8 (ND-2808.1)
TNF-α (pg/ml)	129.5 (ND-410.4)	ND
BALF acute phase proteins:		
CRP (ng/ml)	89.7 (39.5–189.6)	389.7 (192.6–554.4)
Hp (μg/ml)	6.7 (5.2–9.1)	6.2 (5.1–7.5)
BALF Cells:		
Leukocytes ($\times 10^9$/l)	2.9 (1.8–5.1)	**11.4** (7.8–16.9)**
Lymphocytes ($\times 10^9$/l)	0.1 (0–0.3)	[c]2.5 (0.8–6.1)
Alveolar Macrophage ($\times 10^9$/l)	1.7 (1.5–2.3)	[c]6.2 (4.5–10.6)
	Infected (pre-infection)[b]	Infected (8 hpi)
Serum acute phase proteins:		
CRP (μg/ml)	49.7 (18.4–71.5)	**202.2** (93.9–309)*
Hp (mg/ml)	0.7 (0.2–1.1)	0.7 (0.5–1.3)
Saliva acute phase proteins:		
CRP (ng/ml)	3 (1.3–7.4)	27.9 (8.4–37.6)
Hp (μg/ml)	0.4 (0.2–1)	**1.9** (1.3–3.6)*

Results are expressed as median values (interquartile range). [a]Differences between control and infected group in the BALF immediately after death. *$p \leq 0.05$
**$p \leq 0.01$ Wilcoxon rank test. [b]Differences within the infected group between the last time point of sampling (8 hpi) and prior to infection. *$p \leq 0.05$ Wilcoxon signed ranks test. [c]Lymphocytes and alveolar macrophages were not detectable in the BALF of three animals out of the infection group
ND = not detectable because below detection limit
Significant values are marked in bold

These results are in line with previous studies using other *A. pleuropneumoniae* serotypes for experimental infection [16]. The intratracheal infection model used ensures equally distributed lesions and partially overcomes the limitation of the small sample size in this study by a reduction in the variability commonly associated with other routes of infection [16].

After eight hours of infection, the drop in segmented neutrophils in combination with a rise in band cells and metamyelocytes reveals the kinetics of the cellular innate immune response associated with a fast migration of immature band cells from the bone marrow to the blood as well as a migration of mature neutrophils from the blood stream to the site of infection. Rapid neutrophilic infiltration and high levels of IL-8 expression in lung tissue of infected pigs confirm the key role of this neutrophil-chemokine interaction in the pathogenesis of the disease [8, 16].

In serum, no changes in IL-1 concentrations and only slight increases in IL-6 and TNF-α were recorded within the first eight hours after infection, which is in accordance with results of previous studies [8, 36]. Fossum et al. (1998) reported an increase in IL-6, as the earliest detectable pro-inflammatory cytokine, at 20 hpi with *A. pleuropneumoniae* serotype 2 [36]. Recently, a study from Wyns et al. (2015) showed that all three cytokines increased after the experimental infection and the mean peak concentrations of TNF-α and IL-6 in serum were registered at 12 and 10 hpi respectively [37]. In contrast to these findings for pro-inflammatory cytokines, serum CRP concentration raised eight hours after infection. Serum Hp concentration was not affected during the infection trial.

Our findings of a 4-fold increase in serum CRP is in line with the previously described range of a 2- to 9-fold increase after infection. The normal CRP concentrations in the plasma of healthy pigs vary from 11–77 μg/ml with a high individual variation [38, 39], which is also in accordance with our findings. In contrast to CRP, the slow reacting acute phase protein Hp remained at a physiological level (0.19–0.52 mg/ml) [5, 40] in the serum from both groups. In contrast to serum data, IL-6 and IL-1 were increased in BALF from infected animals; leading to the idea that acute bacterial respiratory tract infection might induce localised rather than systemic cytokine responses. However, TNF-α protein was not detectable in infected pigs, even though its mRNA was found to be highly expressed in the lung. The same outcome was observed in a former study [8]. A study in mice showed the ability of surfactant protein A to enhance the production of secretory leukoprotease inhibitor (SLPI), which is known to induce down-regulation of TNF-α production by inhibiting LPS-induced NF-kB activation [41]. Thus, it is tempting to speculate that LPS-induced NF-kB activation might also be involved in the down-regulation of TNF-α detected in BALF of infected pigs compared to control. Nevertheless, further studies are necessary to test the latter hypothesis.

Although the Waldeyer's ring was bypassed by the intratracheal inoculation route the examined innate immune responses were not confined to the lung, but rather disseminated to organs of the upper respiratory tract. While pro-inflammatory cytokines were primarily induced in the lung tissue of all infected animals, the salivary gland was the main site of expression of acute phase proteins, IL-6 and IL-1. The latter finding was unexpected, because it is in contrast to the lack of immune reaction in tonsillar tissue, although both organs might have had pathogen contact at the same time but later than the lung.

Despite their common localisation, the salivary gland and tonsils showed a completely different pattern in the host immune response. Neither acute phase protein nor pro-inflammatory cytokine mRNAs were differentially

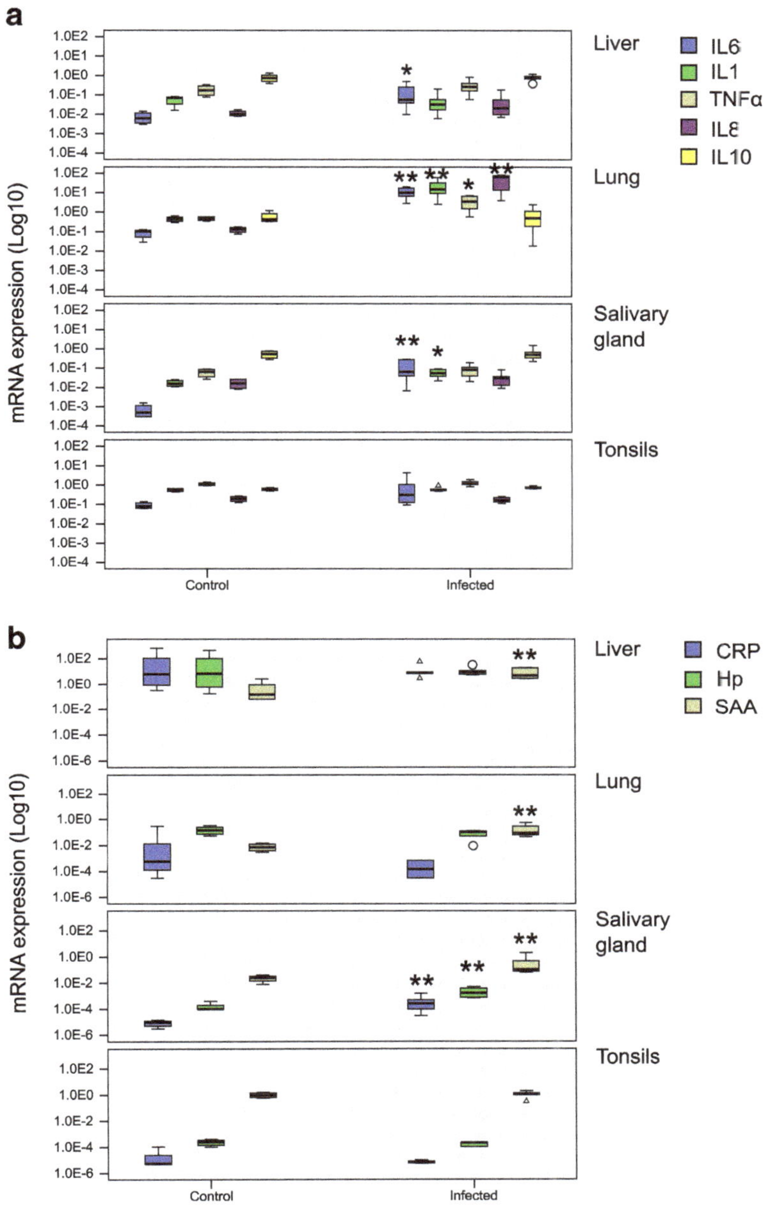

Fig. 3 Cytokine and acute phase protein mRNA analyses. mRNA expression of (**a**) cytokines IL-6, IL-1, TNF-α, IL-8, IL-10 and (**b**) acute phase proteins CRP, C-Reactive Protein; Hp, Haptoglobin and SAA, Serum Amyloid A in different tissues of control ($n = 4$) and infected ($n = 6$) animals. Box-plots show median (line within the box), 25th and the 75th percentiles (box), 1.5 times the interquartile range (whiskers) and outliers (circles and triangles). The results were normalised to reference genes (Actin and Cyclophilin A) and to the internal standard. *$p \leq 0.05$, **$p \leq 0.01$

Table 3 *A. pleuropneumoniae* re-isolated from different tissues of acutely infected animals

Tissue		Animal I1	I2	I3	I4	I5	I6
Lung		x	x	x	x	x	x
Nostril	Left	-	x	-	x	-	-
	Right	-	x	-	-	x	-
Tonsil	Left	-	x	-	x	-	-
	Right	-	-	-	x	-	-

expressed in tonsillar tissue. Acute phase protein extra hepatic production in peripheral lymphoid tissue was previously described during acute *A. pleuropneumoniae* infection [5]. However, the impact of the salivary gland in extra hepatic production of acute phase proteins is largely unknown. Immuno-histochemical findings by Gutierrez et al. (2012) revealed localisation of Hp in the glandular acini and duct epithelial cells of the salivary gland [6]. In our study, not only Hp and SAA, but also CRP was significantly increased in pigs infected with *A.*

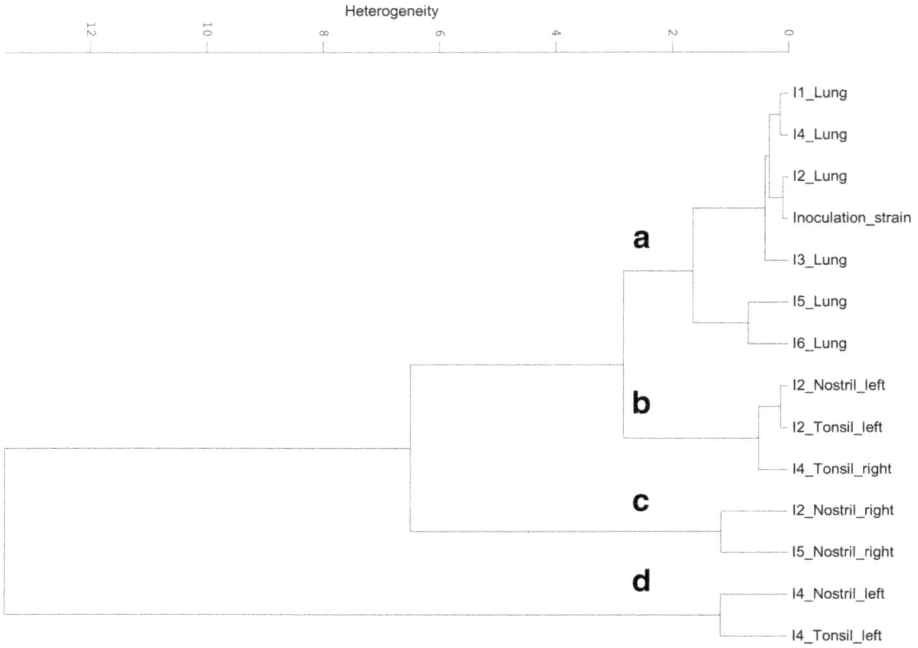

Fig. 4 Hierarchical cluster analysis of FTIR spectra recorded from *A. pleuropneumoniae* serotype 2 re-isolated from different organs of infected pigs. Isolates from different organs of the infected pigs 1–6 (I1-I6) and the strain used for infection were grown for 24 h on PPLO at 37 °C and 5% CO_2, subsequently subjected to FTIR spectroscopy and hierarchical cluster analysis was performed. For calculation of the dendrogram the FTIR spectral regions of 1150 to 1100 cm^{-1} and the Ward's algorithm were used *A. pleuropneumoniae* re-isolated from the lung of all six animals (I1-6) group and the inoculation strain group together in cluster (**a**), while the bacteria isolated from the tonsils and the nostrils group in cluster (**b**–**d**)

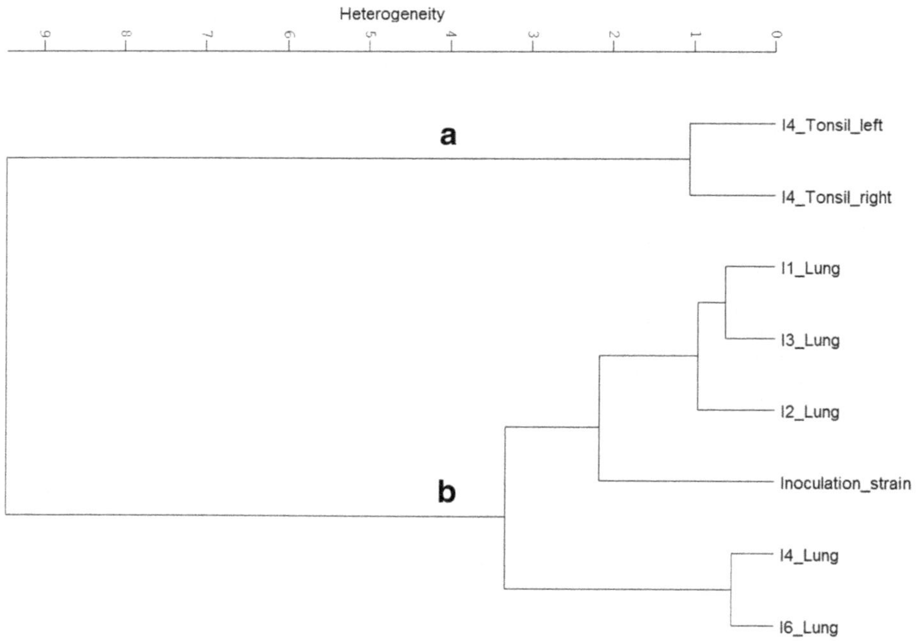

Fig. 5 Hierarchical cluster analyses of FTIR spectroscopic data from CEs of the *A. pleuropneumoniae* serotype 2. Hierarchical cluster analysis was performed using recorded FTIR spectra from the CEs of the infection strain grown *in vitro* and after re-isolation from different organs of the infected pigs 1–4 and 6 (I1-4 and I6): isolates from the lung of I1-4 and 6 as well as the inoculation strain (Cluster **b**), isolates from the left and right tonsil of I4 (Cluster **a**). For calculation of the dendrogram the Ward's algorithm and the FTIR spectral regions of 1200–900 cm^{-1} and 1800–1500 cm^{-1} were used

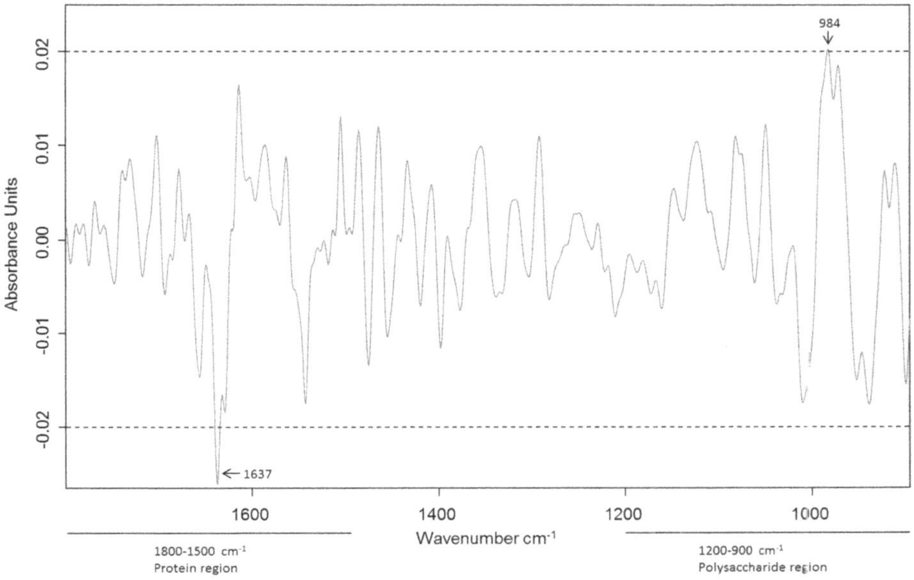

Fig. 6 Differential FTIR spectral analyses. The second derivate, vector-normalised average spectra were calculated from CE of re-isolated *A. pleuropneumoniae* Serotype 2 from the left and right tonsil of the infected pig 4 (I4) and the lung of the infected pigs 1–4 und 6 (I1-4 and I6), respectively. The average spectrum of the lung of I1-4 and 6 was subtracted from the average spectrum of the tonsils of I4. Most pronounced differences could be detected in the frequency area of 1800–900 cm^{-1} and can be related to the protein region (1800–1500 cm^{-1}) and the carbohydrate region (1200–900 cm^{-1})

pleuropneumoniae. This expression was evident both, at a transcriptional level and at the level of the protein, since Hp and CRP reached higher values also in saliva from infected animals. Whether this prominent implication of the salivary gland during acute bacterial infection is linked to the direct presence of *A. pleuropneumoniae* in this site is hitherto unknown. Nonetheless, the detection of the bacterium in the tonsils sited in anatomical proximity, and the reported susceptibility of the salivary gland to *A. pleuropneumoniae* colonisation [42], is a hint that the bacteria could invade this organ. Interestingly, bacteria could be re-isolated from tonsillar tissue, as a consequence of coughing or transport by the mucocillary escalator. However, a host immune response in tonsillar tissue, which would have been indicated by an increase in cytokine or acute phase protein expression, was not detected (Fig. 3).

During the last two decades, FTIR spectroscopy has become a well-established technique for identification of microorganism on the species and subspecies level [11]. Due to its high discriminatory power, FTIR spectroscopy is increasingly employed not only for bacterial identification but also for studying environmental impacts, such as abiotic stress or host genotypes, on the metabolic fingerprints of bacteria [12, 43]. Thus, FTIR spectroscopy represents a suitable tool for exploring the host impacts on *A. pleuropneumoniae* in parallel to the analyses of host reactions in response to the bacterial infection.

In the first step, *A. pleuropneumoniae* re-isolated from different host tissues was subjected to molecular analysis to confirm its genotypic identity with the strain used for inoculation. All isolates were positive in the *A. pleuropneumoniae* serotype 2 specific PCR and showed the same M13-PCR profiles. In contrast to the results from the molecular typing, FTIR spectral analysis revealed a distinct clustering of the isolates. The isolates clustered according to the tissue of re-isolation (Fig 4), reflecting the physiological metabolic adaptation due to their movement from the lower to the upper respiratory tract (Fig. 4–5). This might be indicative for different adaptation strategies, depending on the body compartment of colonisation or infection. Notably, the inoculation strain forms one cluster with the lung isolates while the isolates from the upper respiratory tract formed a separate cluster. This observation fosters out hypothesis that the bacteria are indeed rapidly adapting to the upper respiratory tract, which is reflected in their metabolic fingerprints that are distinct from the ones of the lung isolates and the inoculation strain. Furthermore, our results revealed that the laboratory culture medium (PPLO) and culture conditions used for growth of the inoculation strain mimick the host environment that bacteria are facing during acute infections in the lung (Fig. 4). As shown previously, growth conditions can significantly impact the metabolism and the expression of virulence factors of bacterial pathogens [12] and must be considered when inoculation samples for infection studies are prepared. The observed phenotypical metabolic adaptation of *A. pleuropneumoniae* was reversible, which is in line with recent findings on the loss of host environmentally triggered memory effects over time reported from other bacteria [12, 44, 45]. Since isolation of *A. pleuropneumoniae* from tonsils and nostrils of swine not showing any clinical signs is common, the pathogen is considered to persist at these sites of infection [46]. Thus, when colonizing various host organs, differences in metabolic adaptations may have facilitated a persistence of *A. pleuropneumoniae*. Indeed, the HCA revealed a unique cluster for the lung isolates, while the isolates of the upper respiratory tract were more diverse (Fig. 4). The diversity observed among the latter isolates might reflect the individual appearance of acute disease symptoms, such as coughing.

The most pronounced influence on the metabolic fingerprint during bacterial host organ-specific adaptation was attributed to the spectral range of 1150–1100 cm^{-1}. This frequency area is part of the polysaccharide region (1200–800 cm^{-1}), which is dominated by a complex sequence of peaks associated to stretching ring vibrations of carbohydrates (C—O—C, C—O—P) [47]. Since a comparison of FTIR spectra of the CEs from *A. pleuropneumoniae* from the tonsils with the FTIR spectra recorded from the lung isolates revealed significant differences within their protein and carbohydrate compositions (Fig. 6), it is tempting to speculate that the capsule of the bacteria has an influence on the specific metabolic adaptation of the bacterium to the different host organs. The stronger appearance of β-sheet structures in the CEs from lung isolates indicates a shift towards a higher expression of β-sheet carrying proteins. To decipher the bacterial molecules and mechanisms involved in observed host tissue specific adaptation of *A. pleuropneumoniae* detailed quantitative and qualitative carbohydrate and protein analyses of the capsule are needed, which are clearly beyond the scope of our current work. Preliminary results from an ongoing study also point towards a reduced production of capsule material in the tonsil isolates (Frömbling et al., unpublished) and for *S. aureus* it has already been reported that the loss of capsule expression is advantageous to establish and maintain a chronic infection in humans as well as in animals (e.g. chronic osteomyelitis, bovine mastitis) [48]. Based on our results, it is tempting to speculate that the capsule formation is important for bacterial adaptation to the porcine tonsils as one step towards deciphering persistence of *A. pleuropneumoniae* in infected pig herds.

Conclusions

Altogether, our results indicate an important role of the salivary gland in oral immunity, already eight hours after infection. Contrarily to the lung, *A. pleuropneumoniae* was not able to provoke any immune response in the tonsils. Thus, the specific changes observed in the metabolic fingerprints of *A. pleuropneumoniae* are presumably crucial for bacterial adaptation to porcine tonsils. Further studies will be necessary to decipher the exact role and contribution of the tonsils as a reservoir of host adapted *A. pleuropneumoniae* for the development and establishment of chronic infections.

Additional files

Additional file 1: Information about IL8 primers and optimised qPCR assays. More details about the optimisation and validation of qPCR assays for target gene-specific primers in the pig are included. Particularly in the figure is shown that the suitability of the newly designed primers was verified in separate experiments by performing of a cDNA pool. In melt curve and amplification plots samples are shown in green while controls (no reverse transcription control (NRT) and no template control (NTC)) are shown in yellow and orange respectively. Additionally, an agarose gel electrophoresis of the PCR products of undiluted cDNA pool and controls was performed.

Additional file 2: Hierarchical cluster analysis of FTIR spectroscopic data recorded from A. pleuropneumoniae serotype 2 after 2 and 5 passages under laboratory conditions. After re-isolation from different organs of the infected pigs 1–6 (I1-I6) recorded FTIR spectroscopic data of 2 and 5 passages on laboratory medium were subjected to hierarchical cluster analyses. After two passages nostril and tonsil isolates (upper respiratory tract isolates) cluster apart from all lung isolates, while passaging for five times leads to two intermingled clusters of lung and upper respiratory tract isolates as well as to a decrease in heterogeneity between the samples. For calculation of the dendrogram, the FTIR spectral regions of 900 to 1200 cm^{-1} and 1500 to 1800 cm^{-1} and Ward's algorithm were used.

Acknowledgments
The authors thank K.-H. Waldmann for housing the animals and providing technical equipment.

Funding
Anne Menzel, the design and performance of the animal trial and the animal data collection were supported by the German Research Community (DFG, HE 6419/1-1). Elena L. Sassu and Janna Frömbling as well as all laboratory work, materials, analysis and interpretation of data were supported by the Graduate School for Pig and Poultry Medicine of the University of Veterinary Medicine Vienna, Austria. Elena L. Sassu and Janna Frömbling were supported by the Graduate School for Pig and Poultry Medicine of the University of Veterinary Medicine Vienna.

Authors' contributions
IHP, MES, AS, CD and IM conceived and designed the experiments. AA, IHP, ES and AMe performed infection and clinical examination. MG performed laboratory diagnostic examination. JV produced and verified bacterial inocula. JF and JS performed microbiological analysis of samples. MHT performed histological examination. ES and MP performed cytokine measurements in body fluids. AMG performed acute phase protein quantification in BALF and saliva. AM, ES, CD, and IM carried out analysis of gene expression in tissues. JF and TG performed FTIR and chemometric analysis. ES, JF, MES and IHP wrote the paper. All authors read and critically revised and approved the final manuscript.

Competing interests
The authors declare that they have no competing interests.

Consent for publication
Not applicable.

Author details
[1]University Clinic for Swine, Department of Farm Animals and Veterinary Public Health, University of Veterinary Medicine Vienna, Vienna, Austria. [2]Department of Pathobiology, Functional Microbiology, Institute of Microbiology, University of Veterinary Medicine Vienna, Vienna, Austria. [3]Department of Biomedical Sciences, Institute for Medical Biochemistry, University of Veterinary Medicine Vienna, Vienna, Austria. [4]Department of Animal Medicine and Surgery, University of Murcia, Murcia, Spain. [5]Department of Pathobiology, Institute of Immunology, University of Veterinary Medicine Vienna, Vienna, Austria. [6]Forensic Medicine and Ambulatory Services, Clinic for Swine and Small Ruminants, University of Veterinary Medicine Hannover, Hannover, Germany. [7]Department of Pathology, University of Veterinary Medicine Hannover, Hannover, Germany. [8]Institute for Microbiology, University of Veterinary Medicine Hannover, Hannover, Germany.

References

1. Gottschalk M. Actinobacillosis. In: Zimmerman JJ, Karriker LA, Ramirez A, Schwartz KJ, Stevenson GW, editors. Diseases of Swine. Ames, Iowa, USA: Wiley-Blackwell; 2012. p. 653–69.
2. Chiers K, De Waele T, Pasmans F, Ducatelle R, Haesebrouck F. Virulence factors of Actinobacillus pleuropneumoniae involved in colonization, persistence and induction of lesions in its porcine host. Vet Res. 2010; 41:65.
3. Hellings P, Jorissen M, Ceuppens JL. The Waldeyer's ring. Acta Otorhinolaryngol Belg. 2000;54:237–41.
4. Liebler-Tenorio EM, Pabst R. MALT structure and function in farm animals. Vet Res. 2006;37:257–80.
5. Skovgaard K, Mortensen S, Boye M, Poulsen KT, Campbell FM, et al. Rapid and widely disseminated acute phase protein response after experimental bacterial infection of pigs. Vet Res. 2009;40:23.
6. Gutierrez AM, Yelamos J, Pallares FJ, Gomez-Laguna J, Ceron JJ. Local identification of porcine haptoglobin in salivary gland and diaphragmatic muscle tissues. Histol Histopathol. 2012;27:187–96.
7. Fenwick BW, Osburn BI. Immune responses to the lipopolysaccharides and capsular polysaccharides of Haemophilus pleuropneumoniae in convalescent and immunized pigs. Infect Immun. 1986;54:575–82.
8. Baarsch MJ, Scamurra RW, Burger K, Foss DL, Maheswaran SK, et al. Inflammatory cytokine expression in swine experimentally infected with Actinobacillus pleuropneumoniae. Infect Immun. 1995;63:3587–94.
9. Chen ZW, Chien MS, Chang NY, Chen TH, Wu CM, et al. Mechanisms underlying Actinobacillus pleuropneumoniae exotoxin ApxI induced expression of IL-1beta, IL-8 and TNF-alpha in porcine alveolar macrophages. Vet Res. 2011;42:25.
10. Wenning M SS, Naumann D. Infrared Spectroscopy in the Identification of Microorganisms. In: M Diem PG, JM Chalmers, editor. Handbook of Vibrational Spectroscopy for Medical Diagnosis. Hoboken: John Wiley & Sons; 2008. p. 71–96.
11. Naumann D, Helm D, Labischinski H. Microbiological characterizations by FT-IR spectroscopy. Nature. 1991;351:81–2.
12. Grunert T, Monahan A, Lassnig C, Vogl C, Muller M, et al. Deciphering host genotype-specific impacts on the metabolic fingerprint of Listeria monocytogenes by FTIR spectroscopy. PLoS One. 2014;9:e115959.
13. Wagener K, Grunert T, Prunner I, Ehling-Schulz M, Drillich M. Dynamics of uterine infections with Escherichia coli, Streptococcus uberis and Trueperella pyogenes in post-partum dairy cows and their association with clinical endometritis. Vet J. 2014;202:527–32.
14. Leiner G, Franz B, Strutzberg K, Gerlach GF. A novel enzyme-linked immunosorbent assay using the recombinant Actinobacillus pleuropneumoniae ApxII antigen for diagnosis of pleuropneumonia in pig herds. Clin Diagn Lab Immunol. 1999;6:630–2.
15. Hennig I, Teutenberg-Riedel B, Gerlach GF. Downregulation of a protective Actinobacillus pleuropneumoniae antigen during the course of infection. Microb Pathog. 1999;26:53–63.
16. Baarsch MJ, Foss DL, Murtaugh MP. Pathophysiologic correlates of acute porcine pleuropneumonia. Am J Vet Res. 2000;61:684–90.
17. Hennig-Pauka I, Baltes N, Jacobsen I, Stratmann-Selke J, Gerlach GF, et al. Study of the virulence of Actinobacillus pleuropneumoniae in finishing pigs as a basis for vaccination development. Berl Munch Tierarztl Wochenschr. 2008;121:189 97.
18. Brauer C, Hennig-Pauka I, Hoeltig D, Buettner FF, Beyerbach M, et al. Experimental Actinobacillus pleuropneumoniae challenge in swine: comparison of computed tomographic and radiographic findings during disease. BMC Vet Res. 2012;8:47.
19. Hannan PC, Bhogal BS, Fish JP. Tylosin tartrate and tiamutilin effects on experimental piglet pneumonia induced with pneumonic pig lung homogenate containing mycoplasmas, bacteria and viruses. Res Vet Sci. 1982;33:76–88.
20. Kozlov AV, van Griensven M, Haindl S, Kehrer I, Duvigneau JC, et al. Peritoneal inflammation in pigs is associated with early mitochondrial dysfunction in liver and kidney. Inflammation. 2010;33:295–305.
21. Duvigneau JC, Hartl RT, Groiss S, Gemeiner M. Quantitative simultaneous multiplex real-time PCR for the detection of porcine cytokines. J Immunol Methods. 2005;306:16–27.
22. Soler L, Gutierrez A, Martinez-Subiela S, Ceron JJ. Fast measurement of serum amyloid A in different specimens from swine by using a new one-step time-resolved fluorescent immunoassay. J Vet Diagn Invest. 2011;23:902–8.
23. Soler L, Luyten T, Stinckens A, Buys N, Ceron JJ, et al. Serum amyloid A3 (SAA3), not SAA1 appears to be the major acute phase SAA isoform in the pig. Vet Immunol Immunopathol. 2011;141:109–15.
24. Soler L, Gutierrez A, Mullebner A, Ceron JJ, Duvigneau JC. Towards a better understanding of salivary and meat juice acute phase proteins determination in pigs: an expression study. Vet Immunol Immunopathol. 2013; 156:91–8.
25. Gutierrez AM, Martinez-Subiela S, Ceron JJ. Evaluation of an immunoassay for determination of haptoglobin concentration in various biological specimens from swine. Am J Vet Res. 2009;70:691–6.
26. Gutierrez AM, Escribano D, Fuentes M, Ceron JJ. Circadian pattern of acute phase proteins in the saliva of growing pigs. Vet J. 2013;196:167–70.
27. Hussy D, Schlatter Y, Miserez R, Inzana T, Frey J. PCR-based identification of serotype 2 isolates of Actinobacillus pleuropneumoniae biovars I and II. Vet Microbiol. 2004;99:307–10.
28. Henderson I, Duggleby CJ, Turnbull PC. Differentiation of Bacillus anthracis from other Bacillus cereus group bacteria with the PCR. Int J Syst Bacteriol. 1994;44:99–105.
29. Oberreuter H, Seiler H, Scherer S. Identification of coryneform bacteria and related taxa by Fourier-transform infrared (FT-IR) spectroscopy. Int J Syst Evol Microbiol. 2002;52:91–100.
30. Schabauer L, Wenning M, Huber I, Ehling-Schulz M. Novel physico-chemical diagnostic tools for high throughput identification of bovine mastitis associated gram-positive, catalase-negative cocci. BMC Vet Res. 2014;10:156.
31. Grunert T, Wenning M, Barbagelata MS Fricker M, Sordelli DO, et al. Rapid and reliable identification of Staphylococcus aureus capsular serotypes by means of artificial neural network-assisted Fourier transform infrared spectroscopy. J Clin Microbiol. 2013;51:2261–6.
32. Dubreuil JD, Jacques M, Mittal KR, Gottschalk M. Actinobacillus pleuropneumoniae surface polysaccharides: their role in diagnosis and immunogenicity. Anim Health Res Rev. 2000;1:73–93.
33. Naumann D. Infrared Spectroscopy in Microbiology. In: Meyers RA, editor. Encyclopedia of Analytical Chemistry 102–131 ed. John Wiley & sons: Chichester; 2000.
34. Beekes M, Lasch P, Naumann D. Analytical applications of Fourier transform-infrared (FT-IR) spectroscopy in microbiology and prion research. Vet Microbiol. 2007;123:305–19.
35. Hoeltig D, Hennig-Pauka I, Thies K, Rehm T, Beyerbach M, et al. A novel Respiratory Health Score (RHS) supports a role of acute lung damage and pig breed in the course of an Actinobacillus pleuropneumoniae infection. BMC Vet Res. 2009;5:14.
36. Fossum C, Wattrang E, Fuxler L, Jensen KT, Wallgren P. Evaluation of various cytokines (IL-6, IFN-alpha, IFN-gamma, TNF-alpha) as markers for acute bacterial infection in swine–a possible role for serum interleukin-6. Vet Immunol Immunopathol. 1998;64:161–72.
37. Wyns H, Croubels S, Vandekerckhove M, Demeyere K, De Backer P, et al. Multiplex analysis of pro-inflammatory cytokines in serum of Actinobacillus pleuropneumoniae-infected pigs. Res Vet Sci. 2015;102:45–8.
38. Lauritzen B, Lykkesfeldt J, Skaanild MT, Angen O, Nielsen JP, et al. Putative biomarkers for evaluating antibiotic treatment: an experimental model of porcine Actinobacillus pleuropneumoniae infection. Res Vet Sci. 2003;74: 261–70.

39. Heegaard PM, Klausen J, Nielsen JP, Gonzalez-Ramon N, Pineiro M, et al. The porcine acute phase response to infection with Actinobacillus pleuropneumoniae. Haptoglobin, C-reactive protein, major acute phase protein and serum amyloid A protein are sensitive indicators of infection. Comp Biochem Physiol B Biochem Mol Biol. 1998;119:365–73.
40. Sorensen NS, Tegtmeier C, Andresen LO, Pineiro M, Toussaint MJ, et al. The porcine acute phase protein response to acute clinical and subclinical experimental infection with Streptococcus suis. Vet Immunol Immunopathol. 2006;113:157–68.
41. Ramadas RA, Wu L, LeVine AM. Surfactant protein A enhances production of secretory leukoprotease inhibitor and protects it from cleavage by matrix metalloproteinases. J Immunol. 2009;182:1560–7.
42. Chiers K, Haesebrouck F, van Overbeke I, Charlier G, Ducatelle R. Early in vivo interactions of Actinobacillus pleuropneumoniae with tonsils of pigs. Vet Microbiol. 1999;68:301–6.
43. Alvarez-Ordonez A, Mouwen DJ, Lopez M, Prieto M. Fourier transform infrared spectroscopy as a tool to characterize molecular composition and stress response in foodborne pathogenic bacteria. J Microbiol Methods. 2011;84:369–78.
44. Afroz T, Biliouris K, Kaznessis Y, Beisel CL. Bacterial sugar utilization gives rise to distinct single-cell behaviours. Mol Microbiol. 2014;93:1093–103.
45. Kotula JW, Kerns SJ, Shaket LA, Siraj L, Collins JJ, et al. Programmable bacteria detect and record an environmental signal in the mammalian gut. Proc Natl Acad Sci U S A. 2014;111:4838–43.
46. Sidibe M, Messier S, Lariviere S, Gottschalk M, Mittal KR. Detection of Actinobacillus pleuropneumoniae in the porcine upper respiratory tract as a complement to serological tests. Can J Vet Res. 1993;57:204–8.
47. Yu C, Irudayaraj J. Spectroscopic characterization of microorganisms by Fourier transform infrared microspectroscopy. Biopolymers. 2005;77:368–77.
48. Tuchscherr L, Loffler B, Buzzola FR, Sordelli DO. Staphylococcus aureus adaptation to the host and persistence: role of loss of capsular polysaccharide expression. Future Microbiol. 2010;5:1823–32.

9

Genotyping and comparative pathology of *Spirocerca* in black-backed jackals (*Canis mesomelas*) in South Africa

M. M. Bumby[1*], M. C. Williams[1], J. C. A. Steyl[1], R. Harrison-White[2], H. Lutermann[3], G. T. Fosgate[4], P. J. de Waal[5], J. Mitha[5] and S. J. Clift[1]

Abstract

Background: The pathology of spirocercosis, a disease caused by the infestation of carnivores with the nematode *Spirocerca lupi*, has been extensively described in domestic dogs and coyotes. However, it has not been described in wild carnivores in South Africa. The aim of this study was to evaluate whether black-backed jackals are a host for *Spirocerca* species and to provide a detailed description of the associated pathology. Jackals were also stratified according to age and the *Spirocerca* species recovered were characterized using molecular techniques.

Methods: Standard necropsies were performed on routinely culled jackals from three of the nine provinces of South Africa during the period June 2012 to February 2013. Jackals were screened for the presence of pathognomonic *Spirocerca*-induced lesions and for evidence of aberrant migration. Relevant samples were submitted for histopathology and collected larvae were genotyped at nine microsatellite loci.

Results: *Spirocerca lupi*-associated aortic lesions were found in 16 of 93 (17%) black-backed jackals. Of these, four (25%) were associated with *S. lupi* larvae. Genotyping of the larvae revealed amplification of all nine loci that amplified dog-derived *S. lupi*, with the same level of polymorphism in the allele size ranges. Only 1 of 93 jackals had an esophageal nodule with concurrent *S. lupi*-induced aortic aneurysms. The single esophageal nodule found did not contain adult nematodes, nor did it communicate with the esophageal lumen. None of the jackals that were examined had macroscopically evident spondylitis, which is frequently reported in the dog. Histopathology of the *S. lupi*-induced aortic lesions in the jackal revealed replacement of elastic and smooth muscle fibers by fibrous connective tissue. In cases where inflammation was present, the inflammatory infiltrate consisted predominantly of eosinophils. The single esophageal nodule histologically resembled the early inflammatory nodule described in dogs and consisted of fibrous connective tissue, multifocal accumulation of lymphocytes, plasma cells and rare hemosiderin-laden macrophages.

Conclusions: These lesions suggest that the life cycle of *S. lupi* may not or only rarely be completed in jackals. A possible explanation might be that jackals are relatively resistant to developing significant pathology associated with *S. lupi*-infection. However, before any conclusions can be drawn, many more jackals, including those that die naturally will have to be investigated for evidence of *S. lupi* infection.

Keywords: Aortic aneurysms, Black-backed jackal, Genotyping, Esophageal nodule, Resistance, *Spirocerca lupi*, Spirocercosis

* Correspondence: asteenkamp3@gmail.com
[1]Section Pathology, Department of Paraclinical Sciences, Faculty of Veterinary Science, University of Pretoria, Private bag X04, Onderstepoort 0110, South Africa
Full list of author information is available at the end of the article

Background

Spirocerca lupi is a spirurid nematode of *Canidae*, especially domestic dogs (*Canis familiaris*), which occurs particularly in the tropical and subtropical regions of the world [4]. Dogs become infected by eating the intermediate host (i.e. coprophagous dung beetles), paratenic hosts (e.g. lizards) containing encysted larvae or through coprophagia [14, 42]. Larvae excyst in the stomach, penetrate the gastric mucosa and migrate in the wall of the gastric, gastro-epiploic and celiac arteries to reach the caudal thoracic aorta where they mature to adults. Young adult worms then migrate from the aorta to the caudal esophagus where they develop to mature worms within nodules in the esophageal submucosa and adventitia [42]. Female worms burrow through the esophageal mucosa to establish an opening to the lumen where eggs are deposited, thereby completing the life cycle [42]. Not all ingested larvae reach the aorta; some migrate to aberrant sites, including the kidney, urinary bladder wall, subcutaneous tissues, interdigital skin, trachea, mediastinum, lung and spinal cord [3, 13, 16].

Lesions pathognomonic for spirocercosis in dogs are well documented and include scarring and mineralization of the caudal thoracic aorta with aneurysm formation, spondylitis of the ventral aspect of the caudal thoracic vertebrae and the formation of caudal esophageal nodules [17]. Microscopic aortic lesions that have been reported in dogs include hemorrhage and neutrophil infiltration into vessel walls, smooth muscle and elastic fiber degeneration with replacement by collagen, and occasional foci of mineralization and heterotopic bone formation [15, 42]. Histologically, early esophageal nodules are inflammatory and collagenous. They consist of central necrotic tracts associated with worms and cell debris, surrounded by a collar of degenerate neutrophils, fewer eosinophils and peripheral collagenous stroma with foci of lymphoplasmacytic inflammation. More mature nodules are predominantly fibroblastic with multiple peripheral foci of lymphoplasmacytic inflammation. In 20% of cases the nodules proceed to sarcomatous neoplasia, namely osteosarcoma, fibrosarcoma or anaplastic sarcoma [15, 18]. Esophageal nodules have erroneously been described as granulomas in the past [3, 4], but although scattered macrophages are often present, they rarely predominate as would be expected in granulomatous inflammation [17–19, 42]. Histologically, the spirocercosis-related spondylitic lesion that occurs in close proximity to the peri-aortitis and aortic aneurysms in the caudal thoracic aorta consists of periosteal new woven bone formation perpendicular to and continuous with the underlying mature cortical bone. Scarce lymphoplasmacytic inflammation is observed in tissues adjacent to the periosteum [26].

Spirocercosis has been reported in a variety of wild carnivores, including the coyote (*Canis latrans),* wolf (*Canis lupus*), red fox (*Vulpes vulpes*), grey fox (*Urocyon cinereoargenteus*), neotropical bush dog (*Speothos venaticus*), bobcat (*Felis rufus*) and cheetah (*Acinonyx jubatus)* [4, 12, 30, 32, 35, 38]. *S. lupi*-induced aortic lesions were found in 123 of 150 (82%) coyotes, 23 of 66 (35%) bobcats, one of five (20%) grey foxes and one of two (50%) red foxes examined in West Texas from 1973 to 1977 [32]. The larvae were identified as *S. lupi* by microscopy, which has low specificity [39].

Black-backed jackals are widely distributed throughout southern Africa, are especially prevalent in farming areas and are also closely associated with domestic dogs, particularly in rural and semi-rural areas [37]. The jackal diet includes a large proportion of insects (including beetles), small mammals and lizards and therefore they may represent a reservoir host for *Spirocerca* species [28, 41]. This study reports the results of a survey on 93 black-backed jackals with emphasis on the prevalence of infection, the pathology of infection and the genotype of the parasite in this species.

Methods

Sample population

Black-backed jackals that were routinely culled by farmers in the North West, Gauteng and Mpumalanga provinces of South Africa during the period June 2012 to February 2013 were selected for the study.

Baseline data

Baseline data including age, sex and geographic location were recorded. Based on dentition, jackals were categorized as pups of one to six months of age, juveniles of seven to twelve months of age and adults older than one year, according to a published technique [27], together with R. Harrison-White's personal experience from known age groups of recaptured wild jackals. This technique involves the determination of the amount of wear on the cusps and fissures (grooves) of the first two incisors. One to six month old jackals were classified as such by the presence of deciduous teeth as all of the permanent teeth are present in jackal from the age of six-months [21]. Juvenile jackals were identified by the presence of a full set of permanent teeth with the absence of any wearing of the cusps on both incisor 1 and incisor 2. Jackals older than one year showed variable wear on the cusps and fissures (grooves) of the first two incisors. The proportion of *S. lupi*-associated lesions was compared by age and sex using chi-square or Fisher exact tests in available software (Epi Info, version 6.04, CDC, Atlanta, Georgia, USA). Statistical significance was established at $P < 0.05$.

Gross examination

Necropsies were performed on all jackals following the standard necropsy technique used by the Pathology Section, Department of Paraclinical Sciences, Faculty of Veterinary Science, University of Pretoria. The aorta, vertebrae, esophagus, stomach and intestines were examined for possible *Spirocerca*-associated lesions and other organs / tissues (including the skin, subcutis, mediastinum, kidneys, urinary bladder, spleen, liver, heart, lung and trachea) were carefully examined for signs of aberrant migration. Macroscopically visible lesions were recorded, measured and described in detail. Tissues from macroscopically visible lesions were sampled and preserved in 10% buffered formalin for microscopic evaluation. In the event of aortic pathology being present, the whole aorta and adventitial lymph nodes (*Lnn. Lumbales aortici)* (when present) were collected and placed in 10% buffered formalin. Samples of aortas from an additional six uninfected jackals were collected and fixed in 10% buffered formalin to serve as negative tissue controls to facilitate accurate interpretation of aortic pathology. The thoracic vertebrae were examined for evidence of spondylitis.

Histopathology

Samples collected for light microscopic evaluation were wax-embedded, sectioned and stained with hematoxylin-eosin (H&E) following standard methods [5]. Processing of collected samples was done by the histotechnology laboratory of the Faculty of Veterinary Science, University of Pretoria. Light microscopic evaluation of tissue sections was done by the primary investigator using an Olympus model CX21FS1 light microscope. Aortic sections were additionally stained with Masson's Trichrome and Verhoeff's stain following standard methods for the detection of fibrous connective tissue and elastic fibers, respectively [5].

The severity and duration of inflammation within the sections was graded as mild, moderate or severe and as acute, subacute, chronic or chronic-active, respectively (Table 1).

Genotyping of *Spirocerca* larvae

Larvae that were collected from the subintimal surface of the thoracic aorta as well as from peri-aortic nodules were submitted in 95% ethanol to the Department of Genetics, University of Pretoria, for genotyping. Previously published protocols were used for the deoxyribonucleic acid (DNA) extraction, polymerase chain reaction (PCR) amplification and sequencing [11]. Polymorphic forward primers of nine microsatellite loci for *S. lupi* from domestic dogs were labeled fluorescently. After combining the nine primer sets into a single multiplex reaction, the Quantitect Multiplex PCR kit (Qiagen) was used according to the manufacturer's protocol. An ABI3500xl Genetic Analyser (Applied Biosystems), using GeneScan LIZ500 Internal Size Standard (Applied Biosystems) was used to separate and measure all allele sizes. By evaluating chromatograms in GeneMarker™ version 2.4.0. (SoftGenetics LLC), the genotype of each individual larva was established. Following published protocols, using the program Arlequin version 3.5.1, pairwise F_{ST} values were calculated from larvae collected from jackals and from dogs from three different provinces in South Africa [20].

Results

A total of 51 female and 42 male jackals were examined, of which 67 originated from the North West province, 18 from Gauteng province and 8 from Mpumalanga province of the Republic of South Africa. *S. lupi*-associated aortic lesions were identified in 16 (17%) jackals and did not vary by sex ($P = 0.965$), with 9 being female (56%) and 7 being male (44%). Three of 30 juvenile jackals (10%) and 13 of 48 adult jackals (27%) had *S. lupi*-associated lesions. Thirteen pups were examined, none of which showed any *S. lupi*-associated lesions. Overall, older jackals were more likely than juvenile jackals and pups to have *S. lupi*-associated lesions ($P = 0.018$). A total of 13 larvae were recovered from four of the *S. lupi*-positive cases. A single 4-year-old jackal with *S. lupi*-induced aortic aneurysms also had an esophageal nodule that was devoid of adult nematodes. None had macroscopically evident spondylitis and no lesions suggestive of larval migration were present in the stomach, intestines or other organs.

Gross pathology

Gross lesions in the aorta ranged from plaque-like lesions, intimal pitting consisting of a roughened, irregular intima

Table 1 Grading of inflammation of histopathology tissue sections

Grading of inflammation			
Severity		Duration	
Mild	≤400 inflammatory cells in one high power field (400X magnification)	Acute	Predominance of polymorphonuclear leukocytes (neutrophils and eosinophils), accompanied by prominent inflammatory edema.
Moderate	400–900 inflammatory cells in one high power field (400X magnification)	Subacute	Polymophonuclear inflammatory infiltrate mixed with mononuclear cells (lymphocytes, macrophages and plasma cells). Edema present, but mild.
Severe	>900 inflammatory cells in one high power field (400X magnification)	Chronic	Large numbers of plasma cells, lymphocytes, macrophages and significantly fewer polymorphonuclear leukocytes, accompanied by small blood vessel proliferation and fibroblasts (granulation tissue).
		Chronic - active	Large numbers of plasma cells, lymphocytes, macrophages and polymorphonuclear leukocytes, accompanied by proliferation of small blood vessels and fibroblasts (granulation tissue).

to aortic aneurysms of variable size (Figs. 1 and 2). In two cases, small red *S. lupi* larvae were visible beneath the intimal surface. These were associated with small hemorrhages and hyperemia of the intimal surface. Older aortic lesions showed scarring and thickening of the aorta, with loss of elasticity, and aortic aneurysms were visible from the serosal aspect of the aorta. All aortic lesions were confined to the extra-cardiac, distal thoracic aorta. Observed aneurysms were mostly located in the region of thoracic vertebrae (T) T10 to T13, but ranged from T6-T13. The smallest aneurysm measured 3 mm (mm) in length, 3 mm in breadth and 1 mm in depth, whilst the largest was 12x13x10 mm. The median number of aneurysms was 3 and the range 1–6.

Only one esophageal nodule was present in one of the jackals examined (a 4 year-old female jackal with concurrent aortic aneurysms) (Fig. 3). The sessile, cream-colored nodule was firm and smooth to the touch and mineralization was absent. It was not ulcerated, there was no communication with the esophageal lumen, investigated using a 1 mm diameter blunt probe, and it contained no adult nematodes. The nodule was situated between the 8th and 9th thoracic vertebrae, 58 mm cranial to the diaphragm and measured 25 mm in length, 14 mm in breadth and 12 mm in depth. There was no evidence of esophagitis, esophageal dilatation proximal to the nodule or esophageal stricture formation. No other nodules were identified in that or any other jackal.

Histopathology

Lesions in all aortas from infected jackals were either in a chronic or chronic-active stage of inflammation or there was simply evidence of repair via fibrosis with no concurrent inflammation. The chronic-active cases (Fig. 4) were characterized by large numbers of eosinophils, plasma cells, lymphocytes and fewer neutrophils, hemosiderin-laden macrophages and the occasional mast cell in the tunica adventitia (mainly) and tunica media. The inflammation was severe and predominantly focally-extensive and frequently associated with larvae. Larval migration tracts consisted of necrotic cellular debris, surrounded by the above-mentioned inflammatory cells (especially eosinophils) and copious amounts of fibrin. Also associated with the tracts were large numbers of plump fibroblasts and small caliber blood vessels with hypertrophied endothelial cells (granulation tissue). Following published descriptive techniques, larval cross sections were characterized from the periphery to the interior by a thick, smooth outer cuticle followed by a hypodermis that expanded into the pseudocelom to form two prominent stalked lateral chords, celomyarian-polymyarian musculature, moderate amounts of eosinophilic material in the pseudocelom and a large intestine lined by uninucleate cuboidal epithelial cells with a prominent tall brush border [23]. No mineralization was evident in the larval sections examined. Chronic inflammatory cases were characterized by mild to moderate multifocal inflammation within the tunica media and tunica adventitia. The inflammatory infiltrate consisted predominantly of plasma cells and fewer lymphocytes, hemosiderin-laden macrophages, eosinophils and scant mast cells. Healed aortic lesions (Fig. 5) were characterized by the absence of inflammatory cells and replacement of the elastic and smooth muscle fibers within the tunica intima, –media and -adventitia by fibrous connective tissue compared with the normal aorta (Fig. 5 inset). All 16 cases (100%), however, showed fibrosis and elastic fiber destruction, mainly within the tunica intima and –media and to some extent in the tunica

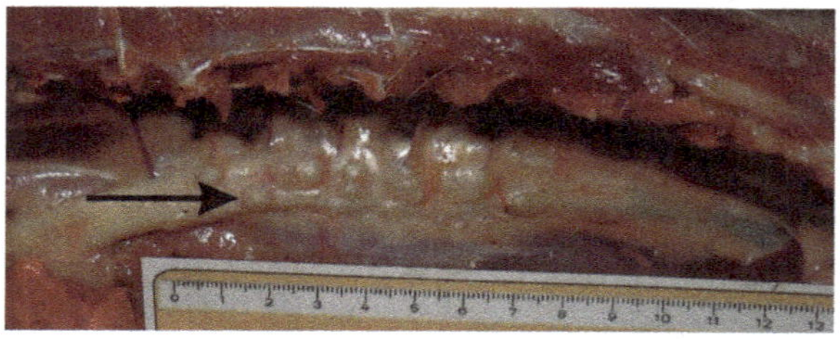

Fig. 1 Macroscopic view of aortic aneurysms in a jackal with *S. lupi* (→)

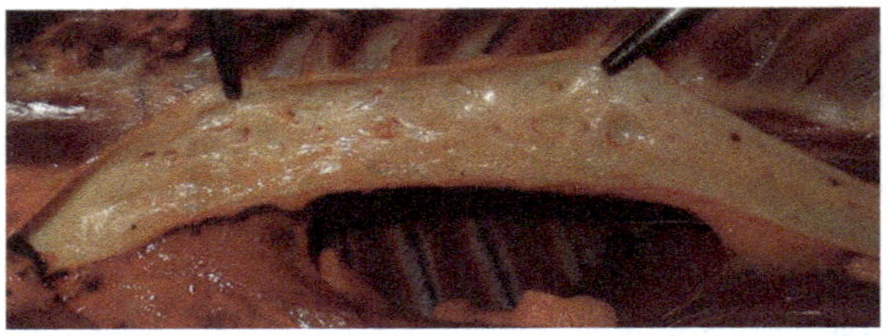

Fig. 2 Macroscopic view of the intimal surface of aortic aneurysms in a jackal with *S. lupi*

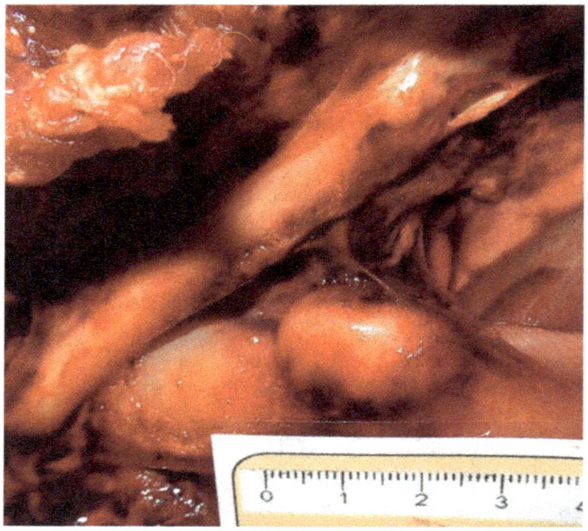

Fig. 3 Macroscopic view of the esophageal nodule in an infected jackal

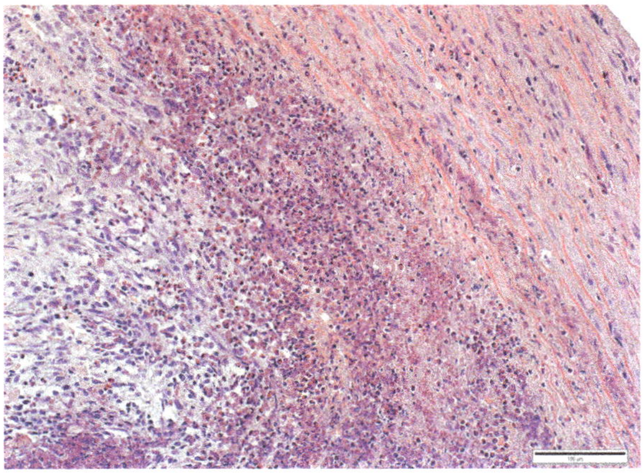

Fig. 4 Histological transverse section of the aorta in the chronic-active inflammatory stage in an infected jackal. Note the abundance of eosinophils. Hematoxylin and eosin (HE)

adventitia, whether inflammation was present or not. Fibrosis ranged from mild to severe, multifocal to coalescing and stained blue with Masson's Trichrome stain. Fibrosis was associated with elastic fiber destruction within the tunica intima, –media and –adventitia (Fig. 6). The internal elastic lamina of the tunica intima was disrupted and the endothelial layer was inconspicuous. The remaining elastic fibers (black with Verhoeff's stain) (Fig. 7) were intermittently dispersed throughout the collagen bundles or were haphazardly arranged in bundles and perpendicularly orientated to the collagen. In severe cases there was complete replacement of elastic fibers within the tunica media by collagen. Eleven cases (69%) had fibroblast metaplasia with mineralization, cartilage and/or heterotopic bone formation

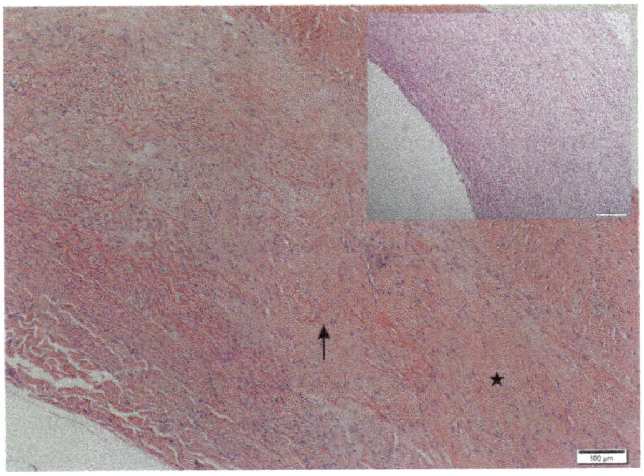

Fig. 5 Histological transverse section of the aorta in the repair via fibrosis stage in an infected jackal. Note the elastic fiber degeneration (↑), mural fibrosis (*) and the absence of inflammatory cells. HE. *Inset:* histological transverse section of a normal aorta in a non-affected jackal at the same magnification. HE

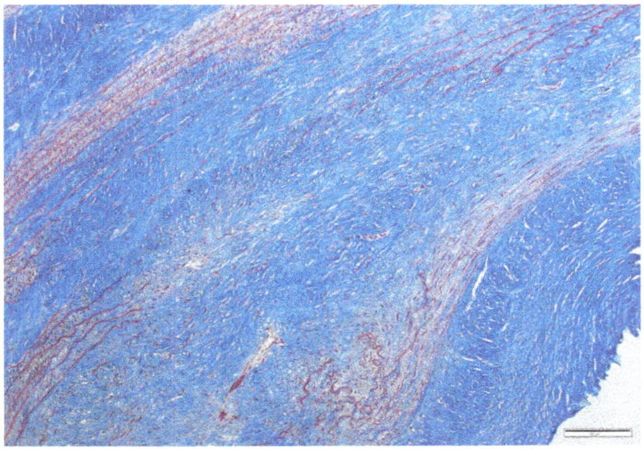

Fig. 6 Histological transverse section of the aorta in an infected jackal. Note the extensive fibrosis (blue). Masson's Trichrome stain

with the occasional presence of hematopoietic cells within the tunica media.

Histologically the esophageal nodule was characterized by large amounts of collagen within the submucosa and extending into the tunica muscularis, with intervening mature fibrocytes and multifocal small clusters of inflammatory cells consisting predominantly of plasma cells and fewer lymphocytes, macrophages and occasional eosinophils. The inflammatory cell infiltrate usually surrounded small foci of necrotic cellular debris, which were often mineralized (Fig. 8). No nematodes or eggs were present in the sections examined.

Genotyping

All nine loci that amplified dog-derived *S. lupi* also produced amplification in larvae that were collected from jackals. All four *S. lupi* populations (three from dogs and one from jackals) showed very small, but significant differentiation from one another. Pairwise F_{ST} values were <0.093, all $P < 0.01$ indicating a single population.

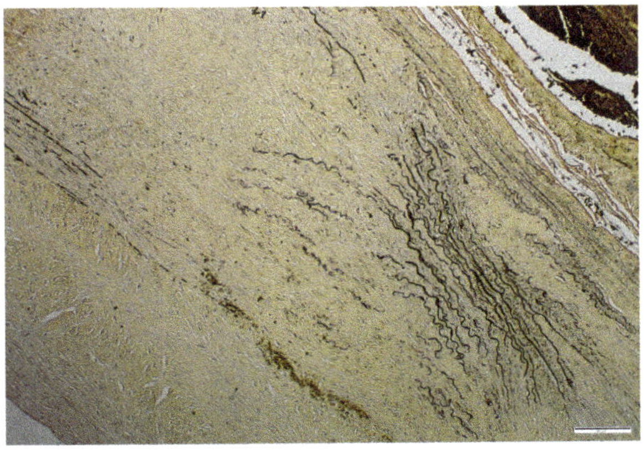

Fig. 7 Histological transverse section of the aorta in an infected jackal. Note the elastic fiber (black) disruption and destruction. Verhoeff's stain

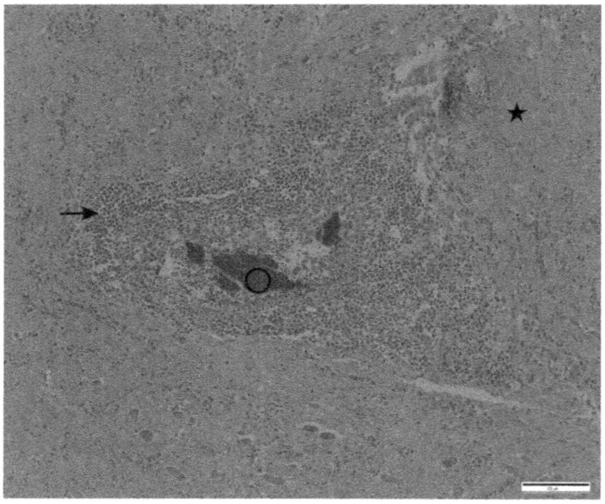

Fig. 8 Histological section of the esophageal nodule in an infected jackal. [inflammatory cells (→), calcified necrotic debris (o), collagen (*)]. HE

Discussion

Our study showed that *S. lupi* is present in the black-backed jackal population in South Africa based on the microsatellite data as well as macroscopic and microscopic findings. The molecular study indicated a close relationship between the *S. lupi* found in dogs and jackals in South Africa. This was illustrated by the amplification of all nine loci in larvae collected from jackals similar to the dog-derived *S. lupi*, with the same levels of polymorphism that were observed as for dogs, where the allele size ranges of the jackal-derived samples fell within the range that was found for dog-derived samples for most loci. The nematodes found in most of the previous studies involving wild carnivores were not molecularly characterized. However, *Spirocerca* species isolated from gastric nodules in a red fox in Denmark was genetically distinct by 7 to 9% from isolates of *S. lupi* from Africa, Europe and Asia, and the authors suggested the existence of a cryptic species within *Spirocerca* [1].

The limitations of this study included the short duration of the study, the relatively small number of animals with *S. lupi*-associated lesions and the possibility that samples were not representative of all jackals, since culls were not randomly selected. This should be addressed in future research. Despite these limitations however, significant data were obtained in this study, namely the genetic classification of *S. lupi* and the presence of *S. lupi*-induced lesions in 16 of 93 jackals. The fact that there was no completion of the parasite's life cycle in any of the 16 infected jackals certainly warrants further investigation.

The *S. lupi*-associated aortic pathology present in jackals is largely similar to that described in dogs, namely intimal thickening, aneurysm formation and dystrophic mineralization as a result of elastic fiber damage within the tunica media, with eventual fibrous replacement and ossification with hematopoietic tissue formation [3, 4, 15, 26]. These characteristics were also described in wild carnivores from the northern hemisphere [32]. The most striking difference between the *S. lupi*-associated aortic pathology in dogs and jackals is the predominance of eosinophils within larval tracts in the jackals' aortas. In the majority of dogs that have been necropsied in South Africa, the larval tracts consist predominantly of neutrophils and far fewer eosinophils [18]. However, most *S. lupi*-induced lesions are in an advanced stage when a necropsy is requested on a dog that has died of spirocercosis, whilst dogs that have died from causes other than *S. lupi* might have incidental and therefore early *S. lupi*-induced lesions, similar to those in jackals. Thus far there has been no systematic study of early lesions in dogs. The *S. lupi*-induced esophageal nodule found in one jackal in this study resembled that of the early inflammatory and collagenous stage in the dog, with no worms or eggs present, no communication with the esophageal lumen and no evidence of neoplastic transformation. None of the jackals examined had caudal thoracic ventral vertebral body spondylitis, which is pathognomonic for *S. lupi* in dogs [17]. In dogs, the larvae frequently show aberrant migration, for which there was no evidence in this study. Various complications following the normal and aberrant migration of larvae in the dog have been described (aortic rupture, esophageal perforation, pneumothorax, pyothorax), none of which were observed in the jackals examined.

Spirocerca-induced lesions in jackals differed from those described in wild carnivores in the northern hemisphere in that larval tracts in the jackal's aortas were dominated by eosinophils and the jackal's esophageal nodule was predominantly fibrous, whereas larval tracts and esophageal nodules in wild carnivores in the northern hemisphere were predominantly described as granulomatous, although in coyotes eosinophils featured prominently in the cellular infiltrate [32]. On the other hand, *Spirocerca*-induced lesions in the red fox (*Vulpes vulpes*) have been reported as gastric and omental nodules characterized microscopically by fibroplasia and an inflammatory infiltrate consisting of lymphocytes, plasma cells, hemosiderin-laden macrophages and fewer neutrophils and eosinophils [1, 22].

Lack of communication of esophageal nodules as observed in the jackal may represent a general trend in wild carnivores. Of 150 coyotes examined in Texas (USA), only 11 (7%) had *S. lupi*-induced esophageal nodules and in only 5 (45%) did the worms establish communication with the esophageal lumen [32]. In a red fox with *Spirocerca*-induced gastric nodules in one study, the worms did establish communication with the gastric lumen, but no *S. lupi* eggs were found in the feces using the fecal flotation egg count technique [29].

Sarcomatous transformation of the esophageal nodule and *S. lupi*-associated spondylitits of the ventral bodies of the caudal thoracic vertebrae were not observed in the jackals in this study and have not been reported in wild carnivores [32]. However, aberrant larval migration has been reported in coyotes, as well as complications of larval migration in a neotropical bush dog (*Speothos venaticus*) and in a red fox [10, 29, 35]. Further studies are needed to establish whether aberrant larval migration or complications of larval migration occur in jackals.

The apparent low pathogenicity found in jackals in this study may suggest that spirocercosis in jackals is merely an incidental finding. However, this is purely speculative as the jackals that were culled in this study were culled for reasons unrelated to illness and the timeline and burden of infection is unknown. Furthermore, unrecorded mortalities may occur in jackals suffering from more severe infestations. Numerous theories exist to explain the differences in pathologies observed in jackals, other wild carnivores (e.g. coyotes) and domestic dogs with spirocercosis, some of which are briefly examined below.

One such theory is that jackals are much older hosts to *S. lupi* and have evolved resistance over time to *S. lupi* infection, whereas dogs might be a far more recent host [33, 43]. The predominance of eosinophils in the jackals' and coyotes' microscopic aortic sections may support the idea that these carnivores may have evolved resistance towards *S. lupi* infection. Eosinophils are potent cells capable of combatting helminth infections and maintaining tissue homeostasis, which significantly influences the efficiency of the innate immune response [6, 36] and presumably helps to minimize the *S. lupi* burden, thus protecting the host at the expense of the parasite [33].

Another theory to consider might be that the dog's immune system is relatively immature and therefore suboptimal for dealing with *S. lupi* infections. During the process of selection and domestication of dogs, many of the structural modifications of modern breeds are evident in changes in the rate of development [9]. These changes are dominated by pedomorphosis (the retention of juvenile morphological characteristics) [24]. It is possible that pedomorphosis has also rendered the dogs' immune system immature.

The difference in the immune response to parasitic infection between urban dogs and jackals might also be due to jackals being scavengers [34], as are coyotes [2]. However, free-ranging or feral dogs are also efficient scavengers, especially in under-resourced communities [8]. Scavengers such as jackals, coyotes, free-ranging and feral dogs have increased exposure to a wider variety and number of microorganisms and/or toxins from decomposed carcasses and refuse [7]. Therefore, they may have evolved an improved innate immune response to infection compared to the domestic dog, which may have an inadequate innate immunity as a result of selective breeding and reduced priming of the immune system. This might explain the abundance of eosinophils in the aortic lesions of the infected jackals examined in this study. Future research should address the immune response against parasitic infections in scavenging (i.e. free-ranging and feral) dogs, versus non-scavenging (i.e. urban) dogs to further evaluate this aspect.

Finally, another aspect worthy of investigation is the composition of the intestinal microflora in jackals, free-ranging and feral dogs and urbanized domestic dogs (i.e. scavengers versus non-scavengers). Various factors such as diet, the use of antibiotics and microbial inoculation can bring about permanent or transient changes in the intestinal microflora and can involve up to 20% of the bacterial strains [25, 31]. Since the main immunological function of gut microflora is the development and maintenance of homeostasis of local and systemic immunity, the composition of the intestinal microflora should influence the immune response [25]. Whereas it is known that antibiotics have a profound effect on the composition of intestinal microflora, the consumption of highly specialized and purified commercial diets by urban dogs is bound to influence the intestinal microflora composition versus the varied diet of jackals, coyotes and scavenger dogs [31]. It seems feasible therefore that specialized diets and antibiotic therapy would impact on the immune response to *S. lupi* infection in urban dogs [31].

Conclusion

It has been established that *S. lupi* is present in the black-backed jackal population in South Africa, but in the sample population in this study the parasite did not appear to complete its life cycle. A possible explanation for this is that jackals may have evolved resistance towards *S. lupi* infection with only moderate immune responses that minimize energetic investment as well as associated pathologies. However, due to the relatively small sample size of this study, there is a clear need to investigate *S. lupi* infestation in a far greater number of jackal. Such an investigation should include necropsies on sick jackals that die and surveys of jackals' feces for the presence of *S. lupi* DNA [40].

Abbreviations

DNA: Deoxyribonucleic acid; et al.: et alia (and others); Fig.: Figure; HE: Haematoxylin and eosin; i.e.: id est. (that is); mm: millimeter; PCR: Polymerase chain reaction; T: Thoracic vertebrae

Acknowledgements

The authors are grateful for Mr. Craig Shepstone for his assistance with transport to culling sites, record keeping and taking of photographs. We thank the staff of the Histopathology Laboratory, Section of Pathology, Department of Paraclinical Sciences, Faculty of Veterinary Science, University of Pretoria, for their careful preparation of tissue sections.

Funding

The University of Pretoria, Faculty of Veterinary Science, Department of Paraclinical Sciences, Section of Pathology were responsible for all costs related to the research and manuscript.

Authors' contributions

MMB collected, analyzed and interpreted data and is the main author of this manuscript. SJC is a major contributor in writing the manuscript and also assisted with the interpretation of data and the histological examination of all tissue sections. MCW is a major contributor in writing of the manuscript and assisted with data interpretation. JCAS and RHW assisted with the collection of data and assisted in data interpretation. HL and GTF contributed in the writing of the manuscript. PJW and JM were responsible for genotyping of the *S. lupi* larvae. All authors read and approved the final manuscript.

Consent for publication

Not applicable.

Competing interests

The authors declare that they have no competing interests with respect to the research, authorship, and/or publication of this article.

Author details

[1]Section Pathology, Department of Paraclinical Sciences, Faculty of Veterinary Science, University of Pretoria, Private bag X04, Onderstepoort 0110, South Africa. [2]Wildlife Damage- Research and Management, North West Parks and Tourism Board, Madikwe and SA Lombard Nature Reserves, North West province, South Africa, P.O. Box 783540, Sandton, Johannesburg 2146, South Africa. [3]Mammal Research Institute, Department of Zoology and Entomology, University of Pretoria, Private Bag X20, Hatfield, Pretoria 0028, South Africa. [4]Department of Production Animal Studies, Faculty of Veterinary Science, University of Pretoria, Private bag X04, Onderstepoort 0110, South Africa. [5]Department of Genetics, University of Pretoria, Pretoria 0002, South Africa.

References

1. Al-Sabi MNS, Hansen MS, Chriel M, Holm E, Larsen G, Enemark HL. Genetically distinct isolates of *Spirocerca* sp. from a naturally infected red fox (*Vulpes vulpes*) from Denmark. Vet Parasitol. 2014;205:389–96.
2. Atwood TC, Gese EM. Coyotes and recolonizing wolves: social rank mediates risk-conditional behaviour at ungulate carcasses. Anim Behav. 2007;75:753–62.
3. Bailey WS. Parasites and cancer: sarcoma in dogs associated with *Spirocerca lupi*. Ann N Y Acad Sci. 1963;108:890–923.
4. Bailey WS. *Spirocerca lupi*: a continuing inquiry. J Parasitol. 1972;58:3–22.
5. Bancroft JD, Gamble M. Theory and practice of histological techniques. 5th ed. London, UK: Churchill Livingstone; 2005.
6. Behm CA, Ovington KS. The role of eosinophils in parasitic helminth infections: insights from genetically modified mice. Parasitol Today. 2000;16:202–9.
7. Blount JD, Houston DC, Møller AP, Wright J. Do individual branches of immune defence correlate? A comparative case study of scavenging and non-scavenging birds. Oikos. 2003;102:340–50.
8. Butler JRA, du Toit JT. Diet of free-ranging domestic dogs (*Canis familiaris*) in rural Zimbabwe: implications for wild scavengers on the periphery of wildlife reserves. Anim Conserv. 2002;5:29–37.
9. Clutton-Brock J. Origins of the dog: domestication and early history. In: Serpell, J., (Ed.)/ the domestic dog: its evolution, behaviour and interactions with people. Cambridge: Cambridge University press; 1995. pp. 7-20.
10. Conder GA, Loveless RM. Parasites of the coyote (*Canis latrans*) in central Utah. J Wildl Dis. 1978;14:247–9.
11. De Waal PJ, Gous A, Clift SJ, Greeff JM. High within-host genetic variation of the nematode *Spirocerca lupi* in a high-density urban dog population. Vet Parasitol. 2012;187:259–66.
12. Diakou A, Karamanavi E, Eberhard M, Kaldrimidou E. First report of *Spirocerca lupi* infection in red fox *Vulpes vulpes* in Greece. Wildl Biol. 2012; 18:333–6.
13. Du Plessis CJ, Keller N, Millward IR. Aberrant extradural spinal migration of *Spirocerca lupi*: four dogs. J Small Anim Pract. 2007;48:275–8.
14. Du Toit CA, Scholtz CH, Hyman WB. Prevalence of the dog nematode *Spirocerca lupi* in populations of its intermediate dung beetle host in the Tshwane (Pretoria) Metropole, South Africa. Onderstepoort J Vet Res, 75. 2008:315–21.
15. Dvir E, Kirberger RM, Malleczek D. Radiographic and computed tomographic changes and clinical presentation of spirocercosis in the dog. Vete Radiol Ultrasound. 2001;42:119–29.
16. Dvir E, Perl S, Loeb E, Shklar-Hirsch S, Chai O, Mazaki-Tovi M, Aroch I, Shamir MH. Spinal intramedullary aberrant *Spirocerca lupi* migration in 3 dogs. J Vet Intern Med. 2007;21:860–4.
17. Dvir E, Kirberger RM, Mukorera V, van der Merwe LL, Clift SJ. Clinical differentiation between dogs with benign and malignant spirocercosis. Vet Parasitol. 2008;155:80–8.
18. Dvir E, Clift SJ, Williams MC. Proposed histological progression of the *Spirocerca lupi*-induced oesophageal lesion in dogs. Vet Parasitol. 2010;168: 61–7.
19. Dvir E, Schoeman JP, Clift SJ, McNeilly TN, Mellanby RJ. Immunohistochemical characterization of lymphocyte and myeloid cell infiltrates in spirocercosis-induced ooesophageal nodules. Parasite Immunol. 2011;33:545–53.
20. Excoffier L, Laval G, Schneider S. Arlequin (version 3.0): an integrated software package for population genetics data analysis. Evol Bioinforma. 2005;1:47–50.
21. Ezemvelo KZN Wildlife. Wildlife management – blackbacked jackal. 2009. Viewed 7 May 2012 from http://www.kznwildlife.com/component/content/article/167-conservation/management/860-blackbacked-jackal.html.
22. Ferrantelli V, Riili S, Vicari D, Percipalle M, Chetta M, Monteverde V, Gaglio G, Giardina G, Usai F, Poglayen G. *Spirocerca lupi* isolated from gastric lesions in foxes (*Vulpes vulpes*) in Sicily (Italy). Polish J Vet Sci. 2010;13:465–71.
23. Gardiner CH, Poynton SL. An atlas of metazoan parasites in animal tissues. Armed forces Institute of Pathology. DC, USA: Washington; 1999.
24. Goodwin D, Bradshaw JWS, Wickens SM. Paedomorphosis affects agonistic visual signals of domestic dogs. Anim Behav. 1997;53:297–304.
25. Guarner F, Malagelada JR. Gut flora in health and disease. Lancet. 2003;361:512–9.
26. Kirberger RM, Clift SJ, van Wilpe E, Dvir E. *Spirocerca lupi*-associated vertebral changes: a radiologic-pathologic study. Vet Parasitol. 2013;195: 87–94.
27. Lombaard LJ. Age determination and growth curves in the black-backed jackal, *Canis mesomelas* Schreber, 1775 (Carnivora: Canidae). Ann Transv Mus. 1971;27:35–181.
28. Loveridge AJ, Nel JAJ. *Canis mesomelas*. In: IUCN 2011. IUCN red list of threatened species. 2008. Version 2011, viewed 11 May 2012, from http://www.iucnredlist.org/details/3755/0.
29. Morandi F, Angelico G, Verin R, Gavaudan S. Fatal spirocercosis in a free-ranging red fox. Vet Rec. 2014;174:228.
30. Murray M, Campbell MH, Jarrett WHF. *Spirocerca lupi* in a cheetah. Afr J Ecol. 1964;2:164.
31. Nover MC, Huffnagel GB. Does the microbiota regulate immune responses outside the gut? Trends Microbiol. 2004;12:562–8.
32. Pence DB, Stone JE. Visceral lesions in wild carnivores naturally infected with *Spirocerca lupi*. Vet Pathol. 1978;15:322–31.
33. Råberg L, Graham AL, Read AF. Decomposing health: tolerance and resistance to parasites in animals. Philos Trans R Soc B. 2009;364:37–49.
34. Richardson PRK. The natural removal of ungulate carcasses, and the adaptive features of the scavengers involved. Pretoria: MSc thesis, University of Pretoria; 1980.
35. Rinas MA, Nesnek R, Kinsella JM, Dematteo KE. Fatal aortic aneurysm and rupture in a neotropical bush dog (*Speothos venaticaus*) caused by *Spirocerca lupi*. Vet Parasitol. 2009;164:347–9.
36. Shamri R, Xenakis JJ, Spencer LA. Eosinophils in innate immunity: an evolving story. Cell Tissue Res. 2011;343:57–83.
37. Skinner JD, Chimimba CT. The mammals of the southern African subregion. 3rd ed. Cape Town, South Africa: Cambridge University Press; 2005.
38. Szczęsna J, Popiolek J. The first record of *Spirocerca lupi* (Rudolphi, 1809) (Spirocercidae, Nematoda) from Poland based on faecal analysis of wolf (*Canis lupus* L.). Helminthologia. 2007;44:230–2.
39. Traversa D, Costanzo F, Iorio R, Aroch I, Lavy E. Mitochondrial cytochrome *c* oxidase subunit 1 (*cox1*) gene sequence of *Spirocerca lupi* (Nematoda, Spirurida): avenues for potential implications. Vet Parasitol. 2007;146:263–70.
40. Traversa D, Avolio S, Modry D, Otranto D, Iorio R, Aroch I, Cringoli G, Milillo P, Albrechtova K, Mihalca A, Lavy E. Copromicroscopic and molecular assays for the detection of cancer-causing parasitic nematode *Spirocerca lupi*. Vet Parasitol. 2008;157:108–16.
41. van de Ven MFN, Tambling CJ, Kerley GIH. Seasonal diet of black-backed jackal in the eastern Karoo, South Africa. J Arid Environ. 2013;99:23–7.

10

Pathological and immunological characteristics of piglets infected experimentally with a HP-PRRSV TJ strain

Zhenguang Li[1,2†], Yanliang He[1†], Xiaoqin Xu[3], Xue Leng[2], Shufen Li[1], Yongjun Wen[2], Fengxue Wang[2], Mingqi Xia[1], Shipeng Cheng[2] and Hua Wu[1,2*]

Abstract

Background: Porcine reproductive and respiratory syndrome (PRRS) remains a major threat to swine industry all over the world. The aim of this study was to investigate the mechanism of pathogenesis and immune responses caused by a highly pathogenic porcine reproductive and respiratory syndrome virus (HP-PRRSV).

Results: All piglets experimentally infected with a HP-PRRSV TJ strain virus developed typical clinical signs of PRRS. The percentages of $CD3^+$, $CD4^+$, and $CD8^+$ lymphocytes significantly decreased in the infected group as compared to the uninfected control animals ($p < 0.01$). Total WBC dropped in the infected animals during the experiment. The level of ELISA antibody against PRRSV increased in 7–10 days after infection and then started to decline. Pathological observations demonstrated various degree lesions, bleeding and necrosis in the lungs of the infected piglets.

Conclusions: These results clearly indicated that HP-PRRSV TJ strain infection would activate host humoral immune response at the early period post infection and cause severe pathological damages on lungs and inhibit cellular immune response after infection.

Keywords: HP-PRRSV, humoral immunity, cell-mediated immunity, immune responses

Background

Porcine reproductive and respiratory syndrome (PRRS) is characterized by reproductive failure in pregnant sows and respiratory distress in pigs of all ages [1]. The disease was first reported in the United States in 1987 and later in the Netherlands and other parts of the world [2]. The PRRS virus (PRRSV) is an enveloped positive-stranded RNA virus which belongs to the family of *Arteriviridae* in the order of the *Nidovirales*. Other related viruses of family *Arteriviridae* include equine arterutus virus, lactate dehydrogenase-elevating virus and simian haemorrhagic fever virus [3].

* Correspondence: wuhua@sinovetah.com
†Equal contributors
[1]Sinovet (Beijing) Biotechnology Co., Ltd., Kaituo Road 5, Haidian District, Beijing 100085, China
[2]State Key Laboratory of Special Economic Animal Molecular Biology, Institute of Special Economic Animal and Plant Sciences, Chinese Academy of Agricultural Sciences,, Juye Street 4899, Changchun, Jilin 130122, China
Full list of author information is available at the end of the article

PRRSV mainly replicates in alveolar macrophages in the lungs and lymphoid organs [4]. Thus, the potential for aerosol spread through respiratory and oropharyngeal excretions within swine confinement units is a distinct possibility. The virus is well- known to stay in lungs and lymphoid organs of infected pigs for a long time. It was reported that an infected sow was able to transmit PRRSV up to 157 days post initial infection [5]. Others had detected PRRSV in lymph organs up to 132 days when the piglets were infected in the uterus [6]. PRRSV was also detected more than 180 days post-infection [7]. The mechanism of PRRSV persistence is not completely understood but is likely related to the emergence of viral variants which can escape host immune response [8].

PRRS has now emerged as the most prevalent disease of swine in the world. In the United States, annual loss due to PRRS is estimated at 560 million dollars [9]. In early 2006, a highly pathogenic disease emerged in some swine farms in Jiangxi province of China, and then spread rapidly to the rest of China [10]. This disease remains a major threat to swine industry all over the world [11]. Infected pigs of all ages presented with clinical signs including continuous high fever of above 41 °C, depression, dyspnea, anorexia, red discoloration of the ears and skin, conjunctivitis, mild diarrhea, shivering and limping. The morbidity rate was 50–100 % with mortality rate of 20–100 % [12]. Studies demonstrated that highly pathogenic porcine reproduction and respiratory syndrome virus (HP-PRRSV) was the major pathogen that caused the outbreak. HP-PRRSV TJ strain was originally isolated from a piglet that died of a "high fever" in Tianjin, China, in 2006, and it had the same characteristics as those of other HP-PRRSV strains observed in China. HP-PRRSV strain TJ was culturally passaged on MARC-145 cells for attenuation so that it could be used for the development of a modified live virus (MLV) vaccine [13]. Genetic analysis indicates that the HP-PRRSV isolated from China has a discontinuous deletion of 30 amino acids (AA) in non-structural protein 2 (Nsp2), compared with the North American type of PRRSV strain. However, the mechanisms contributing to the molecular pathogenesis of the HP-PRRSV have not been elucidated.

Some preliminary studies reported that PRRSV modulates the host immune responses and alters host gene expression [14–17]. In order to further investigate the immunological characteristics of HP-PRRSV, ten five-week-old pigs were experimentally infected with HP-PRRSV TJ strain and pathological changes, humoral and cell-mediated immune responses were evaluated in the present study.

Results

Clinical signs observations post infection

All piglets infected with HP-PRRSV TJ strain virus developed typical clinical signs of HP-PRRS, such as severe depression and anorexia, lameness and shivering, dyspnea, skin cyanosis and death. Four of five PRRSV-infected piglets died of acute respiratory disease. Conversely, no clinical signs were observed in the control ones. Infected animals had persistently high fever (≥41 ° C) at 4 day post infection (dpi), which lasted 9 days (Fig. 1a). In contrast, control piglets remained healthy with normal body temperature throughout the experiment. Animals in group 1 showed significantly higher average clinical scores than the control group (< 0.01) (Fig. 1b). As shown in Fig. 1c, animals infected with HP-PRRSV TJ strain in group 1 lost significantly more body weight than those in control group.

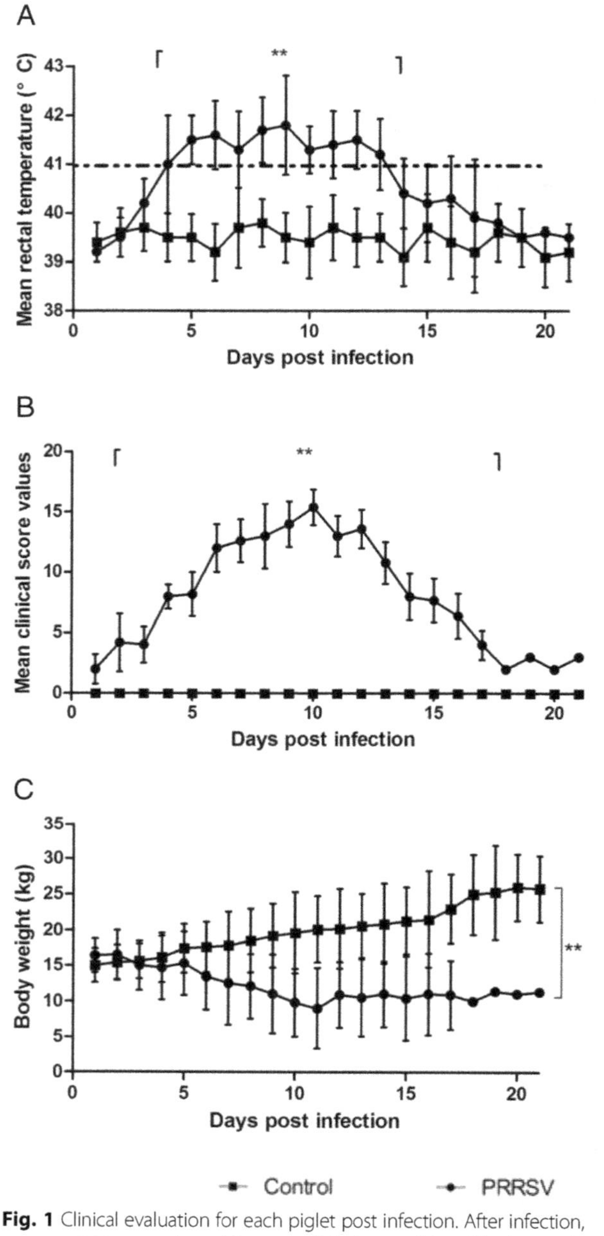

Fig. 1 Clinical evaluation for each piglet post infection. After infection, mean rectal temperatures (**a**), mean clinical score (**b**) and body weight (**c**) of each animal were measured daily in HP-PRRSV inoculation group (PRRSV, $n = 5$) and control group (Control, $n = 5$). Rectal temperatures equal or above 41 °C (≥41 °C) were defined as fever. Data are presented as mean values ± SD. Asterisks indicate significant differences (**$p < 0.01$) between infected and control groups

Gross pathology and histological evaluations of lungs

No macroscopic (gross) lesions were recorded in the lungs collected from the control animals at necropsy (Fig. 2a). In HP-PRRSV-infected group, piglets exhibited severe gross lesions with consolidation and haemorrhage (Fig. 2b). The parenchymas of the infected lungs were firmer and heavier than those of the control group. The average lung lesion score was significantly higher ($p < 0.01$) than that in the control group (Fig. 2c).

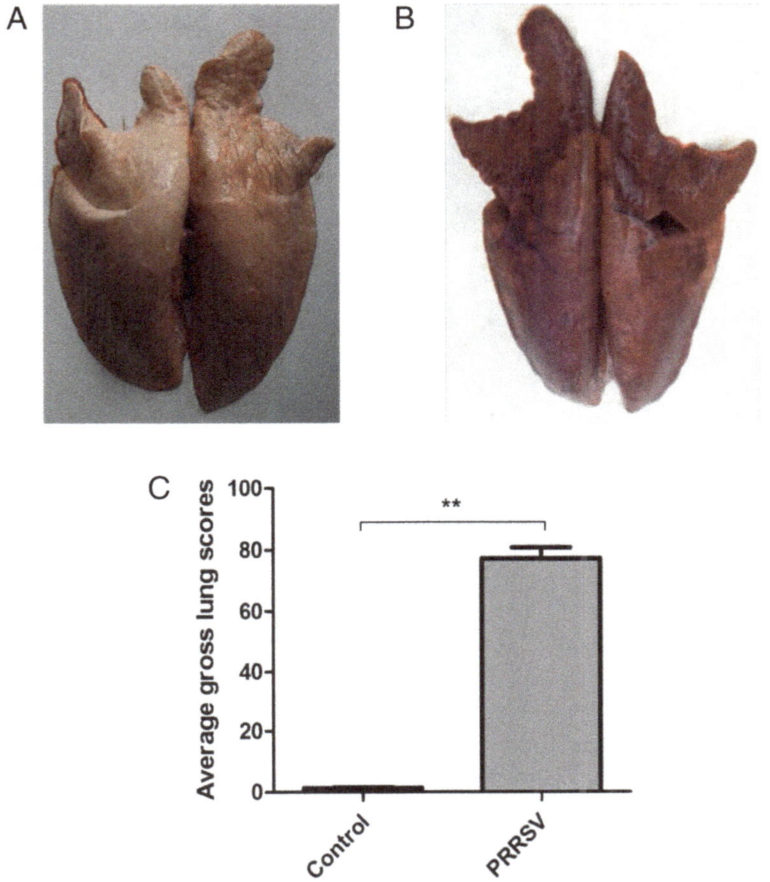

Fig. 2 At necropsy, lungs of the control (**a**) and HP-PRRSV-infected (**b**) animals in the study were examined for macroscopic (gross) pathology. The average lung gross scores were evaluated according to the previous scoring system which estimates the percentage of lung affected by pneumonia in the two groups ($n = 5$). The difference of average lung gross scores between lungs of the control and HP-PRRSV-infected animals was presented (**c**). Data are presented as mean values ± SD. Asterisks indicate significant differences (**$p < 0.01$) between infected and control groups

Under histological examination, all the lungs from control piglets did not exhibit any features that are characteristic of acute PRRSV infection (Fig. 3a). However, the lung tissues collected from PRRSV-infected ones developed interstitial pneumonia with alveolar septa thickened by the infiltration of macrophages and lymphomononuclear cells (Fig. 3b).

Leukocyte (white blood cell) count and antibody detection

The average leukocyte levels during the study are shown in Fig. 4a. Piglets infected with HP-PRRSV TJ strain showed a sharp decrease in white blood cell counts (WBC) on 3 dpi, and reached the lowest level at 7 dpi. Then WBC developed a tendency to increase thereafter till 14 dpi. On 21 dpi, WBC level of the survival one returned to the normal level. In contrast, the WBC level in control group did not show significant change during the course of the experiment (Fig. 4a).

Antibody specific for PRRSV was first demonstrated by ELISA on 3 dpi in the infected group and increased gradually. However, ELISA antibody level showed a decline tendency after peak at 14 dpi. Low S/P ratio can be detected when animals died of infection, with the exception that the surviving one still showed a detectable titre when the experiment terminated. On the contrary, no detectable ELISA titre can be observed throughout the experiment in the control group (Fig. 4b).

Alterations of peripheral T-lymphocyte subpopulations

To investigate the influence of HP-PRRSV infection on peripheral blood T lymphocytes, T-lymphocyte subsets were evaluated using flow cytometry analysis. Before inoculation with the HP-PRRSV TJ strain, there was about 60 % $CD3^+$ T- lymphocytes in the peripheral blood monouclear cells (PBMC) of piglets. As shown in Fig. 5a, the percentage of $CD3^+$ cells significantly decreased at 3 ($p < 0.05$) and 7 dpi ($p < 0.01$), and returned to the similar level as before infection at 10 and 14dpi. However,

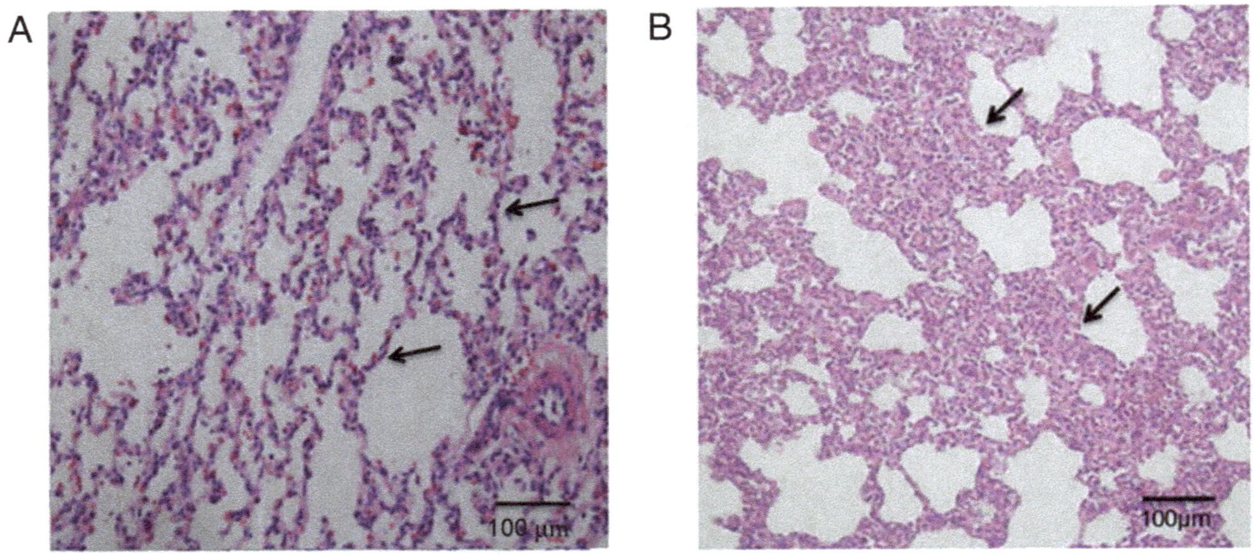

Fig. 3 Histopathological lesions of the lung from HP-PRRSV infected and control piglets. At necropsy, lung samples were collected and processed for histopathology examination following hematoxylin and eosin (H&E) staining. Lungs of piglets infected with HP-PRRSV (**b**) showed severe interstitial pneumonia with thickened the alveolar septa (marked with arrows) accompanied by significant infiltration of mononuclear cells, compared to the lungs of negative control piglets (**a**)

the number of $CD3^+$ cells showed dramatic decline when animals died of disease ($p < 0.01$). No significant change was detected for $CD3^+$cells in the control group (Fig. 5a).

As shown in Fig. 5b, there was about 35 % $CD4^+$ T lymphocyte in the PBMC of infected animals. Then the percentage sharply declined to about 22.7 % at 3 dpi and 15 % at 7 dpi. Interestingly, the proportion of $CD4^+$ cells remained at a low level until 18 dpi in the PRRSV-infected group. Only the surviving one showed a normal level of $CD4^+$ cells at 21 dpi. On the contrary, the control group remained unchanged throughout the experiment.

There was no significant difference of $CD8^+$ cells in the control animals. As shown in Fig. 5c, there was about 19.4 % $CD8^+$ T lymphocytes in PBMC prior to PRRSV infection. However, a transient decrease was observed at 3 dpi. Then there was a gradual increase in the percentage of $CD8^+$ cells at 7–14 dpi. Finally, a slight decrease in the number of $CD8^+$ T lymphocytes occured at 18 dpi, which is still higher than the normal level.

Figure 5d showed the $CD4^+/CD8^+$values in the both groups. The value kept about 1.5 during the study in the control animals. Similarly, in the infected group, the $CD4^+/CD8^+$value remained unchanged at 3 dpi. Nevertheless, the value significantly declined to about 0.6 at 7 dpi and peeked about 0.4 at 10 dpi and remained at a low level until 18 dpi in the PRRSV-infected group. Only the surviving one showed a normal $CD4^+/CD8^+$ value at 21 dpi.

Discussion

PRRS has been a widespread disease in most pig-producing countries since its first emergence two decades ago in the USA [18]. Current studies have indicated that the emergence and epidemic of highly pathogenic PRRSV not only further aggravates the complicated situation of PRRS infection, but also enhances the genetic diversity of PRRSV in China [19]. Since its emergence in 2006, the HP-PRRS has been devastating in China's swine industry. In current study, the newly isolated PRRSV TJ strain was used to experimentally infect piglets and reproduce the disease symptoms in which the clinical signs and mortality were virtually identical to what was seen in the field. The classical PRRS strains induce abortions in pregnant pigs, transient fever, depression and dyspnoea in male and young pigs [4]. Newborn piglets may die, but the mortality rate is generally low in growing pigs. It is intriguing that the new type of PRRSV that recently emerged in China exhibits unusually high mortality in affected pigs of all ages including adults. The pathogenesis of HP-PRRSV needs to be studied in detail in comparison to classical PRRS strains.

Previous studies demonstrated that HP-PRRSV infected pigs exhibited severe clinical symptoms including persistent high fever, red coloration of body, cyanopathy of ears, conjunctivitis, dyspnoea and severe diffuse pulmonary consolidation lesions [20, 21]. Pigs demonstrated significantly reduced numbers of pulmonary alveolar macrophages and peripheral blood monocytes, delayed

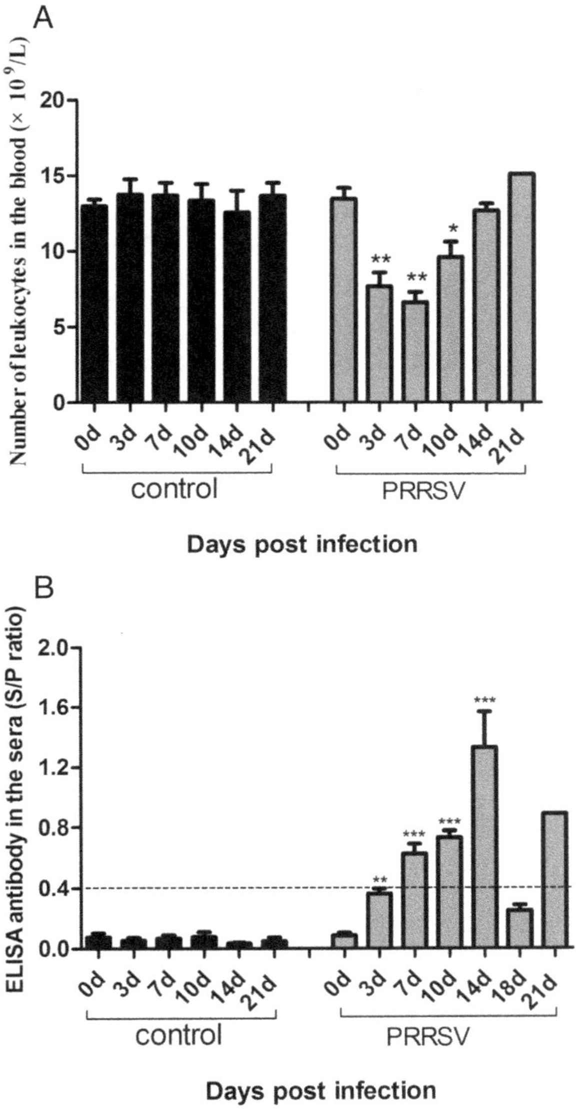

Fig. 4 Leukocyte count and antibody detection in the sera from HP-PRRSV infected and control piglets. The heparinized blood sample from each piglet was collected for white blood cell counts (**a**); ELISA anti-PRRSV antibody titers in the sera were determined with the IDEXX PRRS ELISA kit (**b**). Values represent average titers from five animals. Dashed line at 0.4 S/P ratio designates threshold value above which titers are considered positive for anti-PRRSV antibodies. Data from groups of $n = 5$ piglets are expressed as means ± SD. The horizontal lines represent the geometric mean for each group and statistical analysis was performed and the data are shown as * $p < 0.05$, ** $p < 0.01$, *** $p < 0.001$

neutralizing and non-neutralizing antibody response after PRRSV infection [22–26]. Piglets infected with HP-PRRSV TJ strain in our study developed the typical highly virulent PRRS clinical symptoms reported before. The number of white blood cell counts (WBC) sharply decreased at 3 dpi and peaked at 7 dpi post infection, even though it returned to increase thereafter.

During acute PRRSV infection, pigs developed significantly reduced humoral immune response to classical swine fever modified-live virus vaccine [27]. The immunosuppressive effects are most potent one week after PRRSV infection [28]. It is commonly speculated that HP-PRRSV strains and classical PRRSV strains have similarly destructive effects on the immune system. In present study, the fact that antibody specific for PRRSV was first demonstrated by ELISA at 3 dpi indicated that host humoral immune response was activated at the early period post infection. However, ELISA antibody level showed a dramatic decline after peak at 14 dpi. Undetectable S/P ratio was observed when animals died of disease, which indicated that host humoral immune response may be suppressed by PRRSV infection.

The present study reported the changes of subpopulations of T-lymphocytes in the HP-PRRSV challenged piglets. Pigs were reported to have transient lymphocytopenia of $CD4^+CD8^-$ and $CD4^-CD8^+$ T cells from three days to approximately four weeks after PRRSV infection [29–31]. The T-cell responses to PRRSV are induced 2–8 weeks post-infection [32, 33]. In our study, the percentages of $CD3^+$ T lymphocytes subsets in the PBMCs and $CD8^+$cells in the T lymphocytes both significantly decreased at 3 and/or 7 dpi, then had a tendency to increase until 14 dpi. Similarly, both of $CD3^+$ and CD8 $^+$ cells declined to the low level at 18 dpi when animals died of disease. These results are consistent with Shimizu's report that total lymphocytes, $CD8^+$ cells decreased after PRRS virus infected [31]. Nevertheless, contradictory results showed that restimulation with PRRSV of PBMC derived from PRRSV infected pigs in vitro resulted in an increased percentage of CD3 $^+CD8^{high}$ cells starting from 14 dpi compared to mock-restimulation. On the other hand, the number of $CD4^+$ and $CD4^+/CD8^+$ value showed a similar tendency throughout the experiment period. They both decreased from 3 dpi to 7 dpi and remained the low level before animal died. Interestingly, all the T lymphocytes of the surviving one returned to normal level in the end of the study. These findings agreed with the Shimizu's study. In contrast, previous study demonstrated that PRRSV increased the number of $CD4^+CD8^+CD25^+Foxp3^+$ cells at 14dpi, whereas CD4 $^+CD8^-CD25^+Foxp3^+$ remained constant until 28 dpi [34]. In our study, $CD4^+CD8^+$ cells showed a transient increase from 1 to 3 dpi, though it returned to low level afterward (data not shown).

Results from this study suggest that HP-PRRSV TJ strain has more seriously destructive effects on the immune system than classical PRRSV strains, and induces seriously poor adaptive immune responses on the piglets, and facilitates the invasion of other pathogens.

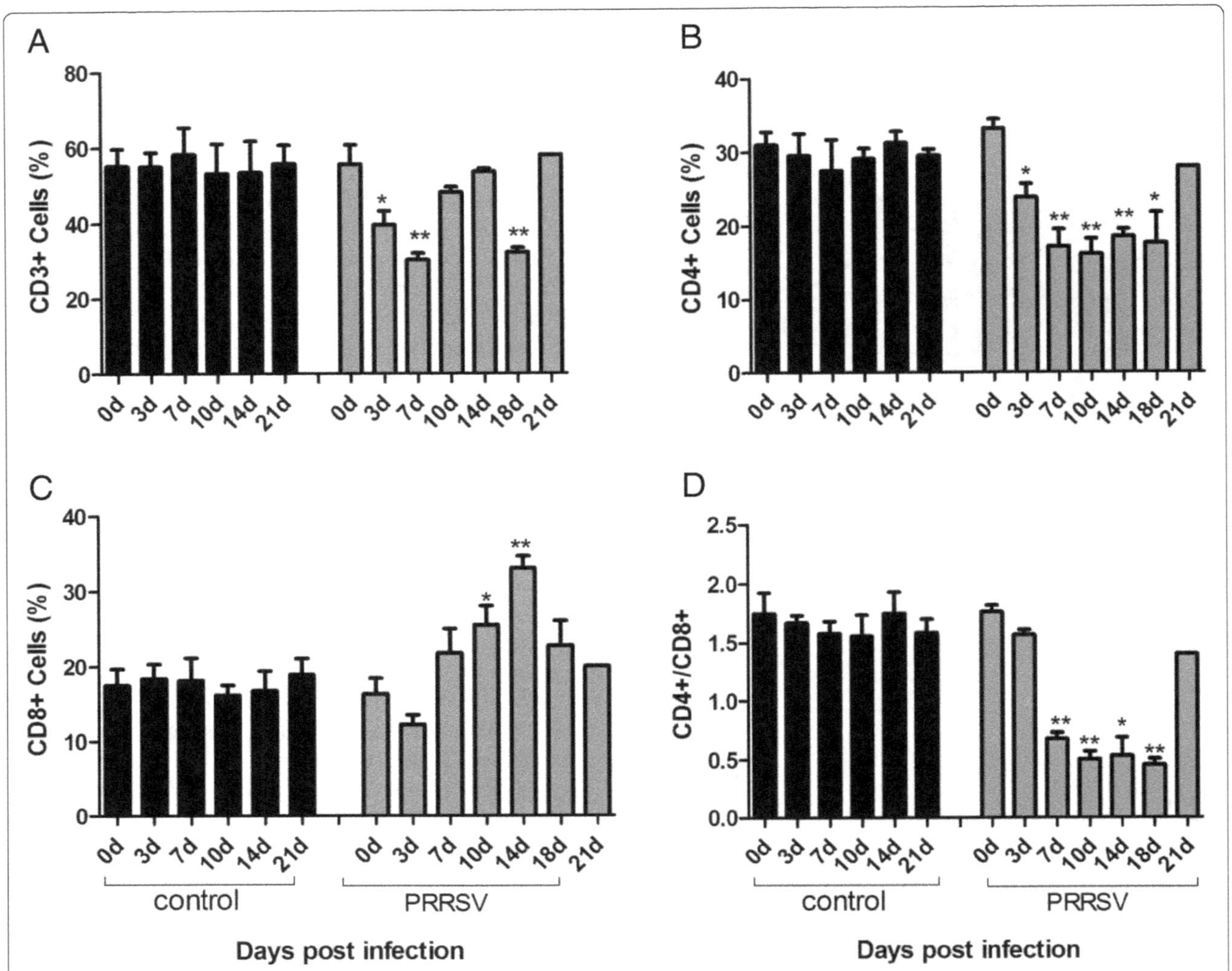

Fig. 5 Percentage of T lymphocyte subsets in peripheral blood of HP-PRRSV infected and non-infected piglets. Piglets were infected with HP-PRRSV and blood was harvested after infection at 0, 3, 7, 10, 14, 18 and 21dpi. Single cell suspensions were prepared and stained with antibodies against T lymphocytes markers CD3, CD4, and CD8 and analyzed by flow cytometry. Representative flow cytometric plots of T lymphocytes are shown in the blood. The detailed analysis for $CD3^+$ T lymphocytes are presented (**a**), $CD4^+$ T lymphocytes (**b**), $CD8^+$ T lymphocytes (**c**) and ratio of $CD4^+/CD8^+$ T lymphocytes (**d**). Data are shown as means ± SD. Asterisks indicate significant differences between the indicated experimental groups (*$p < 0.05$, **$p < 0.01$). Note: The CD4+ and CD8+ population are represented CD4+ CD8-cells and CD8+ CD4- respectively only

Conclusions

In this study, the experimental infection with HP-PRRSV TJ strain has reproduced the disease of high virulence and high mortality compared to the clinical signs seen in classical PRRS. It is indicated that HP-PRRSV TJ strain infection would activate host humoral immune response at the early period post infection and cause severe pathological damages on lungs and inhibit cellular immune response after infection.

However, comparison of pathogenesis between HP-PRRSV and LP-PRRSV infection need to be further investigated.

Methods

Cells, antibodies and viruses

The MARC-145 cell line (derived from African green monkey kidney cells) was employed for viral propagation and titration. MARC-145 cells were maintained in minimum essential medium (MEM) supplemented with 8 % fetal bovine serum (FBS, Hyclone Laboratories Inc, South Logan, UT, USA) at 37 °C, with 5 % CO2. PRRSV strain TJ (GenBank accession no. EU860248) was isolated and maintained in our laboratory as previously described [35]. Antibodies used for flow cytometric analysis, such as anti-CD3 (PE/Cy5-conjugated MAb PPT3), anti-CD4 (PE-conjugated

MAb 74-12-4), and anti-CD8 (FITC-conjugated MAb 76-2-11) were purchased from BD Pharmingen (San Jose, CA).

Animals and experimental design

Ten healthy crossbred piglets from a PRRSV-free herd were obtained, weaned, and transported to the biological safety level 2 (BSL2) facilities at the Teyan Veterinary Biologic Factory at three weeks of age. All animals were confirmed to be free of PRRSV, CSFV, PRV, SIV, *Mycoplasma hyopneumoniae*, and PCV2 infections using methods previously described (Leng et al. [13]). Weaned piglets were collectively housed for several days prior to exposure to virus, and then individually housed in the isolation units from the time of exposure until the end of the observation period. Ten piglets were randomly divided into two groups. Piglets of group 1 ($n = 5$) were inoculated intranasally (i.n.) with $10^{3.0}$ 50 % tissue culture infective doses ($TCID_{50}$) of PRRSV TJ strain. Group 2 ($n = 5$) was inoculated intranasally with supernatant of lysate of MARC-145 cells in a 1-mL volume. All experimental procedures have been reviewed and approved by local Animal Care & Use Committee of Institute of Special Wild Economic Animal and Plant Sciences, Chinese Academy of Agricultural Sciences, Jilin, China.

Clinical observation and sample collection

After infection, animals were monitored twice daily for clinical signs, including depression, anorexia, diarrhea, skin discolorations, conjunctivitis, lameness, coughing, labored and abdominal breathing and respiratory rate. Rectal temperatures were recorded every day throughout the experiment. Clinical signs and food intake were evaluated daily for each animal in both groups. Clinical signs were observed and graded using a scoring system described previously [36], which is shown in Table 1. Blood samples with and without heparin were collected on 0, 3, 7, 10 and 14 days post-infection (dpi). Heparinised blood samples were used to detect $CD3^+$, $CD4^+$, and $CD8^+$ T lymphocytes and white blood cell counts. Serum samples were used to measure the ELISA antibody titers against PRRSV. All the animals were euthanized at day 21 dpi.

Serological examination

PRRSV-specific antibody responses were analyzed with serum collected at 0, 3, 7, 10, 14 and 21 dpi, using a commercial ELISA kit (Idexx Laboratories Inc., Westbrook, ME) according to the manufacturer's instructions. The PRRSV-specific antibody level was reported as an S/P ratio, and the serum samples were considered positive if the S/P ratio was 0.4 or higher.

Table 1 Scores assigned to clinical signs observed in pigs following inoculation of HP-PRRSV

Category of clinical sign	Symptom	Score
Systemic:	Normal	0
	Apathy	1
	Anorexia	2
	Severe depression	5
	Death	10
Respiratory:	Normal	0
	Sneezing, Coughing	1
	Tachypnea	2
	Laboured breathing	3
	Abdominal breathing	5
Other symptoms:	Normal	0
	Diarrhea,	1
	Conjunctivitis	2
	Reddening of the ears	3
	Skin cyanopathy	5

Gross pathology and histological evaluations of lungs

At necropsy, lungs of the animals in the study were examined for macroscopic (gross) pathology, lungs were evaluated and graded using an established scoring system which estimates the percentage of lung affected by pneumonia. On the other hand, lung samples were collected and processed for histopathology examination following hematoxylin and eosin (H&E) staining, as described previously \23].

Leukocyte (white blood cell) counts

Heparinised blood was collected and the leukocyte (white blood cell) counts were determined using an automatic analyzer CA 500 (Sysmex CA-500 automated blood coagulation analyzer, Japan) according to the manufacturer's instructions.

Flow cytometry analysis

Blood was collected and red blood cells were lysed with ACK lysis buffer (BioSource International, Inc., Camarillo, CA) for 1 min at room temperature. Single-cell suspensions (at 106 cells) were prepared in Hanks balanced salt solution (HBSS) (Invitrogen) and stained with antibodies against CD3, CD4, CD8 (BD PharMingen). After incubation on ice for 30 min, cells were washed twice in PBS containing 2 % FBS and 0.02 % NaN3. Then the cells were fixed with 1 % paraformaldehyde. Data collection and analysis were performed with a BD LSR-II flow cytometer, BD FACSDiva software (BD Pharmingen), FlowJo software (TreeStar, San Carlos, CA), Prism software, and Microsoft Excel (Seattle, WA).

Statistical analyses

The significant differences of the in vitro experiment and animal trials were analyzed using a one-way or two-way ANOVA in the GraphPad Prism (version 5.0) software. A *t*-test or F-test was used to estimate the variability among the gross lesion, leukocyte count, antibody level and flow cytometry results. Differences were considered statistically significant at a P value of < 0.05 and extremely significant at a value of $P < 0.01$ or $P < 0.001$.

Abbreviations

BSL2: biological safety level 2; dpi: days post-infection; FBS: fetal bovine serum; FCM: flow cytometry; H&E: Hematoxylin and eosin; HP-PRRSV: Highly pathogenic porcine reproductive and respiratory syndrome virus; MEM: Maintained in minimum essential medium; PBMC: Peripheral blood monouclear cells; PRRSV: Porcine reproductive and respiratory syndrome virus; $TCID_{50}$: Tissue culture infective doses; WBC: White blood cells count

Acknowledgements

We are grateful of Dr. Wenzhi Xue for many helpful suggestions and his critical reading of the manuscript. We also would like to thank Dr. Xuejin Su from Norman Bethune University of Medical Science for the help in the flow cytometry analysis.

Funding

The study was financially supported by the JILIN Science and Technology Development Plan (201505200125JH) and JILIN province project for transformation of scientific and technological achievements (20140307008NY), Technology Innovation Program from Chinese Academy of Agricultural Sciences (20140204066NY) .

Authors' contributions

ZGL and YLH participated in the design of the study, performed the experiments and drafted the manuscript. XQX, SFL helped with the animal experiment. XL and MQX helped with the flow cytometry. YJW, FXW performed the statistical analysis. HW and SPC conceived the study and participated in its design and coordination. All authors read and approved the final manuscript.

Competing interests

The authors declare that they have no competing interests.

Consent for publication

Not applicable.

Consent from client owned animal

Animal experiment and sample collection were obtained the consent from farm owner and approved ethically by local ethics committee of Institute of Special Wild Economic Animal and Plant Sciences, Chinese Academy of Agricultural Sciences, Jilin, China.

Author details

[1]Sinovet (Beijing) Biotechnology Co., Ltd., Kaituo Road 5, Haidian District, Beijing 100085, China. [2]State Key Laboratory of Special Economic Animal Molecular Biology, Institute of Special Economic Animal and Plant Sciences, Chinese Academy of Agricultural Sciences,, Juye Street 4899, Changchun, Jilin 130122, China. [3]Jiangyan Animal Health Inspection Institute, Jiangguan Road 251, Taizhou, Jiangsu 225529, China.

References

1. Rossow KD. Porcine reproductive and respiratory syndrome. Vet Pathol. 1998;35(1):1–20.
2. Paton DJ, Brown IH, Edwards S, Wensvoort G. 'Blue ear' disease of pigs. Vet Rec. 1991;128(26):617.
3. Cavanagh D. Nidovirales: a new order comprising Coronaviridae and Arteriviridae. Arch Virol. 1997;142(3):629–33.
4. Gomez-Laguna J, Salguero FJ, Pallares FJ, Carrasco L. Immunopathogenesis of porcine reproductive and respiratory syndrome in the respiratory tract of pigs. Vet J. 2013;195(2):148–55.
5. Wills RW, Zimmerman JJ, Yoon KJ, Swenson SL, Hoffman LJ, McGinley MJ, Hill HT, Platt KB. Porcine reproductive and respiratory syndrome virus: routes of excretion. Vet Microbiol. 1997;57(1):69–81.
6. Rowland RR, Lawson S, Rossow K, Benfield DA. Lymphoid tissue tropism of porcine reproductive and respiratory syndrome virus replication during persistent infection of pigs originally exposed to virus in utero. Vet Microbiol. 2003;96(3):219–35.
7. Bilodeau R, Archambault D, Vezina SA, Sauvageau R, Fournier M, Dea S. Persistence of porcine reproductive and respiratory syndrome virus infection in a swine operation. Can J Vet Res. 1994;58(4):291–8.
8. Rowland RR, Kervin R, Kuckleburg C, Sperlich A, Benfield DA. The localization of porcine reproductive and respiratory syndrome virus nucleocapsid protein to the nucleolus of infected cells and identification of a potential nucleolar localization signal sequence. Virus Res. 1999;64(1):1–12.
9. Neumann EJ, Kliebenstein JB, Johnson CD, Mabry JW, Bush EJ, Seitzinger AH, Green AL, Zimmerman JJ. Assessment of the economic impact of porcine reproductive and respiratory syndrome on swine production in the United States. J Am Vet Med Assoc. 2005;227(3):385–92.
10. Li Y, Wang X, Bo K, Tang B, Yang B, Jiang W, Jiang P. Emergence of a highly pathogenic porcine reproductive and respiratory syndrome virus in the Mid-Eastern region of China. Vet J. 2007;174(3):577–84.
11. Tian K, Yu X, Zhao T, Feng Y, Cao Z, Wang C, Hu Y, Chen X, Hu D, Tian X, et al. Emergence of fatal PRRSV variants: unparalleled outbreaks of atypical PRRS in China and molecular dissection of the unique hallmark. PLoS One. 2007;2(6), e526.
12. Tong GZ, Zhou YJ, Hao XF, Tian ZJ, An TQ, Qiu HJ. Highly pathogenic porcine reproductive and respiratory syndrome. China Emerg Infect Dis. 2007;13(9):1434–6.
13. Leng X, Li Z, Xia M, He Y, Wu H. Evaluation of the efficacy of an attenuated live vaccine against highly pathogenic porcine reproductive and respiratory syndrome virus in young pigs. Clinical and vaccine immunology : CVI. 2012; 19(8):1199–206.
14. Albina E, Carrat C, Charley B. Interferon-alpha response to swine arterivirus (PoAV), the porcine reproductive and respiratory syndrome virus. J Interferon Cytokine Res. 1998;18(7):485–90.
15. Lopez OJ, Osorio FA. Role of neutralizing antibodies in PRRSV protective immunity. Vet Immunol Immunopathol. 2004;102(3):155–63.
16. Meier WA, Galeota J, Osorio FA, Husmann RJ, Schnitzlein WM, Zuckermann FA. Gradual development of the interferon-gamma response of swine to porcine reproductive and respiratory syndrome virus infection or vaccination. Virology. 2003;309(1):18–31.
17. Beura LK, Sarkar SN, Kwon B, Subramaniam S, Jones C, Pattnaik AK, Osorio FA. Porcine reproductive and respiratory syndrome virus nonstructural protein 1beta modulates host innate immune response by antagonizing IRF3 activation. J Virol. 2010;84(3):1574–84.
18. Albina E. Epidemiology of porcine reproductive and respiratory syndrome (PRRS): an overview. Vet Microbiol. 1997;55(1–4):309–16.
19. Zhou L, Yang H. Porcine reproductive and respiratory syndrome in China. Virus Res. 2010;154(1–2):31–7.
20. Feng Y, Zhao T, Nguyen T, Inui K, Ma Y, Nguyen TH, Nguyen VC, Liu D, Bui QA, To LT, et al. Porcine respiratory and reproductive syndrome virus variants, Vietnam and China, 2007. Emerg Infect Dis. 2008;14(11):1774–6.

21. Zhou YJ, Hao XF, Tian ZJ, Tong GZ, Yoo D, An TQ, Zhou T, Li GX, Qiu HJ, Wei TC, et al. Highly virulent porcine reproductive and respiratory syndrome virus emerged in China. Transbound Emerg Dis. 2008;55(3–4):152–64.
22. Rossow KD, Bautista EM, Goyal SM, Molitor TW, Murtaugh MP, Morrison RB, Benfield DA, Collins JE. Experimental porcine reproductive and respiratory syndrome virus infection in one-, four-, and 10-week-old pigs. J Vet Diagn Invest. 1994;6(1):3–12.
23. Halbur PG, Paul PS, Frey ML, Landgraf J, Eernisse K, Meng XJ, Lum MA, Andrews JJ, Rathje JA. Comparison of the pathogenicity of two US porcine reproductive and respiratory syndrome virus isolates with that of the Lelystad virus. Vet Pathol. 1995;32(6):648–60.
24. Halbur PG, Paul PS, Meng XJ, Lum MA, Andrews JJ, Rathje JA. Comparative pathogenicity of nine US porcine reproductive and respiratory syndrome virus (PRRSV) isolates in a five-week-old cesarean-derived, colostrum-deprived pig model. J Vet Diagn Invest. 1996;8(1):11–20.
25. Done SH, Paton DJ. Porcine reproductive and respiratory syndrome: clinical disease, pathology and immunosuppression. Vet Rec. 1995;136(2):32–5.
26. Charerntantanakul W, Platt R, Johnson W, Roof M, Vaughn E, Roth JA. Immune responses and protection by vaccine and various vaccine adjuvant candidates to virulent porcine reproductive and respiratory syndrome virus. Vet Immunol Immunopathol. 2006;109(1–2):99–115.
27. Suradhat S, Kesdangsakonwut S, Sada W, Buranapraditkun S, Wongsawang S, Thanawongnuwech R. Negative impact of porcine reproductive and respiratory syndrome virus infection on the efficacy of classical swine fever vaccine. Vaccine. 2006;24(14):2634–42.
28. Thanawongnuwech R, Brown GB, Halbur PG, Roth JA, Royer RL, Thacker BJ. Pathogenesis of porcine reproductive and respiratory syndrome virus-induced increase in susceptibility to Streptococcus suis infection. Vet Pathol. 2000;37(2):143–52.
29. Lamontagne L, Page C, Larochelle R, Magar R. Porcine reproductive and respiratory syndrome virus persistence in blood, spleen, lymph nodes, and tonsils of experimentally infected pigs depends on the level of CD8high T cells. Viral Immunol. 2003;16(3):395–406.
30. Samsom JN, de Bruin TG, Voermans JJ, Meulenberg JJ, Pol JM, Bianchi AT. Changes of leukocyte phenotype and function in the broncho-alveolar lavage fluid of pigs infected with porcine reproductive and respiratory syndrome virus: a role for CD8(+) cells. J Gen Virol. 2000;81(Pt 2):497–505.
31. Shimizu M, Yamada S, Kawashima K, Ohashi S, Shimizu S, Ogawa T. Changes of lymphocyte subpopulations in pigs infected with porcine reproductive and respiratory syndrome (PRRS) virus. Vet Immunol Immunopathol. 1996;50(1–2):19–27.
32. Xiao Z, Batista L, Dee S, Halbur P, Murtaugh MP. The level of virus-specific T-cell and macrophage recruitment in porcine reproductive and respiratory syndrome virus infection in pigs is independent of virus load. J Virol. 2004;78(11):5923–33.
33. Bautista EM, Molitor TW. Cell-mediated immunity to porcine reproductive and respiratory syndrome virus in swine. Viral Immunol. 1997;10(2):83–94.
34. Silva-Campa E, Mata-Haro V, Mateu E, Hernandez J. Porcine reproductive and respiratory syndrome virus induces CD4 + CD8 + CD25 + Foxp3+ regulatory T cells (Tregs). Virology. 2012;430(1):73–80.
35. Xue Leng, Zhenguang Li, Mingqi Xia, Xiyu Li, Fengxue Wang, Wei Wang, Xiuhua Zhang, Hua Wu, Xue Leng, Zhenguang Li, Mingqi Xia, Xiyu Li, Fengxue Wang, Wei Wang, Xiuhua Zhang, Hua Wu. Mutations in the genome of the highly pathogenic porcine reproductive and respiratory syndrome virus potentially related to attenuation. Veterinary Microbiology. 2012;157(1-2):50–60.
36 Prieto C, Martinez-Lobo FJ, Diez-Fuertes F, Aguilar-Calvo P, Simarro I, Castro JM. Immunisation of pigs with a major envelope protein sub-unit vaccine against porcine reproductive and respiratory syndrome virus (PRRSV) results in enhanced clinical disease following experimental challenge. Vet J. 2011; 189(3):323–9.

11

Evaluation of different nested PCRs for detection of *Anaplasma phagocytophilum* in ruminants and ticks

Jifei Yang[1], Zhijie Liu[1], Qingli Niu[1], Junlong Liu[1], Jingying Xie[1], Qiuyu Chen[1], Ze Chen[1], Guiquan Guan[1], Guangyuan Liu[1], Jianxun Luo[1*] and Hong Yin[1,2*]

Abstract

Background: *Anaplasma phagocytophilum* is a causative agent of granulocytic anaplasmosis in mammals, which has a broad geographical distribution and a high degree of clinical diversity. Currently, numerous PCR assays have been developed and used for the detection of *A. phagocytophilum* in various specimens. However, their performance varies. The aim of this study was to evaluate the performance of five nested PCR assays by detection of 363 ruminant and tick samples, and to select the most appropriate methods for the sensitive detection of *A. phagocytophilum* in environmental or clinical samples.

Results: Positive PCR results for *A. phagocytophilum* were obtained in 75 (20.7 %), 42 (11.6 %) and 19 (5.2 %) specimens with primer sets EC (EC9/EC12a and SSAP2f/SSAP2r), EE (EE1/EE2 and EE3/EE4) and ge (ge3a/ge10r, ge9f/ge2), respectively. The amplification of template DNA with the primer set MSP (MAP4AP5/MSP4AP3, msp4f/msp4r) could not be obtained in both ruminants and ticks, and a low specificity of the EL primers [EL(569)F/EL(1193)R, EL(569)F/EL(1142)R] in tick samples was observed. Our results revealed that the nested PCR with primer set EC complementary to the *16S rRNA* gene was the most sensitive assay for detection of *A. phagocytophilum* in ruminant and tick specimens. *A. phagocytophilum* was detected in 47 (35.1 %) sheep, 12 (10.4 %) cattle, and 17 (14.9 %) ticks. Two *A. phagocytophilum* genotypes were identified, that varied between sheep and cattle in sample collection sites.

Conclusions: This report provides more valuable information for the diagnosis and management of granulocytic anaplasmosis in China.

Keywords: *A. phagocytophilum*, Diagnosis, PCR, Ruminants, Tick, Prevalence

Background

HGA (Human granulocytic anaplasmosis) is an emerging tick-borne zoonosis caused by the obligate intracellular bacterium *Anaplasma phagocytophilum* (formerly known as *Ehrlichia phagocytophila*, *Ehrlichia equi* or the HGE agent) [1, 2]. The organism is commonly maintained in nature through an enzootic cycle involving ticks and vertebrate hosts [3, 4]. Several *Ixodes* ticks are known or suspected vectors of *A. phagocytophilum*, including *Ixodes scapularis* and *Ixodes pacificus* in North America, *Ixodes ricinus* in Europe, and *Ixodes persulcatus* in Russia and Asian [3, 5–8]. *A. phagocytophilum* infects a variety of hosts and causes granulocytic anaplasmosis in humans but also in wild and domestic animals [9, 10]. Since the first suspected human case was reported in Anhui province in 2006, more than 90 cases of HGA have been recorded in Beijing, Tianjin, Shandong, Henan, Hubei and Inner Mongolia in China [11, 12]. The actual number of human cases may be much higher due to the poor diagnostic tools, non-specificity of the reported symptoms and lack of awareness of public health professionals [13].

Rapid and sensitive detection of *A. phagocytophilum* is an essential step for the control and prevention of HGA in endemic areas. *A. phagocytophilum* was initially

* Correspondence: luojianxun@caas.cn; yinhong@caas.cn
[1]State Key Laboratory of Veterinary Etiological Biology, Key Laboratory of Veterinary Parasitology of Gansu Province, Lanzhou Veterinary Research Institute, Chinese Academy of Agricultural Science, Xujiaping 1, Lanzhou, Gansu 730046, P. R. China
Full list of author information is available at the end of the article

identified as a human agent using molecular methods rather than culture or serological tests [1, 14]. Since then, PCR assays have played an important role in the laboratory diagnosis of HGA in clinical and environmental specimens for their rapidity and relative ease of performance. However, their performance varies significantly [15, 16]. Most studies have always focused on the analytical sensitivity or specificity of those PCR assays, and the ability to detect small amounts of nucleic acid and specific nucleic acid fragments, to enable distinction of closely related strains [15, 16]. However, considerable variation within *A. phagocytophilum* strains has been described, and isolates from various hosts or geographic locations have displayed genetic diversity and divergence within frequently used PCR-target genes, such as *groESL*, *ankA* and *msp4* [17–19]. Some assays could not detect all the variants or ecotypes of *A. phagocitophilum*. Thus, it is critical to evaluate the performance of prospective assays in certain species and in a given geographic area in order to obtain more reliable results. The objective of this study was to evaluate five nested PCRs for detection of *A. phagocytophilum* in ruminants and tick specimens from northwest China.

Methods

EDTA–K^{2+} anticoagulated blood samples were taken from the jugular vein of 249 asymptomatic domestic ruminants (134 sheep and 115 cattle) and collected in a sterile tube in May 2015 from Ili Kazakh Autonomous Prefecture, in northern Xinjiang, China. One hundred and fourteen ticks were collected from sheep, cattle and other livestock within same herds. Five species of ticks were identified in accordance with the standard taxonomic keys [20]. Seventy-two ticks collected from cattle were identified as *Dermacentor marginatus*; 35 ticks collected from sheep were identified as *Haemaphysalis punctata* ($n = 28$), *Haemaphysalis concinna* ($n = 3$) and *Hyalomma asiaticum* ($n = 4$); and seven ticks collected from horses were identified as *Hyalomma detritum*. The samples collection in the present study was consented by animals owners. All animal treatments and handling complied with Ethical Guidelines and were approved by the Animal Ethics Committee of Lanzhou Veterinary Research Institute, Chinese Academy of Agricultural Sciences.

DNA was extracted from blood and tick samples using a Gentra Puregene DNA Purification kit (Qiagen) as described previously [9]. All DNA samples were examined for the presence of *A. phagocytophilum* by nested PCRs. The PCR primers are listed in Table 1. The reaction was performed in an automatic thermocycler (Bio-Rad, Hercules, CA, USA) in a total volume of 25 μL containing 2.5 μL of 10× PCR buffer (Mg^{2+} Plus), 2.0 μL of each dNTP at 2.5 mM, 1.25 U of *Taq* DNA polymerase

Table 1 Oligonucleotide primers used for detection of *A. phagocutophilum*

Target gene	Primer name	Primer Sequence (5′-3′)	Annealing temp (°C)	Amplicon size (bp)	Reference
16S rRNA	ge3a	CACATGCAAGTCGAACGGATTATTC	55	932	[25]
	ge10r	TTCCGTTAAGAAGGATCTAATCTCC			
	ge9f	AACGGATTATTCTTTATAGCTTGCT	55	546	
	ge2	GGCAGTATTAAAAGCAGCTCCAGG			
Msp4	MAP4AP5	ATGAATTACAGAGAATTGCTTGTAGG	54	849	[24, 27]
	MSP4AP3	TTAATTGAAAGCAAATCTTGCTCCTATG			
	msp4f	CTATTGGYGGNGCYAGAGT	55	381	
	msp4r	GTTCATCGAAAATTCCGTGGTA			
16S rRNA	EE-1	TCCTGGCTCAGAACGAACGCTGGCGGC	50	1433	[23]
	EE-2	AGTCACTGACCCAACCTTAAATGGCTG			
	EE-3	GTCGAACGGATTATTCTTTATAGCTTGC	50	926	
	EE-4	CCCTTCCGTTAAGAAGGATCTAATCTCC			
groEL	EL(569)F	ATGGTATGCAGTTTGATCGC	62	624	[26, 34]
	EL(1193)R	TCTACTCTGTCTTTGCGTTC			
	EL(569)F	ATGGTATGCAGTTTGATCGC	56	573	
	EL(1142)R	TTGAGTACAGCAACACCACCGGAA			
16S rRNA	EC9	TACCTTGTTACGACTT	55	1462	[35]
	EC12a	TGATCCTGGCTCAGAACGAACG			
	SSAP2f	GCTGAATGTGGGGATAATTTAT	55	641	
	SSAP2r	ATGGCTGCTTCCTTTCGGTTA			

(TaKaRa, Dalian, China), 2.0 μL of template DNA, 1.0 μL of each primer (20 pmol) and 16.25 μL of distilled water. DNA from sheep infected with *A. phagocytophilum* validated by sequencing (Gene accession no. JN558811) was used as a positive control, and sterile water was used as the blank control for each run. The cycling conditions for the first and second round amplification involved 4 min of denaturation at 94 °C, 35 cycles at 94 °C for 30 s, annealing for 30 s at a temperature dependent on the primers applied (annealing temperatures shown in Table 1), and 72 °C for 1 to 1.5 min (dependent on the length of target fragments), with a final extension step at 72 °C for 10 min. The PCR products were visualized by UV transillumination in a 1.5 % agarose gel following electrophoresis and staining with ethidium bromide.

A. phagocytophilum positive samples were selected randomly and verified by sequencing. The PCR products were cloned into the pGEM-T Easy vector (Promega, Shanghai, China) and subjected to bidirectional sequencing (Sangon Biotech, Shanghai, China). The sequences obtained were compared with reference sequences from GenBank (see Additional file 1). A phylogenetic tree was then constructed using the neighbor-joining (NJ) algorithm with the Kimura two-parameter model of the Mega 4.0 Software [21]. The GenBank accession numbers for the partial 16S rRNA gene sequences obtained in this study were as follows: KT944028-KT944029 and KT951192.

The results were analyzed using a Chi-square test in Predictive for Analytics Software (PASW) Statistics version 18. A difference was considered statistically significant at $P < 0.05$.

Results

Of the total 363 ruminant and tick specimens that were included in our evaluation of the five nested PCR assays, positive PCR results for *A. phagocytophilum* were obtained in 75 (20.7 %), 42 (11.6 %) and 19 (5.2 %) specimens with primer sets EC (EC9/EC12a and SSAP2f/SSAP2r), EE (EE1/EE2 and EE3/EE4) and ge (ge3a/ge10r, ge9f/ge2), respectively (Table 2). DNA of *A. phagocytophilum* was found in only two cattle specimens using primer set EL [EL(569)F/EL(1193)R, EL(569)F/EL(1142)R]. However, unspecific products were obtained in tick specimens with EL primers as a result of two bands between 250 and 500 bp (data not shown). Under the PCR conditions outlined, amplification of the template DNA with the primer set MSP (MAP4AP5/MSP4AP3, msp4f/msp4r) could not be obtained (Table 2). Apart from the primer sets EL and MSP, the assays showed that the positive rates of *A. phagocytophilum* infection in ruminant and tick specimens ranged from 5.6 to 20.7 %. The highest positive rate (20.7 %, 75/363) was observed using the EC primer set (Table 2). The PCR with EC primer set was more sensitive than the ones with EE and ge primer sets (Chi2 = 39.944, df = 2, $P < 0.001$); and the PCR with EE primer set was more sensitive than that with ge primer set (Chi2 = 9.468, df = 1, $P < 0.01$). Moreover, an additional tick sample (2–21) was negative with EC primers but positive with EE, which gave an overall positivity rate of 20.9 % in our sample population. As shown in Table 2, the infection rates of *A. phagocytophilum* were 35.1 %, 10.4 % and 14.9 % in sheep, cattle and ticks, respectively. Of those tick samples, *A. phagocytophilum* was detected in *D. marginatus* collected from cattle and *H. punctata* collected from sheep.

The specificity of the assay was controlled by sequencing. Considering the highest sensitivity of the assay with EC primers in this study, 20 samples (four from cattle, seven from sheep, five from *D. marginatus* and four from *H. punctata*) positive for EC primers and the tick sample (*D. marginatus*, sample ID: 2–21, negative for EC but positive for EE) were selected for sequencing. Sequence analyzed by a BLASTn search in GenBank confirmed the presence of *A. phagocytophilum* in those samples. Four sequences (GenBank accession no. KT944028) identified in cattle showed 99.7 % identity to the isolate KS20 (GenBank accession no. KJ782390) from cattle in Kashgar, Xinjiang province. The remaining 16 sequences (GenBank accession no. KT944029) identified in sheep and ticks were identical to each other and showed 99.2 % identity to strain YC38

Table 2 *A. phagocytophilum* in ruminants and ticks detected by nested PCRs

Host (No. tested)	No. (%) positive with:					
	EC9/EC12a SSAP2f/SSAP2r	EE1/EE2 EE3/EE4	ge3a/ge10r ge9f/ge2	EL(569)F/EL(1193)R EL(569)F/EL(1142)R	MAP4AP5/MSP4AP3 msp4f/msp4r	At least one primer
Sheep ($n = 134$)	47 (35.1)	31 (23.1)	9 (6.7)	0 (0)	0 (0)	47 (35.1)
Cattle ($n = 115$)	12 (10.4)	6 (5.2)	3 (2.6)	2 (1.7)	0 (0)	12 (10.4)
Tick ($n = 114$)	16 (14)	5 (4.4)	7 (6.1)	NA[a]	0 (0)	17 (14.9)
Total ($n = 363$)	75 (20.7)	42 (11.6)	19 (5.2)	NA[a]	0 (0)	76 (20.9)

[a]: not applied

(GenBank accession no. KJ782381) from sheep in Yecheng, Xinjiang province. Moreover, one sequence (GenBank accession no. KT951192) identified in *D. marginatus* tick (2–21) had 98.9 % identity to the BL102-7 strain (GenBank accession no. KJ410249) derived from *Hyalomma asiaticum* in Xinjiang. Phylogenetic analyses revealed that the *A. phagocytophilum* isolates identified in this study are placed on two separate clades (Fig. 1).

Discussion

A. phagocytophilum is an emerging tick-borne zoonotic agents of public health significance [1]. The disease presents as a clinical syndrome, ranging from asymptomatic to fatal disease [22]. Nonspecific symptoms and signs are manifested in the disease state, and most commonly manifested by fever, chills, headache, and myalgias, which are difficult to differentiate from those of other febrile illness [15, 22]. PCR-based methods are powerful tools and play an important role in the confirmation of *A. phagocytophilum* infection in clinical and environmental specimens. Since the first identification of the HGA agent in 1994, numerous PCR amplification assays and primer sets have been described for detection of *A. phagocytophilum* [1, 23–27]. However, their performance varies [16, 28]. Thus, a choice of PCR methods with appropriate primers that target different DNA segments of *A. phagocytophilum* is crucial for obtaining the best possible results, and this affects the sensitivity and specificity of the diagnostic assays significantly.

A. phagocytophilum infection has been reported in humans, wild and domestic animals in China, and the infection rates were variable in different hosts or geographic locations [9, 12, 29, 30]. In this study, the positive rate was significantly higher in sheep than in cattle (Chi2 = 20.781, df = 1, $P < 0.001$), similar result has been described in previous report [29]. Of those tick samples, *A. phagocytophilum* infection was found in *D. marginatus* and *H. punctata* ticks. However, we could not conclude that the role of *D. marginatus* and *H. punctata* as reservoirs or vectors of *A. phagocytophilum* because of the agent detected in this study could be from the hosts, which warrants further investigation.

In the present study, five primer sets, designed to amplify *16S rRNA*, the heat shock gene operon *groESL* and major surface protein gene *msp4*, were used to evaluate the applicability of nested PCR for detection of *A. phagocytophilum* DNA in ruminant and tick specimens. Considerable differences were observed in the performance of these five assays. The results indicated that the nested PCR with EC primer set targeting the 16S rRNA gene is the most sensitive method (Chi2 = 39.944, df = 2, $P < 0.001$). The assay with MSP primer set appeared less useful for detection of *A. phagocytophilum* in ruminants and ticks, and the EL primer set was less effective for detection of tick specimens. The primer sets EE was more sensitive than ge, MSP and EL, but significantly less useful than EC (Chi2 = 11.096, df = 1, $P < 0.01$). However, a previous evaluation of several different published methods for PCR amplification of specific DNA in *A. phagocytophilum*-infected HL-60 cells showed that the ge primer set provided the highest analytical sensitive and specificity, which could detect the equivalent of 0.25 infected cells [16]. Beyond the optimization of the nucleic acid amplification conditions, the PCR amplification efficiency could be influenced by the concentration of DNA templates in this

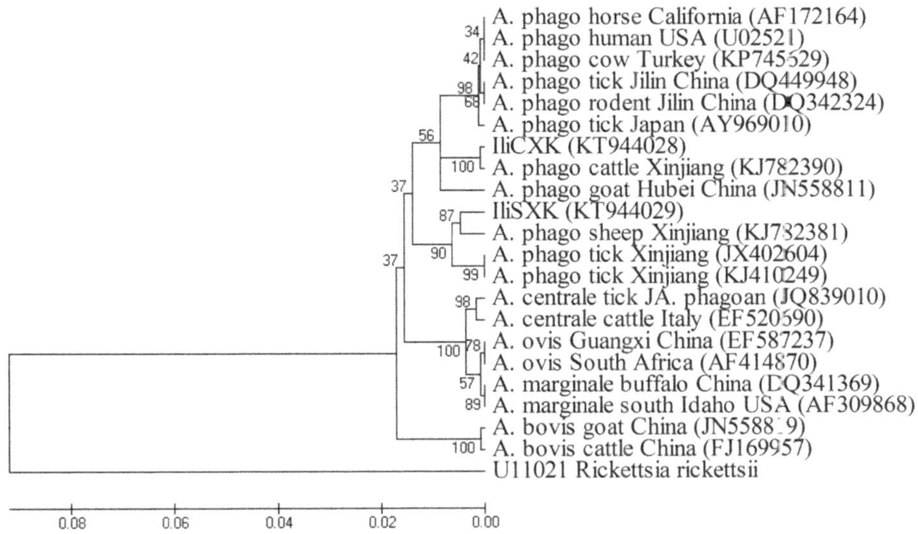

Fig. 1 Phylogenetic analysis of *A. phagocytophilum* (*A. phago*) based on 16S rRNA gene partial sequences (599 bp). *Rickettsia rickettsii* is used as an outgroup

comparative analysis study. Although one tick sample (2–21) was negative for EC but positive for EE, the assay with the EC primer set showed high sensitivity in ruminants and ticks. Sequence analysis of EC–positive samples verified the specificity of the assay. Based on the comparative analysis of those five assays, the nested PCR with EC primer set would provide more reliable results for *A. phagocytophilum* detection in ruminant and tick specimens.

Phylogenetic analysis of the obtained *A. phagocytophilum* 16S rRNA gene sequences in this study showed that they were variable from the sequence from the positive control (Gene accession no. JN558811), excluded possible contamination and indicated the complexity of the genotype of the *A. phagocytophilum* in the field (Fig. 1). The *A. phagocytophilum* strain one (GenBank accession no. KT944028) identified in cattle was most closely related to the isolate detected in cattle from Kashgar (GenBank accession no. KJ782390) (Fig. 1). The strain two (GenBank accession no. KT944029) identified in sheep and ticks were most closely related to the isolate detected in sheep from Yecheng (GenBank accession no. KJ782381) (Fig. 1). These results suggested that *A. phagocytophilum* genotypes are vary between sheep and cattle in sample collection sites.

The results of the present study support the use of nested PCR with primer set EC (EC9/EC12a and SSAP2f/SSAP2r) targeting the *16S rRNA* gene, which was the most sensitive assay for the detection of *A. phagocytophilum* DNA in ruminants and ticks in the region investigated in China. Although this assay was more sensitive than others, it could also miss positive samples for unknown reasons. Given that no test is actually 100 % sensitive or specific, an important consideration is that two or more assays should always be used in parallel to achieve maximum sensitivity for the molecular detection of *A. phagocytophilim.*

There are numerous factors involved in the optimization of PCR assays, and the potential discrepancies make it difficult to ensure the performance of a given assay in different laboratories. *A. phagocytophilum* displayed a high degree of genetic diversity, host tropisms and variation in pathogenicity [31]. Considerable strain variation of *A. phagocytophilum* has been reported in different hosts or geographic locations, and the organism can be genetically divided into several subclusters using *groESL*, *ankA* and *msp4* [17–19]. Recently, four distinct ecological clusters correlate with host species have been established based on *ankA* gene [32], four geographically dispersed ecotypes were identified based on *groESL* gene and showed significantly different host ranges in Europe [33]. Thus, each laboratory should determine the efficacy of those assays under local conditions, and the choice of appropriate assays could yield accurate results for the detection of *A. phagocytophilum* in ticks and animals.

Conclusions

The performance of five nested PCR assays was accessed by parallel detection of field-collected samples. The nested PCR with primer set EC (EC9/EC12a and SSAP2f/SSAP2r) targeting the *16S rRNA* gene was the most sensitive assay for the detection of *A. phagocytophilum* DNA in ruminants and ticks. *A. phagocytophilum* was detected in 47 (35.1 %) sheep, 12 (10.4 %) cattle, and 17 (14.9 %) ticks collected from Ili Kazakh Autonomous Prefecture in northern Xinjiang, and two *A. phagocytophilum* genotypes were identified. These findings not only provide valuable information for the control of *A. phagocytophilum* infection, but also indicate potential implications for public health.

Competing interests

The authors declare that they have no competing interests.

Authors' contributions

HY and JY designed this study and critically revised the manuscript. JL participated in its design, coordination and manuscript revision. JY, ZL, QC, ZC and QN participated in sample collection and identification. JY, JX, JL, GL and GG performed the experiments, data analysis, and drafted the manuscript. All authors read and approved the final manuscript.

Acknowledgements

This study was financially supported by the NSFC (№31372432, №31201899, №31272556, №31402189, №31471967), ASTIP, FRIP (2014ZL010), CAAS; Creative Research Groups of Gansu Province (№1210RJIA006); NBCIS CARS-38, Special Fund for Agro-scientific Research in the Public Research (№201303035, №201303037), MOA; 973 Program (2015CB150300), Supporting Program (2013BAD12B03, 2013BAD12B05), MOST, China; Jiangsu Co-innovation Center programme for Prevention and Control of Important Animal Infectious Diseases and Zoonoses, State Key Laboratory of Veterinary Etiological Biology Project. The research was also facilitated by CRP No. 16198/R0 IAEA.

Author details

[1]State Key Laboratory of Veterinary Etiological Biology, Key Laboratory of Veterinary Parasitology of Gansu Province, Lanzhou Veterinary Research Institute, Chinese Academy of Agricultural Science, Xujiaping 1, Lanzhou, Gansu 730046, P. R. China. [2]Jiangsu Co-innovation Center for Prevention and Control of Important Animal Infectious Diseases and Zoonoses, Yangzhou 225009, P. R. China.

References

1. Chen SM, Dumler JS, Bakken JS, Walker DH. Identification of a granulocytotropic Ehrlichia species as the etiologic agent of human disease. J Clin Microbiol. 1994; 32(3):589–95.
2. Zhan L, Cao WC, Chu CY, Jiang BG, Zhang F, Liu W, Dumler JS, Wu XM, Zuo SQ, Zhang PH. Tick-borne agents in rodents, China, 2004–2006. Emerg Infect Dis. 2009;15(12):1904.
3. Bown KJ, Begon M, Bennett M, Woldehiwet Z, Ogden NH. Seasonal dynamics of *Anaplasma phagocytophila* in a rodent-tick (*Ixodes trianguliceps*) system, United Kingdom. Emerg Infect Dis. 2003;9(1):63–70.
4. Dumler JS, Barbet AF, Bekker CP, Dasch GA, Palmer GH, Ray SC, Rikihisa Y, Rurangirwa FR. Reorganization of genera in the families Rickettsiaceae and Anaplasmataceae in the order Rickettsiales: unification of some species of *Ehrlichia* with *Anaplasma*, *Cowdria* with *Ehrlichia* and *Ehrlichia* with *Neorickettsia*, descriptions of six new species combinations and designation of *Ehrlichia equi* and 'HGE agent' as subjective synonyms of *Ehrlichia phagocytophila*. Int J Syst Evol Microbiol. 2001;51(Pt 6):2145–65.
5. Cao WC, Zhao QM, Zhang PH, Yang H, Wu XM, Wen BH, Zhang XT, Habbema JD. Prevalence of *Anaplasma phagocytophila* and *Borrelia burgdorferi* in *Ixodes persulcatus* ticks from northeastern China. Am J Trop Med Hyg. 2003;68(5):547–50.

6. Liz JS, Anderes L, Sumner JW, Massung RF, Gern L, Rutti B, Brossard M. PCR detection of granulocytic ehrlichiae in *Ixodes ricinus* ticks and wild small mammals in western Switzerland. J Clin Microbiol. 2000;38(3):1002–7.
7. Shpynov S, Fournier PE, Rudakov N, Tarasevich I, Raoult D. Detection of members of the genera *Rickettsia*, *Anaplasma*, and *Ehrlichia* in ticks collected in the Asiatic part of Russia. Ann N Y Acad Sci. 2006;1078:378–83.
8. Telford 3rd SR, Dawson JE, Katavolos P, Warner CK, Kolbert CP, Persing DH. Perpetuation of the agent of human granulocytic ehrlichiosis in a deer tick-rodent cycle. Proc Natl Acad Sci U S A. 1996;93(12):6209–14.
9. Yang J, Liu Z, Guan G, Liu Q, Li Y, Chen Z, Ma M, Liu A, Ren Q, Luo J, et al. Prevalence of *Anaplasma phagocytophilum* in ruminants, rodents and ticks in Gansu, north-western China. J Med Microbiol. 2013;62(Pt 2):254–8.
10. Foley JE, Nieto NC, Adjemian J, Dabritz H, Brown RN. *Anaplasma phagocytophilum* infection in small mammal hosts of *Ixodes* ticks, western United States. Emerg Infect Dis. 2008;14(7):1147–50.
11. Zhang L, Liu Y, Ni D, Li Q, Yu Y, Yu XJ, Wan K, Li D, Liang G, Jiang X, et al. Nosocomial transmission of human granulocytic anaplasmosis in China. JAMA. 2008;300(19):2263–70.
12. Fang LQ, Liu K, Li XL, Liang S, Yang Y, Yao HW, Sun RX, Sun Y, Chen WJ, Zuo SQ, et al. Emerging tick-borne infections in mainland China: an increasing public health threat. Lancet Infect Dis. 2015;15(12):1467–79.
13. Jin H, Wei F, Liu Q, Qian J. Epidemiology and control of human granulocytic anaplasmosis: a systematic review. Vector Borne Zoonotic Dis. 2012;12(4): 269–74.
14. Bakken JS, Dumler JS, Chen SM, Eckman MR, Van Etta LL, Walker DH. Human granulocytic ehrlichiosis in the upper Midwest United States. A new species emerging? JAMA. 1994;272(3):212–8.
15. Dumler JS, Brouqui P. Molecular diagnosis of human granulocytic anaplasmosis. Expert Rev Mol Diagn. 2004;4(4):559–69.
16. Massung RF, Slater KG. Comparison of PCR assays for detection of the agent of human granulocytic ehrlichiosis, *Anaplasma phagocytophilum*. J Clin Microbiol. 2003;41(2):717–22.
17. Morissette E, Massung RF, Foley JE, Alleman AR, Foley P, Barbet AF. Diversity of *Anaplasma phagocytophilum* strains, USA. Emerg Infect Dis. 2009;15(6): 928–31.
18. Strasek Smrdel K, Tozon N, Duh D, Petrovec M, Avsic Zupanc T. Diversity of *groESL* sequences of *Anaplasma phagocytophilum* among dogs in Slovenia. Clin Microbiol Infect. 2009;15 Suppl 2:79–80.
19. Strasek Smrdel K, von Loewenich FD, Petrovec M, Avsic Zupanc T. Diversity of *ankA* and *msp4* genes of *Anaplasma phagocytophilum* in Slovenia. Ticks Tick Borne Dis. 2015;6(2):164–6.
20. Deng GF, Jiang ZL. Economic insect fauna of China, Fasc 39 Acari: Ixodiate. Beijing: Science Press; 1991.
21. Tamura K, Dudley J, Nei M, Kumar S. MEGA4: Molecular Evolutionary Genetics Analysis (MEGA) software version 4.0. Mol Biol Evol. 2007;24(8):1596–9.
22. Bakken JS, Dumler JS. Clinical diagnosis and treatment of human granulocytotropic anaplasmosis. Ann N Y Acad Sci. 2006;1078:236–47.
23. Barlough JE, Madigan JE, DeRock E, Bigornia L. Nested polymerase chain reaction for detection of *Ehrlichia equi* genomic DNA in horses and ticks (*Ixodes pacificus*). Vet Parasitol. 1996;63(3–4):319–29.
24. Bown KJ, Lambin X, Ogden NH, Petrovec M, Shaw SE, Woldehiwet Z, Birtles RJ. High-resolution genetic fingerprinting of European strains of *Anaplasma phagocytophilum* by use of multilocus variable-number tandem-repeat analysis. J Clin Microbiol. 2007;45(6):1771–6.
25. Massung RF, Slater K, Owens JH, Nicholson WL, Mather TN, Solberg VB, Olson JG. Nested PCR assay for detection of granulocytic ehrlichiae. J Clin Microbiol. 1998;36(4):1090–5.
26. Reye AL, Hubschen JM, Sausy A, Muller CP. Prevalence and seasonality of tick-borne pathogens in questing *Ixodes ricinus* ticks from Luxembourg. Appl Environ Microbiol. 2010;76(9):2923–31.
27. de la Fuente J, Massung RF, Wong SJ, Chu FK, Lutz H, Meli M, von Loewenich FD, Grzeszczuk A, Torina A, Caracappa S, et al. Sequence analysis of the *msp4* gene of *Anaplasma phagocytophilum* strains. J Clin Microbiol. 2005;43(3):1309–17.
28. Schotthoefer AM, Meece JK, Ivacic LC, Bertz PD, Zhang K, Weiler T, Uphoff TS, Fritsche TR. Comparison of a real-time PCR method with serology and blood smear analysis for diagnosis of human anaplasmosis: importance of infection time course for optimal test utilization. J Clin Microbiol. 2013;51(7):2147–53.
29. Yang J, Li Y, Liu Z, Liu J, Niu Q, Ren Q, Chen Z, Guan G, Luo J, Yin H. Molecular detection and characterization of *Anaplasma* spp. in sheep and cattle from Xinjiang, northwest China. Parasit Vectors. 2015;8:108.
30. Liu Z, Ma M, Wang Z, Wang J, Peng Y, Li Y, Guan G, Luo J, Yin H. Molecular survey and genetic identification of *Anaplasma* species in goats from central and southern China. Appl Environ Microbiol. 2012;78(2):464–70.
31. Barakova I, Derdakova M, Carpi G, Rosso F, Collini M, Tagliapietra V, Ramponi C, Hauffe HC, Rizzoli A. Genetic and ecologic variability among *Anaplasma phagocytophilum* strains, northern Italy. Emerg Infect Dis. 2014;20(6):1082–5.
32. Scharf W, Schauer S, Freyburger F, Petrovec M, Schaarschmidt-Kiener D, Liebisch G, Runge M, Ganter M, Kehl A, Dumler JS, et al. Distinct host species correlate with *Anaplasma phagocytophilum ankA* gene clusters. J Clin Microbiol. 2011;49(3):790–6.
33. Jahfari S, Coipan EC, Fonville M, van Leeuwen AD, Hengeveld P, Heylen D, Heyman P, van Maanen C, Butler CM, Foldvari G, et al. Circulation of four *Anaplasma phagocytophilum* ecotypes in Europe. Parasit Vectors. 2014;7:365.
34. Alberti A, Zobba R, Chessa B, Addis MF, Sparagano O, Pinna Parpaglia ML, Cubeddu T, Pintori G, Pittau M. Equine and canine *Anaplasma phagocytophilum* strains isolated on the island of Sardinia (Italy) are phylogenetically related to pathogenic strains from the United States. Appl Environ Microbiol. 2005;71(10):6418–22.
35. Kawahara M, Rikihisa Y, Lin Q, Isogai E, Tahara K, Itagaki A, Hiramitsu Y, Tajima T. Novel genetic variants of *Anaplasma phagocytophilum*, *Anaplasma bovis*, *Anaplasma centrale*, and a novel *Ehrlichia* sp. in wild deer and ticks on two major islands in Japan. Appl Environ Microbiol. 2006;72(2):1102–9.

12

Effects of selected Palestinian plants on the in vitro exsheathment of the third stage larvae of gastrointestinal nematodes

Rana Majed Jamous[1], Mohammed Saleem Ali-Shtayeh[1*], Salam Yousef Abu-Zaitoun[1], Alex Markovics[2] and Hassan Azaizeh[3,4]

Abstract

Background: Gastrointestinal parasites are one of the main restrictions to small ruminant production. Their pathological importance is primarily related to the major production losses, in quantity or quality, induced by the direct action of worms. Control of these parasites is based exclusively on the frequent use of anthelmintic drugs. However, the resistance to anthelmintics in worm populations after commercialisation of chemical drugs is now widespread. Therefore, there is a need to find new natural resources to ensure sustainable and effective treatment and control of these parasites. The aim of this study was to evaluate the anthelmintic activity, as minimum inhibitory concentration (IC_{50} mg/mL), of different plant extracts using larval exsheathment inhibition assay using a two-species but steady population of parasitic nematodes (ca. 20% *Teladorsagia circumcinta* and 80% *Trichostrongylus colubriformis*).

Results: The study showed that the ethanolic extracts of 22 out of the 48 plant extracts, obtained from 46 plant species, have an inhibitory effect >50% (at concentrations of 100 mg/mL) on the third stage larvae (L3) of the nematodes exhibited the strongest inhibition activity (94%) with IC_{50} of 0.02 mg/mL, where other members of the Rhamnaceae family have shown to possess strong anthelmintic activity (70–89%).

Conclusions: Plant extracts are potential rich resources of anthelmintics to combat helminthic diseases. Our results suggest that extracts from *Rhamnus elaternus, Epilobium hirsutum, Leucaena leucocephala* and *Rhamnus palaestinus* have promising anthelmintic activity, with potential applications in animal therapeutics and feed.

Keywords: Anthelmintics, Exsheathment inhibition assay (LEIA), Medicinal plants, Polyphenolic compounds, Tannins, Palestinian flora

Background

Infections of the gastrointestinal tract of ruminants with parasitic nematodes represent a major pathology associated with outdoor production of sheep and goats worldwide [1–4]. Small ruminant are infected with the same prominent gastrointestinal parasites, which induce similar pathological symptoms and economic consequences [5]. Gastrointestinal nematodes are one of the main restrictions to sheep and goats production and may cause more than 20% loss for marketable products [6]. Their pathological importance is primarily related to the major production losses, in quantity or quality, induced by the direct action of worms. However, other studies suggested that the host's immune-mediated response in grazing meat-breed lambs infected with *T. colubriformis* is the major component of production loss [7].

Control of gastrointestinal parasites is based exclusively on the frequent use of anthelmintic drugs. However, this apparently exclusive reliance on synthetic molecules is not sustainable and currently faces several limitations. The first one is the rapid development of resistance to anthelmintics in worm populations after commercialisation of chemical drugs and the occurrence, in some regions, of multi-resistant strains strongly challenges the control of these parasites with drugs nowadays [8–11]. Second, is the increased concern of consumers over drug residues in meat and milk

* Correspondence: msshtayeh@yahoo.com
[1]Biodiversity& Environmental Research Center –BERC, Til, Nablus, Palestine
Full list of author information is available at the end of the article

products, and a potential risk for environmental contamination [12]. In the attempt to reduce the use of chemicals due to the concern about human health and environmental toxicology, new and safer food control approaches such as the use of natural compounds are nowadays being developed [13–15].

In vivo and in vitro studies have shown that plants containing secondary metabolites, such as tannins, sesquiterpene lactones and flavone glycosides, are a promising option for use in integrated nematode control in farm production systems [16–18]. Tannin-rich plant extracts have shown in vitro to prevent eggs hatching of nematodes, and hinder development, motility, and exsheathment of larvae [19–21]. In addition, feeding of goats and sheep with tanniferous plants has led to reduction of nematode egg excretion and worm burden [22–25]. Some differences in activity of the same tannin-rich resource might be depending on the tested parasite species.

Natural compounds from plants provide a remarkable opportunity in the search for new, effective and safe anthelmintic products [26–28]. In Palestine, medicinal plants have been reported to play a vital role in the treatment of many disease conditions in humans [29–32]. A recent study has revealed that around 140 medicinal plant species are still in use in traditional medicine in Palestine for the treatment of several livestock diseases including gastro-intestinal infections (causing diarrhea, colic, flatulence, constipation, digestive system, and anthelmintic) [33]. This research also showed the gastrointestinal disorders is the disease group in the study area that scored the highest informant consensus factor (ICF) value (0.90), followed by urinary, and reproductive disorders (0.89) [33]. However, these plants have not been experimentally evaluated for their anthelmintic activity to justify their use in the treatment of such infections. The current study was therefore aimed at: collection of potential local plant species from Palestine, extraction of the bioactive ingredients, and determining the total phenolic and tannin contents; evaluation of the anthelmintic activity of different plant extracts using larval exsheathment inhibition assay (LEIA), and determination of the minimum inhibitory activity (IC_{50}) of the most active plants extracts.

Methods

Preparation of plant extracts for exsheathment tests.

Areal parts of 46 plant species belonging to 26 families were collected from open fields during the period from June 2015 to February 2016 from Palestine, where plant species were identified by Prof. M. S. Ali-Shtayeh from the Biodiversity and Environmental Research Center, BERC, Til Village, Nablus (Table 1). Voucher specimens are deposited in the Herbarium of BERC. Plant parts were dried at 50 °C for 24 h, then ten grams from each dried material was grinded and incubated separately with 100 mL of 70% ethanol at 35 °C for 3 h. The extracts were then filtered and dried using rotary evaporator at 50 °C to remove the ethanol followed by freeze drying. The powdered extracts were stored at – 20 °C for further analysis [18]. Extraction yield was calculated as g extract per g dried matter (DM) of plant leaves.

Determination of total phenolic content

Total phenols in plant extracts were measured by a colorimetric assay following the Folin-Ciocalteu method [34]. In brief, 0.5 mL of each sample dissolved in methanol (1 mg/mL) was transferred to test tube and mixed with 2.5 mL of a 10 fold dilute Folin-Ciocalteu reagent and 2 mL of 7.5% sodium carbonate. The tubes were allowed to stand for 30 min at room temperature. Then the absorbance was recorded spectrometrically at 760 nm versus gallic acid as blank, and total phenolic content was expressed as mg gallic acid equivalent (GAE)/g dry weight. All samples were analyzed in three replicates.

Determination of tannin contents

Tannin content in each plant sample was measured using the polyvinylpyrrolidone (PVP) following the method described by Makkar et al. [35]. In brief, 0.5 mL of extract dissolved in methanol (1 mg/mL) was mixed with 0.5 mL (100 mg /mL) of PVP, vortexed for few seconds, stand for 15 min at 4 °C and then centrifuged for 10 min at 3000 rpm. The non-tannin phenolics were determined in the clear supernatant in the same way as for total phenolic content. Total phenols in plant extracts were measured by the colorimetric assay following the Folin-Ciocalteu method as described above. Tannin content was calculated as the difference between total phenolic and non-tannin phenolic contents in the plant extracts.

Larval exsheathment inhibition assays (LEIA)

We used one donor goat that was parasitized by two nematode species, *Teladorsagia circumcincta* and *Trichostrongylus colubriformis* which are considered the main species at our region and usually found in the same animal. Species were identified as described by Van Wyk et al. [36]: their proportions in the suspension were steady throughout the year: 25, 75; 25, 75; 20, 80; and 18, 82%; in winter, spring, summer, and fall, respectively. The LEIA assay was performed according to Bahuaud et al. [37]. The extracts were diluted in phosphate buffer solution (PBS), and the tested concentration was 1 mg/mL. The test was performed on three replicate samples of each plant extract as well as of samples of the PBS solution, which served as a negative control. Approximately 200 L3 larvae (150 µl) were mixed with

Table 1 List of local flora analyzed for their exsheathment inhibition activity (LEIA) of the third stage larvae (L3) of a mixture of nematodes species

Scientific name (Family) (Voucher specimen)	English Name	Plant part	Total phenolic content (GAE-mg/g)	Tannins (GAE-mg/g)	% Exsh. inhibition (60 min)	IC50 (mg/mL)
Rhamnus alaternus L. (Rhamnaceae) (BERC-BX-C-0124)	Italian Buckthorn	Leaves	68.1	46.35	94	0.02
Rhamnus palaestinus Boiss. (Rhamnaceae) (BERC-BX-C-0150)	Palestine Buckthorn	Leaves	126.85	86.6	89	0.22
Epilobium hirsutum L. (Onagraceae) (BERC-BX-C-0250)	Great Willowherb	Leaves	234.58	98.68	84	0.03
Pistacia palaestina Boiss. (Anacardiaceae) (BERC-BX-C-0010)	Palestinian Pistachio, Terebinth	Leaves	121.63	58.93	84	0.50
Laurus nobilis L. (Lauraceae) (BERC-BX-C-0061)	Laurel, Sweet Bay	Leaves	96.98	84.58	79	0.37
Ziziphus sativa Gaetn. (Rhamnaceae) (BERC-BX-C-0231)	Jujube	Leaves	136.75	86.75	76	2.09
Leucaena leucocephala (Lam.) (Fabaceae) (BERC-BX-C-0264)	Leucaena	Leaves	136.85	69.45	74	0.10
Ziziphus spina-christi (L.) Desf. (Rhamnaceae) (BERC-BX-C-0186)	Christ's Thorn Jujube	Leaves	131.23	80.8	70	1.78
Myrtus communis L. (Myrtaceae) (BERC-BX-C-0051)	Common Myrtle	Leaves	143.93	72.43	69	0.73
Juglans regia L. (Juglandaceae) (BERC-BX-C-0230)	Wallnut	Leaves	90.58	42.55	68	1.23
Sarcopoterium spinosum (L.) Spach. (Rosaceae) (BERC-BX-C-0084)	Shruppy Barnet	Areal Parts	215.93	103.48	65	0.37
Dittrichia viscosa (L.) Greuter (Asteraceae) (BERC-BX-C-0032)	Inula	Areal Parts	162.8	73.4	63	0.40
Rhus coriaria L. (Anacardiaceae) (BERC-BX-C-0037)	Sicilian Sumach	Leaves	256.78	19.68	62	0.30
Olea europaea L. (Oleaceae) (BERC-BX-C-0086)	Olives	Leaves	80.43	47.6	60	2.02
Acacia saligna (Labill.) Wendl. f. (Mimosaceae) (BERC-BX-C-0042)	Blue-Leafed Wattle	Leaves	154	74.9	55	
Carthamus tenuis (Boiss. & Blanche) Bornm. (Asteraceae) (BERC-BX-C-0582)	Safflower	Areal Parts	41.8	19.15	55	
Satureja thymbra L. (Lamiaceae) (BERC-BX-C-0206)	Summer Savory	Areal Parts	97.45	31.4	53	
Quercus calliprinos Webb (Fagaceae) (BERC-BX-C-0016)	Kermes Oak	Leaves	211.4	102.45	52	
Cistus creticus L. (Cistaceae) (BERC-BX-C-0157)	Cretan Rock Rose	Leaves	219.85	84.65	51	
Nicotiana glauca Graham (Solanaceae) (BERC-BX-C-0193)	Tobacco Tree	Leaves	31.2	11.15	50	
Rosmarinus officinalis L. (Lamiaceae) (BERC-BX-C-0018)	Rosemary	Areal Parts	201.85	153.15	50	
Vitis vinifera L. (Vitaceae) (BERC-BX-C-0111)	Grape	Leaves	81.93	51.05	50	
Capparis spinosa L. (Capparaceae) (BERC-BX-C-0106)	Caper Bush, Egyptian Caper	Fruits	65.15	33	49	
Eucalyptus camaldulensis Dehn. (Myrtaceae) (BERC-BX-C-0039)	Red River Gum	Leaves	197.23	131.05	49	
Leucaena leucocephala (Lam.) (Fabaceae) (BERC-BX-C-0264)	Leucaena	Fruits	39.75	14.28	49	
Cupressus sempervirens L. (Cupressaceae)	Cypress	Leaves	106.4	70.8	48	

Table 1 List of local flora analyzed for their exsheathment inhibition activity (LEIA) of the third stage larvae (L3) of a mixture of nematodes species *(Continued)*

Scientific name (Family) (Voucher specimen)	English Name	Plant part	Total phenolic content (GAE-mg/g)	Tannins (GAE-mg/g)	% Exsh. inhibition (60 min)	IC50 (mg/mL)
Capparis spinosa L. (Capparaceae) (BERC-BX-C-0106)	Caper Bush, Egyptian Caper	Leaves	18.9	0.35	46	
Solanum luteum Mill. (Solanaceae) (BERC-BX-C-118)	Hairy Nightshade	Leaves	40.2	11.65	45	
Ceratonia siliqua L. (Caesalpiniaceae) (BERC-BX-C-0137)	Carob	Leaves	215.15	104.6	44	
Heliotropium europaeum L. (Boraginaceae) (BERC-BX-C-0161)	Common Heliotrope	Leaves	26.15	8.2	43	
Helianthemum syriacum (Jacq.) Dum (Cistaceae) (BERC-BX-C-0482)	Common Rock -Rose	Areal Parts	162.55	71.5	41	
Atriplex halimus L. (Chenopodiaceae) (BERC-BX-C-0014)	Shruppy Saltbush, Sea Orache	Leaves	19.8	9.48	39	
Salvia fruticosa Mill. (Lamiaceae) (BERC-BX-C-0006)	White Sage, Common Sage	Leaves	130.4	65.65	39	
Teucrium capitatum L. (Lamiaceae) (BERC-BX-C-0167)	Cat Thyme	Areal Parts	60.18	28.08	37	
Pinus halepensis Mill. (Pinaceae) (BERC-BX-C-0015)	Aleppo Pine	Leaves	81.08	53.93	36	
Rubus sanctus Schreb. (Rosaceae) (BERC-BX-C-0113)	Brandle, Blackberry	Leaves	154.05	72.15	34	
Crataegus aronia (L.) DC. (Rosaceae) (BERC-BX-C-0059)	Hawthorn, Azarole	Leaves	106.5	69.83	33	
Cupressus arizonica Greene (Cupressaceae)	Arizona Cypress	Leaves	126.13	68.33	32	
Ruta chalepensis L. (Rutaceae) (BERC-BX-C-0008)	Rue	Leaves	41.3	21.93	30	
Teucrium creticum L. (Lamiaceae) (BERC-BX-C-0173)	Cretan Germander	Areal Parts	52.4	19.8	29	
Varthemia iphionoides Boiss. & Blanche (Asteraceae) (BERC-BX-C-0135)	Common Verthemia	Areal Parts	94.3	45.58	29	
Elaeagnus angustifolia L. (Elaeagnaceae) (BERC-BX-C-0050)	Narrow-Leaved Oleaster	Leaves	50.23	33.95	27	
Origanum syriacum L. (Lamiaceae) (BERC-BX-C-0026)	Wild Thyme, Mother Of Thyme	Areal Parts	91.23	40.83	25	
Euphorbia hierosolymitana Boiss. (Euphorbiaceae) (BERC-BX-C-0170)	Spurge	Areal Parts	42.53	18.9	21	
Lantana camara L. (Verbenaceae) (BERC-BX-C-0134)	Lantana	Areal Parts	84.65	44.78	17	
Thuja occidentalis L. (Cupressaceae) (BERC-BX-C-0040)	Tree Of Life	Areal Parts	71.98	42.38	12	
Retama raetam (Forssk.) Webb (Fabaceae) (BERC-BX-C-0043)	Retama, White Broom	Areal Parts	99.48	72.7	8	
Ficus carica L. (Moraceae) (BERC-BX-C-0048)	Fig Tree	Leaves	35.3	13.25	7	

30 μl of PBS, and 150 μl of diluted plant extract (at a concentration of 1 mg/mL). The mixture was incubated for 3 h at 37 °C. After the incubation period, larvae were washed with PBS and centrifuged at 3000 rpm; this step was repeated three times. Artificial exsheathment was induced in vitro by adding a solution of sodium hypochlorite (2% *w*/*v*) and sodium chloride (16.5% w/v), diluted 1:300 in PBS, to the larval suspension. The kinetics of larval exsheathment process was determined by removing an aliquot containing about less than one-fifth of the larvae content at time intervals of 0, 15, 30, 45, and 60 min from exposure, and counting the number of

exsheathed and ensheathed individuals under Olympus microscope CX31 (400×). Counts were averaged within each time point.

Minimum inhibitory concentration (IC_{50})

The minimum inhibitory concentration (IC_{50}), which is defined as the amount of the extract necessary to decrease the larval exsheathment by 50%, was determined by the regression between the percentage of exsheathment inhibition and concentration of the extracts (mg/mL) after 45 min incubation using Microsoft Excel Program 2010. Plant extract concentrations used were 1, 0.5, 0.25, and 0.125 (mg/mL). PBS was used as a negative control.

Statistical analyses

The percentage of larval exsheathment in each plant extract and negative control was calculated as follow [38]:

$$\%\text{of Exsheated Larvae} = \left[\frac{\text{Number of exsheated L3 larvae}}{\underset{\text{Ensheated Larvae}}{\text{Number of}} + \underset{\text{Exsheated larvae}}{\text{Number of}}}\right] \text{X } 100$$

Values of semi-log slopes for the percentages of exsheathed larvae at each of the five time intervals were calculated and subjected to analysis of variance using the General Linear Model procedure of SAS (1989). For LEIA, the model comprised treatment with 50 levels (48 plant extracts × 1 extraction method, and a PBS control).

Results

Polyphenolic compounds and tannins

Extraction yields ranged between 13 and 37% depending on the plant species. The polyphenols concentration expressed as gallic acid equivalent are shown in Table 1 and Fig. 1. Total polyphenols levels in plant extracts were ranged from 18.9 mg/g GAE in *Capparis spinosa* leaves to 256.8 mg/g GAE in *Rhus coriaria* (Fig. 1, Table 1). On the other hand tannin levels were ranged from 0.35 mg/g GAE in *C. spinosa* leaves to 153.2 mg/g GAE in *Rosmarinus officinalis* (Fig. 1, Table 1). It is worth noting that, although *Capparis spinosa* possess very low levels of total phenols and tannins it showed moderate exsheathment inhibition activity (46%).

Larval exsheathment inhibition assay (LEIA)

The exsheathment of the infective third stage larvae (L3) of the mixed-species nematodes in the control groups was similar in all assays with more than 90% of exsheathment obtained after 60 min of incubation. In the tested plant extracts, after 3 h of contact with each plant extract, the percentage of exsheathment inhibition activity, obtained after 60 min, ranged between 7 and 94% where *Rhamnus elatarnus, Rhamnus. palaestinus, Pistacia palaestina,* and *Epilobium hirsutum* showed the highest percentage of exsheathment inhibition activity of 94, 89, 84, and 84%, respectively (Table 1).

Out of the 48 plant extracts tested, 22 extracts showed exsheathment inhibitory activity of ≥50%, where 17 exhibited LEIA of ≥30% - < 50%, and 9 plant extracts showed <30% LEIA. The minimum inhibitory concentration IC_{50} was calculated for the 14 plant extracts that showed ≥60% exsheathment inhibition activity (Table 1). *Rhamnus alaternus* extracts which possess relatively moderate levels of total phenols (68.1 mg/g) and tannins (46.35 mg/g), have shown the highest LEIA (94%) and lowest IC_{50} (0.02 mg/mL, Table 1 and Fig. 2). On the other hand, some plant extracts showed low exsheathment inhibition activity despite having relatively high total phenolic content. Examples of those were: *Crataegus aronia*, (106.5 mg/g, 33% LEIA), *Cupressus arizonica* (126.13, 32), *Salvia fruticosa* (130.4, 39), and *Rubus sanctus* (154.1, 34). However, no significant correlation was detected in this study between total phenolic or tannin contents and the % of exsheathment inhibition activity.

Discussion

The eggs of parasitic strongyles are excreted in the animal faeces, hatch under suitable environmental conditions especially on pasture, producing two non-parasitical larval stages followed by a third-stage infective larvae (L3) that is ensheathed, i.e., retaining the shed cuticle from the previous moult for protection. L3 exsheathment is therefore a critical process in the life cycle, being a transitionary step from the free-living to the parasitic stages where its exsheathment inhibition is considered as a crucial stage of its control [39]. Using a two-species but steady population of parasitic nematodes (ca. 20% *Teladorsagia circumcinta* and 80% *Trichostrongylus colubriformis*) was used in different works since both are found in the same animal [40].

In our results the Rhamnaceae family was represented by 4 species (*Rhamnus alaternus, Rh. palaestinus, Ziziphus spina-christi, Z. sativa*). The four species were among the 10 plant extracts with highest LEIA (Table 1). Different parts of the plants (leaves, aerial parts, seeds, fruits, and roots) belonging to the Rhamnaceae family are traditionally used in traditional medicine for the treatment of many illnesses such as inflammation, fever, insomnia, relieve pain, anthelmintic, weakness, hepatic disorders, obesity, urinary problems, muscle spasm and viral infections [41–44]. The Biological activity studies on these species revealed different medicinal features including antioxidant [45, 46], antimicrobial [46–48], anti-diabetic [49] and antifungal [50] activities. In addition, some of these species are grazed by animals including goats and sheep where polyphenol content may affect larval reproduction.

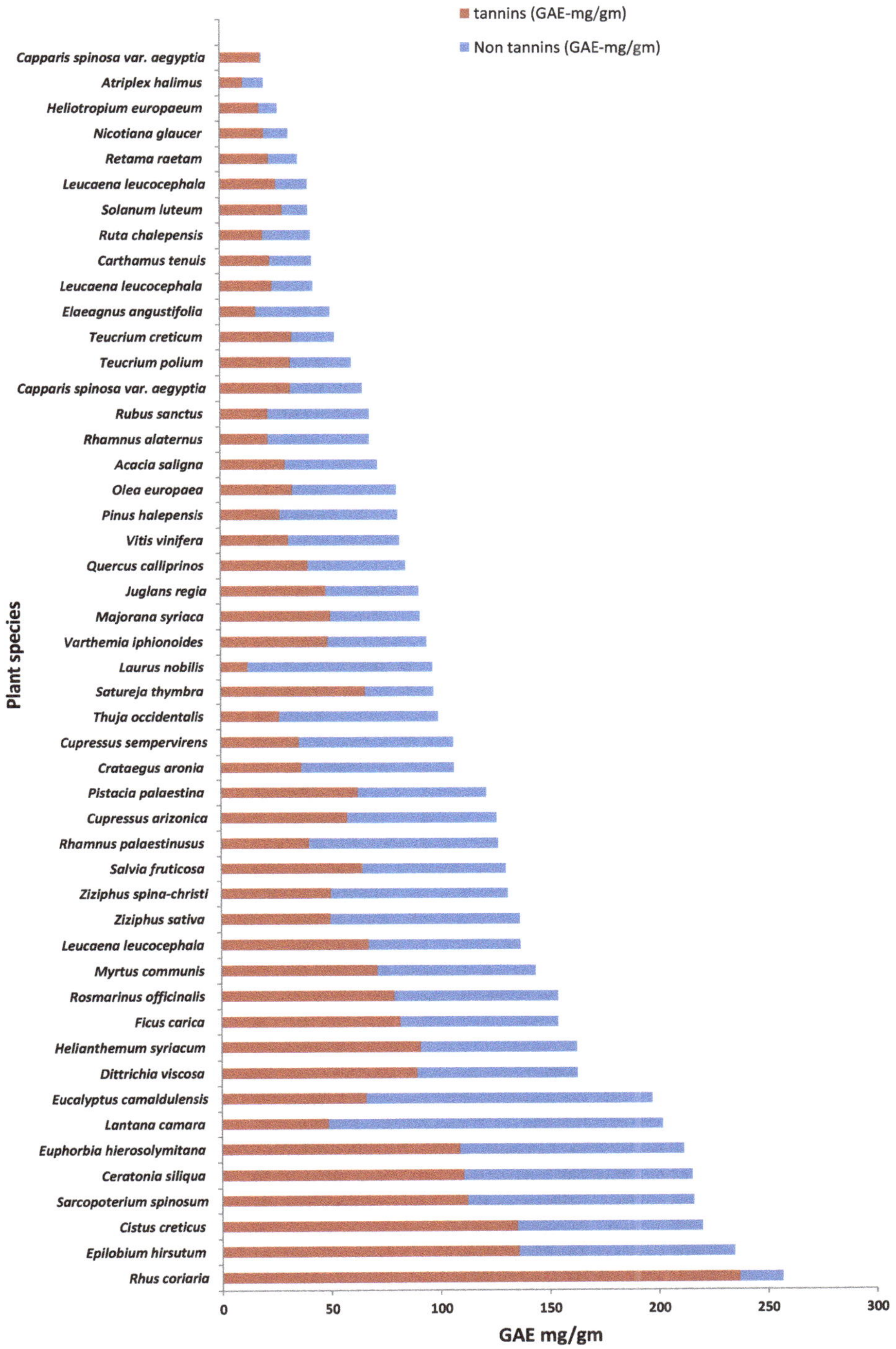

Fig. 1 Total tannins and non-tannin contents of the tested plant extracts

The Rhamnaceae species are known to produce a variety of characteristic secondary compounds including triterpenes, cyclopeptides alkaloids, benzylisoquinoline alkaloids (BIAs), and flavonoids [51]. Several studies have mentioned the importance of some phytochemicals like alkaloids, glycosides, terpenoids, tannins and flavonoids for showing anthelmintic activity of plant extracts [52, 53]. In this study we assume that the polyphenols and flavonoids were responsible for the anthelmintic activity of the Rhamnaceae plants which needs further investigation. We acknowledge that the value of the Folin-Ciocalteu to determine total phenolics is controversial. The extraction

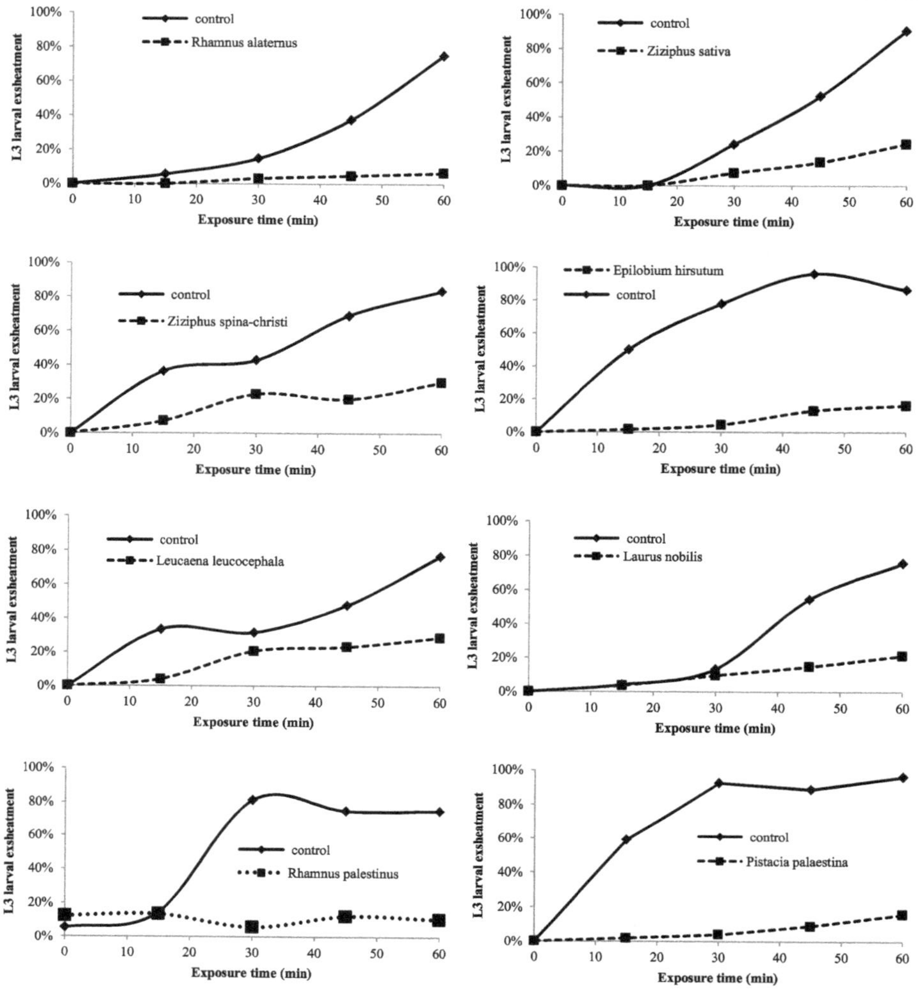

Fig. 2 Minimum inhibitory concentration (IC_{50}) of 8 plant extracts which exhibited >70% exsheathment inhibition activity

of phenolic compounds from plant materials is influenced by different factors including: chemical structure, mineral nutrients, physiological processes, the extraction method, the solvent of extraction, the size of the particles forming samples, the time of sampling, extraction time, the conditions of storage as well as the presence of interfering compounds. Inorganic substances may also interact with Folin-Ciocalteu reagent giving varying results; in addition the structural features of phenolics are another parameter that should be considered when this assay is applied. However, it is the most straightforward measurement of phenolics and enables comparison of published data. In addition, we used PVP method in order to test total tannins out of the total phenols despite we know there are other methods to precipitate tannins from plant extracts such as alkaline ethanol [54].

Other plants which have shown LEIA >70% included *Epilobium hirsutum* (84), *Pistacia palaestina* (84), *Laurus nobilis* (79), and the leaves of *Leucaena leucocephala* (74).

Epilobium hirsutum has shown to possess a strong antioxidant and anticandidal activity [55], the plant contains polyphenols including steroids (especially β-sitosterol and its esters), tannins (gallic, protocatechuic, ellagic and p-coumaric acids) and flavonoids (in particular myricetin, isomyricetin, quercetin, and 5-quercetin-3-O-β-d-glucuronide) [56–58]. The isolated β-sitosterol from the methanolic extract of rhizomes of *Hedychium spicatum* has shown to possess a strong anthelmintic activity [59], thus the presence of β-sitosterol and tannins in *E. hirsutum* might explain its strong LEIA in this study.

Pistacia palaestina is used in traditional Palestinian herbal medicine for weight loss, and for the treatment of diabetes, urinary tract infections, kidney gallstone, and neuropathic pain [42]. In this study the plant exhibited strong LEIA (84%) with IC_{50} of 50 µg /mL. A strong

LEIA was also reported to *P. atlantica* of the same genus and family with very low IC_{50}value of 3.5 µg /mL [18].

Laurus nobilis leaves are used as a spice for cooking purposes, the plant is used traditionally for the treatment of gastric diseases [42, 60]. The plant leaves have been reported to possess wound healing, neuroprotective, antioxidant, antiulcerogenic, anticonvulsant, antimutagenic, antiviral, anticholinergic, antibacterial, and antifungal activities [61]. The anthelmintic activity of the plant can be associated with the presence of various sesquiterpene lactones which have been reported to be present in the plant [62]. Williams et al., [63], have attributed the anthelmintic activity of *Cichorium intybus* to its sesquiterpene lactones composition.

Leucaena leucocephala is often used as feed for livestock [64, 65]. Leucaena possesses anthelmintic properties against both *Haemonchus contortus* [66] and *Trichostrongylus colubriformis* [67]. In our study the leaves of *Leucaena* have shown strong LIEA with IC_{50} of 100 µg/mL. The anthelmintic activity of the plant might be attributed to the protease inhibitor activity of the plant extracts [68]. Another study conducted in 2015 [69] performed a bio-guided fractionation of an aqueous extract of *Leucaena leucocephala* leaves using the egg hatch assay (EHA) to identify the phytochemicals present in fresh leaves with anthelmitic activity. The isolation procedures used led to the identification of an active fraction mainly composed of quercetin (82.21%) and caffeic acid (13.42%) which inhibited the egg hatching of *Cooperia* spp. by 90.49 ± 2.8% of ($P < 0.05$).

Tannins are the most studied compounds for anthelmintic activity, however, some researchers have shown that the ethanolic extracts of *Pistacia lentiscus* still possess some anthelmintic activity remains after all tannins are bound by polyethyleneglycol [70]. In this study, some plants possess low levels of total phenols and tannin content, e.g., *Nicotiana glauca*, and *Capporis spinosa*, however these plants exhibited a moderate LEIA. *Nicotiana glauca* is an herbaceous plant with high toxicity due to its primary alkaloid anabasine content [71]. Although *N. glauca* possesses a low total phenolic and tannin contents the plant exhibited 50% EIA, the anthelmintic activity of the plant might be attributed to its toxicity. However, the aqueous and methanolic extracts of plants of the same genus (*N. tabacum*) have shown to possess anthelmintic activity when administrated orally for sheep naturally infected with mixed species of gastrointestinal nematodes [72].

Capparis spinosa fruits and leaves have been tested in this study for their LEIA, the tannin content ranged between 0.35 mg/g in leaves to 33 mg/g in fruits, with LEIA of 46, and 49%, respectively. The anthelmintic activity of ethanolic extract of root bark of *C. spinosa* was evaluated against earthworm, and the activity was found to be dose dependent [73]. Traditional medicine plays a vital role in the development of new drugs; a lot of plant-originated drugs in clinical medicine today were derived from traditional medicine [74–76]. Fifteen of the plant species analyzed in this study for their LEIA were mentioned to be used traditionally in ethnoveterinary medicine in Palestine for the treatment of several animal ailments [33]. Nine of these plants were reported to be used for the treatment of gastrointestinal diseases including diarrhea, and anthelmintic (Table 2). Our results

Table 2 Ethnoveterinary uses of plants used in Traditional Arabic Palestinian Herbal medicine (TAPHM) [33]

Plant	Ethnoveterinary uses
Ceratonia siliqua	Nourishment, anthelmintic, scabies, eye inflammation, cleaning uterus, delay in giving birth, diarrhea
Crataegus aronia	Urine retention, constipation, inflammation, coccidia, pregnancy poisoning
Cupressus sempervirens	Diarrhea
Dittrichia viscosa	Expectorant, appetizer, flatulence, postpartum inflammation
Eucalyptus camaldulensis	Fever & malaria, flatulence, bees anaesthetization, diarrhea, scabies, inflammation
Ficus carica	Ulcers, insects bites, constipation, nourishment
Myrtus communis	Diarrhea, ulcers
Olea europaea	Eye diseases, bone fractures, anthelmintic, bruises, nourishment, injuries, scabies, colic, flatulence, diarrhea
Origanum syriacum	Flatulence, inflammation, Bites, cold, appetizer
Rosmarinus officinalis	Animal fertility, arthritis, inflammation, constipation
Salvia fruticosa	Appetizer, cleaning the uterus, colic, flatulence, poisoning, colc, diarrhea, satiety
Solanum luteum	Dimples, scabies, injuries
Teucrium capitatum	Diarrhea, colic, bleeding, scabies, flatulence
Varthemia iphionoides	Colic, scabies diarrhea, fever, flatulence, pregnancy poisoning, udder infections
Ziziphus spina-christi	Diarrhea, nourishment, anthelmintic, inflammation, carbuncles

support these ethnoveterinary studies and using these plants as grazing pasture or feed additives might contribute to a sustainable control of these nematodes in small ruminants.

Conclusion

Our results suggest natural resources that possess strong larval exsheathment inhibition activity with potential applications in animal therapeutics and feed. In our study the calculated IC_{50} values for the most active extracts of *Rhamnus alaternus,* and *Epilobium hirsutum* were 20, and 30 μg /mL, respectively. This is a strong indication of the high anthelmintic potential of these plants. Future studies are needed for screening in-depth phytochemical, clinical and possible studies on molecular mechanism of action. At the same time efforts should be made to normalize the plant extracts with potent anthelmintic activity and formulate best alternative herbal products to either substitute or supplement man-made drugs which are presently in use.

Abbreviations

DM: Dry matter; EIA: Exsheathment inhibition activity; GAE: Gallic acid equivalents; IC_{50}: Minimum inhibitory concentration; LEIA: Larval exsheathment inhibition assays; PBS: Phosphate buffered saline; PVP: Polyvinylpyrrolidone

Acknowledgments

Not applicable.

Funding

This research was supported in part by BARD-MARD Facilitating Grant Reference Number FG-9513-14 to the first author.

Authors' contributions

RMJ, and SYAZ carriedout laboratory work and data analyses. HA suggested the project, and revised the manuscript. AM supplied the parasites, suggested the project and contributed to conception and design. MSAS, RMJ, and SYAZ coordinated plant collection and prepared plant extracts. MSAS and RMJ wrote the manuscript. All authors read the final version of the manuscript. All authors read and approved the final manuscript.

Consent for publication

Not Applicable.

Competing interests

The authors declare that they have no competing interests.

Author details

[1]Biodiversity& Environmental Research Center –BERC, Til, Nablus, Palestine. [2]Kimron Veterinary Institute, Ministry of Agriculture and Rural Development, Jerusalem, Israel. [3]The Institute of Applied Research, The Galilee Society, P.O.B. 437, 20200 Shefa-Amr, Israel. [4]Tel Hai College, Department of Environmental Science, 2208 Upper Galilee, Israel.

References

1. Knox MR, Torres-Acosta JFJ, Aguilar-Caballero AJ. Exploiting the effect of dietary supplementation of small ruminants on resilience and resistance against gastrointestinal nematodes. Vet Parasitol. 2006;139:385–93.
2. Roeber F, Jex AR, Gasser RB. Impact of gastrointestinal parasitic nematodes of sheep, and the role of advanced molecular tools for exploring epidemiology and drug resistance - an Australian perspective. Parasites & Vectors. 2013;6:153. doi:10.1186/1756-3305-6-153.
3. Hoste H, Torres-Acosta JF. Non chemical control of helminths in ruminants: adapting solutions for changing worms in a changing world. Veterinary Parasitology. 2011;180(1-2):144–154.
4. Badran I, Abuamsha R, Aref R, Alqisi W, Alumor J. Prevalence and diversity of gastrointestinal parasites in small ruminants under two different rearing systems in Jenin District of Palestine. An - Najah Univ. J. Res. (N. Sc.). 2012; 26:1-18.
5. Hoste H, Sotiraki S, Landau SY, Jackson F, Beveridge I. Goat-nematode interactions: think differently. Trends in Parasitology. 2010;26(8):376–381.
6. Bellani L, Mantovani A, Mordenti A, Restani R. Socio-Economic Effects of Parasitic Disease of Animals. Veterinaria Italiana. 1974;11-12:501-520.
7. Jackson F, Coop RL. The development of anthelmintic resistance in sheep nematodes. Parasitol. 2000;120:95–107.
8. Papadopoulos E, Himonas C, Coles GC. Anthelmintic Resistance of Sheep and Goat Gastrointestinal Nematodes, Proceedings of the 7th Hellenic Veterinary Congress, Thessaloniki, 28 November-1 December, 1996, p. 149.
9. Gilleard J. Understanding anthelmintic resistance: the need for genomics and genetics. Int J Parasitol. 2006;36(12):1227–39.
10. Kaplan RM. Drug resistance in nematodes of veterinary importance: a status report. Trends Parasitol. 2004;20(10):477–81.
11. Wolstenholme AJ, Fairweather I, Prichard RK, von Samson-Himmelstjerna G, Sangster NC. Drug resistance in veterinary helminths. Trends Parasitol. 2014; 20(10):469–76.
12. Waller PJ, Thamsborg SM. Nematode control in "green" ruminant production systems. Trends Parasitol. 2004;20:493–7.
13. Kyriazakis I, Houdijk J. Immunonutrition: nutritional control of parasites. Small Rum Res. 2006;62:79–82.
14. Abushelaibi AA, Al Shamsi MS, Afifi H. Use of Antimicrobial Agents in Food Processing Systems. Recent Pat Food, Nutr Agric. 2012;4(1):2–7.
15. Cheng G, Hao H, Sh X, Wang X, Dai M, Huang L, Yuan Z. Antibiotic alternatives: the substitution of antibiotics in animal husbandry? Front Microbiol. 2014;13(5):217. https://doi.org/10.3389/fmicb.2014.00217.
16. Brunet S, Jackson F, Hoste H. Effects of sainfoin (*Onobrychis viciifolia*) extract and monomers of condensed tannins on the association of abomasal nematode larvae with fundic explants. Int J Parasitol. 2008;38:783–90.
17. Hoste H, Jackson F, Athanasiadou S, Thamsborg SM, Hoskin SO. The effects of tannin rich plants on parasitic nematodes in ruminants. Trends Parasitol. 2006;22:253–61.
18. Azaizeh H, Halahleh F, Abbas N, Markovics A, Muklada H, Ungar ED, Landau SY. 2013. Polyphenols from *Pistacia lentiscus* and *Phillyrea latifolia* impair the exsheathment of gastro-intestinal nematode larvae. Vet Parasitol. 2013;191:44–50.
19. Barrau E, Fabre N, Fouraste I, Hoste H. Effect of bioactive compounds from sainfoin (*Onobrychis viciifolia* Scop.) on the in vitro larval migration of *Haemonchus contortus*: role of tannins and flavonol glycosides. Parasitology. 2005;131:531–8.
20. Brunet S, Aufrère J, El Babili F, Fouraste I, Hoste H. The kinetics of exsheathment of nematode larvae is disturbed in presence of tannin-rich plant (sainfoin) both in vitro and in vivo. Parasitology 2007;134:1253–1262.
21. Molan AL, Faraj AM. The effects of condensed tannins extracted from different plant species on egg hatching and larval development of *Teladorsagia circumcincta* (Nematoda: Trichostrongylidae). Folia Parasitol. 2010;57(1):62–8.
22. Lange KC, Olcott DD, Miller JE, Mosjidis JA, Terrill TH, Burke JM, Kearney MT. Effect of sericea lespedeza (*Lespedeza cuneata*) fed as hay, on natural and experimental *Haemonchus contortus* infections in lambs. Vet Parasitol. 2006;141:273–8.
23. Heckendorn F, Haring DA, Maurer V, Senn M, Hertzberg H. Individual administration of three tanniferous forage plants to lambs artificially infected with *Haemonchus contortus* and *Cooperia curticei*. Veterinary Parasitology. 2007;146:123–34.
24. Minho AP, Bueno ICS, Louvandini H, Jackson F, Gennari SM, Abdalla AL. Effect of acacia tannin extract in the control gastrointestinal parasites in sheep. Anim Feed Sci Technol. 2008;147(1–3):172–81.

25. Minho AP, Filippsen LF, Francisco A, Amarante T, Abdalla AL. Efficacy of condensed tannin presents in acacia extract on the control of *Trichostrongylus colubriformis* in sheep. Ciência Rural. 2010;40(6):1360–5.
26. Hammond JA, Fielding D, Bishop SC. Prospects for plant anthelmintics in tropical veterinary medicine. Vet Res Commun. 1997;21(3):213–28.
27. Waller PJ, Bernes G, Thamsborg SM, Sukura A, Richter SH, Ingebrigtsen K, Höglund J. Plants as de-worming agents of livestock in the Nordic countries: historical perspective, popular beliefs and prospects for the future. Acta Vet Scand. 2001;42(1):31–44.
28. Kumarasingha R, Preston S, Yeo TC, Lim DSL, Tu CL, Palombo EA, Shaw JM, Gasser RB, Boag PR. Anthelmintic activity of selected ethno-medicinal plant extracts on parasitic stages of *Haemonchus contortus*. Parasites & Vectors. 2016;9:187. https://doi.org/10.1186/s13071-016-1458-9.
29. Ali-Shtayeh MS, Jamous Rana M, Jamous RM. Complementary and alternative medicine use amongst Palestinian diabetic patients. Complementary Therapies in Clinical Practice. 2011a; https://doi.org/10.1016/j.ctcp.2011.09.001.
30. Ali-Shtayeh MS, Jamous Rana M, Jamous RM. Herbal preparation use by patients suffering from cancer in Palestine. Complementary Therapies in Clinical Practice. 2011b;17(04):235–40. https://doi.org/10.1016/j.ctcp.2011.06.002.
31. Ali-Shtayeh MS, Jamous Rana M, Jamous Rania M, Salameh NM. Complementary and alternative medicine (CAM) use among hypertensive patients in Palestine. Complement Ther Clin Pract. 2013;19(4):256–63.
32. Ali-Shtayeh MS, Jamous Rana M, Salameh NM, Jamous Rania M, Hamadeh AM. Complementary and alternative medicine use among cancer patients in Palestine with special reference to safety- related concerns. J Ethnopharmacol. 2016a;187:104–22.
33. Ali-Shtayeh MS, Jamous Rana M, Jamous RM. Traditional arabic Palestinian ethnoveterinary practices in animal health care: a field survey in the West Bank (Palestine). J Ethnopharmacol. 2016b;182:35–49.
34. Singh R, Kumar P, Singh G. Total phenolic, flavonoids and tannin contents in different extracts of *Artemisia absinthium*. J Intercultural. 2012;1(2):101–4.
35. Makkar HPS, Blümmel M, Borowy NK, Becker K. Gravimetric determination of tannins and their correlations with chemical and protein precipitation methods. J Sci Food Agric. 1993;61:161–5.
36. Van Wyk JA, Cabaret J, Michael LM. Morphological identification of nematode larvae of small ruminants and cattle simplified. Vet Parasitol. 2004;119:277–306.
37. Bahuaud D, Martinez-Ortiz de Montellano C, Chauveau S, Prevot F, TorresAcosta F, Fouraste I, Hoste H. Effects of four tanniferous plant extracts on the in vitro exsheathment of third-stage larvae of parasitic nematodes. Parasitology. 2006;132(4):545–54.
38. Oliveira LM, Bevilaqua CM, Macedo IT, Morais SM, Monteiro MV, Campello CC, Ribeiro WL, Batista EK. Effect of six tropical tanniferous plant extracts on larval exsheathment of *Haemonchus contortus*. Rev Bras Parasitol. 2011;20:155–60.
39. Hertzberg H, Huwyler U, Kohler L, Rehbein S, Wanner M. Kinetics of exsheathment of infective ovine and bovine strongylid larvae in vivo and in vitro. Parasitol. 2002;125:65–70.
40. Azaizeh H, Mreny R, Markovics A, Muklada H, Glazer I, Landau SY. Seasonal variation in the effects of Mediterranean plant extracts on the exsheathment kinetics of goat gastro-intestinal nematode larvae. Small Ruminant Res. 2015;131:130–5.
41. Lee SM, Min BS, Lee C-G, Kim K-S, Kho YH. Cytotoxic triterpenoids from the fruits of *Zizyphus jujube*. Planta Med. 2003;69:1051–4.
42. Ali-Shtayeh MS, Jamous RM. Traditional Arabic Palestinian herbal medicine, TAPHM. Til, Nablus, Palestine: Biodiversity and Environmental Research Center, BERC; 2008.
43. Kirtikar KR, Basu B. Indian Medicinal Plants. 2nd ed. Periodical expert book Agency: Delhi; 1984.
44. Han BH, Park MH. Folk Medicine: The Art and the Science. 6th ed. Washington, DC: The American Chemical Society; 1986.
45. Boussahel S, Dahamna S, Ruberto G, Siracusa L, Harzallah D. Phytochemical Study and antioxidant activities of leaves extracts from *Rhamnus alaternus* L. Pharmacogn Commun. 2013;3:46–53.
46. Boussahel S, Speciale A, Dahamna S, Amar Y, Bonaccorsi I, Cacciola F, Cimino F, Donato P, Ferlazzo G, Harzallah D, Cristani M. Flavonoid profile, antioxidant and cytotoxic activity of different extracts from Algerian *Rhamnus alaternus* L. bark. Pharmacognosy Magazine. 2015;11Suppl 1:S102–9.
47. Elsadig Karar MG, Quiet L, Rezk A, Jaiswal R, Rehders M, Ullrich MS, Brix K, Kuhnert N. Phenolic profile and *in vitro* assessment of cytotoxicity and antibacterial activity of *Ziziphus spina-christi* Leaf Extracts. Medicinal Chemistry. 2016;6(3):143–56.
48. Moghadam MS, Maleki S, Darabpour E Motamedi H, Nejad SMS. Antibacterial activity of eight Iranian p ant extracts against methicillin and cefixime resistant *Staphylococcous aureus* strains. Asian J Trop Med 2010;3: 262-262.
49. Michel CG, Nesseem DI, Ismail MF. Anti-diabetic activity and stability study of the formulated leaf extract of *Zizyphus spina-christi* (L.) Willd with the influence of seasonal variation. J Ethnopharmacol. 2011:133:53–62.
50. Hadizadeh I, Peivastegan B, Kolahi M. Antifungal activity of nettle (*Urtica dioica* L.), colocynth (*Citrullus colocynthis* L. Schrad), oleander (*Nerium oleander* L.) and konar (*Ziziphus spina-christi* L.) extracts on plants pathogenic fungi. Pakistan J Biol Sci. 2009;12:58–63.
51. Alarcón J, Cespedes CL. Chemical constituents and biological activities of South American Rhamnaceae. Phytochem Rev. 2015;14:389. https://doi.org/10.1007/s11101-015-9404-6.
52. Acharya S, Dash GK, Brahman DK, Chhetri RR. Preliminary phytochemical investigation and anthelmintic activity of *Acacia suma* (Roxb) barks. International Research Journal of pharmacy. 2011;2(1):136–141.
53. Dash S, Das C, Sahoo DC. Phytochemical and anthelmintic screening of crud barck of *Adenanthera pavovina* Lim. Pharmacie Globalen (IJCP). 2010;2(10):1–4.
54. Xingchu GX, Li Y, Qu H. Removing tannins from medicinal plant extracts using an alkaline ethanol precipitation process: A case study of danshen injection. Molecules. 2014;19:18705–20.
55. Jamous RM, Abu Zaitoun SY, Husein AI, Qasem IBY, Ali-Shtayeh MS. Screening for Biological Activities of Medicinal Plants Used in Traditional Arabic Palestinian Herbal Medicine. Eur J Med Plants. 2015;9(1):1–13.
56. Barakat HH, Hussein SAM, Marzouk MS, Merfort I, Linscheid M, Nawwar MAM. Polyphenolic metabolites of *Epilobium hirsutum*. Phytochemistry. 1997;46(5):935–41.
57. Gruenwald J, Brendler T, Jaenicke C. PDR for herbal. New Jersey: Medical Economics Company; 2000.
58. Ivancheva S, Manolova N, Serkedjieva J, Dimov V, Ivanovska N. Polyphenols from Bulgarian medicinal plants with anti-infectious activity. Basic Life Sciences. 1992;59:717–28.
59. Sravani T, Paarakh PP, Shruthi SD. In silico and in vitro anthelmintic activity of B-sitosterol isolated from rhizomes of *Hedychium spicatum* Buch.-Ham. Ind J Narutal Prod Resour. 2014;5(3):258–61.
60. Dall'Acqua S, Cervellati R, Speroni E, Costa S, Guerra MC, Stella L, Greco E, Innocenti G. Phytochemical composition and antioxidant activity of *Laurus nobilis* L. leaf infusion. J Med Food. 2009;12(4):869–76.
61. Patrakar R, Mansuriya M, Patil P. Phytochemical and Pharmacological Review on *Laurus nobilis*. International Journal of Pharmaceutical and Chemical Sciences. 2277–5005;1 (2):595–602.
62. Fang F, Sang S, Kuang YC, Alexander G, Chi-Tang H, Robert TR. Isolation and identification of cytotoxic compounds from Bay leaf (*Laurus nobilis*). Food Chemistry. 2005;93:497–501.
63. Williams AR, Peña-Espinoza MA, Boas U, Simonsen HT, Enemark HL, Thamsborg SM. Anthelmintic activity of chicory (*Cichorium intybus*): in vitro effects on swine nematodes and relationship to sesquiterpene lactone composition. Parasitology. 2016;143(6):770–7.
64. Prasad JVNS, Korwar GR, Rao KV, Mandal UK, Rao GR, Srinivas I, et al. Optimum stand density of for wood production in Andhra Pradesh, Southern India. *leucaena leucocephala* Biomass Bioenergy 2011;35(1):227–235.
65. Pandey VC, Kumar A. *leucaena leucocephala*: an underutilized plant for pulp and paper production. Genet Resour Crop Evol. 2013;60(3):1165–71.
66. Oliveira LMB, Bevilaqua CML, Macedo ITF, Morais SM, Monteiro MVB, Campello CC, Ribeiro WLC, Batista EKF. Effect of six tropical tanniferous plant extracts on larval exsheathment of Haemonchus contortus. Rev Bras Parasitol Vet. 2011;20(2):155–60.
67. Cunha FR, Oliveira DF, Campos VP. Extratos vegetais com propriedades nematicidas e purificação do princípio ativo do extrato de *Leucaena leucocephala*. Fitopatol Bras. 2003;28(4):438–41.
68. Soares AMS, Araújo SA, Lopes SG, Costa Junior LM. Anthelmintic activity of *Leucaena leucocephala* protein extracts on *Haemonchus contortus*. Revista Brasileira de Parasitologia Veterinária. 2015;24(4):396–401.
69. von Son-de Fernex E, Alonso-D'iaz MA, Mendoza-de Gives P, Valles-de la Mora B, Gonz' alez-' Cortazar M, Zamilpa A, Epigmenio CG. Elucidation of *Leucaena leucocephala* anthelmintic- ike phytochemicals and the

ultrastructural damage generated to eggs of Cooperia spp. Veterinary Parasitology. 2015; https://doi.org/10.1016/j.vetpar.2015.10.005
70. Landau S, Azaizeh H, Muklada H, Glasser T, Ungar ED, Baram H, Abbas N, Markovics A. 2010. Anthelmintic activity of *Pistacia lentiscus* foliage in two Middle Eastern breeds of goats differing in their propensity to consume tannin-rich browse. Veterinary Parasitology. 2010;173(2010):280–6.
71. Fekih Hassen M, Ben Sik Ali H, Jaoued O, Ayed S, Tilouche N, Gharbi R, Elatrous S. Severe *Nicotiana glauca* poisoning: a case report. J Clin Toxicol. 2014;4:–216. https://doi.org/10.4172/2161-0495.1000216.
72. Iqbal Z, Lateef M, Jabbar A, Muhammad G, Gilani HA. In vitro and in vivo anthelmintic activity of *Nicotiana tabacum* Linn. leaves against gastrointestinal nematods of sheep. Phytothr Res. 2006;20(1):46–8.
73. Mali RG, Mahajan S, Patil KS. Anthelmintic activity of root bark of *Capparis spinosa*. Ind J Nat Prod. 2005;21:50–1.
74. Fabricant DS, Farnsworth NR. The value of plants used in traditional medicine for drug discovery. Environ Health Perspect. 2001;109:69–75.
75. Li-Weber M. New therapeutic aspects of flavones: The anticancer properties of *Scutellaria* and its main active constituents Wogonin, Baicalein and Baicalin. Cancer Treat Rev. 2009;35:57–68.
76. Yuan H, Ma Q, Ye L, Piao G. The Traditional medicine and modern medicine from natural products. Molecules. 2016;21(5):559. https://doi.org/10.3390/molecules21050559.

13

Harmonizing methods for wildlife abundance estimation and pathogen detection in Europe—a questionnaire survey on three selected host-pathogen combinations

Jana Sonnenburg[1,2*], Marie-Pierre Ryser-Degiorgis[3], Thijs Kuiken[4], Ezio Ferroglio[5], Rainer G. Ulrich[6], Franz J. Conraths[1], Christian Gortázar[7], Christoph Staubach[1] and APHAEA project partners

Abstract

Background: The need for wildlife health surveillance as part of disease control in wildlife, domestic animals and humans on the global level is widely recognized. However, the objectives, methods and intensity of existing wildlife health surveillance programs vary greatly among European countries, resulting in a patchwork of data that are difficult to merge and compare. This survey aimed at evaluating the need and potential for data harmonization in wildlife health in Europe. The specific objective was to collect information on methods currently used to estimate host abundance and pathogen prevalence. Questionnaires were designed to gather detailed information for three host-pathogen combinations: (1) wild boar and Aujeszky's disease virus, (2) red fox and *Echinococcus multilocularis*, and (3) common vole and *Francisella tularensis*.

Results: We received a total of 70 responses from 19 European countries. Regarding host abundance, hunting bags are currently the most widely accessible data source for widely distributed mid-sized and larger mammals such as red fox and wild boar, but we observed large differences in hunting strategies among countries as well as among different regions within countries. For small rodents, trapping is the method of choice, but practical applications vary among study sites. Laboratory procedures are already largely harmonized but information on the sampled animals is not systematically collected.

Conclusions: The answers revealed that a large amount of information is available for the selected host-pathogen pairs and that in theory methods are already largely harmonized. However, the comparability of the data remains strongly compromised by local differences in the way, the methods are applied in practice. While these issues may easily be overcome for prevalence estimation, there is an urgent need to develop tools for the routine collection of host abundance data in a harmonized way. Wildlife health experts are encouraged to apply the harmonized APHAEA protocols in epidemiological studies in wildlife and to increase cooperation.

Keywords: Animal abundance, Diagnostic methods, Europe, Harmonization, Questionnaire, Wildlife

* Correspondence: janson@vet.dtu.dk
[1]Federal Research Institute for Animal Health, Friedrich-Loeffler-Institut, Institute of Epidemiology, Südufer 10, 17493 Greifswald, Insel Riems, Germany
[2]National Veterinary Institute, Technical University of Denmark, Bülowsvej 27, Building 1-6, 1870 Frederiksberg C, Denmark
Full list of author information is available at the end of the article

Background

The need for wildlife health surveillance as part of disease control in wildlife, domestic animals and humans on the global level is now widely recognized. Increasing efforts are made to implement wildlife health surveillance schemes in various parts of the world. The Working Group on Wildlife of the World Organization for Animal Health (OIE) biannually collects, compiles and distributes information on a global scale. In Europe, the objectives, methods and intensity of existing wildlife health surveillance programs vary greatly among countries [1]. This results in a patchwork of data, which are difficult to merge and compare. Harmonized methods could allow a more reliable description of the disease status in populations on regional and continental scales. Efficient communication and coordination beyond national borders are required for effective early warning, because the migration of wildlife populations is usually not limited by borders between countries and globalization dramatically increases the risk of pathogen movements. Also, the understanding of factors influencing pathogen maintenance and spread in populations requires the application of similar investigation methods allowing reliable comparisons among regions with different patterns of pathogen occurrence [2].

The setup of a European wildlife health surveillance network under the umbrella of the European Wildlife Disease Association (EWDA [3]) in autumn 2009 represented an important first step to improve communication and data exchange among institutions involved in wildlife health surveillance in Europe [1]. In 2012, an EMIDA ERA-NET [4] project "harmonized Approaches in monitoring wildlife Population Health, and Ecology and Abundance" (acronym APHAEA, [5]) was started in close association with EWDA activities. The project aimed to develop a European wildlife disease surveillance network capable of providing reliable estimates on abundance of wildlife species and pathogen distribution and occurrence in key wildlife species in order to improve wildlife health surveillance in general. First, literature reviews on methods for estimating wildlife population abundance (leading to the production of 'Species cards') and for wildlife disease diagnostics ('Diagnosis cards') were conducted with the aim to propose selected methods for data harmonization on a large scale (APHAEA protocols [5]). The second step in the APHAEA project consisted in evaluating the willingness of wildlife health experts throughout Europe to participate in harmonization efforts and to contribute to case studies on host abundance and pathogen prevalence, using the three following host-pathogen combinations as examples: (1) wild boar (*Sus scrofa*) and Aujeszky's disease virus (ADV; pseudorabies virus, *Suid herpesvirus 1*), (2) red fox (*Vulpes vulpes*) and *Echinococcus multilocularis* (*E. multilocularis*; alveolar echinococcosis), and (3) common vole (*Microtus arvalis*) and *Francisella tularensis* (*F. tularensis*; tularemia). Thus, the selection included an ungulate, a carnivore and a rodent as hosts as well as a virus, a parasite and a bacterium with economic or zoonotic importance as pathogens. Pathogens, for which diagnostic standards already exist by legislation of the European Union (EU), were deliberately excluded.

This article reports the results of a questionnaire survey performed among wildlife health experts who volunteered to participate in the APHAEA project. The survey aimed at describing the current situation and discussing the needs and potential of harmonizing methods in wildlife health research in Europe. More specifically, information was collected on: (1) the methods used to estimate host abundance and the availability of such data and (2) the methods used for pathogen detection and the availability of laboratory results together with sample metadata, for the three above-mentioned host-pathogen combinations in European countries.

Methods

From summer 2012 to early 2013, wildlife health experts throughout Europe were informed about APHAEA by an oral presentation at the EWDA 2012 conference, written documents distributed through wildlife health internet forums and individual email contacts. The contacted experts were asked to forward the information to any potentially concerned colleagues in their respective countries. Altogether, 53 persons from 25 institutions in 18 European countries registered as external APHAEA project partners during that time period.

Questionnaires were designed to collect detailed information on the abundance of each selected host and on prevalence estimates for each corresponding pathogen. Information based on historical records was asked for as well as currently available data or information potentially accessible in the future. There was one questionnaire per host-pathogen combination [Additional files 1, 2 and 3].

The questionnaires included questions on the considered region (name, size), the existing data sources for animal abundance, the performed hunting schemes (for wild boar and fox), the temporal and regional scales, for which the data were available, and the recorded animal metadata. In addition, information was gathered on the occurrence of the selected pathogens or diseases in animal hosts (epidemic vs. endemic status or disease freedom) and in humans (for tularemia). Description of the geographical origin of samples was based on the Nomenclature of Territorial Units for Statistics (NUTS), a geocode standard for referencing subdivisions of countries for statistical purposes. There are three NUTS levels, with two more detailed levels of local administrative units (LAUs) [6]. Participants were also asked, whether data from former, on-going or future investigations were available.

APHAEA recommended the following protocols for wild animal abundance: hunting bag data on a large scale and more accurate density estimates (such as thermal imaging and distance sampling, camera-trapping or drive counts) on a local scale for wild boar; spot light counts for red fox; and snap trapping for common vole (APHAEA protocols [5]). For pathogen prevalence estimation the following diagnostic protocols were recommended by APHAEA: enzyme-linked immunosorbent assay (ELISA) for ADV; the sedimentation and counting technique (SCT) for *E. multilocularis*; and polymerase chain reaction (PCR) for *F. tularensis* (APHAEA protocols [5]).

The questionnaires were circulated among experts from the five APHAEA core partner countries (Spain, Italy, Switzerland, Germany and The Netherlands) and sent to all registered external partners in October 2013. All partners were invited to pass the questionnaires to other colleagues active in the wildlife field in their respective countries.

Results

We received a total of 70 completed questionnaires from 19 European countries (Fig. 1 and Acknowledgements). Responses were obtained on all three host-pathogen pairs from seven countries, on two host-pathogen pairs from five countries, and on one host-pathogen pair from six countries. Seventeen of 53 experts, who had registered as APHAEA partners (33%), answered at least to one questionnaire. In addition, 31 non-registered experts filled in questionnaires. A total response ratio could not be calculated because the number of experts who finally received the questionnaires was not known.

Wild boar and Aujeszky's disease virus

We received 31 completed questionnaires for the host-pathogen combination wild boar and ADV. The size of the considered study areas within countries ranged from 28 to 640,679 km^2 (mean = 71,195 km^2; median = 10,391 km^2; Fig. 2).

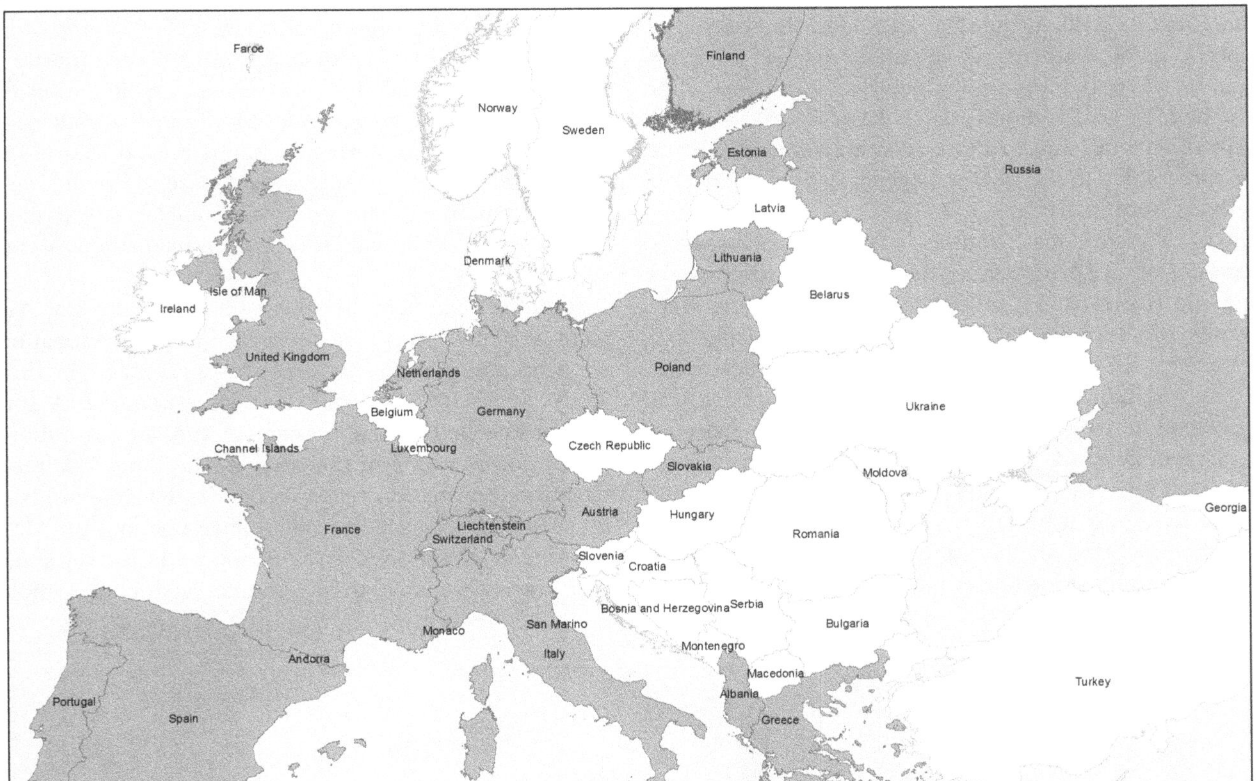

Fig. 1 Map of Europe showing the countries for which a questionnaire was completed for at least one host-pathogen combination (*dark grey areas*)

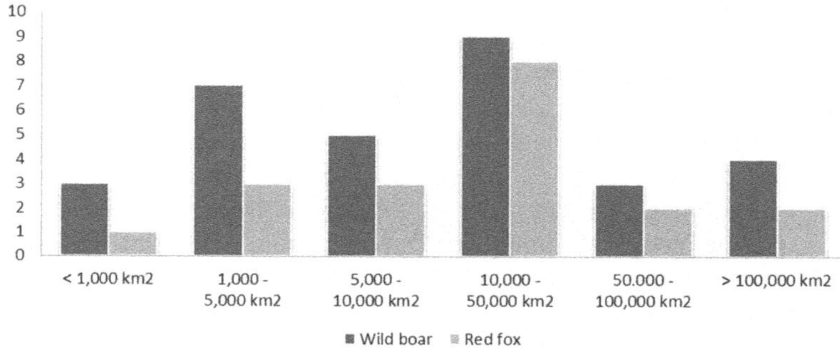

Fig. 2 Number of study areas categorized by size of study area in km2 reported by the questionnaire respondents for wild boar and Aujeszky's disease virus ($n = 31$) and for red fox and Echinococcus multilocularis ($n = 18$)

Host abundance-related questions

The reported data sources for wild boar abundance are shown in Fig. 3a. More accurate methods such as drive counts, snow tracking, kilometric abundance index, pellet counts, capture-mark-recapture and photo-trapping were applied by academic groups for research purposes. Other data sources included crop and car damage statistics, the wild boar surveillance database of the EU reference laboratory for Classical Swine Fever/African Swine Fever (EURL CSF/ASF-WB-DB, [7]), predictions obtained by modelling hunting bags and interviews of hunters, game wardens or veterinarians. For 16 study areas (52%), only hunting bag data were available. Nine respondents (29%) indicated to have access to both hunting statistics and to more accurate abundance data. For three study areas, only data generated by alternative methods were available.

In most study areas, hunting was allowed in specific season(s) or performed year-round with seasonal peaks (Fig. 4). However, 11 different hunting seasons were mentioned. Hunting was allowed at least from October to December, but never in April in 21 of 22 study areas. In one questionnaire, it was reported that hunting was performed in the opposite year period, i.e. from February to September and not in the usual autumn/winter months. Other management schemes such as selective culling by official game managers for population reduction were reported for five study areas in addition to the regular hunting periods or as independent measures.

The regional and temporal scale as well as additional information from the accessible wild boar data is shown in Table 1. Overall, data accuracy and specifications varied considerably among countries and study areas.

Four of the 31 respondents (15%) declared that hunting statistics were recorded in the EURL CSF/ASF-WB-DB for their countries.

Pathogen-related questions

The status of ADV in wild boar as reported by the survey participants is presented in Fig. 5. The source of information was stated in 14 cases and consisted mostly of research data (71%), but also of information available from official ADV surveillance (partly in domestic pigs) or from annual monitoring programs in wild boar (29%). Diagnostic findings of Aujeszky's disease in hunting dogs and information from veterinary officials were mentioned as an additional source of information for one study area.

Seventeen partners (55%) stated that historical data were available, in 21 study areas (68%) investigations were on-going at the time of the survey and in three study areas (10%) investigations were planned. A total lack of information and absence of studies was only reported for one (3%) of the study areas. Table 2 summarizes the information that was or may become available for wild boar samples from these investigations on ADV.

Eighteen laboratories participating in the survey stated that they were able to investigate wild boar samples

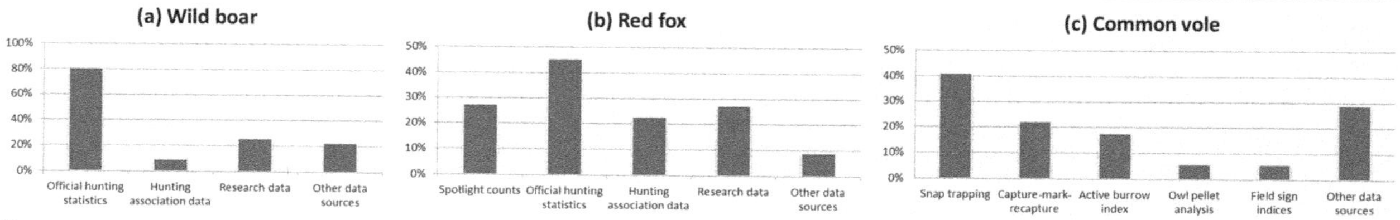

Fig. 3 Existing data sources on the abundance of **a** wild boar ($n = 31$), **b** red foxes($n = 22$) and **c** common voles ($n = 17$) as reported by questionnaire respondents (multiple answers were possible)

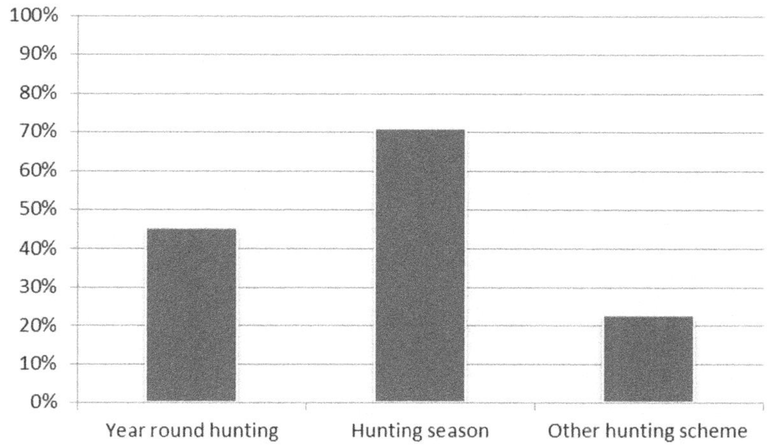

Fig. 4 Wild boar hunting scheme for wild boar in the considered study areas as reported by questionnaire respondents ($n = 31$, multiple answers were possible). Other management schemes include e.g. selective culling by official game managers for population reduction

Table 1 Regional scale, time scale and additional information from the accessible wild boar data as reported by questionnaire respondents

	Official hunting statistics ($n = 25$)	Hunting association data ($n = 3$)	Research data ($n = 8$)	Other*** ($n = 7$)
Regional scale				
NUTS 1*	10	1	0	1
NUTS 2*	13	2	1	1
NUTS 3*	17	2	2	0
LAU 1*	8	1	6	0
LAU 2*	12	2	5	1
Other (e.g. hunting grounds, hunting estates, 10 × 10 km)	10	0	1	1
Time scale				
Month	2	1	2	0
Quarter	0	1	1	0
Year	23	3	6	3
Other (e.g. hunting season, daily)	9	0	1	1
Additional information				
Age class	13	1	9	3
Weight	7	1	9	1
Sex	12	1	9	3
Cause of death**	12	2	7	2
Others (e.g. *Trichinella* testing, fecundity, general health)	0	0	0	1

* See [7] for more information
** E.g. found dead, shot sick, road traffic accident, regular hunting
*** e.g. EURL CSF/ASF-WB-DB

serologically and 12 were capable of detecting the virus or its genome (four by PCR, two by virus isolation and one by immunofluorescence assay). Laboratories without a possibility to test samples in their own country stated that they were willing to send serum samples (12 partners) or tissue samples (five partners) to a foreign laboratory.

Red fox and *E. multilocularis*

We received 22 completed questionnaires for the host-pathogen combination red fox and *E. multilocularis*. The size of the considered study areas ranged from 865 to 239,000 km^2 (mean = 45,290 km^2, median = 23,861 km^2, Fig. 2).

Host abundance-related questions

The sources of information on red fox abundance are shown in Fig. 3b. These data sources were even more heterogeneous than for wild boar, but hunting statistics were also the main data source for fox abundance. Furthermore, hunting statistics regarding foxes were available for longer time periods (up to 80 years, median = 15 years) than data generated by other methods (up to 9 years, median = 3 years).

Ten study areas (45%) practice year-round hunting with seasonal peaks ($n = 3$) and a protection period for females with pups ($n = 1$). For seven study areas, the hunting season was indicated to last from September until January/February (32%), while hunting took place in the opposite season, i.e. from July to February, in one study area (5%).

Table 3 show the regional and temporal scale, at which information on red fox abundance was available for the considered study areas. Like for wild boar, the available metadata are very inconsistent among countries and areas.

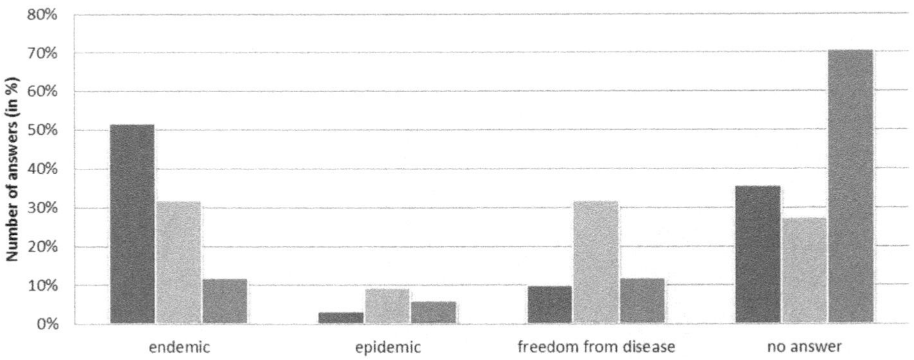

Fig. 5 Disease status regarding Aujeszky's disease in wild boar (*dark grey bars*, $n = 31$), *Echinococcus multilocularis* in red foxes (*light grey bars*, $n = 22$) and *Francisella tularensis* in common voles (*middle grey bars*, $n = 17$) in the considered study areas as reported by questionnaire respondents

Only eleven partners (50%) mentioned that they could record data by spotlight counting in the framework of future studies.

Pathogen-related questions

The status of the occurrence of *E. multilocularis* reported by the survey participants is shown in Fig. 5.

Numerous studies on *E. multilocularis* in red fox have been performed, are on-going or planned, with very variable sample sizes. Eight survey participants (36%) stated that they were able to investigate samples by the intestinal scraping technique in their own laboratory. Seven laboratories (32%) could perform SCT, 13 laboratories offered PCR (59%) and 4 laboratories applied other techniques (18%), including EmsB microsatellite analysis ($n = 3$) and a copro-antigen ELISA ($n = 1$) One participant did not specify the applied methods. Seven participants (32%) confirmed that they were able to send sera and tissue samples (intestines, intestinal mucosa, carcasses, feces or isolated specimens of *E. multilocularis*) to another laboratory, while seven participants (32%) denied that they could do so.

Table 2 Information available for wild boar samples from ongoing, historical or planned investigations on Aujeszky's disease virus as reported by questionnaire respondents

	Ongoing ($n = 21$)	Historical ($n = 17$)	Planned ($n = 3$)
Age class	15	12	3
Sex	15	12	3
Date	15	11	3
Location	16	13	3
Cause of death [a]	10	4	2
Results of serological investigations	16	12	3
Results of genetic and virological investigations	6	7	3

[a] E.g. found dead, shot sick, road traffic accident, regular hunting

Table 4 presents the potentially available information on samples from ongoing, historical or planned studies.

Common vole and *F. tularensis*

We received 17 completed questionnaires for the host-pathogen combination common vole and *F. tularensis.*

Table 3 Regional scale, time scale and additional information available from the red fox data as reported by questionnaire respondents

	Spotlight counts ($n = 6$)	Official hunting statistics ($n = 10$)	Hunting association data ($n = 5$)	Research data ($n = 6$)
Regional scale				
NUTS 1 [a]	0	2	0	0
NUTS 2 [a]	1	3	1	1
NUTS 3 [a]	1	4	1	2
LAU 1 [a]	1	0	1	2
LAU 2 [a]	1	0	2	1
Other (e.g. experimental field area)	5	4	3	2
Time scale				
Month	1	0	1	2
Quarter	1	0	1	1
Year	6	11	5	1
Other not specified by the participants)	1	0	0	3
Additional information				
Age class	0	3	1	4
Sex	0	4	1	4
Cause of death [b]	0	7	4	3

[a]See [7] for more information
[b]Type of carcass, e.g. found dead, shot sick, road traffic accident, regular hunting

Table 4 Information available for samples from ongoing, historical or planned investigations on *Echinococcus multilocularis* as reported by questionnaire respondents

	Ongoing ($n = 8$)	Historical/finished ($n = 11$)	Planned ($n = 5$)
Age class[a]	7	7	3
Sex	8	7	3
Collection date	8	9	3
Location	8	9	3
Cause of death[b]	3	5	2
Results of intestinal scraping technique	2	5	0
Results of sedimentation and counting technique	2	4	0
Results of PCR	4	6	2
Results of other investigations	1	4	1
Other[c]	1	2	0

[a]Age categorization, e.g. juvenile, adult
[b]Type of carcass, e.g. found dead, shot sick, road traffic accident, regular hunting
[c]additional intestinal parasites, reproduction status, body condition and size estimates

Host abundance-related questions

The source of information on common vole abundance is shown in Fig. 3c. Again, data sources were heterogeneous. The snap trapping method (recommended APHAEA protocol) is currently applied by only 7% of the respondents (2–20 plots). Nevertheless, abundance data from snap trapping were available for 6 to 72 years (median = 20 years). Active burrow index data and data from owl pellet analyses were available for 20 or 6 years, respectively, while field sign indices were available for only 1 to 2 years.

Seven participants (41%) stated that it would be possible to survey populations by snap trapping for common voles following the APHAEA protocol, whereas four participants (24%) denied due to animal welfare issues.

Pathogen-related questions

Tularemia was mentioned as a notifiable disease in 14 of the participating countries (82%). Of these 14 countries, 10 (59%) reported human cases of tularemia in 2012, whereas three (18%) did not register any human cases and four (24%) failed to provide the relevant information. The reported tularemia status of *F. tularensis* in the considered study areas is shown in Fig. 5.

Few studies were performed in the past, five were ongoing and more were planned at the time of the survey. Five participants (29%) indicated to have the possibility to investigate samples in their own laboratory by culture methods and other tests (isolation and typing, special nutrient media resistance, biological test with the subsequent growth of material on special media). Nine partners (53%) could perform PCR in their laboratories and six (35%) use serological techniques like the microagglutination test, ELISA, Western blot or the immunofluorescence antibody assay. Ten partners (59%) with access to common vole samples, but without possibility to test them for *F. tularensis*, were able to send tissue samples to another laboratory, and eight respondents (47%) could send serum samples.

In four study areas (24% of the respondents), data on *F. tularensis* were available for other rodents belonging to the families Cricetidae, and Muridae.

The available information on common vole samples from ongoing and permanent, historical or planned studies is shown in Table 5. Host information was collected only in the framework of snap trapping and included species (6 of 7 studies), age class (4 of 7 studies) and sex (6 of 7 studies).

Discussion

Effective wildlife disease surveillance and investigations of disease dynamics in wildlife populations requires knowledge of wildlife population sizes, their dynamics and changes in the geographical distribution over time. Such information is required to design appropriate sampling protocols for pathogen/disease surveys, to develop disease contingency plans, to assess the risk of pathogen transmission among different species and to guide wildlife management strategies in general [8]. However, for coordinated health surveillance efforts on a large scale, methods for assessing host population abundance and for detecting pathogen occurrence need to be harmonized in order to obtain comparable data [9].

The aim of this questionnaire survey was to clarify the potential for harmonizing methods in wildlife health research and population monitoring on the continental scale in Europe. Attempts to describe host abundance or disease/pathogen occurrence across countries were previously performed using available data, but they focused mostly on the host or the pathogen, on pooled data

Table 5 Available information on common vole samples in ongoing, historical or planned studies as reported by questionnaire respondents

	Ongoing ($n = 5$)	Historical ($n = 8$)	Planned ($n = 6$)
Age class	3	4	4
Sex	3	4	4
Date	3	4	5
Results of culture methods and tests [a]	1	1	2
Results of PCR	1	2	5
Results of serological investigations [a]	1	1	2

[a]Specified as IFA in one case

without information on their heterogeneity or underlined the difficulty to perform reliable comparisons [10–14]. To our knowledge, this article is the first to report the heterogeneity of the existing data in detail and the resulting limitations concerning their use for meta-studies. This is illustrated by the types of data available for three pairs of key host species and disease agents.

Wildlife experts showed a strong willingness to participate in the APHAEA project in general and in the questionnaire survey in particular. The participation of only a few European countries might have led to an incomplete and biased picture of the situation in Europe. Scandinavian and numerous Eastern European countries had registered as APHAEA partners and participated in networking activities concerning wildlife health, although they were not represented in the survey (Fig. 1). Scandinavia is known to carry out general wildlife health surveillance [1] and there are published data on *F. tularensis* and *E. multilocularis* in wildlife from Scandinavia and Eastern Europe [15, 16]. Therefore, the non-participation of countries in this specific survey does not necessarily reflect a lack of interest or a lack of activity.

However, our study included 68% of the EU member states and the three host-pathogen combinations referred to very different hosts and pathogens. The results obtained for each combination highlighted various challenges regarding the harmonization of methods for estimating host abundance or detecting pathogen occurrence. Some of these challenges were common for most or all studied regions, others were specific for individual areas or countries. Other host-pathogen combinations might have shown different levels of harmonization end even more difficulties; nevertheless, we believe that our results provide in principle an adequate overview on already performed harmonization efforts and the problematic lack of harmonization in other areas.

The present questionnaire survey revealed hunting bags are currently the most widely accessible data source that or hunted mid-sized and large mammals such as red fox and wild boar. While hunting bags may generate interesting data on a large scale [10, 14], their use remains controversial, because they are not readily comparable among countries and even among study areas within the same country due to different hunting efforts and hunting regulations [14]. However, more accurate methods for wildlife abundance estimation, i.e. those generating animal density estimations rather than hunting-based estimations, are time-consuming and costly. This makes it more difficult to applied them on a large scale and on the long term [17–20]. Therefore, the few data at the moment, available on live animal densities need to be combined with alternative data sources including hunting bags to model wildlife host abundances. In parallel, improved collaboration between experts in wildlife health and in wildlife ecology is required to develop tools for host abundance estimations which fulfill the need of epidemiological investigations.

For small mammals, which are not hunted, such as common voles, methods for abundance estimations vary widely, which poses even more severe challenges for comparing study areas. Due to the absence of relatively easily accessible data such as hunting bags, damage statistics and traffic accidents, which can deliver helpful information on population trends when combined, harmonization efforts are even more urgent to enable work at the continental scale.

By contrast, methods for pathogen detection are largely harmonized for all three considered pathogens due to a limited number of available techniques. Furthermore, EU regulations already exist for the selection of diagnostic methods for numerous pathogens and represent invaluable support towards harmonized procedures. Nevertheless, the collection of metadata on the samples is not yet sufficiently systematic. Information on the animals, from which the samples originate, is essential for data interpretation and comparisons among regions and countries [21]. It is therefore important to strive for a better harmonization of diagnostic data beyond laboratory procedures in the future.

The proposed APHAEA protocols have the potential to contribute to a more comprehensive harmonization on a European scale. Nevertheless, their application is not mandatory and implementing new methods require human and financial resources, which are usually limited. Overall, harmonization needs a common will to strive to a common goal, whether it concerns host abundance or pathogen detection, research or monitoring. We ultimately need to build a baseline for European-wide co-operations in disease surveillance and control, where wildlife management plays an essential role. The EURL CSF/ASF-WB DB is a good example on how data on wild boar hunting bags and disease surveillance could be standardized and combined on large scale.

Conclusions

A solid basis for a harmonized wildlife disease surveillance scheme exists in Europe, which integrates information on host populations and pathogens. The situation regarding the harmonization of methods for pathogen diagnosis is encouraging, but there are still opportunities for improvement. Importantly, much work needs to be done regarding the harmonization of wildlife abundance estimation methods. Therefore, we urge wildlife health experts to consider the recommended methods for harmonization for both pathogen detection and species abundance estimation in future studies (so-called

APHAEA protocols, www.aphaea.org or www.ewda.org) to collect metadata on the animals concerned and to collaborate in the development of practice-oriented tools for wildlife abundance estimations.

Abbreviations

ADV: Aujeszky's disease virus; APHAEA: harmonized Approaches in monitoring wildlife Population Health, and Ecology and Abundance; *E. multilocularis*: *Echinococcus multilocularis*; ELISA: Enzyme-linked immunosorbent assay; EURL CSF/ASF-WB-DB: European Union reference laboratory Classical Swine Fever/African Swine Fever wild boar surveillance database; EWDA: European Wildlife Disease Association; *F. tularensis*: *Francisella tularensis*; IST: Intestinal scraping technique; LAU: Local administrative unit; NUTS: Nomenclature of Territorial Units for Statistics; PCR: Polymerase chain reaction; SCT: Sedimentation and counting technique

Acknowledgements

We thank Mandy Herzig, Christian Imholt, Thomas Müller, Sabine Schwarz and Astrid Sutor for their feedbacks on the questionnaire design. We are particularly indebted to all partners who answered the questionnaires (see detailed list below). We are very grateful to Matthias Merboth and Thorsten Schrapps for their continuous excellent technical support.

APHAEA project partners who participated in the survey:

Pelayo Acevedo (Spain), Andreas Agreiter (Italy), Anna Bajer (Poland), Alex Barlow (United Kingdom), Charalambos Billinis (Greece), Franck Boue (France), Andrea Cadamuro (Italy), Maria S. Calabrese (Italy), Gioia Capelli (Italy), Isabel Lopes de Carvalho (Portugal), Adriano Casulli (Italy), Ermanno Cetto (Italy), Mario Chiari (Italy), Leo J. M. Dekkers (The Netherlands), Peter Deplazes (Switzerland), J. Paul Duff (United Kingdom), Javier Millán Gasca (Spain), Walter Glawischnig (Austria), Irina Golovljova (Estonia), Roland Grunow (Germany), Jean Hars (France), Marja Isomursu (Finland), Jens Jacob (Germany), Kastriot Korro (Albania), Antonio Lavazza (Italy), Jane Learmount (United Kingdom), Annick Linden (Belgium), Andrzej Lipowski (Poland), Miriam Maas (The Netherlands), Ignasi Marco (Spain), Roman Meier (Switzerland), Marcos Miñarro Prado (Spain), Viacheslav Morozov (Russia), Sofia Núncio (Portugal), Riccardo Orusa (Italy), Thomas Romig (Germany), Sophie Rossi (France), Francisco Ruiz-Fons (Spain), Gianmaria Sommavilla (Italy), Michal Stanko (Slovakia), Adolf Steinrigl (Austria), Herbert Tomaso (Germany), Jurga Turcinaviciene (Lithuania), Umberto Zamboni (Italy)

Funding

Funding was provided by the EMIDA ERA-NET project APHAEA (grant no. 2811ERA117).

Authors' contributions

JS carried out the survey, analyzed the data and drafted the manuscript. MR contributed to study design and recruitment of participants, delivered data for the survey and drafted the manuscript. CS designed and coordinated the study and delivered data for the survey. FJC delivered data for the survey. RGU recruited participants. TK, CG and EF contributed to study design. All authors participated in the development of the three questionnaires, critically read and approved the final version of the manuscript.

Competing interests

The authors declare that they have no competing interests.

Consent for publication

Not applicable.

Author details

[1]Federal Research Institute for Animal Health, Friedrich-Loeffler-Institut, Institute of Epidemiology, Südufer 10, 17493 Greifswald, Insel Riems, Germany. [2]National Veterinary Institute, Technical University of Denmark, Bülowsvej 27, Building 1-6, 1870 Frederiksberg C, Denmark. [3]Centre for Fish and Wildlife Health, Department Infectious Diseases and Pathobiology, Vetsuisse Faculty, University of Bern, Länggass-Str. 122, Postfach 8466, CH-3001 Bern, Switzerland. [4]Department of Viroscience, Erasmus Medical Centre, P.O. Box 2040Ee1726, 3000, CA, Rotterdam, The Netherlands. [5]Dipartimento di Scienze Veterinarie, Università degli Studi di Torino, Largo Paolo Braccini, 2 (già Via L. DaVinci, 44), 10095 Grugliasco, TO, Italy. [6]Federal Research Institute for Animal Health, Institute of Novel and Emerging Infectious Diseases, Friedrich-Loeffler-Institut, Südufer 10, 17493 Greifswald, Insel Riems, Germany. [7]SaBio Instituto de Investigaciónen Recursos Cinegéticos IREC Universidad de Castilla—La Mancha & CSIC, Ronda de Toledo s/n, 13071 Ciudad Real, Spain.

References

1. Kuiken T. Establishing a European network for wildlife health surveillance. Rev Sci. 2011;30:755–61.
2. Patz JA, Daszak P, Tabor GM, Aguirre AA, Pearl M, Epstein J, et al. Unhealthy landscapes: Policy recommendations on land use change and infectious disease emergence. Environ Health Perspect. 2004;112:1092–8.
3. European Wildlife Disease Association (EWDA). 2016. Available from: www.ewda.org. Accessed Apr 2016.
4. Coordination of European Research on Emerging and major Infectious Diseases of Livestock. 2016. Available from: http://era-platform.eu/. Accessed Apr 2016.
5. Harmonised approaches in monitoring wildlife population health, and ecology and abundance. 2016. Available from: http://www.aphaea.org/. Accessed Apr 2016.
6. CSF/ASF wild boar surveillance database. 2016. Available from: http://public.surv-wildboar.eu. Accessed Apr 2016.
7. Acevedo P, Ruiz-Fons F, Vicente J, Reyes-García AR, Alzaga V, Gortázar C. Estimating red deer abundance in a wide range of management situations in Mediterranean habitats. J Zool. 2008;276:37–47.
8. Salman MD. Animal disease surveillance and survey systems: methods and applications. 1st ed. Ames: Iowa State Press; 2003. p. xii–222.
9. Vetter SG, Ruf T, Bieber C, Arnold W. What is a mild winter? Regional differences in within-species responses to climate change. PLoS One. 2015;10:1–17.
10. Gortázar C, Delahay RJ, Mcdonald RA, Boadella M, Wilson GJ, Gavier-Widen D, et al. The status of tuberculosis in European wild mammals. Mamm Rev. 2012;42:193–206.
11. Schöning JM, Cerny N, Prohaska S, Wittenbrink MM, Smith NH, Bloemberg G, et al. Surveillance of bovine tuberculosis and risk estimation of a future reservoir formation in wildlife in Switzerland and Liechtenstein. PLoS One. 2013;8.
12. Meier RK, Ruiz-Fons F, Ryser-Degiorgis M-P. A picture of trends in Aujeszky's disease virus exposure in wild boar in the Swiss and European contexts. BMC Vet Res. 2015;11:277.
13. Massei G, Kindberg J, Licoppe A, Gacic D, Sprem N, Kamler J, et al. Wild boar populations up, numbers of hunters down? A review of trends and implications for Europe. Pest Manag Sci 2015;71:492–500.
14. Hestvik G, Warns-Petit E, Smith LA, Fox NJ, Uhlhorn H, Artois M, et al. The status of tularemia in Europe in a one-health context: a review. Epidemiol Infect. 2015;143:2137–60.
15. Wahlström H, Enemark HL, Davidson RK, Oksanen A. Present status, actions taken and future considerations due to the findings of E. multilocularis in two Scandinavian countries. Vet Parasitol. 2015;213:172–81.
16. Keuling O, Greiser G, Grauer A, Strauß E Bartel-Steinbach M, Klein R, et al. The German wildlife information system (WILD): Population densities and den use of red foxes (Vulpes vulpes) and badgers (Meles meles) during 2003-2007 in Germany. Eur J Wildl Res. 2011;57:95–105.
17. Vos A. Population dynamics of the red fox (Vulpes vulpes) after the disappearance of rabies in county Garmisch-Partenkirchen, Germany, 1987-1992. Ann Zool Fenn. 1995;32:93–7.
18. Acevedo P, Vicente J, Höfle U, Cassinello J, Ruiz-Fons F, Gortazar C. Estimation of European wild boar relative abundance and aggregation: a novel method in epidemiological risk assessment. Epidemiol Infect. 2006; 135:519–27.
19. Acevedo P, Quiras-Fernandez F, Casal J, Vicente J. Spatial distribution of wild boar population abundance: Basic information for spatial epidemiology and wildlife management. Ecol Indic. 2014;36:594–600.

14

Techniques for thoracic duct cannulation without thoracotomy in piglets

Hung-Hsun Yen* and Helen M. S. Davies

Abstract

Background: Pigs are the natural hosts of many zoonotic pathogens such as influenza viruses and *Staphylococcus aureus* and thus have advantages over non-natural hosts when studying these zoonotic diseases. In addition, pulmonary infections are a key issue in the pig industry, for example: porcine reproductive and respiratory syndrome virus infection. Exploration of the pathogenesis of swine pulmonary infections, in particular at the onset of disease, will provide valuable information for the development of vaccines against these diseases. Therefore, there is need to develop a methodology that allows for in vivo sampling of efferent pulmonary lymph with minimum damage to the target tissues for studying the pathogenesis of swine pulmonary infections.

Results: We introduce the surgical procedures for cannulating the thoracic duct at its point of entry into the external jugular vein cranial to the first rib on the left in pigs. Using this methodology, we monitored the amounts of triglyceride and cholesterol in the lymph collected from the thoracic duct following 30 h fasting and at multiple time points after meals. It was found that the levels of triglyceride rather than cholesterol corresponded to the milky appearance of the lymph samples.

Conclusions: Our techniques provide a strategy for collecting lymph including pulmonary lymph from the thoracic duct without thoracotomy. A pig model for collecting in vivo, in situ efferent lymph draining the lower respiratory tract and its local lymph nodes in real-time with minimal tissue damage to the target tissues opens a new door for studying disease processes in pulmonary infections. Techniques described here are the key to this door.

Keywords: Lymphatic cannulation, Thoracic duct, Pulmonary lymph, Swine

Background

Obtaining pulmonary lymph draining the lungs and the local lymph nodes (i.e. tracheobronchial lymph nodes) from the natural hosts of lung pathogens provides a strategy for monitoring in vivo, in situ pulmonary immunobiology and screening the biomarkers following pulmonary infections. Pigs are the natural hosts of several zoonotic pathogens for example influenza viruses (H1N1, H3N2, and H1N2) [1], Japanese encephalitis virus [2, 3] and *Staphylococcus aureus* [4], and thus are suitable for studying disease processes in these infections. Indeed, interest in using pigs as a model for influenza virus infection has increased since the outbreak of the swine-origin influenza A (H1N1) 2009 virus infection in humans [5, 6].

* Correspondence: hyen@unimelb.edu.au
Faculty of Veterinary and Agricultural Sciences, The University of Melbourne, Parkville, Victoria 3010, Australia

Pulmonary infections are a key issue in humans and in the pig industry [7]. For example, the economic loss to the pork producers caused by porcine reproductive and respiratory syndrome virus (PRRSV) infection was estimated to be US $664 million per annum [8]. To explore the pathogenesis of swine pulmonary infections, in particular at the onset of these diseases, will provide valuable information for the development of vaccines against these diseases. Real-time in vivo pulmonary lymph collection provides the chance to monitor the progress of an infection from the first contact of a pathogen with the host to the induction of illness. To achieve effective monitoring of pulmonary responses, a strategy for accessing in vivo pulmonary lymph samples in pigs is needed.

The structure of porcine lymph nodes is inverted compared to other species. Pabst and Binns also reported that most porcine lymphocytes leave lymph nodes via high endothelial venules (HEVs) instead of the efferent lymph [9]. However, the report by Binns in 1980 [10], indicates that, "In spite of the low cell numbers, efferent lymph responds to antigenic stimulation of the lymph node.". Binns also mentioned that, '...efferent lymph flow and contents are normal in other respects...'. According to these previous findings, the efferent lymph supernatant of pigs will provide a useful source of samples for studying the components and immunity of the local lymph node and its draining tissues even though the numbers of white cells are relatively low. However, studies on the changes to the cells in porcine efferent lymph to infections at the draining tissues may be limited since it is unclear what type of lymphocyte egresses from lymph nodes via efferent lymph.

Techniques for cannulating the thoracic duct following thoracotomy by approaching its segment within the thoracic cavity have been described in pigs [11, 12]. However, surgical incisions into the chest wall result in severe tissue damage that can also induce immune responses other than those triggered by the pathogen in a pulmonary infection study. Due to this consideration, a model for harvesting pulmonary lymph without inducing severe tissue damage to the chest wall would be beneficial for respiratory studies.

From the anatomical layout, pulmonary afferent lymph from the lungs, in particular the caudal lobes of the lungs, drains into the tracheobronchial lymph centres and then enters the thoracic duct directly or through the cranial mediastinal lymph centre [13]. Anatomical dissection demonstrated that the thoracic duct extends cranially beyond the first rib, prior to terminating in the external jugular vein on the left in 12 of a group of 15 Large White piglets [14]. Therefore, procedures for catheterizing the thoracic duct can be developed by approaching the region where the thoracic duct joins the external jugular vein at the thoracic inlet.

Although techniques for thoracic duct cannulation without thoracotomy using different approaches have been developed in sheep [15, 16], the surgical approaches in pigs need to be re-developed due to noticeable anatomical variations [17]. For example, pigs have a prominent subclavian muscle lateral to the ampulla of the thoracic duct on the left. The porcine subclavian muscle arises from the second to fourth costal cartilage, courses dorsolaterally passing over the shoulder joint and joins with the aponeurosis of the supraspinatus muscle whereas the subclavian muscle of sheep is a narrow band, which joins the tendon of insertion of the brachiocephalic muscle. In addition, pigs have dorsal, middle and ventral superficial cervical lymph nodes in the caudal cervical region whereas only the superficial cervical lymph nodes are present in sheep. The locations of these lymph nodes also vary in these two species. Considering the anatomical variations between sheep and pigs, surgical procedures for thoracic duct annulation in sheep cannot be directly applied to pigs. Surgical procedures to achieve an approach to the thoracic duct with minimum damage to local tissues in pigs need to be studied and tailored based on porcine anatomy.

Here, we describe the surgical procedures developed for cannulating the thoracic duct with minimum tissue damage and without thoracotomy in pigs.

Methods

Experimental animals

The University of Melbourne Animal Experimentation Ethics Committee approved all experimental procedures. The methods were carried out in accordance with the approved guidelines.

Four female Large White piglets (aged 4–9 weeks, live weight range 9.3 to 17.1 kg) were housed in pens within the Faculty of Veterinary and Agricultural Sciences animal facility. These pigs were fed with commercial pellets (1 kg/day) and allowed access to water ad libitum. Following surgery, one pig was housed in a metabolic cage to reduce the possibility of wound damage and cannula removal. The other pigs were housed in pens post-surgery. At the end of the study, they were euthanized by intravenous injection of Lethabarb (Pentobarbitone) into the external jugular vein.

One pig was euthanized to obtain the anatomical images of the thoracic duct and the left tracheal trunk at their points of entry into the external jugular vein at the cervico-thoracic junction. Three pigs of different ages were used to develop the surgical procedures for thoracic duct cannulation without thoracotomy.

General surgical procedures

Anaesthetic protocol

Prior to surgery, pigs were fasted overnight and provided water ad libitum. Anaesthesia was induced by intramuscular injection of Atropine (0.054 mg/kg) + Ketamine (15 mg/kg) + Xylazil (1 mg/kg) and then maintained with isoflurane (1.5–2.5 %) and oxygen using a mask. To prevent hypothermia, the pigs were placed on a heating pad in surgery. Each pig received an intramuscular injection of procaine penicillin (1 mL dose) and analgesic (Temgesic, 0.1 mg/kg) while under anaesthesia. Another dose of analgesic was given at day one post-surgery.

Cannulas

We used cannulas, SV28 (internal diameter 0.40 mm; external diameter 0.80 mm; CBAS-coated, Carmeda AB, Stock-holm, Sweden) and SV45 (internal diameter 0.58 mm; external diameter 0.96 mm) of different bores for pigs of different body weights [16]. The SV28 cannula was only applied to the cannulation surgery in a 5-week-old pig that weighed 9.3 kg. For an 8-week old pig, which weighed 17.1 kg and a 7-week old pig, which weighed 14.7 kg, we used the SV45 cannulas for the surgeries.

Triglyceride and cholesterol measurement

Quantitation of triglycerides and cholesterol was carried out by Gribbles Veterinary Pathology (Melbourne, Australia).

Results

Other than the information provided in Fig. 1, the detailed anatomical structures in the left cervicothoracic region and the left forelimb in pigs were acquired from textbooks [13, 18, 19]. The basic technique for inserting a cannula into a lymphatic has been described in previous publications [16, 20, 21]. As a result, unless the procedures were essential for this surgery, they are not repeated here.

The animal was positioned in right lateral recumbency. After a surgical incision in the skin cranial to the prescapular region, dissections were conducted towards the thoracic inlet to approach and isolate the thoracic duct. The skin incision of about 13 cm in these pigs was commenced from the cranial boundary of the subclavian muscle and its junction with the omotransversarius muscle and extended ventrally to about 2 cm cranial to the shoulder joint. After cutting through the superficial fascia, dissection was required to penetrate through the subcutaneous tissue and fat to separate the subclavian muscle from the cleidooccipitalis part of brachiooccipitalis muscle. This was mostly performed through blunt dissection to avoid damaging the main blood vessels, nerves, lymphatics and muscles.

Branching from the superficial cervical artery and vein, there were generally two blood vessels that coursed caudally in the subcutaneous tissue and fat to the supraspinatus region. Consequently, care was required to isolate these large blood vessels and ligate them. Transecting these blood vessels provided more space to approach the deeper tissues. After transecting these blood vessels, two self-retained retractors were placed in

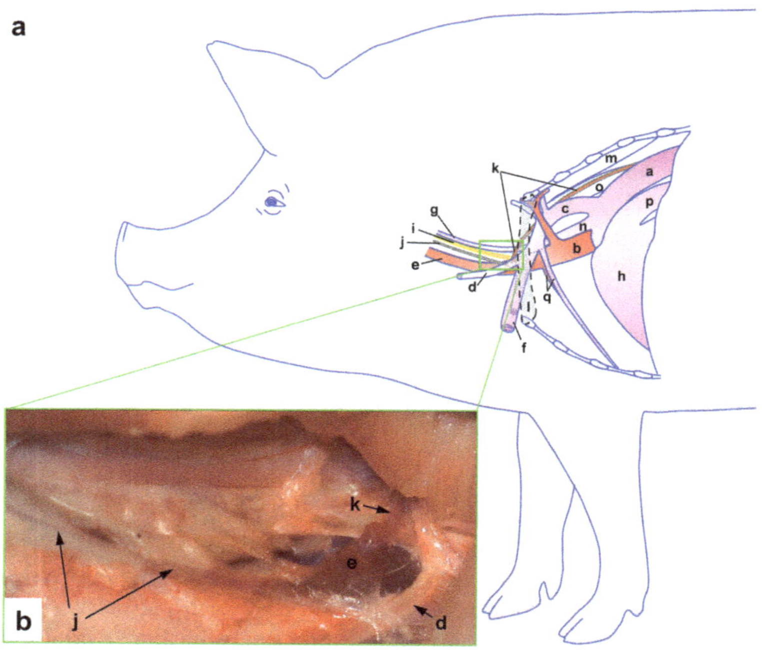

Fig. 1 Schematic view (**a**) and photograph (**b**) of the thoracic duct and the tracheal trunk in the cervicothoracic region on the left side. (**a**) The thoracic duct containing lymph draining the lungs emerging from the thoracic cavity joins the external jugular vein at the cranial thoracic inlet. The ampulla of the thoracic duct is located craniomedially to the first rib (l). The thoracic duct (k) is medial to the subclavian and superficial cervical arteries (c & d respectively) and lateral to the common carotid artery (g) and vagosympathetic trunk (i). (a) thoracic aorta; (b) cranial vena cava; (c) subclavian artery; (d) superficial cervical artery; (e) external jugular vein; (f) axillary artery; (g) common carotid artery; (h) heart; (i) vagosympathetic trunk; (j) tracheal trunk; (k) thoracic duct; (l) first rib; (m) longus colli; (n) brachiocephalic trunk; (o) oesophagus; (p) pulmonary trunk. (**b**) Dissections were performed from the cranial border of the left forelimb to expose the cranial thoracic inlet. The superficial cervical artery (d) was retracted to reveal the thoracic duct (k) and its point of entry into the left external jugular vein (e). The tracheal trunk (j) coursing caudally from the medial retropharyngeal lymph centre also entered the left external jugular vein (e). The image was taken from a euthanized 7-week old Large White pig

the skin opening to generate an operating area and to improve access to the thoracic duct.

Blunt dissection was then used to penetrate the connective tissues and locate the superficial cervical artery and vein, the dorsal superficial cervical lymph nodes (SCLD) and the efferent lymphatic of the SCLD. The efferent lymphatic of the SCLD drains into the external jugular vein and the point of its entry to the external jugular vein was next to the ampulla of the thoracic duct. Consequently, one approach to find the junction of the thoracic duct and the external jugular vein was to follow the efferent lymphatic of the SCLD as well as the superficial cervical artery that runs parallel to it. The other key lymphatic that needed to be identified in this region was the tracheal trunk. The tracheal trunk lies deeper in the fat and the connective tissues between the forelimb and the trachea. From our experience in pig dissections, the tracheal trunk was obviously bigger than the efferent lymphatic of the SCLD. Pigs might sometimes have double tracheal trunks [22]. When approaching and isolating the thoracic duct and its ampulla, we avoided damaging the tracheal trunk and the efferent lymphatic of the SCLD. Leaking lymph in the surgical area would have increased the difficulties in structure identification and cannula insertion.

The brachial plexus had nerve branches crossing the axilla from the neck musculature to the forelimb on the left. Great care was needed to avoid cutting the nerve branches of the brachial plexus when doing blunt dissections to isolate the thoracic duct and its ampulla. In particular, muscular nerve branches from the cervical nerve, C6/C7 to the subscapular region crossed the region of dissection. We opted to make space to approach the thoracic duct from the connective tissues and fat dorsal to the first big nerve branch that crossed to the subscapular region (usually a branch of C6/C7 that innervated the subscapular muscles). At day one post-surgery, all pigs were able to actively move around including climbing on the fences of the metabolic cage using the leg on the surgical (left) side. This outcome supported the conclusion that the surgical procedures we opted for did not result in damage to these nerve branches.

When the thoracic duct and its ampulla were identified, a segment of the lymphatic vessel was isolated that was enough to place two overhead knots around it. Isolation of this segment of the lymphatic was a critical step and there were some structures near the thoracic duct that ought to be noticed and should not be damaged. Figure 1 illustrates a schematic view (a) and a photograph (b) of the thoracic duct and its relationships to the adjacent structures in the cervicothoracic region on the left. As indicated in Fig. 1a, the left vagosympathetic trunk and common carotid artery were medial to the thoracic duct and they ran together with the thoracic duct through the thoracic inlet into the thorax. In addition, the superficial cervical artery was directly on the top of the thoracic duct and the ventral portion of the thoracic duct contacted the wall of the external jugular vein (Fig. 1a & Fig. 2). Figure 1b presents the thoracic duct and the tracheal trunk at the cranial thoracic inlet with the superficial cervical artery retracted to expose their points of entry into the external jugular vein on the left side of a euthanized animal. In addition, the placement of the suture around the thoracic duct had to be conducted with care. We used long forceps with blunt ends to separate the thoracic duct from the external jugular vein underneath and to place the suture. At least, two pre sutures were required to be placed around the thoracic duct. One was to ligate the thoracic duct to prevent bleeding from the external jugular vein. The other was to secure the cannula after its insertion into the thoracic duct. If there was enough space to do so it would be helpful to add an additional suture to secure the cannula. An intra-operative image of the surgical field with pre sutures around the thoracic duct is presented in Fig. 2. In this image, the superficial cervical artery was retracted ventrally using a pair of forceps to reveal a fragment of the thoracic duct and its ampulla for cannula insertion.

The cannula was inserted into the thoracic duct from a cut made in the upstream end of the ampulla (Fig. 3).

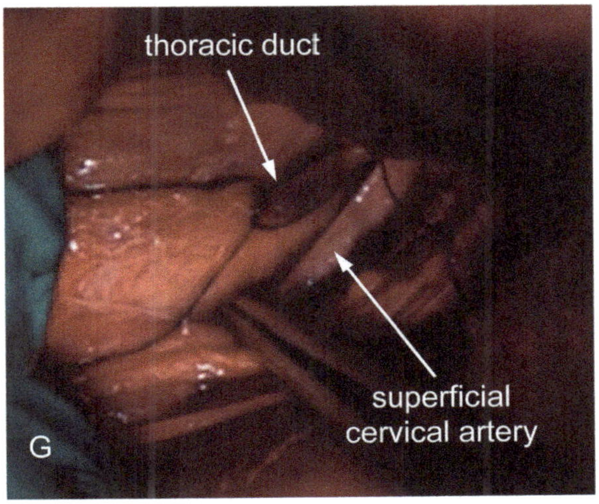

Fig. 2 Intraoperative photograph of the surgical field. Surgery was conducted to separate a segment of the thoracic duct and its ampulla at the cranial thoracic inlet. The thoracic duct was gently isolated and two pre sutures were placed around it (Only one pre suture that is around the ampulla is shown in this image). The superficial cervical artery was retracted ventrally using a pair of forceps to reveal the thoracic duct. The size of the ampulla changed depending on the amount of blood in it. The ampulla is in a collapsed state in this image (G: gloves)

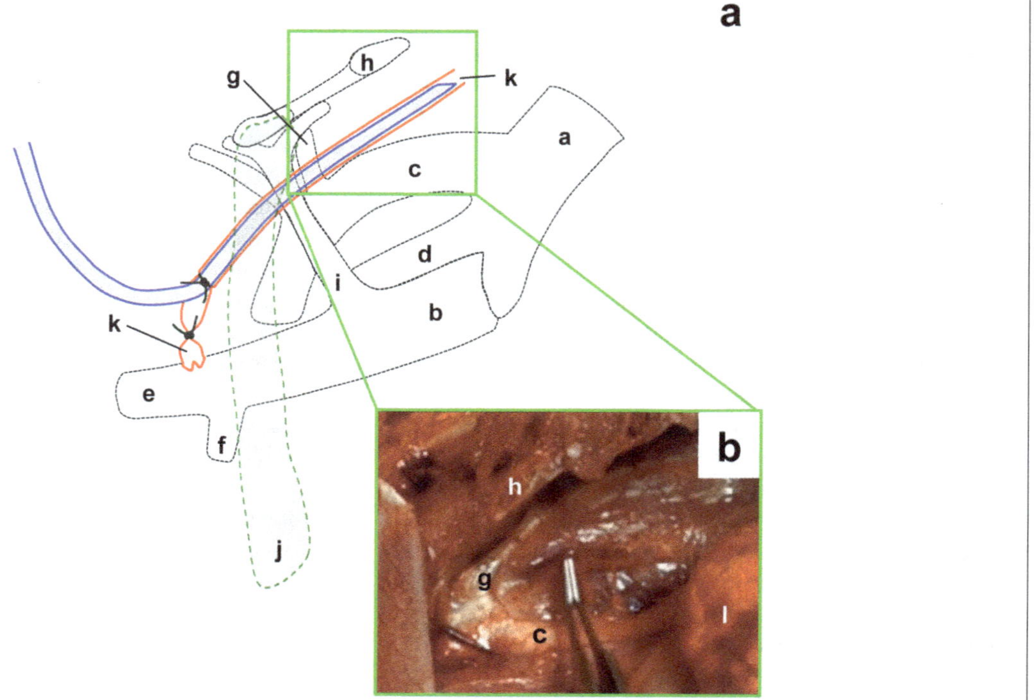

Fig. 3 Sketch of thoracic duct cannulation (**a**) and a photograph (**b**) of a cannula in the thoracic duct at the cranial thorax on the left side. The cannula was inserted into the thoracic duct from a cut into the upstream end of the ampulla. After inserting the cannula into the thoracic duct, the cannula was then gently pushed forward until its bevelled leading end passed the junction of the costocervical trunk and subclavian artery. The bevelled end of the cannula is placed in the segment of the thoracic duct medial to the second to third rib as this position has more space and is free of major blood vessels. (**b**) Dissections were performed to confirm the insertion of a cannula in the thoracic duct following a thoracic duct cannulation surgery. This photograph of the cranial thorax shows a cannula in a segment of the thoracic duct elevated by a pair of forceps. Since the cannula was in the thoracic duct, the pressure of lifting it up did not cause the lymphatic to collapse where it was supported by the forceps. The cannula could be pushed gently far enough so that its bevelled leading end reached the segment of the thoracic duct medial to the 2nd to 3rd ribs. (a) thoracic aorta; (b) cranial vena cava; (c) subclavian artery; (d) brachiocephalic trunk; (e) external jugular vein; (f) subclavian vein; (g) costocervical trunk; (h) 2nd rib; (i) costocervical vein; (j) first rib; (k) thoracic duct; (l) lung

After inserting the cannula into the thoracic duct, the cannula was then gently pushed forward until its bevelled end passed the junction of the costocervical trunk and subclavian artery. The bevelled end (lead) of the cannula is best placed in a position with more space and free of major blood vessels in the cranial thorax. The segment of the thoracic duct medial to the second and the third ribs was a suitable position for the lead of the cannula. An autopsy was performed to confirm the insertion of a cannula into the thoracic duct as well as the location of the lead of a cannula in the thoracic duct immediately after the cannulation surgery. Figure 3b shows a cannula within the thoracic duct in the cranial thorax that has been elevated by a pair of forceps. Since the cannula was within the thoracic duct, the pressure of lifting the duct up did not result in a collapsed lymphatic at the contact point of the forceps Additional file 1: Video S1 and Additional file 2: Video S2.

After cannula insertion into the lymphatic, a small coil of the cannula was left subcutaneously. The cannula was secured using a purse-string suture at its skin opening dorsocranial to the cranial angle of the scapula [23]. For the first surgery in a 5-week-old pig, the end of the cannula external to the animal was protected in a SILASTIC® Foley catheter (16G) that was sutured to the skin at the cannula's exit to the skin and attached to a step-in harness (PETstock, Victoria, Australia). The use of a Foley catheter provided additional protection to the cannula and possibly the protection resulted in a longer period of lymph collection during the post-operative period. However, active movements of the pig induced more tissue damage at the skin opening since the calibre of the Foley catheter was much bigger than that of the SV28 and SV45 cannulas. In the 8-week old pig, we did not suture the Foley catheter to the cannula's skin opening. Instead, the Foley catheter was sutured to the skin near the cannula's skin opening. Only minor tissue responses were found at the cannula's skin opening in this pig. The step-in harness together with the Foley catheter was secured on the animal with tubular elastic net bandages (size 3, Surgifix®). The tube for lymph collection was secured in a plastic bottle that was tightly tethered to the harness on the left side of the pig. An opening on the side of the bottle was made to allow convenient changing of the collecting tube.

The success of the thoracic duct cannulation surgery was confirmed by observing the colour of fluid collected. As presented in Fig. 4a, the supernatant of lymph samples (samples 2–4) collected from the thoracic duct at different time points after meals post-surgery were all milky. The colour of the "milky" or turbid lymph resembled that of the body fat of the animal. We also collected lymph (sample 1) from the animals during the period after successful cannulation and before the animal woke up. It was found that the supernatant of this lymph sample did not show the milky appearance of the later samples. The level of triglyceride was obviously lower in this sample (Fig. 4b) compared to the milky samples. However, no apparent differences of cholesterol levels were found between the milky and non-milky samples. Compatible results were found in another cannulated pig showing that the levels of triglyceride rather than cholesterol corresponded to the milky appearance of the lymph samples (Fig. 4). Before surgery, the animals did not have food intake for about 30 h. It was likely due to this reason that the lymph supernatant in sample 1 was not milky. When the cannula came out of the thoracic duct at day three post-surgery in this pig, the fluid collected from the cannula was not milky (sample 5). The colour of the supernatant of this sample (sample 5) looked like that of porcine sera.

The levels of triglyceride and cholesterol in the lymph from the thoracic duct of a 5-week old pig were assayed for six days (Fig. 5). It was found that the amount of cholesterol was at a constant level between 0.4 and 1.6 mmol/mL. The level of triglyceride varied depending on the time for sampling in each day following unknown variations in food consumption. With regular food intake, the amount of triglyceride was between 8 and 10 mmol/mL (days 3–6). The amount of triglyceride peaked after meals and dropped dramatically without recent food intake.

It was found that lymph flow went smoothly when a cannula with a bigger calibre was placed in the thoracic duct. The rate of lymph flow was about 7 mL per hour

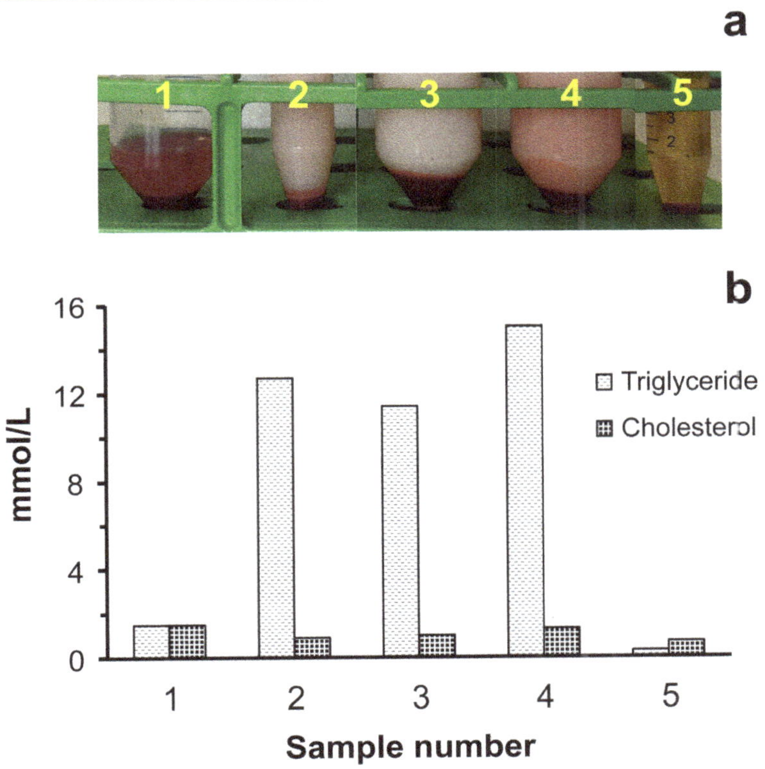

Fig. 4 The appearance of thoracic duct lymph and interstitial fluid samples (**a**) and their corresponding levels of triglyceride and cholesterol (**b**). A cannula with an internal diameter of 0.58 mm and an external diameter of 0.96 mm (code: SV45) was inserted into the thoracic duct of an 8-week old pig. Lymph and interstitial fluid samples collected from this animal at different stages post-surgery were collected (**a**) and the levels of triglyceride and cholesterol in these samples are shown in (**b**). The sample labels are: 1: lymph from the thoracic duct, collected after about 30 h of fasting; 2–4: lymph from the thoracic duct after meals; 2: lymph harvested from 11 to 13 h post-surgery (14 mL of lymph in 2 h); 3: lymph harvested from 16 to 22 h post-surgery (42 mL of lymph in 5.5 h); 4: 23–33 h post-surgery; 5: interstitial fluid, cannula came out of the thoracic duct

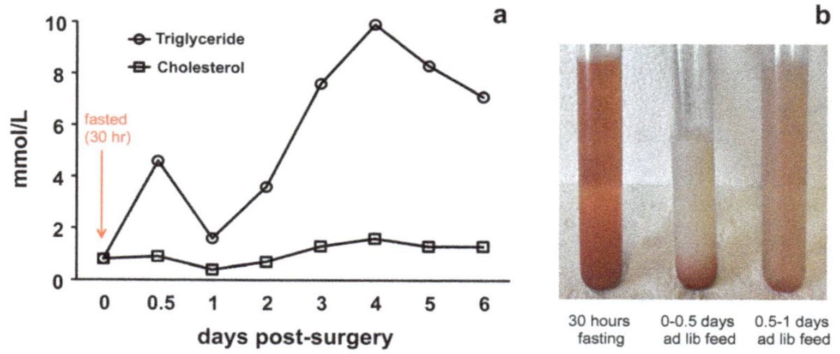

Fig. 5 The level of triglyceride and cholesterol in the lymph collected from the thoracic duct following cannulation surgery. Triglyceride and cholesterol levels (**a**) and appearance (**b**) of lymph samples harvested from the thoracic duct of a 5-week old pig at different time points post-surgery

with an SV45 cannula (internal diameter 0.58 mm; external diameter 0.96 mm) in an 8-week old pig, which weighed 17.1 kg at day one post-surgery. We also successfully inserted an SV45 cannula into the thoracic duct of a 7-week old pig, which weighed 14.7 Kg (Fig. 3b, pig euthanized after cannula insertion). Considering the smaller body size of the animal, we chose to use a smaller SV28 cannula (internal diameter 0.40 mm; external diameter 0.80 mm) in a 5-week-old pig, which weighed 9.3 kg (Fig. 5). The thoracic duct of the smaller pigs was generally smaller. It would require less skill to insert a smaller calibre cannula for animals of small sizes. However, cannula blocking by clot formation occurred frequently (once daily, always at night) in the 5-week-old pig with the smaller SV28 cannula. With intermittent cannula clotting and blocking, the total lymph volume harvested from a 5-week-old pig using an SV28 cannula from day 2 to day 5 post-surgery was 18.7, 46.5, 23.5, 16.6 and 18.0 mL respectively.

From previous experience severe cannula blocking occurred only occasionally where the SV45 cannulas were regularly applied to lymphatic cannulation surgeries in sheep, which weighed over 30 kg. We recognise that the SV45 cannulas are a more suitable choice than the SV28 cannula for the thoracic duct cannulation surgery in piglets even though the piglets only weighed around 10 Kg.

Discussion

This is a pilot study to develop the surgical procedures for cannulating the thoracic duct at its point of entry into the external jugular vein cranial to the first rib on the left in pigs. The results in this study demonstrated that it was possible to catheterize the thoracic duct without thoracotomy and without damaging the major blood vessels, nerves and muscle bellies in 5 to 8-week old pigs. This model offers a strategy for accessing pulmonary lymph in real time and will provide a chance for evaluating in vivo pulmonary host-pathogen interplay with further modifications.

Though this surgery was successfully developed, there is still room to improve this model. In particular, to design and test a harness that can protect the external segment of the cannula from being destroyed by the animals would further ensure more robust application of the techniques described here. That is also what we will try to achieve in the subsequent studies. Pigs are strong and intransigent animals and thus additional procedures are required for protecting the cannula from any damage created by the pigs' behaviours. Approaches such as having an external canvas pouch ("12 × 17 cm") sutured to the skin [24] or simply by putting a solid vest on the pig are all good strategies for cannula protection. The outcome of catheter protection by applying an external custom-made canvas pouch to keep the catheters for medicine infusion in the study [24] by Swindle et al. was promising. However, many sutures were required to secure the canvas pouch to the animal. We tried a Foley catheter, which is soft and stretchy, tethered to a commercial harness for cannula protection. Compared to the application of a canvas pouch, our approach only required 2–3 sutures. Both methods were useful since they achieved the purpose of cannula protection. Our approach of using a Foley catheter for cannula protection did achieve its purpose, although the method of securing the Foley catheter to the skin at the cannula's exit requires improvement. The success of cannula protection for long-term lymph collection using a Foley catheter should be confirmed in more animals.

This porcine thoracic duct cannulation model was primarily developed for use in pulmonary studies. However, the application of this model is not limited to pulmonary studies alone. The model could also be useful for studying diseases in which multiple organs are infected by the pathogen under study. For example, the reproductive and the respiratory tracts are the two major target organs for the porcine reproductive and respiratory syndrome virus. This model would also be a considerable boost for studying a few human diseases such as

Staphylococcus aureus and rotavirus infections in which pigs have already been used as an animal model [4]. Catheterisation of the thoracic duct in pigs allowing for continuous in vivo, and real-time lymph sampling will also be useful in studies involving gastro-enterology and pharmacokinetics. For example, to collect lymph samples draining the cardiac region of the stomach, especially the esophagogastric junction caudal to the diaphragm, our thoracic duct cannulation model is so far the only available choice without thoracotomy. It was found that myeloid cells and T cells infiltrate into the cardiac region of porcine stomachs in *Helicobacter pylori* infection [25].

To expand the application of this model in biomedical research, we can combine this model with other methods. There were plenty red blood cells in the thoracic duct of pigs [26]. In order to avoid removing too many RBCs from the animal by continuous sampling, a lymphatico-venous shunt can be performed to drain lymph back to the circulation, similar to those described previously [11, 27]. For some studies such as those on the pharmacokinetics of medicines, molecules i.e. exosomes [28, 29] and cytokines in the body fluids in which supernatants are the target samples, we can collect lymph using a three-way valve (stopcock) that links the catheters. By draining lymph back to the circulation and using three-way stopcocks to control lymph flow, it is possible to collect lymph samples at specific arranged time points. Using this strategy, lymph samples draining the tissues may be collected at multiple time points post-treatment from the same animal instead of euthanizing a sequence of animals to obtain the tissues at each single time point.

Considering the low numbers of white cells in the peripheral afferent and efferent lymph [10], the approach we developed will be more helpful in studying the changes of components in the supernatants of efferent lymph before and after treatments. The contaminations of lipids in the lymph samples should not hinder the detection of components such as ovalbumin in the lymph supernatants when suitable methods are applied to assaying the lymph samples. Ovalbumin that was delivered to the lungs of sheep could be detected in the lymph collected from the thoracic duct using protein-specific ELISA [16]. Other components such as nitric oxide (NO), RNA and DNA can be purified using the commercially available products, such as reversed phase C18 columns [30], SV Total RNA Isolation System (Promega) and TRIzol LS Reagent (Invitrogen) depending on the aims of the research. Methods such as PCR and next-generation sequencing technologies allowing single cell sequencing are useful and sensitive tools for analyzing samples with low quantity. These technologies now make it possible to detect more information from the limited numbers of efferent lymph cells, which responded to antigen stimulation in a way that is qualitatively similar to that in sheep but smaller in magnitude [10].

Conclusions

To obtain the kinetics of the components in the lymph would boost our understanding of the immunobiology of the draining tissues or pathobiology of the draining tissues in infections. Here, we provide a new approach to monitor the lymphatic kinetics of the thoracic duct in real-time in piglets. With further modifications of our method to achieve long-term lymph collections, we believe that this method will be a useful approach in investigating the processes of diseases such as that induced by PRRSV or *Mycoplasma hyopneumoniae* in pigs.

Abbreviations

PRRSV: Porcine reproductive and respiratory syndrome virus; RBCs: Red blood cells

Acknowledgements

The Early Career Researcher Grant, The University of Melbourne, supported this work. The authors thank Mr Bob Geyer and Ms Ai Fen Huan for their care of experimental animals and assistances in surgery. The authors also thank
Dr Wayne Kimpton for providing the surgical instruments and cannulas for this study.

Funding

The Early Career Researcher Grant, The University of Melbourne, supported this work.

Authors' contributions

HHY conceived of the method, developed the surgical procedures, conducted surgery, analysed the results, annotated the structures, drew the schematic pictures and drafted the manuscript. HD analysed and interpreted the results, annotated the structures and helped to draft the manuscript. Both authors read and approved the final manuscript.

Competing interests

The authors declare that they have no competing interests.

References

1. Van Reeth K. Avian and swine influenza viruses: our current understanding of the zoonotic risk. Vet Res. 2007;38(2):243–60.
2. Khan SU, Salje H, Hannan A, Islam MA, Bhuyan AA, Islam MA, Rahman MZ, Nahar N, Hossain MJ, Luby SP, et al. Dynamics of Japanese encephalitis virus transmission among pigs in Northwest Bangladesh and the potential impact of pig vaccination. PLoS Negl Trop Dis. 2014;8(9):e3166.
3. van-den-Hurk AF, Ritchie SA, Johansen CA, Mackenzie JS, Smith GA. Domestic pigs and Japanese encephalitis virus infection, Australia. Emerg Infect Dis. 2008;14(11):1736–8.
4. Meurens F, Summerfield A, Nauwynck H, Saif L, Gerdts V. The pig: a model for human infectious diseases. Trends Microbiol. 2012;20(1):50–7.
5. van der Laan JW, Herberts C, Lambkin-Williams R, Boyers A, Mann AJ, Oxford J. Animal models in influenza vaccine testing. Expert Rev Vaccines. 2008;7(6):783–93.
6. Itoh Y, Shinya K, Kiso M, Watanabe T, Sakoda Y, Hatta M, Muramoto Y, Tamura D, Sakai-Tagawa Y, Noda T, et al. In vitro and in vivo characterization of new swine-origin H1N1 influenza viruses. Nature. 2009;460(7258):1021–5.

7. Opriessnig T, Gimenez-Lirola LG, Halbur PG. Polymicrobial respiratory disease in pigs. Anim Health Res Rev. 2011;12(2):133–48.
8. Holtkamp D, Kliebenstein J, Neumann EJ, Zimmerman J, Rotto H, Oder T, Wang C, Yeske P, Mowrer C, Haley C. Assessment of the economic impact of porcine reproductive and respiratory syndrome virus on United States pork producers. J Swine Health Prod. 2013;21(2):72–84.
9. Pabst R, Binns RM. Heterogeneity of lymphocyte homing physiology: several mechanisms operate in the control of migration to lymphoid and non-lymphoid organs in vivo. Immunol Rev. 1989;108:83–109.
10. Binns RM. Pig lymphocytes - behaviour, distribution and classification. Monogr Allergy. 1980;16:19–37.
11. Chanoit G, Ferre PJ, Lefebvre HP. Chronic lymphatico-venous bypass: surgical technique and aftercare in a porcine model. Interact Cardiovasc Thorac Surg. 2007;6(6):705–7.
12. Jensen LT, Olesen HP, Risteli J, Lorenzen I. External thoracic duct-venous shunt in conscious pigs for long term studies of connective tissue metabolites in lymph. Lab Anim Sci. 1990;40(6):620–4.
13. Saar LI, Getty R. Porcine lymphatic system. In: Getty R, editor. Sisson and Grossman's the anatomy of the domestic animals, vol. 2. Philadelphia: W B Saunders Company; 1975. p. 1343–58.
14. Yen HH, Murray CM, Davies HMS. Anatomical basis for the development of a thoracic duct cannulation model without thoracotomy in Large White pigs. BMC Vet Res. 2015;11:109.
15. Kassai T, Shnain A, Kadhim J, Altaif K, Jabbir M. Collection of lymph from sheep by the cannulation of the thoracic duct and an application of the method in hosts infected with Dictyocaulus filaria. Magyar Allatorvosok Lapja. 1972;27:691–6 (in Hungarian).
16. Yen HH, Wee JL, Snibson KJ, Scheerlinck JP. Thoracic duct cannulation without thoracotomy in sheep: a method for accessing efferent lymph from the lung. Vet Immunol Immunopathol. 2009;129(1–2):76–81.
17. König HE, Liebich H-G. Veterinary anatomy of domestic mammals. Stuttgart: Schattauer; 2009.
18. Schummer A, Wilkens H, Vollmerhaus B, Habermehl K-H. The circulatory system, the skin, and the cutaneous organs of the domestic mammals / translation by Walter G. Siller and Peter A. L. Wight, vol. 3. Berlin: Verlag Paul Parey; 1981.
19. Dyce KM, Sack WO, Wensing CJG. Textbook of veterinary anatomy. 4th ed. St. Louis: Saunders/Elsevier; 2010.
20. Yen HH, Scheerlinck JP, Gekas S, Sutton P. A sheep cannulation model for evaluation of nasal vaccine delivery. Methods. 2006;38(2):117–23.
21. Schwartz-Cornil I, Epardaud M, Bonneau M. Cervical duct cannulation in sheep for collection of afferent lymph dendritic cells from head tissues. Nat Protoc. 2006;1(2):874–9.
22. Gomercic MD, Vukicevic TT, Gomercic T, Galov A, Fruk T, Gomercic H. The cisterna chyli and thoracic duct in pigs (Sus scrofa domestica). Vet Med. 2010;55(1):30–4.
23. Swindle MM. Swine in the laboratory: surgery, anesthesia, imaging, and experimental techniques. New York: CRC Press, Taylor & Francis Group; 2007.
24. Swindle MM, Wiest DB, Smith AC, Garner SS, Case CC, Thompson RP, Fyfe DA, Gillette PC. Fetal surgical protocols in Yucatan miniature swine. Lab Anim Sci. 1996;46(1):90–5.
25. Kronsteiner B, Bassaganya-Riera J, Philipson C, Viladomiu M, Carbo A, Pedragosa M, Vento S, Hontecillas R. Helicobacter pylori infection in a pig model is dominated by Th1 and cytotoxic CD8+ T cell responses. Infect Immun. 2013;81(10):3803–13.
26. Binns RM, Hall JG. The Paucity of lymphocytes in the Lymph of Unanaesthetised Pigs. Br J Exp Pathol. 1966;47(3):275–80.
27. Mendenhall HV, Horvath C, Piechowiak M, Johnson L, Bayer K. An external thoracic duct venous shunt to allow for long term collection of lymph and blood in the conscious pig in advances in Swine in Biomedical Research: Volume 2, edited by Mike E. Tumbleson, Lawrence B. Schook, vol. 2. Boston: Springer US; 1996.
28. Vlassov AV, Magdaleno S, Setterquist R, Conrad R. Exosomes: current knowledge of their composition, biological functions, and diagnostic and therapeutic potentials. Biochim Biophys Acta. 2012;1820(7):940–8.
29. Chen T, Xi QY, Ye RS, Cheng X, Qi QE, Wang SB, Shu G, Wang LN, Zhu XT, Jiang QY, et al. Exploration of microRNAs in porcine milk exosomes. BMC Genomics. 2014;15:100.
30. Wu A, Duan T, Tang D, Xu Y, Feng L, Zheng Z, Zhu J, Wang R, Zhu Q. Determination of nitric oxide-derived nitrite and nitrate in biological samples by HPLC coupled to nitrite oxidation. Chromatographia. 2013;76:1649–55.

15

Molecular typing of *Leptospira interrogans* serovar Hardjo isolates from leptospirosis outbreaks in Brazilian livestock

Maria Raquel V. Cosate[1*], Tetsu Sakamoto[1], Tiago Antônio de Oliveira Mendes[1], Élvio C. Moreira[3], Carlos G. Regis da Silva[2], Bruno S. A. F. Brasil[4], Camila S. F. Oliveira[3], Vasco Ariston de Azevedo[5], José Miguel Ortega[1], Rômulo C. Leite[3] and João Paulo Haddad[3]

Abstract

Background: Leptospirosis is caused by pathogenic spirochetes of the genus *Leptospira* spp. This zoonotic disease is distributed globally and affects domestic animals, including cattle. *Leptospira interrogans* serogroup Sejroe serovar Hardjo and *Leptospira borgpetersenii* serogroup Sejroe serovar Hardjo remain important species associated with this reproductive disease in livestock production. Previous studies on Brazilian livestock have reported that *L. interrogans* serovar Hardjo is the most prevalent leptospiral agent in this country and is related to clinical signs of leptospirosis, which lead to economic losses in production. Here, we described the isolation of three clinical strains (Norma, Lagoa and Bolivia) obtained from leptospirosis outbreaks that occurred in Minas Gerais state in 1994 and 2008.

Results: Serological and molecular typing using housekeeping (*secY* and 16SrRNA) and *rfb* locus (ORF22 and ORF36) genes were applied for the identification and comparative analysis of *Leptospira* spp. Our results identified the three isolates as *L. interrogans* serogroup Sejroe serovar Hardjo and confirmed the occurrence of this bacterial strain in Brazilian livestock. Genetic analysis using ORF22 and ORF36 grouped the *Leptospira* into serogroup Sejroe and subtype Hardjoprajitno. Genetic approaches were also applied to compare distinct serovars of *L. interrogans* strains by verifying the copy numbers of the IS1500 and IS1533 insertion sequences (ISs). The IS1500 copy number varied among the analyzed *L. interrogans* strains.

Conclusion: This study provides evidence that *L. interrogans* serogroup Sejroe serovar Hardjo subtype Hardjoprajitno causes bovine leptospirosis in Brazilian production. The molecular results suggested that *rfb* locus (ORF22 and ORF36) could improve epidemiological studies by allowing the identification of *Leptospira* spp. at the serogroup level. Additionally, the IS1500 and IS1533 IS copy number analysis suggested distinct genomic features among closely related leptospiral strains.

Background

Leptospirosis is one of the most significant bacterial zoonotic diseases. It is caused by pathogenic species of the genus *Leptospira* and results in high mortality and morbidity [1, 2]. Rodents are the main reservoirs of spirochetes, and different species can function as maintenance hosts. Humans are usually infected through contaminated water or direct contact with the infected urine or abortion fluids of rodents and livestock animals [3, 4]. The most prevalent subtypes in cattle herds are *Leptospira borgpetersenii* serovar Hardjo and *Leptospira interrogans* serovar Hardjo. Differences among these subtypes are related to the geographic areas of isolation, genomic patterns and pathogenic features [5]. Hardjoprajitno isolates have been described in Australia, the United States of America (USA), the United Kingdom, Mexico, and Canada [6]. In South America, this *Leptospira* subtype was first reported in Argentina [7], and serological analyses showed a high prevalence of serogroup Sejroe in livestock in Brazil [8].

The identification and characterization of new bacterial strains have enhanced epidemiological studies of disease and improved general knowledge of the isolates [4].

* Correspondence: raquelcosate@ymail.com
[1]Instituto de Ciências Biológicas, Departamento de Bioquímica e Imunologia, Universidade Federal de Minas Gerais, Belo Horizonte, MG, Brazil
Full list of author information is available at the end of the article

However, the *Leptospira* genus presents a different taxonomic classification among the bacterial phyla, with both its serological and genetic features useful for phylogenetic identification [9]. *Leptospira* spp. taxonomic classification involves genomic features and serological analyses and comprises approximately 300 serovars grouped into 24 serogroups and several species. In the clinical setting, microscopic agglutination testing (MAT) is the serologic method used for leptospirosis diagnosis. However, because this technique is difficult and laborious, new molecular approaches are relevant candidates for improvement of the classification of *Leptospira* species isolates in routine samples.

Bovine leptospirosis infections cause clinical conditions associated with reproductive failure, including abortion, mastitis and a reduction in milk production [10]. The pathogenic and clinical evolution of these infections could be associated with the *Leptospira* subtype [11]. Serological characteristics are based on differences in the structure of the exposed lipopolysaccharide (LPS), which is synthesized by proteins at the *rfb* locus [12–14]. This locus was first identified in the *L. interrogans* serovar Copenhageni [12]. Subsequent studies reported that *L. borgpetersenii* serovar Hardjo contained 32 open read frames (ORFs) and serovar Copenhageni contained 31 ORFs inside the *rfb* locus [13, 14]. An additional ORF found in *L. interrogans* serovar Hardjo was named ORF36 [15]. Previous analyses suggested that ORF1-ORF14 and ORF21-ORF22 of the *rfb* locus in *L. interrogans* serovar Hardjo were acquired by lateral gene transfer from *L. borgpetersenii* serovar Hardjo and that ORF15-ORF20 and ORF23-ORF31 were acquired by lateral gene transfer from *L. interrogans* serovar Copenhageni [15].

Different methodologies have been applied in *Leptospira* spp. genetic studies to improve the characterization of leptospirosis, including quantitative real-time PCR techniques, which have been used for diagnostic and taxonomic purposes and the comparative analysis of *Leptospira* strains for epidemiological studies [16, 17]. The determination of insertion sequences and copy numbers has also been used for molecular bacterial typing [18, 19, 20]. For instance, the IS1500 and IS1533 mobile elements, which are classified in the IS3-like and IS110 families, respectively, were more frequent in the genomes of the major pathogenic species *Leptospira interrogans* and *Leptospira borgpetersenii*, respectively [21–23].

In the present study, we describe three clinical strains of *Leptospira* spp. from two leptospirosis outbreaks in livestock that occurred in the state of Minas Gerais, Brazil, in 1994 and 2009. To identify the isolates, we performed MAT and applied genotyping approaches using housekeeping (*secY* and 16S rRNA) and *rfb* locus (ORF22 and ORF36) genes. Furthermore, real-time quantitative PCR was performed to compare the relative copy numbers of IS1500 and IS1533 among the clinical and reference leptospiral strains. Our data suggested that *rfb* loci (ORF22 and ORF36) could be useful for serovar and serogroup identification and that mobile elements might indicate differences among *Leptospira* strains.

Methods

Leptospira spp. reference strains

We used 14 *Leptospira* strains belonging to *Leptospira interrogans* and *Leptospira borgpetersenii* for the genotyping analysis (Table 1). The reference strains were obtained from the Pan American Health Organization, Argentina and the Royal Tropical Institute, the Netherland, Holland, Amsterdam. The *Leptospira* spp. were cultured in liquid Ellinghausen and McCullough (EMJH) medium modified under aerobic conditions at 28 °C in the absence of light [9].

Epidemiological characterization of leptospirosis outbreaks

Blood and urine were collected from 316 and 326 animals, respectively, from two dairy farms in the state of Minas Gerais, Brazil, where leptospirosis outbreaks in livestock occurred in May 1994 and May 2009. All of the selected animals presented clinical signs compatible with leptospirosis, such as abortions, reduction in milk production and stillbirths [10]. The collected blood samples were submitted to MAT [24]. We collected the urine of MAT-positive animals to proceed with *Leptospira* isolation.

Microscopic agglutination test (MAT)

To confirm the leptospirosis diagnosis, MAT was used to detect antibodies to *Leptospira* according to the method of Faine et al. [9]. MAT was also used for serological bacterial typing of isolates according to the Leptospirosis Reference Centre (KIT, the Netherlands). Live cultures of 13 *Leptospira* spp. reference strains representing eight *L. interrogans* serogroups and four *L. borgpetersenii* serogroups (sensu *lato* qualification) were used (Additional file 1). The sera were screened at 1:100 dilutions and further diluted on a two-fold basis to determine the final titer. *Leptospira* spp. interpretation based on the MAT was performed by the identification of an agglutination index ≥50% per microscopic field at a given dilution, which was considered a positive reaction.

Leptospira spp. isolation procedure

Ten-fold serial dilutions of urine samples directly obtained from MAT-positive farm animals were inoculated into tubes containing 5 ml of EMJH medium supplemented with 10% bovine serum albumin and 5% rabbit

Table 1 List of *Leptospira* spp. reference strains

Species	Serogroup	Serovar	Strain
L. interrogans	Canicola	Canicola	Hond Utrecht IV
	Pomona	Pomona	Pomona
	Icterohaemorrhagiae	Lai	Lai
	Icterohaemorrhagiae	Copenhageni	M-20
	Bataviae	Bataviae	Van Tienen
	Sejroe	Hardjo	Hardjoprajitno (OMS)
	Hebdomadis	Hebdomadis	Hebdomadis
	Australis	Bratislava	Jez Bratislava
	Sejroe	Wolffi	Wolffi
L. borgpetersenii	Tarassovi	Tarassovi	Perepelicin
	Mini	Mini	Sari
	Sejroe	Sejroe	M-84
	Sejroe	Hardjo	Hardjobovis-Sponselee
	Mini	Swazizak	Swajizak

serum. The cultures were incubated at 28 °C and examined weekly for 10 weeks using dark-field microscope [9]. Five hamsters were inoculated intraperitoneally with 500 μl of positive culture. Their kidneys were obtained 21 days after inoculation and cultured in EMJH medium [9]. Clinical isolates were typed with the monoclonal antibodies (mABs) F16C28 and F106C1, which were specific for serogroup Sejroe and serovar Mini, respectively, in the agglutination reaction. The monoclonal antibodies were produced and screened at the Royal Tropical Institute (KIT), Amsterdam, the Netherlands.

DNA isolation, conventional PCR and gene sequencing

A total of 10^6 cells were collected by centrifugation at 13,000 g and incubated overnight at 50 °C in 200 μl of lysis buffer (50 mM Tris/HCl, pH 8.0, 50 mM EDTA, 100 mM NaCl, and 1% SDS) containing 100 μg/ml proteinase K. Genomic DNA was extracted by the phenol/chloroform method and precipitated with ethanol [25].

PCR was performed with a total volume of 25 μl, including 200 μM dNTPs, 1.5 mM $MgCl_2$, 10 mM KCl, 10 mM Tris-HCl, 10 pM of each primer, 20 ng of genomic DNA and 500 U of Taq polymerase. The primer sequences and the expected product sizes are shown in Table 2. The reaction mixtures were subjected to the following amplification protocol for all of the genes analyzed: 3 min at 95 °C, followed by 29 cycles consisting of 95 °C for 1 min, a target-specific annealing temperature for 1 min and 72 °C for 1 min, and a final extension at 72 °C for 10 min (Table 2). The PCR products were analyzed by 1% agarose gel electrophoresis and stained with ethidium bromide. The PCR products were sequenced

Table 2 List of primers used for PCR detection, sequencing and qRT-PCR assays

Gene target	Sequence (5'-3')	Melting temp. (°C)	Amplicon length (bp)
16S rDNA	F: ACT AAC GCT GGC GGC GCG R: TAC CCA CGC TTT CGT GCC	56	1500
secY (1)	F: GCG ATT CAG TTT AAT CCT G R: GCG ATT CAG TTT AAT CCT GC	58	245
ORF22	F: ATT ATT GAG ACA GAG ATA R: AAG CGG AAC GGG ACG AAT	56	561
ORF36	F: AGT CGG GGT TCG ATA CTG R: GGT CAG TCC TGT AAC TGC	54	489
IS1500[a]	F: TAC GGA GCA AGA ACG GTT R: AGA TCC GAT TCT TAT GAT TC	56	143
IS1533[a]	F: TTG TAA TCC CTG TGT TGT TT R: TTA AAT AGT CCA CTC CTC G	56	130
secY (2)[a]	F: CTG AAT CGC TGT ATA AAA GT R: GAA GGC TGG TAA ACA AAA G	58	130

[a]for qRT-PCR

using a BigDye 3.1 Terminator Sequencing Kit (Applied Biosystems) and an ABI Prism 3130 automated sequencer [26].

Real-time PCR

Real-time PCR was performed in a total volume of 20 μl containing 50 ng of *Leptospira* spp. genomic DNA, 250 nM each of the forward and reverse primers, and 10 μl of 2× SYBR Green Master Mix (Applied Biosystems). The primer sequences and melting temperatures are described in Table 2. All of the reactions were performed in triplicate and were run on an ABI/PRISM 7500 Fast Sequence Detection System (Applied Biosystems) under the following conditions: 98 °C for 2 min, followed by 40 cycles of denaturation at 95 °C for 15 s and annealing/elongation for 15 s at 56 °C. DNA sequencing of the PCR products confirmed their specificity. The relative quantification of the IS1500 and IS1533 copy numbers was calculated by the $2^{-\Delta\Delta Ct}$ method [26] using the *secY* gene as the endogenous control [16]. The reference strain *L. interrogans* serovar Lai was used as the calibrator strain for the quantification of both IS1500 and IS1533. A BLAST search using each primer pair was performed to determine the number of amplifiable regions in the genome. In this analysis, we determined the presence of seven and two regions amplifiable by the primer pairs designed for IS1500 and IS1533, respectively.

Molecular phylogenetic analysis

Homologous sequences of each genomic region of interest in other *Leptospira* spp. were retrieved from the GenBank database through a BLAST search [27]. This search was performed on the NCBI web server (http://blast.ncbi.nlm.nih.gov/Blast.cgi) by submitting the nucleotide sequences obtained from our isolates as queries against the refseq_genomic and refseq_rna databases. The search was conducted in October 2015. Then, we manually selected representative *Leptospira* species and serovar sequences (Additional files 2 and 3, according to the specific genomic region analyzed) from the BLAST results and conducted the phylogenetic analysis. The selected sequences together with the sequences obtained in this work were aligned using MUSCLE [28] implemented in MEGA 6 [29]. All of the phylogenetic trees in this work were inferred by the neighbor-joining method (model: maximum composite likelihood; bootstrap replications: 1000) implemented in MEGA 6 [29] and visualized using FigTree [http://tree.bio.ed.ac.uk/software/figtree/].

Results

Leptospirosis outbreaks from Minas Gerais were mainly caused by serovar Hardjo subtype Hardjoprajitno

The evaluation of the two leptospirosis outbreaks was performed using serological MAT to identify the prevalent *Leptospira* serogroups. A total of 132 out of 316 bovine serum samples from the first outbreak (41.8%) and 125 out of 258 samples from the second outbreak were MAT positive. Serovar Hardjo (Hardjoprajitno) showed a high positive reaction frequency [132 samples (41.8% of the positive samples) from the first outbreak and 125 samples (48.4% of the positive samples) from the second outbreak, followed by Wolffi (38.6–33.7%), Bratislava (35.1–33.7%) and Bataviae (21.8–24%). A small number of samples from the two leptospirosis outbreak reacted with serovars Canicola (two samples), Hebdomadis (five samples), Pyrogens (one sample) and Pomona (one sample). Analysis of the antibody titers showed that the highest titers at both farms were observed with serovar Hardjo (Additional file 1).

We isolated one *Leptospira* strain from the urine samples of seropositive animals from the first outbreak, which was referred to as "Norma", and two strains from the second outbreak, which were referred to as "Lagoa" and "Bolivia". The serological identification of these clinical isolates was assessed using two monoclonal antibodies (mAB) (F16C28 and F106C9, provided by the Royal Tropical Institute, Amsterdam, the Netherlands). For these analyses, MAT was applied to evaluate the agglutination titers of the monoclonal antibodies and clinical samples. The mAB F16C28 could distinguish *Leptospira* from serogroup Sejroe serovar Sejroe from *Leptospira* from serogroup Sejroe serovar Hardjo. The expected agglutination titer for serovar Sejroe was 80 and for serovar Hardjo was greater than 80 [30]. In contrast, mAB F106C9 showed a positive agglutination titer only for serovar Mini. The antibody analysis for all three isolates showed agglutination titers of 200 with mAB F16C28 and negative agglutination with mAB F106C9. These results indicated that Norma, Bolivia and Lagoa belonged to serogroup Sejroe serovar Hardjo.

Phylogenetic analysis of the 16S rDNA and *secY* gene sequences

Because serovar Hardjo was encountered in three *Leptospira* species (*L. interrogans*, *L. borgpetersenii* and *L. meyeri*), we sequenced the 16S rDNA and *secY* gene genomic regions of our isolates (Norma, Lagoa and Bolivia) and applied phylogenetic methods for each genomic region to classify them taxonomically into one of these species. The sequences obtained from our isolates were identical to one another in both cases (16S rDNA and *secY*); thus, we sampled these sequences as one sample (Norma/Lagoa/Bolivia) in our phylogenetic analysis. In both phylogenetic trees (inferred by the neighbor-joining method; bootstrap: 10,000; model: maximum composite likelihood) generated using the 16S rDNA and *secY* sequences, all of the clinical isolates clustered together and were classified as *L. interrogans* (Fig. 1). In the 16S

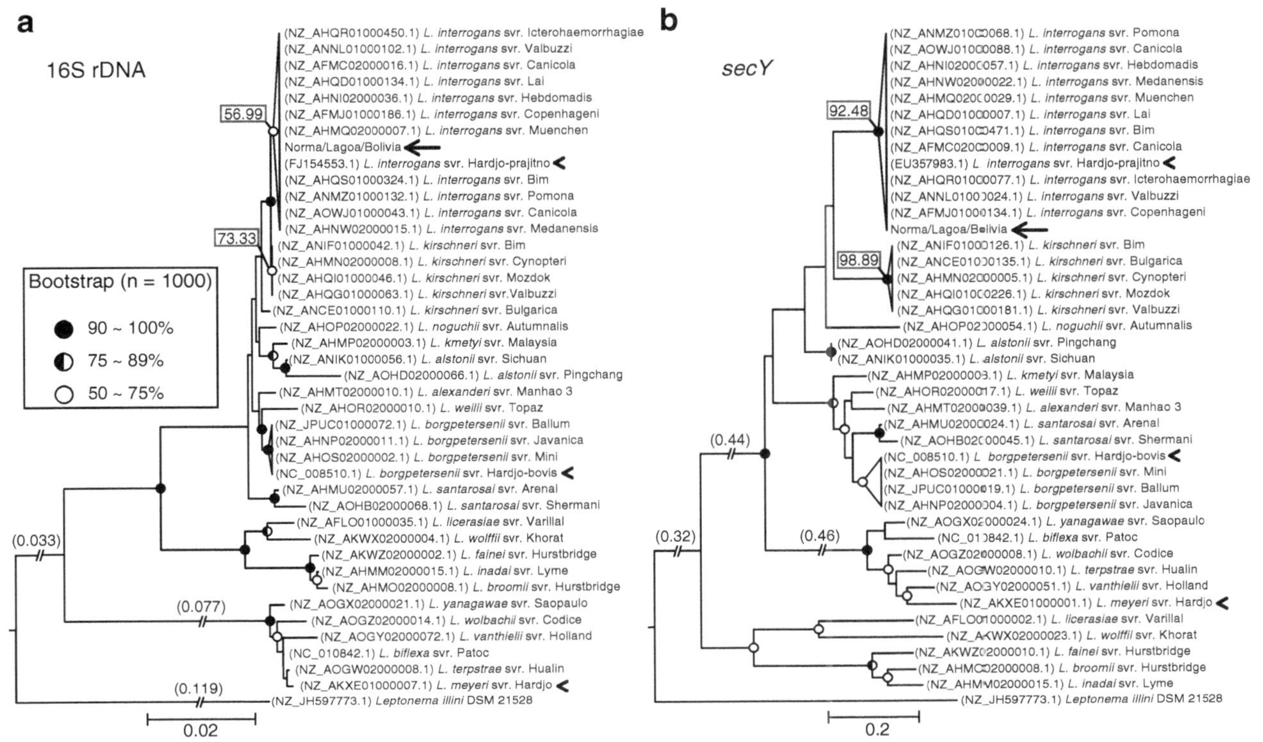

Fig. 1 Phylogenetic trees of *Leptospira* spp. using (**a**) 16S rDNA and (**b**) *secY* sequences. The nucleotide sequences were aligned using Muscle, and the trees were generated using the neighbor-joining method (bootstrap: 1.000, model maximum composite l kelihood). The clinical isolates from this work are indicated with *arrows*. *Leptospira* strains of the Hardjo serovar are indicated with *arrowheads*. *Circles* at nodes reflect the bootstrap support. An ancestral node without a circle indicates a bootstrap value below 50%. The bootstrap values of the nodes that group *L. interrogans* or *L. kirschneri* are located on these nodes in *rectangles*. Long branches are broken, and the real lengths are displayed on these branches in *parenthesis*. In both trees, orthologous sequences from *Leptonema illini* DSM 21528 were used as the outgroup

rDNA analysis, the cluster formed by *L. interrogans* serovars was supported by a low bootstrap value (56.99%) due to the high sequence similarity between the *L. interrogans* and *L. kirschneri* samples (90%–100%). In contrast, the phylogenetic analysis of the *secY* gene showed well-supported branches clustering both *L. interrogans* (bootstrap value: 92.48%) and *L. kirschneri* (bootstrap value: 98.89%) species, as shown in Fig. 1. Furthermore, the other *Leptospira* species of serovar Hardjo included in the analysis clustered together with their respective species in both phylogenetic trees. These results allowed us to identify our three isolates (Norma, Lagoa and Bolivia) as belonging to the *L. interrogans* species.

Occurrence and molecular evolution of ORF22 and ORF36 of the *rfb* locus in *Leptospira* spp.

The *rfb* locus is largely used for the identification of different *Leptospira* serogroups. The ORF22 sequences of the *Leptospira* species of serovar Hardjo were highly similar to one another, whereas ORF36 was specific to *L. interrogans* serovar Hardjo [15]. To further classify our clinical isolates taxonomically, these ORFs were amplified by PCR. Reference strains of the *L. interrogans* and *L. borgpetersenii* species (Additional file 2) were used as the controls.

For ORF22, PCR amplification with the primers Orf22–1 and Orf22–2 (Table 1) produced a primary 561-bp PCR product in samples with the genomic material of the *L. interrogans* serovars Hardjo, Hebdomadis, and Mini, the *L. borgpetersenii* serovar Tarassovi and the Hardjo strain Sponselee (Fig 2a). Following the PCR amplification assay, the full-length ORF22 from all of the positive amplicons was sequenced. By retrieving orthologs of ORF22 from other *Leptospira* strains from the GenBank database, we observed that almost all of the *L. interrogans* strains in the database had ORF22 in their genomes. Nevertheless, the phylogenetic analysis demonstrated that some ORF22 sequences from *L. interrogans* strains clustered together with the ORF22 sequences from *L. borgpetersenii*, indicating that an ORF22 replacement event occurred in these *L. interrogans* strains (Fig. 2b). The clinical isolates (Norma/Lagoa/Bolivia), *L. interrogans* strain Brem 329 (NZ AKXA02000046.1) and serovars Bataviae (NZ AHQV01000071.1), Hebdomadis (NZ AHNI02000062.1) and Medanensis (NZ AHNW02000148.1) are examples of *L.*

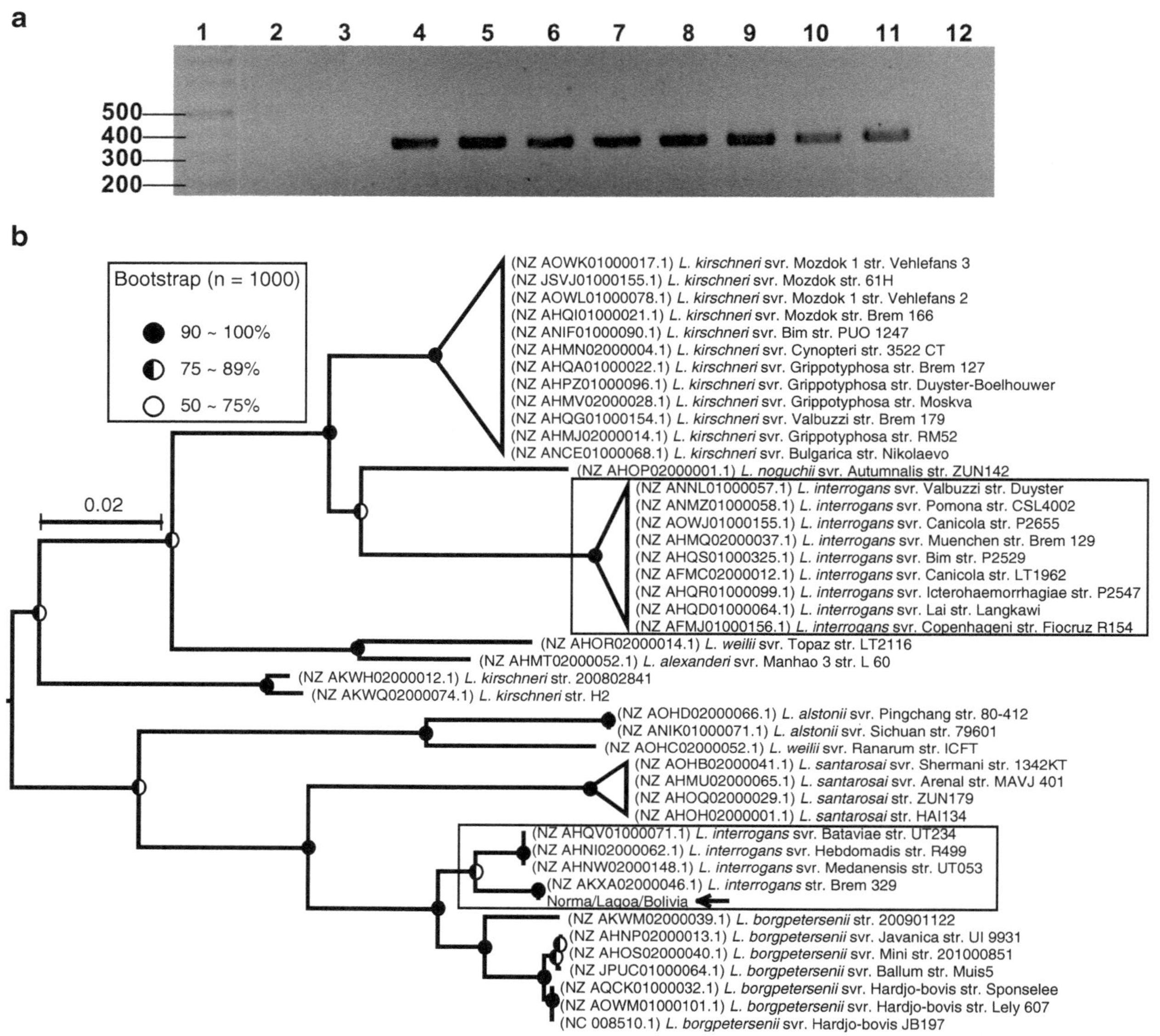

Fig. 2 **a** PCR detection in *Leptospira* isolates and reference strains and (**b**) phylogenetic analysis of ORF22. The lanes in the gel (**a**) correspond to (1) molecular size marker, (2) svr. Lai, (3) svr. Copenhageni, (4) svr. Hardjo (OMS), (5) isolate Norma, (6) isolate Lagoa, (7) isolate Bolivia, (8) svr. Tarassovi, (9) svr. Mini, (10) svr. Hebdomadis, (11) svr. Sponselee and (12) negative control. The phylogenetic tree (**b**) was inferred using the neighbor-joining method (bootstrap: 1000, model: maximum composite likelihood) and rooted in the midpoint. The ORF22 sequences of the *L. interrogans* strains are separated into two clusters (*gray rectangle*). The *L. kirschneri* strains are separated into two clusters, and *L. borgpetersenii* is shown in one cluster. Samples representing our clinical isolates are indicated with *arrows*. *Circles* at nodes reflect the bootstrap support

interrogans strains that contained ORF22 substitutions. Our data also showed two clades for the *L. kirschneri* bacterial strains, which suggested that this ORF had great potential for leptospiral molecular typing. The bootstrap values supporting the clade information from our clinical isolates and the retrieved sequences are shown in Fig. 2b.

The occurrence of ORF36 in our isolates and the reference *Leptospira* strains was also characterized by PCR amplification and partial sequencing using the primer pair Orf36–1 and Orf36–2 (Table 2). In this case, positive amplification was observed only in the clinical isolates Norma, Bolivia and Lagoa and the reference strain OMS, which belonged to *L. interrogans* serogroup Sejroe serovar Hardjo (Fig. 3a). DNA sequencing and a BLAST search for similar sequences in the refseq genomic database also indicated the specificity of ORF36 to the Hardjoprajitno subtype. The BLAST search retrieved a single genome accession with high identity (96%) from *L. interrogans* strain Brem 329 (NZ_AKXA02000046.1).

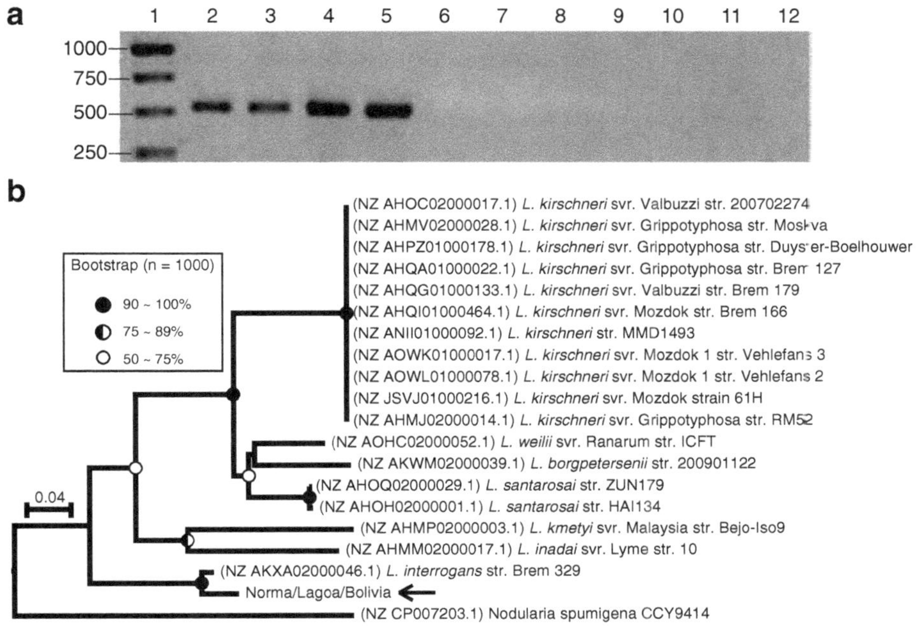

Fig. 3 a PCR detection in *Leptospira* isolates and reference strains and (**b**) phylogenetic analysis of ORF36. The lanes in the gel (**a**) correspond to (1) molecular size marker, (2) svr. Hardjo (OMS), (3) isolate Norma, (4) isolate Lagoa, (5) isolate Bolivia, (6) svr. Lai, (7) svr. Copenhageni, (8) svr. Mini, (9) svr. Hebdomadis, (10) svr. Tarassovi, (11) svr. Sponselee and (12) negative control. The phylogenetic tree (**b**) was inferred using the neighbor-joining method (bootstrap: 1000, model: maximum composite likelihood) and rooted in the midpoint. Samples representing our clinical isolates are indicated with *arrows*. *Circles* at the nodes reflect the bootstrap support. An ancestral node without a *circle* indicates a bootstrap value below 50%

The other *Leptospira* genome accessions retrieved by the BLAST algorithm were from *L. borgpetersenii* (one sample), *L. kirschneri* (ten samples), *L. weilii* (1 sample), *L. santarosai* (two samples), *L. inadai* (one sample) and *L. kmetyi* (one sample), but their identities with the query were 74% (Fig. 3b). Despite the phylogenetic proximity of the *L. interrogans* and *L. kirschneri* species demonstrated in the 16S rDNA and *secY* gene sequences by the phylogenetic analysis (Fig. 1), the tree topology generated from ORF36 split the sequences from *L. interrogans* close to the root instead of clustering them together with the sequences from *L. kirschneri*. This finding could be an indication of gene acquisition by lateral gene transfer in these *L. interrogans* strains. However, we could also hypothesize that ORF36 underwent several mutation events and acquired a novel function while other *L. interrogans* strains lost this ORF.

The accession numbers of the sequences, the alignment positions and the predicted sequence information are shown in Additional file 2. All of the sequenced nucleotide sequences cited here were submitted to the GenBank database under accession numbers JQ765 630.1-JQ765634 for 16S rRNA, KU2167449-KU216751/ FJ667608 for *secY*, JQ965147- JQ965150 for ORF22 and JQ765636- JQ765639.1 for ORF36.

Insertion sequence copy numbers in *Leptospira interrogans* serovars

Studies of IS1500 and IS1533 using the hybridization technique have suggested that the copy numbers of these mobile elements can be used as a tool for epidemiological purposes in strains classified as *L. interrogans* and *L. borgpetersenii*, respectively [31, 32]. In this study, we used quantitative real-time PCR to estimate and compare the copy numbers of the IS1500 and IS1533 insertion sequences in the *L. interrogans* strains classified as serovar Hardjo to enhance the molecular characterization of these clinical isolates. For copy number calibration, we used the *L. interrogans* serovar Lai strain 56,601 genome (NC_004342) and determined the number of amplifiable regions for each primer pair via sequence similarity analysis using the BLAST algorithm. These analyses determined that serovar Lai had seven and two amplifiable regions in its genome using the primer pairs for IS1500 and IS1533, respectively (Additional file 3).

For IS1500, *Leptospira* strains belonging to serogroup Sejroe (Norma, Lagoa, Bolivia, reference strain OMS and Wolffi) showed higher copy numbers (from ten to 28 copies) than the other two serogroups [Icterohaemorrhagiae (serovars Lai and Copenhageni) and Pomona]. In serogroup Sejroe, strains belonging to serovar Hardjo

(Norma, Lagoa, Bolivia and OMS) showed large variations in their copy numbers (Fig. 4). Our results determined the existence of at least ten copies for strain Norma, 28 for strain Bolivia, 18 for strain Lagoa and 20 for reference strain OMS. The sample from serovar Wolffi showed a copy number comparable to the Lagoa strain, with 16 copies. In the other *L. interrogans* isolates, we identified 7 copies in the Copenhageni strain and 6 copies in the Pomona strain (Fig. 4).

In contrast to IS1500, the IS1533 mobile element analysis demonstrated little variation in the copy numbers. In serovar Hardjo, at least three copies were present in Bolivia and two copies in Lagoa, Norma and the reference strain OMS. Of the other *L. interrogans* strains, at least three copies were present in serovar Wolffi, one copy in serovar Copenhageni and no copies in serovar Pomona. The standard deviation represented the Ct value analysis from three independent experiments, as show in Fig. 4.

To check the consistency of our results, we also retrieved the genome sequence of *L. interrogans* serovar Copenhageni from the GenBank database (NC_005823.1) and verified whether the copy number obtained by each primer pair determined by real-time PCR in this serovar matched the number of amplifiable regions determined in silico by the BLAST search. We identified seven amplifiable regions using the IS1500 primer pair as the queries and a single amplifiable region using the IS1533 primer pair as the queries (Additional file 3). These results corroborated the results obtained from the real-time PCR analysis.

Discussion

MAT is considered the standard serological test for leptospirosis diagnosis, but cross-reactivity frequently occurs, which raises questions concerning correct serovar identification [22]. Although the isolation of *Leptospira* spp. from infected animals or patients and molecular characterization are accurate diagnostic procedures for the taxonomic and serovar identification of a *Leptospira* strain, these procedures are laborious and expensive.

Another issue with leptospirosis serovars is that their classification based on genomic regions often does not correspond to their classification based on serological analysis [2]. This lack of correspondence prevents serological correlations because the genomic regions selected for the analysis represent ribosomal regions and housekeeping genes. To overcome this limitation, approaches based on molecular biology techniques, including restriction fragment length polymorphism (RFLP) analysis [33] and multiple locus sequence typing (MLST;[34]), have been proposed to render the serovar identification procedure more rapid and less expensive. Additionally, PCR-based approaches using variable number tandem repeats (VNTR; [35]) and the *rfb* locus [36] have demonstrated promise in distinguishing *Leptospira* serovars. Here, we characterized two leptospirosis outbreaks at dairy farms in the state of Minas Gerais, Brazil, using a conventional serological analysis (MAT) in combination with molecular biology approaches.

Serological analysis using MAT in a total of 642 animals from two dairy farms in the state of Minas Gerais determined that approximately half of the animals were seropositive and that Hardjo was the prevalent serovar. We also observed cross-reactivity between the Hardjo and Wolffi serovars, which could be explained by both serovars belonging to the Sejroe serogroup [37]. Previous bovine leptospirosis epidemiological studies of livestock

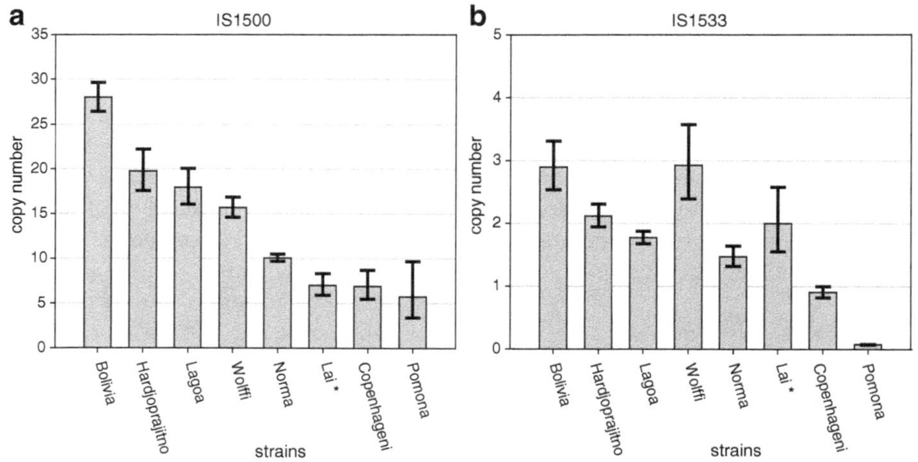

Fig. 4 Copy number quantification of (**a**) IS1500 and (**b**) IS1533 by qRT-PCR in the *Leptospira* isolate and reference strain genomes. *Bars* represent the mean values of three replicates (±SD). IS copy number inference in other *Leptospira* spp. samples was performed using *secY* as the endogenous control and svr. Lai as the calibrator (*asterisk*)

from different Brazilian regions have also shown the seroprevalence of the Hardjo serovar [38, 39], demonstrating a high incidence of this serovar in leptospirosis outbreaks in Brazil.

The three clinical isolates obtained in this work (Norma, Lagoa and Bolivia) were classified as the Sejroe serogroup by the monoclonal antibody analysis and as *L. interrogans* species by the phylogenetic analysis of the 16S rDNA and *secY* gene sequences. We also achieved a more detailed taxonomic classification by analyzing ORF22 and ORF36 of the *rfb* locus. All of the clinical isolates contained an ORF22 with high similarity to the reference strain Hardjoprajitno and positive amplification of ORF36, which is a specific ORF encountered in *L. interrogans* serovar Hardjo. Due to the high specificity of these molecular markers for subtype Hardjoprajitno, we classified all of the clinical isolates as belonging to *Leptospira interrogans* serogroup Sejroe serovar Hardjo based on the serological and molecular data.

The *rfb* locus was previously described in different works as a genomic region acquired by *Leptospira* spp. from lateral gene transfer. Thus, we presume that differences can occur among bacterial strains, especially in microorganisms isolated from different geographical areas and from different hosts.

Previous studies have described sequence dissimilarities in some ORFs of the *rfb* locus between *L. interrogans* serovar Copenhageni and *L. interrogans* serovar Hardjo, including ORF22 and ORF36 [14, 15]. In the PCR analysis, amplification using our primers for ORF22 was observed in serovars classified in the serogroups Sejroe, Hebdomadis, Mini and Tarassovi. Conversely, the Lai, Copenhageni and Canicola serovars were negative in this analysis. Using sequencing and phylogenetic methods, we observed that the PCR-positive serovars were clustered in a branch with the *L. interrogans* and *L. borgpetersenii* species. Although the Lai, Copenhageni and Canicola serovars were PCR-negative for our primers, ORF22 was present in their genomes and clustered in another branch with only the *L. interrogans* species (Fig. 2b). The tree topology clearly demonstrated a lateral gene transfer event in which the ORF from *L. borgpetersenii* replaced the ORF22 of some *L. interrogans* species. The phylogenetic tree also showed a close relationship between the ORF22 sequences from our isolates from serogroup Sejroe serovar Medanensi and the Hebdomadis and Mini serogroups. Historically, the Hebdomadis, Mini and Sejroe serogroups belonged to the same serogroup (Hebdomadis) and displayed a similar antigenic profile [40]. Our data from the ORF22 analysis were in disagreement with previous studies related to the *rfb* locus in *L. interrogans* serovar Hardjo because our isolates were similar to *L. interrogans* serovar Hebdomadis. This finding suggested that ORF22 might play an important role in shaping the antigenic profiles of these serogroups because they had the same origin.

ORF36 was previously described as an extra ORF present in *L. interrogans* serovar Hardjo [15]. PCR analysis of this ORF demonstrated positive amplification only in the *L. interrogans* serovar Hardjo reference strain and our clinical isolates (Norma, Bolivia and Lagoa), as show in Fig. 3a. To evaluate the distribution of the ORF36 sequence throughout the available *Leptospira* genomes, we queried this ORF against the NCBI genome database. This query retrieved a single strain of the *L. interrogans* species with high similarity (Brem 329) and other *Leptospira* species with low similarity, including *L. borgpetersenii*, *L. kirschneri*, *L. weilii*, *L. santarosai*, *L. inadai* and *L. kmetyi* (Fig. 3b). In the phylogenetic analysis, the tree topology generated by the ORF36 sequences was contrasted with the topologies generated by the 16S rDNA and *secY* sequences when we compared the closeness between the *L. interrogans* and *L. kirschneri* samples, which again suggested an evolutionary event that escaped the neutral models. ORF36 was likely deleted early in the *L. interrogans* lineage and was acquired later by horizontal gene transfer in some species. We could also hypothesize that this ORF was subfunctionalized and deleted in almost all of the *L. interrogans* serovars, whereas the other serovars neofunctionalized ORF36 and maintained it in their genomes. Here, our analyses are in agreement with previous discussions of the *rfb* locus and indicate that this ORF may be unique to *L. interrogans* serovar Hardjo strains. We also emphasize the high similarity between the ORF22 and ORF36 sequences of our clinical isolates and *L. interrogans* strain Brem 329. The latter strain was isolated in Germany from horses and was classified in the Sejroe serogroup but had no serovar classification. Based on our analysis, we suggest that strain Brem 329 also belongs to the Hardjo serovar, but this suggestion requires serological analysis for confirmation. Here, we designed primers to search for the genomic regions described in a previous work [14] that discussed *L. interrogans* serovar Hardjo and showed that this bacterial type had the *rfb* locus obtained from *L. interrogans* serovar Copenhageni and *L. borgpetersenii* serovar Hardjobovis. In this work, we searched for this information in our isolates because a comparison of bacterial strains obtained from different geographic regions worldwide could reveal different genomics features. We designed primers for these regions, sequenced these specific regions and compared the sequences with the available data. Our analysis showed that ORF22 in our isolates was similar to ORF22 in *L. interrogans* serovar Hebdomadis, which differed from the data described by De La Peña et al., and that ORF36 could be found in other *L. interrogans* serovars. Previous works related to the *rfb* locus theme mentioned that this genomic region was acquired from bacteria classified in this genus. Based on these statements, we attempted to verify the presence of these genes in our isolates.

Next, we performed an IS analysis of the *Leptospira* reference strains and our samples. In this bacterial phylum, mobile elements represent an important region that is directly involved in genomic diversity among microorganisms [41, 42]. Moreover, information about IS copy numbers in the genome has been demonstrated to be useful in epidemiological studies of the *Leptospira* genus [26, 31, 43]. We found considerable variation in the copy numbers among the serovars and even among isolates of the same serovar, which allowed us to identify each strain by the IS copy number profile [21, 31, 32, 44]. One methodology used to determine the IS copy number is Southern blotting using IS fragments as probes [21, 31, 32]. Here, we recommend quantitative real-time PCR as an alternative to determine the copy number of a mobile element with greater precision. We selected the insertion sequences IS1500 and IS1533, which are used for the taxonomic and serovar classification of *L. interrogans* and *L. borgpetersenii*, respectively [31, 32]. The copy number estimations determined here were shown to be consistent, with the number determined in the Copenhageni strain almost the same as the number determined by the in silico analysis using the genome sequence of this strain.

The quantitative PCR assays for IS1500 demonstrated significant copy number variation among the *L. interrogans* serovars (copy number range: 6 to 28) and even among our clinical isolates (copy number range: 10 to 28). From these results, we classified the samples containing more IS1500 copies as belonging to the Sejroe serogroup and the samples with seven or six copies as belonging to the Icterohaemorrhagiae or Pomona serogroups. Experiments with more samples are needed to determine how well the quantification of IS1500 can distinguish among *L. interrogans* serovars or serogroups, but the large variation in the IS1500 copy number and good precision of the method in determining the copy number are indicative of its potential for epidemiological studies. IS1533 is well distributed in the *L. borgpetersenii* genome and can reach almost one hundred copies; in contrast, this mobile element is present in *L. interrogans* at a low copy number, as indicated in previous studies. Our results showed a low number and variation of IS1533 among the sampled *L. interrogans* serovars (copy number range: 0 to 4), suggesting that the transference and recombination of genetic material between the two species occurred in punctual regions of the *L. interrogans* genome and might not have interfered with its IS1533 copy number. Moreover, the difference in the IS contents of the Lagoa and Bolivia strains isolated at the same time represent clear genetic variability that suggests the co-circulation of different strains during an outbreak.

Leptospira spp. identification is an essential procedure to aid in the selection of the best means to control the disease. In this work, we endorse the importance of molecular characterization for the identification of *Leptospira* spp. by analyzing ORF22 and ORF36 from the *rfb* locus and the copy numbers of mobile elements (IS1500 and IS1533). Phylogenetic analysis based on *rfb* locus genes suggested the great potential of this region for the generation of taxonomic information. IS analysis also helps address other questions concerning the genomic organization of *Leptospira* strains because differences in copy numbers may be associated with genetic rearrangements and pseudo-gene formation. Finally, we succeeded in isolating three *Leptospira* samples from livestock from the state of Minas Gerais, Brazil, which were classified as *L. interrogans* serogroup Sejroe serovar Hardjo. Therefore, this study enhanced epidemiological research and suggested different vaccine formulations to contribute to bovine leptospirosis control in this endemic region. Research to analyze distinct genomic features among *Leptospira* spp. using molecular approaches and bioinformatics studies should be undertaken to improve our knowledge of their pathogenicity, evolution and epidemiology.

Conclusion

The present study described the occurrence of *L. interrogans* serovar Hardjo subtype Hardjoprajitno in livestock production through the isolation of bacterial strains. Partial genetic analysis using *rfb* locus genes (ORF22 and ORF36) suggested that these genes could be useful for taxonomic studies. Genetic comparative analyses among *Leptospira* spp. propose differences among clinical strains, which may contribute to new studies within these microorganisms. Moreover, this work may improve knowledge about the most prevalent serovar in Brazilian herds of cattle. An efficient vaccine should contain local isolates, and periodic molecular analysis of circulating isolates may contribute to the identification of important genetic variants that should be included in new vaccine formulations for leptospirosis control.

Acknowledgments

The Escola de Veterinária- Universidade Federal de Minas Gerais is acknowledged for the manufacture and supply of the *Leptospira* spp. culture and the technical help of Antonio Benjamin. This work was funded by Conselho Nacional de Desenvolvimento Científico e Tecnológico (CNPq), FAPEMIG, CAPES.

Funding

This study was supported by Conselho Nacional de Desenvolvimento Científico e Tecnológico (CNPq) and Instituto Nacional de Ciência e Tecnologia (INCT) de Informação Genético-Sanitária da Pecuária Brasileira.

Authors' contributions

All authors read and approved the final manuscript. Conceived and designed the experiments: MRVC, ECM, CGRS, BSAF, and JPH. Performed the experiments: MRVC, CGRS, BSAF, and CSFO. Analyzed the data: MRVC, TAOM,

CGRS, TS, BSAF, and JPH. Contributed reagents/materials/analysis tools: JMO, RCL, and JPH. Wrote the paper: MRVC, TAOM, TS, CGRS, VACA and JPH.

Competing interests
The authors declare that they have no competing interests.

Consent for publication
Not applicable.

Author details
[1]Instituto de Ciências Biológicas, Departamento de Bioquímica e Imunologia, Universidade Federal de Minas Gerais, Belo Horizonte, MG, Brazil. [2]Laboratório de Biologia Parasitária, Centro de Pesquisas Gonçalo Moniz-Fiocruz, Salvador, BA, Brazil. [3]Departamento de Medicina Veterinária Preventiva, Escola de Veterinária, Universidade Federal de Minas Gerais, Belo Horizonte, MG, Brazil. [4]Embrapa Agroenergia, Brasília, Brazil. [5]Universidade Federal de Minas Gerais, Departamento de Genética - Instituto de Ciências Biol'ogicas de Minas Gerais, Belo Horizonte, Brazil.

References

1. Ko AI, Goarant C, Picardeau M. Leptospira: the dawn of the molecular genetics era for an emerging zoonotic pathogen. Nat. Rev. Microbiol. 2009;7:736.
2. Levett PN. Leptospirosis. Clin Microbiol Rev. 2001;14:296–326.
3. Scolamacchia F, Handel IG, Fèvre EM, Morgan KL, Tanya VN, Bronsvoort BM de C. Serological patterns of brucellosis, leptospirosis and Q fever in *Bos indicus* cattle in Cameroon. PLoS One. 2010;5:e8623.
4. Bourhy P, Collet L, Clément S, Huerre M, Ave P, Giry C, et al. Isolation and characterization of new Leptospira genotypes from patients in Mayotte (Indian Ocean). PLoS Negl Trop Dis. 2010;4:e724.
5. Ellis WA, Thiermann AB, Montgomery J, Handsaker A, Winter PJ, Marshall RB. Restriction endonuclease analysis of *Leptospira interrogans* serovar hardjo isolates from cattle. Res Vet Sci. 1988;44:375–9.
6. Chappel RJ, Millar BD, Adler B, Hill J, Jeffers MJ, Jones RT, et al. *Leptospira interrogans* Serovar hardjo is not a major cause of bovine abortion in Victoria. Aust Vet J. 1989;66:330–3.
7. Myers DM, Caparo AC, Moreno JP. Isolation of serotype hardjo and other leptospirae from armadillos in Argentina. Bull Pan Am Health Organ. 1977; 11:131–9.
8. Cosate MRV, Barouni AS, Moreira EC, Veloso IF, Gomes MTR, Salas CE. Molecular characterization by LSSP-PCR and DNA sequencing of a pathogenic isolate of *Leptospira interrogans* from Brazil. Zoonoses Public Health. 2012;59:379–88.
9. Faine S, Adler B, Bolin C, Perolat P. *Leptospira* and Leptospirosis. Melbourne: Med Science; 1999.
10. Ellis WA, O'Brien JJ, Bryson DG, Mackie DP. Bovine leptospirosis: some clinical features of serovar hardjo infection. Vet Rec. 1985;117:101–4.
11. Kingscote BF. Diagnosis of Leptospira serovar hardjo infection in cattle in Canada. Can Vet J Rev Vét Can. 1985;26:270–4.
12. Mitchison M, Bulach DM, Vinh T, Rajakumar K, Faine S, Adler B. Identification and characterization of the dTDP-rhamnose biosynthesis and transfer genes of the lipopolysaccharide-related rfb locus in *Leptospira interrogans* serovar Copenhageni. J Bacteriol. 1997;179:1262–7.
13. Kalambaheti T, Bulach DM, Rajakumar K, Adler B. Genetic organization of the lipopolysaccharide O-antigen biosynthetic locus of Leptospira borgpetersenii serovar Hardjobovis. Microb Pathog. 1999;27:105–17.
14. de la Peña-Moctezuma A, Bulach DM, Adler B. Genetic differences among the LPS biosynthetic loci of serovars of *Leptospira interrogans* and Leptospira borgpetersenii. FEMS Immunol Med Microbiol. 2001;31:73–81.
15. de la Peña-Moctezuma A, Bulach DM, Kalambaheti T, Adler B. Comparative analysis of the LPS biosynthetic loci of the genetic subtypes of serovar Hardjo: *Leptospira interrogans* subtype Hardjoprajitno and Leptospira borgpetersenii subtype Hardjobovis. FEMS Microbiol Lett. 1999;177:319–26.
16. Ahmed A, Engelberts MFM, Boer KR, Ahmed N, Hartskeerl RA. Development and validation of a real-time PCR for detection of pathogenic leptospira species in clinical materials. PLoS One. 2009;4:e7093.
17. Thaipadungpanit J, Thaipadunpanit J, Chierakul W, Wuthiekanun V, Limmathurotsakul D, Amornchai P, et al. Diagnostic accuracy of real-time PCR assays targeting 16S rRNA and lipL32 genes for human leptospirosis in Thailand: a case-control study. PLoS One. 2011;6:e16236.
18. Zhong C, Peng D, Ye W, Chai L, Qi J, Yu Z, et al. Determination of plasmid copy number reveals the total plasmid DNA amount is greater than the chromosomal DNA amount in bacillus thuringiensis YBT-1520. PLoS One. 2011;6:e16025.
19. Moreno Switt AI, den Bakker HC, Cummings CA, Rodriguez-Rivera LD, Govoni G, Raneiri ML, et al. Identification and characterization of novel Salmonella Mobile elements involved in the dissemination of genes linked to virulence and transmission. PLoS One. 2012;7:e41247.
20. Cerqueira GM, McBride AJA, Picardeau M, Ribeiro SG, Moreira AN, Morel V, et al. Distribution of the leptospiral immunoglobulin-like (lig) genes in pathogenic Leptospira species and application of ligB to typing leptospiral isolates. J Med Microbiol. 2009;58:1173–81.
21. Zuerner RL, Ellis WA, Bolin CA, Montgomery JM. Restriction fragment length polymorphisms distinguish Leptospira borgpetersenii serovar hardjo type hardjo-bovis isolates from different geographical locations. J Clin Microbiol. 1993;31:578–83.
22. Zuerner RL, Bolin CA. Differentiation of *Leptospira interrogans* isolates by IS1500 hybridization and PCR assays. J Clin Microbiol. 1997;35:2612–7.
23. Mahillon J, Chandler M. Insertion Sequences. Microbiol Mol Biol Rev. 1998; 62:725–74.
24. Bulach DM, Kalambaheti T, de la Peña-Moctezuma A, Adler B. Lipopolysaccharide biosynthesis in Leptospira. J Mol Microbiol Biotechnol. 2000;2:375–80.
25. Ryu E. Rapid microscopic agglutination test for Leptospira without non-specific reaction. Bull Off Int Épizooties. 1970;73:49–58.
26. Tamai T, Sada E, Kobayashi Y. Restriction endonuclease DNA analysis of *Leptospira interrogans* serovars Icterohaemorrhagiae and Copenhageni. Microbiol Immunol. 1988;32:887–94.
27. Koidl C, Bozic M, Burmeister A, Hess M, Marth E, Kessler HH, et al. J Clin Microbiol. 2007;45:347–50.
28. Altschul SF, Gish W, Miller W, Myers EW, Lipman DJ. Basic local alignment search tool. J Mol Biol. 1990;215:403–10.
29. Edgar RC. MUSCLE: multiple sequence alignment with high accuracy and high throughput. Nucleic Acids Res. 2004;32:1792–7.
30. Tamura K, Peterson D, Peterson N, Stecher G, Nei M, Kumar S. MEGA5: molecular evolutionary genetics analysis using maximum likelihood, evolutionary distance, and maximum parsimony methods. Mol Biol Evol. 2011;28:2731–9.
31. Terpstra WJ, Korver H, van Leeuwen J, Klatser PR, Kolk AH. The classification of Sejroe group serovars of *Leptospira interrogans* with monoclonal antibodies. Zentralblatt Für Bakteriol Mikrobiol Hyg Ser Med Microbiol Infect Dis Virol Parasitol. 1985;259:498–506
32. Zuerner RL, Alt D, Bolin CA. IS1533-based PCR assay for identification of *Leptospira interrogans* Sensu Lato serovars. J Clin Microbiol. 1995;33:3284–9.
33. Chirathaworn C, Kongpan S. Immune responses to Leptospira infection: roles as biomarkers for disease severity. Braz J Infect Dis Off Publ Braz Soc Infect Dis. 2014;18:77–81.
34. Zakeri S, Khorami N, Ganji ZF, Sepahian N, Malmasi A-A, Gouya MM, et al. Leptospira Wolffii, a potential new pathogenic Leptospira species detected in human, sheep and dog. Infect Genet Evol J Mol Epidemiol Evol Genet Infect Dis. 2010;10:273–7.
35. Ahmed A, Ferreira AS, Hartskeerl RA. Multilocus sequence typing (MLST): markers for the traceability of pathogenic Leptospira strains. Methods Mol Biol Clifton NJ. 2015;1247:349–59.
36. Majed Z, Bellenger E, Postic D, Pourcel C, Baranton G, Picardeau M. Identification of variable-number tandem-repeat loci in *Leptospira interrogans* Sensu Stricto. J Clin Microbiol. 2005;43:539–45.
37. Bezerra da Silva J, Carvalho E, Hartskeerl RA, Ho PL. Evaluation of the use of selective PCR amplification of LPS biosynthesis genes for molecular typing of leptospira at the serovar level. Curr Microbiol. 2011;62:518–24.
38. Aguiar DM, et al. Seroprevalence of Leptospira spp in cattle from Monte Negro municipality, western Amazon. Pesq. Vet. Bras. 2006;26:102–4.
39. Figueiredo A de O, Pellegrin AO, Gonçalves VSP, Freitas EB, Monteiro LARC, Oliveira JM de, et al. Prevalence and risk factors for bovine leptospirosis in Mato Grosso do Sul, Brazil. Pesqui. Veterinária Bras. 2009;29(5):375–81.
40. Silva FJ, Conceição WLF, Fagliari JJ, Girio RJS, Dias RA, Borba MR, et al. Prevalence and risk factors of bovine leptospirosis in the state of Maranhão, Brazil. Pesqui Veterinária Bras. 2012;32:303–12.
41. Kmety E, Dikken H. Classification of the species *Leptospira interrogans* and history of its serovars. Groningen: University Press Groningen; 1993.
42. Ochman H, Lawrence JG, Groisman EA. Lateral gene transfer and the nature of bacterial innovation. Nature. 2000;405:299.

16

Clinical, diagnostic and pathologic features of presumptive cases of *Chlamydia pecorum*-associated arthritis in Australian sheep flocks

Evelyn Walker[1,2], Cecily Moore[2], Patrick Shearer[3], Martina Jelocnik[1], Sankhya Bommana[1], Peter Timms[1] and Adam Polkinghorne[1*]

Abstract

Background: Arthritis is an economically significant disease in lambs and is usually the result of a bacterial infection. One of the known agents of this disease is *Chlamydia pecorum*, a globally recognised livestock pathogen associated with several diseases in sheep, cattle and other hosts. Relatively little published information is available on the clinical, diagnostic and pathologic features of *C. pecorum* arthritis in sheep, hindering efforts to enhance our understanding of this economically significant disease. In this case series, a combination of standard diagnostic testing used routinely by veterinarians, such as the *Chlamydia* complement fixation text (CFT), veterinary clinical examinations, and additional screening via *C. pecorum* specific qPCR was used to describe putative chlamydial infections in five sheep flocks with suspected ovine arthritis.

Case presentation: Five separate cases involving multiple lambs (aged six to ten months) of different breeds with suspected *C. pecorum* arthritis are presented. In two of the five cases, arthritic lambs exhibited marked depression and lethargy. Arthritis with concurrent conjunctivitis was present in four out of five lamb flocks examined. *Chlamydia* CFT demonstrated medium to high positive antibody titres in all flocks examined. *C. pecorum* shedding was evident at multiple sites including the conjunctiva, rectum and vagina, as determined via qPCR. Two of the five flocks received antimicrobials and all flocks recovered uneventfully regardless of treatment.

Conclusion: This case series highlights the features a field veterinarian may encounter in cases of suspected ovine chlamydial arthritis. Our analysis suggests a presumptive diagnosis of chlamydial arthritis in lambs can be made when there is evidence of joint stiffness with or without synovial effusion and elevated chlamydia antibody titres. *C. pecorum*-specific qPCR was found to be a useful ancillary diagnostic tool, detecting *Chlamydia* positivity in low or negative CFT titre animals. Variables such as symptom duration relative to sampling, sheep breed and farm management practices were all factors recorded that paint a complex epidemiological and diagnostic picture for this disease. These case studies serve to provide a platform for further research to improve diagnostic testing and new treatment and control strategies for *C. pecorum* infections in sheep.

Keywords: *Chlamydia pecorum*, Ovine, Arthritis, Conjunctivitis, CFT, qPCR

Abbreviations: CFT, Complement fixation test; qPCR, Quantitative polymerase chain reaction; rRNA, Ribosomal RNA

* Correspondence: apolking@usc.edu.au
[1]Centre for Animal Health Innovation, Faculty of Science, Health, Education & Engineering, University of the Sunshine Coast, Maroochydore, QLD, Australia
Full list of author information is available at the end of the article

Background

Australia is one of the largest global players in sheep production and exports. In the Australian sheep industry, arthritis ($30 M) is ranked as the leading economic cost of lameness, followed by footrot ($18.4 M) [1]. Economic losses due to arthritis are incurred through on farm costs (e.g. loss of production from weight loss, treatment and culling) and condemnations at abattoirs. Arthritis in lambs has a number of potential aetiological agents such as *Erysipelothrix rhusiopathiae* (*E. rhusiopathiae*) [2], *Histophilus somni* (*Hemophilus somnus*) *Mycoplasma* spp. and *Chlamydia pecorum*, [3] but unfortunately these are not well documented in Australia.

C. pecorum is an obligate intracellular bacterial pathogen with a capacity to infect a wide range of animal hosts including sheep, goats, pigs, cattle [4] and wildlife such as the koala [5]. Although *C. pecorum* is believed to be ubiquitous in Australia, only a few case reports of chlamydiosis have been described by district veterinarians in sheep producing areas of New South Wales (NSW) [4, 6–8]. Worldwide, the presence of *C. pecorum* in rectal and conjunctival swabs from both symptomatic and asymptomatic livestock appears to be a common finding. In European countries, a high prevalence of *C. pecorum* shedding has been reported in clinically healthy sheep [9, 10] and in sheep flocks with overt disease, such as conjunctivitis [11] and enteritis [12]. In sheep, *C. pecorum* is most commonly associated with polyarthritis and keratoconjunctivitis [13–17]. *C. pecorum* has also been implicated in a few sporadic cases of respiratory disease [18] and abortions [19] in sheep. *C. pecorum* appears to be commonly excreted in the faeces of healthy sheep [5], with recent estimates that 30 % of Australian sheep flocks may be shedding *C. pecorum* [20]. The major route of transmission of *C. pecorum* is believed to be faecal-oral, through ingestion or inhalation of infective *Chlamydia* [21]. The implications of this faecal-shedding and its pathogenic potential to induce arthritis is unclear. Recent molecular typing studies suggest that different strains of *C. pecorum* isolated from disease affected sites, or from non-affected tissues within the same host, have different pathogenic potential [22–24].

Despite recent advances in molecular typing, which are still largely restricted to research use only, veterinarians in Australia continue to diagnose *C. pecorum* infections in sheep based on history, clinical examination findings and serological testing using the complement fixation test (CFT) [4, 25]. Histopathology is not routinely performed as it requires sacrifice of the affected animal. New validated molecular diagnostics are also becoming available, however, they are not widely used in veterinary diagnostic testing laboratories [4]. As it stands, diagnosis of chlamydial arthritis infections in sheep is difficult, as presentation is variable from flock to flock in terms of severity and clinical symptoms. The lack of definitive diagnostic tests to distinguish chlamydial arthritis from other possible causes of arthritis in lambs and the inability to discriminate pathogenic and non-pathogenic strains of *C. pecorum* further complicates the diagnostic picture. The paucity of epidemiological and risk factor studies also hampers efforts to diagnose and manage this disease.

To assist in improving the diagnosis of these infections and in understanding their biology and epidemiology, we present the various historical, clinical and diagnostic findings of five separate cases of suspected chlamydiosis diagnosed in lamb flocks across the Central West district of New South Wales (NSW), Australia.

Case presentation

The presenting complaint in all cases, as reported by the sheep producer was arthritis affecting weaned lambs. These cases were spread across the year with lambing and weaning in sheep in this region dependent on seasonality and individual on farm management practices. The age of the lambs ranged between 6 and 10 months. An overview of the major flock history findings is summarised in Table 1. The majority of affected lambs displayed clinical signs consistent with arthritis. Common clinical signs amongst the cases included joint stiffness and depression, although a range of other clinical signs were also reported (Table 2). The diagnostic laboratory findings from each set of cases is presented in Table 3. A case-by-case description follows.

Table 1 Summary of flock history in presumptive cases of chlamydial arthritis

History	Flock 1	Flock 2	Flock 3	Flock 4	Flock 5
Age (months)	6	6	10	8	10
Breed	X-bred	X-bred	White Suffolk	X-bred	Border Leicester
Sex	Mixed	Mixed	Mixed	Mixed	Mixed
Homebred	N	Y	Y	N	Y
Flocksize	450	150	500	22	101
No affected [n (%)]	96 (21)	20 (13)	9 (1.8)	2 (9.1)	3 (3.0)
Duration of symptoms (days)	14	4	Unknown	7	Unknown

Table 2 Summary of clinical signs observed in presumptive cases of chlamydial arthritis

Clinical signs	Flock 1	Flock 2	Flock 3	Flock 4	Flock 5
Lethargy	++	++	–	–	–
Gait abnormality	–	++	–	++	–
Joint stiffness	++	++	++	++	+
Joint swelling	+	++	++	+	+
Depression	++	++	–	–	–
Tucked up	–	–	–	++	–
Recumbency	++	++	–	+	–
Conjunctivitis	++	–	+	+	++
Pyrexia	++	++	–	++	–
Weight loss	–	–	–	–	–

+ present, ++ common, – not reported

Flock 1

The clinical details of animals from Flock 1 are described in Tables 1 and 2. Animals presented with a 2 week history of severe lethargy and ongoing joint stiffness. The owner first observed symptoms 1 week after weaning. At weaning, all lambs were treated for internal parasites (Cydectin® Oral, Virbac), received their second vaccination for clostridial diseases (Glanvac®6, Zoetis) and were moved onto fresh dryland lucerne (*Medicago sativa*). Approximately 4 % (out of 450) of lambs were affected at the time of examination. The affected lambs were the progeny of introduced ewes that displayed no signs of ill health. The owner reported that other lamb mobs born to homebred ewes were not affected. No formal diagnosis of chlamydial arthritis was made prior to this clinical investigation. However, the owner stated that he had a similar outbreak in his lambs 3 to 4 years ago, 1 to 2 weeks after their second clostridial vaccination.

At examination, lambs displayed extreme lethargy and depression (Fig. 1a), pyrexia (average rectal temperature of 40.5 °C) and preferred to lie down in the sheep yards. When the lambs were forced to move, they moved slowly and stiffly. Ten of the poorest lambs were examined. Seven out of ten arthritic lambs had a concurrent bilateral conjunctivitis (Fig. 1b). Only one lamb had a palpable joint swelling involving the front fetlock.

Serum and swab samples (conjunctival, rectal and vaginal) were collected from the ten affected lambs. Serum samples were analysed for anti-*Chlamydia* antibodies using the CFT by the State Veterinary Diagnostic Laboratory in NSW. The *Chlamydia* CFT used in this laboratory detects antibodies to *C. pecorum* elementary bodies [25]. A serum sample was considered positive with a titre of 16 or greater.

C. pecorum-specific qPCR was performed on swab samples collected and processed as previously described [26]. Briefly, the qPCR assay detects the 202 base pair region of the *C. pecorum* 16S ribosomal RNA (rRNA) gene. Specific primers used were 16Sf (5′AGTCGAAC GGAATAATGGCT3′) and 16Sr (5′CCAACAAGCTGA TATCCCAC3′). DNA from processed swabs was extracted using a QIamp DNA Mini kit (Qiagen). The presence of *C. pecorum* DNA from each swab site was analysed using the average number of *C. pecorum* DNA copies (in replicate) per microliter of template. A sample was considered positive when 10 or more copies of *C. pecorum* DNA were present.

Laboratory test results are described in Table 3. All ten lambs were positive on both conjunctival and rectal qPCR. Seven lambs were positive on vaginal qPCR. Seven out of ten lambs had a positive antibody titre of 16 or greater with five of these seven having a titre of 32 or greater.

Affected lambs were treated with a single intramuscular injection of oxytetracycline long-acting 300 mg/mL at a dose rate of 1 mL per 10 kg bodyweight and repeated 7 days later. The owner reported significant improvement in affected lambs within 48 h following initial and subsequent treatments. A follow up visit was

Table 3 Summary of laboratory results from flocks with suspected chlamydial arthritis

Laboratory Test	Result	Flock 1	Flock 2	Flock 3	Flock 4	Flock 5
		N = 10	*N* = 6	*N* = 30	*N* = 22	*N* = 101
Chlamydia CFT	Positive	7	6	4	7	31
	Negative	3	0	26	15	70
Conjunctival qPCR	Positive	10	5	1	0	11
	Negative	0	0	29	22	90
Rectal qPCR	Positive	10	5	9	1	2
	Negative	0	1	21	21	99
Vaginal qPCR	Positive	7	2	0	0	2
	Negative	0	3	16	14	50
E. rhusiopathiae joint culture	Positive	–	–	1	–	–
	Negative	–	–	1	–	–

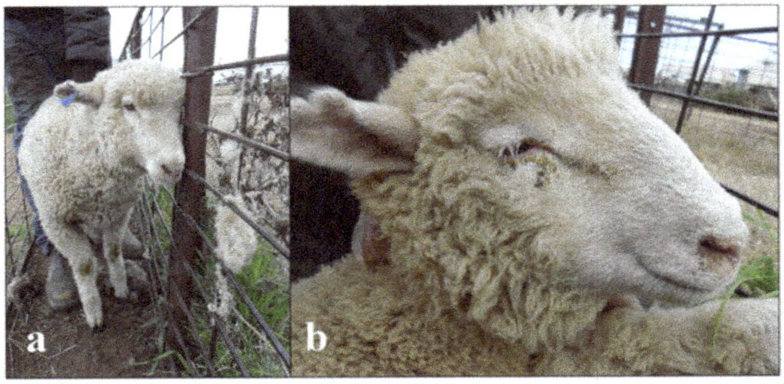

Fig. 1 Affected lambs from flock 1 demonstrating severe depression and requiring assistance to stand (**a**) and concurrent bilateral conjunctivitis (**b**)

conducted 19 days after presentation. The owners treated a total of 96 affected lambs out of 450. Affected lambs were isolated in a lucerne paddock away from other lamb mobs. Lambs examined in the sheep yards displayed significant improvement such that they appeared bright, alert and responsive as opposed to extreme lethargy and depression previously observed. There were still obvious clinical signs of stiffness and resolving conjunctivitis in the affected lamb mob however. The palpable joint swelling detected in one lamb had completely resolved. There were no palpable joint swellings in the remaining lambs. Seven months later, the owner reported another outbreak of arthritis with similar symptoms as previously described in a new mob of weaned lambs.

Flock 2

The owner reported a 4 day history of a hopping gait when sheep were driven in the morning. The gait abnormalities would resolve transiently the longer they were forced to move as if "they warmed themselves out of it," as reported by the owner. Affected lambs also spent more time away from the rest of the mob and preferred to lie down near the water troughs. The lamb mob consisted of 800 homebred weaners made up of 150 X-bred lambs and the remaining consisting of Merinos. Only X-bred lambs were affected at this point (Tables 1 and 2).

All lambs were weaned a week prior to the clinical investigation onto fresh dryland lucerne (*Medicago sativa*). Prior to weaning, lambs were grazing on wheat crop, received booster vaccinations against clostridial disease (Glanvac®6, Zoetis) and treated for internal parasites (Genesis™ Xtra Drench, Ancare). The owner reported a 4 year history of post-mulesing arthritis on farm and had been managing the problem by vaccinating only the Merinos against Erysipelothrix (Eryvac®, Zoetis) at marking since they were mulesed while the X-bred lambs were not. Approximately 20 out of 150 X-bred lambs were affected (13 %).

The hopping gait reported by the owner was not observed at the time of examination. The owner had drafted six of the worst affected animals in the flock for examination. All six lambs appeared stiff, depressed and lethargic, and preferred to lie in sternal recumbency in the sheep yards. There were no signs of conjunctivitis observed. Five out of six lambs had pyrexia with rectal temperatures averaging 40.5 °C. Two out of six lambs had a swelling present in one front carpal joint. A paddock muster of the overall lamb flock revealed additional stiff moving lambs.

As outlined in Table 3, all six lambs had positive CFT antibody titres of 64 or greater with four of these lambs demonstrating high positive titres of 128. Five lambs were positive at both conjunctival and rectal sites and two lambs were positive at the vaginal site by qPCR. In addition to *Chlamydia* antibodies, serum was also analysed for phosphorus, calcium, magnesium, copper and vitamin D to exclude vitamin and mineral deficiencies and/or toxicoses that could be triggering the gait abnormalities. However, these findings were unremarkable.

The owner elected not to treat affected lambs and instead chose to let them rest and recover in their own time. Extended withholding periods, costs and time associated with mustering, mass treatment and the need for follow up treatments meant that it was not an economically viable option. The lambs recovered uneventfully.

Flock 3

Ten month old homebred White Suffolk mixed sex lambs were examined after the owner reported an ongoing history of arthritis affecting a small percentage of his lamb flock every year (Table 1). Lambs had been grazing dryland lucerne a month prior and leading up to the day of presentation. Out of 30 lambs examined (Table 2), nine lambs exhibited clinical signs of arthritis with palpable swellings of single and multiple joints. None of these lambs with arthritis exhibited a concurrent conjunctivitis. However, there were seven lambs that had conjunctivitis only. Serum and swabs were collected from the 16 affected lambs and 14 clinically healthy lambs from the same flock.

In total, four lambs demonstrated a positive antibody titre of 16 or greater with three of these having titres of 32. Among these seropositive animals, two had arthritis present in one or more joints with no concurrent conjunctivitis. A total of eight lambs were positive by *C. pecorum* qPCR from rectal swabs, with three of these having arthritis present in one or more joints. One lamb with an antibody titre of 32 had no clinical symptoms of conjunctivitis nor arthritis, however, both conjunctival and rectal swabs were qPCR positive. In addition, one out of two sacrificed lambs was positive for *E. rhusiopathiae* on joint culture.

Flock 4

Two out of twenty-two 8 month old, recently purchased mixed sex X-bred lambs were presented with a 7 day history of lameness (Table 1). Lambs were grazing a combination of native pasture and dryland lucerne. On physical examination, both affected lambs were hunched, tucked up and stiff legged. They were quiet and preferred to spend more time lying down in comparison to the other lambs within the same flock.

Both affected lambs had pyrexia (both with rectal temperatures of 40.3 °C) despite cold temperatures on the day of examination. One lamb had a swelling involving the front fetlock joint and intermittently held this affected leg up (Fig. 2b). This lamb did not have any other palpable joint swellings but appeared to have a shifting lameness in the back legs, holding either leg up at intermittent intervals. The second lamb examined was very lethargic, hunched when standing and preferred to lay down in sternal recumbency whenever possible (Fig. 2a and b). There were no palpable joint swellings in this affected lamb.

Twenty additional lambs from the same flock were examined, with none of these displaying symptoms of arthritis and only one showing signs of a mild conjunctivitis (Table 2). Serum and swab samples were collected from affected and clinically healthy individuals as described previously. Seven lambs were *Chlamydia* antibody positive, with titres of 16 or greater; the two affected lambs had the highest titres of 64 and 128. All conjunctival and vaginal swabs were qPCR negative for *C. pecorum*. Only one lamb (clinically normal) had a qPCR positive rectal swab (Table 3).

The owner elected to pursue antimicrobial therapy for the two affected lambs. Single intramuscular injections of long-acting oxytetracycline (300 mg/mL at a dose rate of 1 mL per 10 kg bodyweight) were administered to affected lambs a week apart. The owner reported significant improvement within 24 h, reporting that affected lambs spent less time recumbent and more time standing and grazing with the rest of the flock. One week later, the owner reported that one lamb had no clinical signs of arthritis and the other lamb still had clinical signs of arthritis, but was improving.

Flock 5

A mixed sex, homebred Border Leicester lamb flock was followed up after previously diagnosed annual cases of chlamydiosis in their lambs (Table 1). Out of 101 ten month old lambs examined, three had joint abnormalities involving swellings of the carpal and hock joints (Table 2). Clinical symptoms of arthritis were absent in the remaining lambs. Fifty percent of the lamb flock had ongoing conjunctivitis throughout the previous 2 months. Serum and swab samples were collected as described previously from clinically affected and unaffected lambs within the same flock. A total of 31 lambs had positive *Chlamydia* CFT titres of 16 or greater (Table 3). Eleven lambs were *C. pecorum* qPCR positive from rectal swabs, with two having positive conjunctival and vaginal swabs. Three lambs had evidence of arthritis present in one or more joints. Two lambs were sacrificed for joint histopathology. Both of the sacrificed lambs were initially identified at 6 months of age with palpable joint effusions involving one or more joints and (i) rising

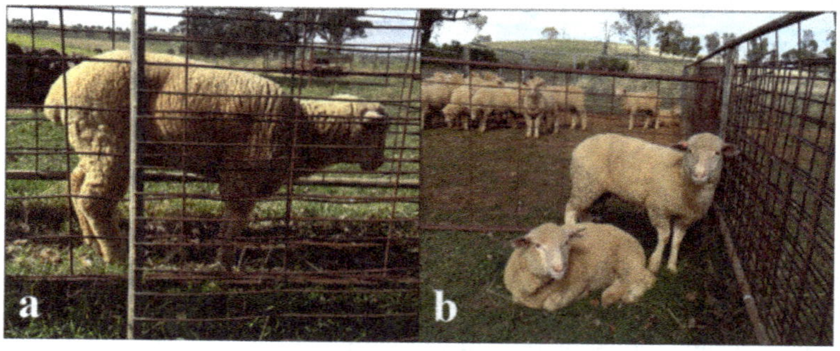

Fig. 2 Affected lambs from flock 4 demonstrating tucked up appearance (**a**) and sternal recumbency (**b**) and minimal weight bearing in right front affected leg when standing (**b**)

16 fold positive antibody titres; (ii) a bilateral conjunctivitis; and (iii) qPCR positivity at the rectal sites (both lambs) and conjunctival site (one lamb). At 10 months of age, the joint effusions resolved partially in one lamb with only one joint demonstrating a palpable carpal joint lesion (Fig. 3a). Histopathology of both carpal and hock joints for this affected lamb demonstrated a chronic, multifocal lymphoplasmacytic synovitis (Fig. 3b and c). The bilateral conjunctivitis identified previously had resolved completely. The joint effusion resolved completely in the other lamb at 10 months of age. On joint histopathology, this lamb demonstrated a mild, multifocal hyperplasia of synoviocytes affecting only one carpal joint (Fig. 4). Bilateral mucopurulent conjunctivitis was still present in this lamb.

At the time of sacrifice, both of these lambs were qPCR negative at rectal and conjunctival sites and antibody titres had declined to 32 and 8.

Conclusions

The clinical and laboratory findings described in each of these cases highlight the relatively complex clinical picture for these presumptive cases of chlamydial polyarthritis (Tables 2 and 3).

As with all clinical investigations, the presumptive diagnosis of chlamydial arthritis began on-farm. While the clinical presentation of animals across all case studies varied (Table 2), the common denominator amongst affected animals was the presence of joint stiffness and/or swelling (5/5 flocks; 100 %). Other signs such as lethargy, gait abnormalities, depression or recumbency were more variable and indeed, transitory amongst animals even on individual properties. Interestingly, in four out of the five flocks, signs of arthritis were also accompanied by evidence of conjunctivitis. Although many aetiologic agents may cause conjunctivitis in sheep, *C. pecorum* is recognised as a potential cause and, indeed, genetic typing has suggested that *C. pecorum* strains associated with arthritis may also be the same strains that cause conjunctivitis [22].

In terms of the laboratory diagnosis, *Chlamydia* CFT was found to be a more reliable indicator of chlamydial positivity at the flock level rather than for diagnosis of individual animals. Across all five flocks, 33 % (55/169) of serum samples were positive. The severity of clinical symptoms in individual animals did not necessarily correlate with individual antibody titre levels, however. Individual animals with severe disease involving multiple joints (e.g. flock three) did not have greater antibody titres. Conversely, individual animals (e.g. flocks one and two) with extreme lethargy, joint stiffness and pyrexia did have greater antibody titres. Similarly, some affected lamb flocks had positive *Chlamydia* CFT antibody titres as well as *C. pecorum* qPCR positivity at multiple sites (e.g. conjunctival, rectal and vaginal) while other lamb flocks had positive *Chlamydia* CFT antibody titres but were *C. pecorum* qPCR negative at multiple sites. These observations are similar to other reports in cattle where there was little association between chlamydial shedding and seropositivity [27, 28].

C. pecorum specific qPCR findings appeared to be useful in detecting chlamydial infections in flocks and in individuals with low or negative CFT titres, such as in flock three. The *C. pecorum* qPCR positivity detection

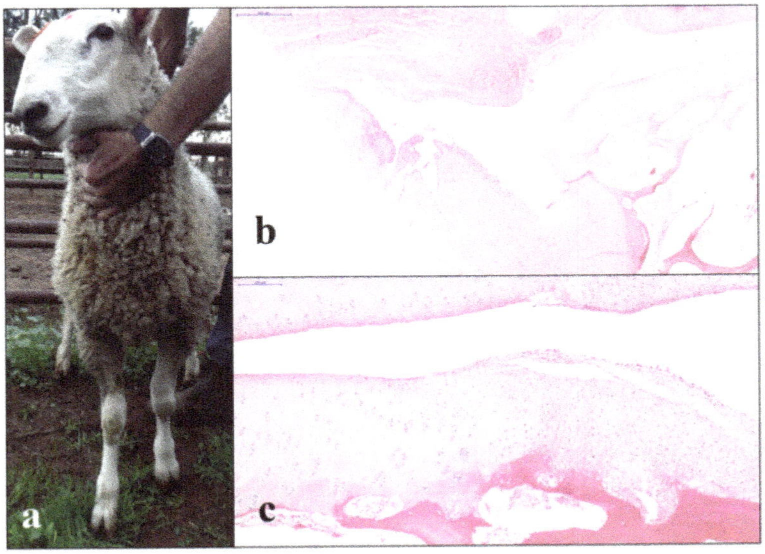

Fig. 3 Affected lambs from flock 5 demonstrating carpal swelling (**a**). Within all joints, there is diffuse, mild lymphoplasmacytic synovitis (**b**). Haematoxylin and eosin, 5×. And, focally extensive degeneration and necrosis of chondrocytes (**c**). Haematoxylin and eosin, 20×

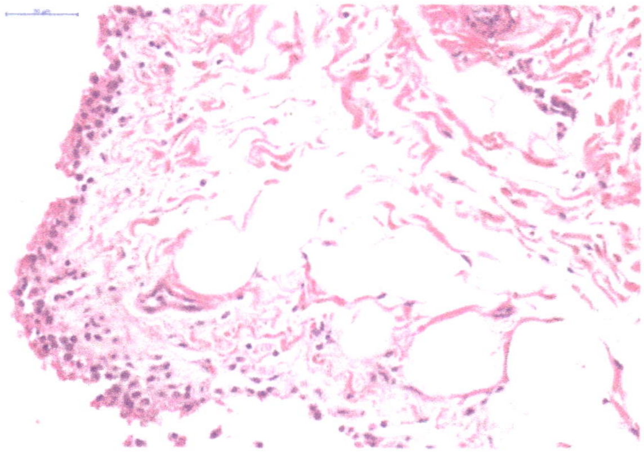

Fig. 4 Focally extensive synovial cell hyperplasia. Haematoxylin and eosin, 40×

rate of total conjunctival, rectal and vaginal swabs collected across all five flocks was 15 % (65/431). In *C. pecorum* positive animals, the conjunctival and rectal sites had equal detection rates with 27/168 (16 %) and 27/169 (16 %) positive swabs, respectively.

The duration of clinical symptoms and the sampling time point are factors that likely influenced the results of the chlamydial CFT and qPCR testing. In flocks one and two for example, the affected lambs were sampled within 1 to 2 weeks of manifestation of clinical signs and subsequently had greater serotitres and qPCR positive rates. In flocks three and five where there was a chronic history of arthritis and the exact duration of symptoms was unknown, there was a much lower rate of seropositivity and/or positive qPCR. In flock five, individual animals with arthritis were sampled at 6 months of age with high CFT titres and positive qPCR rates and later sampled at 10 months of age with declining antibody and qPCR positive rates despite still having arthritic symptoms in the flock. In other animals, CFT positivity was found in the absence of qPCR positivity which, presumably indicated recent past exposure rather than current infection.

While more detailed studies are clearly required to establish baseline data on the relationship between chlamydial CFT, chlamydial qPCR and clinical signs of chlamydial polyarthritis, based on the cases presented in this study, we nevertheless believe that a presumptive diagnosis of chlamydial arthritis in lambs can be made when there is evidence of joint stiffness with or without synovial effusion and elevated *Chlamydia* antibody titres. Ancillary testing such as *C. pecorum* specific qPCR can also be used to determine the presence of acute infection at a given point in time in the absence of complete microbiological testing for other agents.

These case studies also highlight other factors that may influence the pathogenesis of *Chlamydia*-related polyarthritis. One example of this is the breed of sheep. All sheep in this study were either X-bred, White Suffolk or Border Leicester breeds. Previous reports have suggested that rapid growth rates afforded by high meat producing British breeds and their crosses may play a role in the development of arthritis [6–8]. It should also be noted that these breeds are not routinely mulesed. Wounds generated from mulesing and shearing potentially act as entry points for the bacteria, *E. rhusiopathiae* and subsequently increase the prevalence of arthritis [2]. Flock 3 had evidence of both *E. rhusiopathiae* (in one lamb) and *C. pecorum* (in several lambs) without a history of mulesing, which would suggest that, unlike with *E. rhusiopathiae*, this farming practice is not likely to be a risk factor for chlamydial arthritis.

Another factor that has been linked to the onset of chlamydial arthritis is grazing. In Central NSW, dryland lucerne is commonly fed to finishing lambs because of its relatively high protein content availability. An association between this common feeding practice and the incidence of chlamydial infection has previously been postulated [6], with the suggestion that lambs grazing irrigated lucerne potentially carried a higher risk of developing clinical disease by infectious agents targeting tissues and joints in rapidly growing lambs. In the case of *C. pecorum*, one possible explanation is that the high protein content of lucerne coupled with the high metabolic rate of cells of rapidly growing lambs could potentially result in higher replication rates of intracellular *Chlamydia* [29]. However, the authors have seen cases of chlamydial conjunctivitis in Merino lambs grazing native pastures (unpublished observations). Anecdotal evidence also exists to support treatment of endemic chlamydiosis in lambs by removing affected lambs from lucerne and spelling them on native pastures to aid in the recovery of arthritic lambs (unpublished observations). Further investigation into the epidemiology of this disease is necessary, to explore whether different types of grazing are indeed risk factors for this disease in sheep.

In terms of treatment, although two owners in this study reported significant improvement after antimicrobial intervention with oxytetracycline, there is evidence suggesting that antimicrobial therapy may trigger chlamydial infection latency rather than completely eliminating the infection [30–32]. Relapses after treatment, development of chronic persistent infections [8, 17, 33] and return to chlamydial pre-treatment levels based on quantitative real-time PCR at the cessation of short term antimicrobial therapy [34] have all been reported. In the author's experience, individual lambs may benefit from antimicrobial treatment, but mass treatment of lambs does not enhance overall flock performance in comparison to flocks without antimicrobial intervention.

These case reports present an overview of the different clinical and diagnostic presentations of lambs with chlamydial arthritis. The major findings of this case series are:

1) a presumptive flock diagnosis of chlamydial arthritis in lambs can be made by assessment of clinical signs (joint stiffness with or without synovial effusion) and chlamydial CFT positivity;
2) in individual animals, there is often a discrepancy between chlamydial CFT and/or chlamydial PCR positivity and the presence of clinical signs;
3) timing of sampling relative to the presence of clinical signs is probably a major factor in the discrepancies between different diagnostic approaches used in this study;
4) other factors such as breed, grazing history and treatment are all factors that potentially influence the pathogenesis of chlamydial arthritis in lambs.
5) co-infections with other agents known to cause arthritis in sheep (e.g. *E. rhusiopathiae* and others) are possible and should be considered as differential diagnoses.

These conclusions highlight the need for additional on-farm studies to better understand the diagnosis, epidemiology and impact of chlamydial polyarthritis on the Australian sheep industry but also in other sheep-producing nations globally. Further experimental infection studies would also provide insight into disease pathogenesis especially with respect to "pathogenic" and "non-pathogenic" *C. pecorum* strains that have been recently proposed [22–24]. Antimicrobial therapy with questionable efficacy ideally needs to be replaced with whole farm management tools and/or the development of a vaccine that may minimise the risk of disease spread and development. A continued focus on this disease is anticipated to make these breakthroughs possible.

Funding

This work was funded by an Australian Research Council Linkage Project Grant (LP140100315) awarded to AP, PT and EW. The funding body had no role in the design of the study and collection, analysis, and interpretation of data and in writing the manuscript.

Authors' contributions

EW performed field work, assisted with laboratory analysis and drafted the manuscript. CM performed field work and assisted with diagnosis and case definitions. PS performed histopathology and assisted with drafting the manuscript. MJ and SB were primarily responsible for laboratory analysis and assist with drafting the manuscript. PT and AP conceived the study and assisted with drafting of the manuscript. All authors read and approved the final manuscript.

Competing interests

The authors do not have any competing interests.

Consent for publication

Not applicable.

Author details

[1]Centre for Animal Health Innovation, Faculty of Science, Health, Education & Engineering, University of the Sunshine Coast, Maroochydore, QLD, Australia. [2]Central West Local Land Services, Dubbo & Coonabarabran, NSW, Australia. [3]State Veterinary Diagnostic Laboratory, Elizabeth Macarthur Agricultural Institute, Menangle, NSW, Australia.

References

1. Sackett D, Holmes P, Abbott K, Jephcott S, Barber, M. Assessing the economic cost of endemic disease on the profitability of Australian beef cattle and sheep producers. In: Meat and Livestock Australia. 2006. http://www.mla.com.au/CustomControls/PaymentGateway/ViewFile.aspx?mFDUp1AYI9VUf+h/ZH4CYhopVLs5O3WvID8Tvjx4WwqlhJCS8/UdRwc9AKswn/HN3EYMKKAfsht7d1Tnt3BqiA==. Accessed 1 Nov 2014.
2. Paton MW, Rose IR, Sunderman FM, Holm MM. Effect of mulesing and shearing on the prevalence of *Erysipelothrix rhusiopathiae* arthritis in lambs. Aust Vet J. 2003;81:694–7.
3. Haskell SRR. Polyarthritis. In: Blackwell s five minute veterinary consult: ruminant. 1st ed. Iowa: Wiley-Blackwell; 2008. p. 722–3.
4. Walker E, Lee EJ, Timms P, Polkinghorne A. *Chlamydia pecorum* infections in sheep and cattle: a common and under-recognised infectious disease with significant impact on animal health. Vet J. 2015;206:252–60.
5. Polkinghorne A, Hanger J, Timms P. Recent advances in understanding the biology, epidemiology and control of chlamydial infections in koalas. Vet Microbiol. 2013;165:214–23.
6. Kemp JB. Chlamydial disease in sheep and cattle. In: 1986 Proceedings 69th Annual Conference. 1986. http://flockandherd.net.au/archive/1986.html. Accessed 11 Aug 2014.
7. Watt B. Chlamydial infection in sheep. In: 2011 District Veterinarian Conference Proceedings. 2011. http://www.flockandherd.net.au/sheep/reader/chlamydial-infection.html. Accessed 11 Aug 2014.
8. Walker E. *Branhamella ovis* and *Chlamydia pecorum* isolated from a case of conjunctivitis (with some polyarthritis) in lambs. In: 2013 District Veterinarian Conference Proceedings. 2013. http://www.flockandherd.net.au/sheep/reader/conjunctivitis-branhamella-chlamydia.html. Accessed 11 Aug 2014.
9. Clarkson MJ, Philips HL. Isolation of faecal chlamydia from sheep in Britain and their characterization by cultural properties. Vet J. 1997;153:307–11.
10. Lenzko H, Moog U, Henning K, Lederbach R, Diller R, Menge C, Sachse K, Sprague LD. High frequency of chlamydial co-infections in clinically healthy sheep flocks. BMC Vet Res. 2011;7:29.
11. Polkinghorne A, Borel N, Becker A, Lu ZH, Zimmerman DR, Brugnera E, Pospischil A, Vaughan L. Molecular evidence for chlamydial infections in the eyes of sheep. Vet Microbiol. 2009;135:142–6.
12. Osman KM, Ali HA, ElJakee JA, Galal HM. *Chlamydophila psittaci* and *Chlamydophila pecorum* infections in goats and sheep in Egypt. Rev Sci Tech. 2011;30:939–48.
13. Dickinson L, Cooper BS. Contagious conjunctivo-keratitis of sheep. J Pathol. 1959;78:257–66.
14. Mendlowski B, Segre D. Polyarthritis in sheep. I. Description of the disease and experimental transmission. Am J Vet Res. 1960;21:68–73.
15. Cutlip RC, Smith PC, Page LA. Chlamydial polyarthritis of lambs: a review. J Am Vet Med Assoc. 1972;161:1213–6.
16. Storz J, Spears P. Pathogenesis of chlamydial polyarthritis in domestic animals: characteristics of causative agent. Ann Rheum Dis Suppl. 1979;38:111–5.
17. Andrews AH, Goddard PC, Wilsmore AJ, Dagnell GJR. A chlamydial keratoconjunctivitis in a British sheep flock. Vet Rec. 1987;120:238 9.
18. Biberstein EL, Nisbet DI, Thompson DA. Experimental pneumonia in sheep. J Comp Pathol. 1967;77:181–92.

19. Seaman J. Chlamydia isolated from abortion in sheep. Aust Vet J. 1985;62:436.
20. Yang R, Jacobson C, Gardner G, Carmichael I, Campbell AJD, Ryan U. Longitudinal prevalence and faecal shedding of *Chlamydia pecorum* in sheep. Vet J. 2014;201:322–6.
21. Storz J, Kaltenboeck B. Diversity of *Chlamydia*-induced diseases. In: Zerai W, Miodrag R, editors. Rickettsial and chlamydial diseases of domestic animals. Oxford: Pergamon Press; 1993.
22. Jelocnik M, Walker E, Pannekoek Y, Ellem J, Timms P, Polkinghorne A. Evaluation of the relationship between Chlamydia pecorum sequence types and disease using a species-specific multi-locus sequence typing scheme (MLST). Vet Microbiol. 2014;174:214–22.
23. Yousef Mohamad K, Roche SM, Myers G, Bavoil PM, Laroucau K, Magnino S, Laurent S, Rasschaert D, Rodolakis A. Preliminary phylogenetic identification of virulent *Chlamydophila pecorum* strains. Infect Genet Evol. 2008;8:764–71.
24. Yousef Mohamad K, Kaltenboeck B, Rahman KS, Magnino S, Sachse K, Rodolakis A. Host adaptation of *Chlamydia pecorum* towards low virulence evidence in co-evolution of the *ompA*, *incA*, and ORF663 loci. PLoS One. 2014;9:e103615.
25. Sachse K, Vretou E, Livingstone M, Borel N, Pospischil A, Longbottom D. Recent developments in the laboratory diagnosis of chlamydial infections. Vet Microbiol. 2009;135:2–21.
26. Mathew M, Beagley KW, Timms P, Polkinghorne A. Preliminary characterisation of tumor necrosis factor alpha and interleukin-10 responses to *Chlamydia pecorum* infection in the koala (*Phascolarctos cinereus*). PLoS One. 2013;8(3):e59958.
27. Wehrend A, Failing K, Hauser B, Jäfer C, Bostedt H. Production, reproductive, and metabolic factors associated with chlamydial seropositivity and reproductive tract antigens in dairy herds with fertility disorders. Theriogenology. 2005;63:923–30.
28. Kauffold J, Henning K, Bachmann R, Hotzel H, Melzer F. The prevalence of chlamydiae of bulls from six bull studs in Germany. Anim Reprod Sci. 2007;102:111–21.
29. Harper A, Pogson CI, Jones ML, Pearce JH. Chlamydial development is adversely affected by minor changes in amino acid supply, blood plasma amino acid levels, and glucose deprivation. Infect Immun. 2000;68:1457–64.
30. Mårdh PA, Löwing C. Treatment of chlamydial infections. Scand J Infect Dis Suppl. 1990;68:23–30.
31. Hogan RJ, Mathews SA, Mukhopadhyay S, Summersgill JT, Timms P. Chlamydial persistence: beyond the biphasic paradigm. Infect Immun. 2004;72:1843–55.
32. Goellner S, Schubert E, Liebler-Tenorio E, Hotzel H, Saluz HP, Sachse K. Transcriptional response patterns of *Chlamydophila psittaci* in different in vitro models of persistent infection. Infect Immun. 2006;74:4801–8.
33. Aiello SE, Moses MA. Chlamydial polyarthritis-serositis in large animals. In: The Merck Veterinary Manual. 2012. http://www.merckvetmanual.com/mvm/musculoskeletal_system/arthropathies_in_large_animals/chlamydial_polyarthritis-serositis_in_large_animals.html. Accessed 30 Dec 2015.
34. Reinhold P, Liebler-Tenorio E, Sattler S, Sachse K. Recurrence of *Chlamydia suis* infection in pigs after short-term antimicrobial treatment. Vet J. 2011;187:405–7.

17

Antibiotic susceptibility profiles of *Mycoplasma synoviae* strains originating from Central and Eastern Europe

Zsuzsa Kreizinger[1], Dénes Grózner[1], Kinga M. Sulyok[1], Kristin Nilsson[1], Veronika Hrivnák[1], Dušan Benčina[2] and Miklós Gyuranecz[1*]

Abstract

Background: *Mycoplasma synoviae* causes infectious synovitis and respiratory diseases in chickens and turkeys and may lead to egg shell apex abnormalities in chickens; hence possesses high economic impact on the poultry industry. Control of the disease consists of eradication, vaccination or medication. The aim of the present study was to determine the in vitro susceptibility to 14 different antibiotics and an antibiotic combination of *M. synoviae* strains originating from Hungary and other countries of Central and Eastern Europe.

Results: Minimal inhibitory concentration (MIC) values of a total of 41 *M. synoviae* strains were determined by the microbroth dilution method. The strains were collected between 2002 and 2016 and originated from Hungary ($n = 26$), Austria ($n = 3$), the Czech Republic ($n = 3$), Slovenia ($n = 3$), Ukraine ($n = 3$), Russia ($n = 2$) and Serbia ($n = 1$). Tetracyclines (with MIC_{50} values of 0.078 μg/ml, ≤0.25 μg/ml and 0.5 μg/ml for doxycycline, oxytetracycline and chlortetracycline, respectively), macrolides (with MIC_{50} values of ≤0.25 μg/ml for tylvalosin, tylosin and tilmicosin), pleuromutilins (with MIC_{50} values of 0.078 μg/ml and ≤0.039 μg/ml for tiamulin and valnemulin) and the combination of lincomycin and spectinomycin (MIC_{50} 1 μg/ml (0.333/0.667 μg/ml)) were found to be the most effective antibiotic agents against *M. synoviae* in vitro. High MIC values were detected in numerous strains for fluoroquinolones (with MIC_{50} values of 1.25 μg/ml and 2.5 μg/ml for enrofloxacin and difloxacin), neomycin (MIC_{50} 32 μg/ml), spectinomycin (MIC_{50} 2 μg/ml), lincomycin (MIC_{50} 0.5 μg/ml) and florfenicol (MIC_{50} 4 μg/ml). Nevertheless, strains with elevated MIC values were detected for most of the applied antibiotics.

Conclusions: In the medical control of *M. synoviae* infections the preliminary in vitro antibiotic susceptibility testing and the careful evaluation of the data are crucial. Based on the in vitro examinations doxycycline, oxytetracycline, tylvalosin, tylosin and pleuromutilins could be recommended for the therapy of *M. synoviae* infections in the region.

Keywords: Antibiotic resistance, Chicken, Turkey, MIC, Microbroth dilution, *Mycoplasma synoviae*

Background

Mycoplasma synoviae is a cell wall-less pathogen which has significant economical impact in the poultry industry [1]. Clinical signs caused by this bacterium comprise synovitis and respiratory diseases in chickens and turkeys, and mainly in commercial egg layers the reduction of egg production and hatchability, and egg shell apex abnormalities [2]. The severity of the clinical signs may vary from sub-clinical to severe forms and is aggravated by the presence of other pathogens (e.g. infectious bronchitis virus, Newcastle disease virus, influenza A virus, *Escherichia coli* or other mycoplasmas) and inadequate housing conditions [3, 4].

The three main approaches for the control of the disease are eradication followed by prevention, vaccination or medication. While eradication and vaccination provide long-term solution for the control of mycoplasmosis, medication can be a prompt and effective tool to reduce the economic losses by mitigating egg transmission and clinical signs [1]. However, antibiotic susceptibility

* Correspondence: m.gyuranecz@gmail.com
[1]Institute for Veterinary Medical Research, Centre for Agricultural Research, Hungarian Academy of Sciences, Hungária körút 21, Budapest 1143, Hungary
Full list of author information is available at the end of the article

profile should first be determined to maximize treatment efficacy [5].

Due to their cell wall-less characteristic mycoplasmas are readily resistant to ß-lactam antibiotics and as they do not synthesize folic acid sulphonamides, sulfones or trimethoprim are ineffective against these pathogens also [6]. Natural resistance to erythromycin and other 14-membered ring macrolides was described in *M. synoviae* [7]. Mycoplasmas showed susceptibility to tetracyclines, fluoroquinolones and macrolides both in vitro and in vivo, and the efficacy of tiamulin and the combination of lincomycin and spectinomycin against *M. synoviae* under experimental conditions had been proved long before [5, 7–14]. In vitro determination of antibiotic susceptibility of *M. synoviae* is an essential tool for the choice of the appropriate antibiotic agent in the therapy with taking in consideration the factors which may influence the antimicrobial effect in vivo (e.g. biofilm synthesis) [15]. However, the performance of the in vitro tests in the case of mycoplasmas is time-consuming and requires special techniques, thus usually it is not carried out in routine diagnostics and comparable data about the antibiotic susceptibility of *M. synoviae* strains originating from Europe are scarce in the literature also [5, 7, 13, 16, 17].

In the present study the antibiotic susceptibility profile of *M. synoviae* strains originating from Central and Eastern Europe was determined by microbroth dilution method in the case of antibiotics commonly used in veterinary practice and which have potential to be used against avian mycoplasmosis.

Methods

M. synoviae strains were isolated from trachea swabs collected from turkeys and chickens originating from the Central and Eastern European region between 2014 and 2016. Production phase of the sampled chickens varied among breeders, commercial layers and broilers, while only meat-type turkeys were examined in the study (Table 1). Ethical approval and specific permission were not required for the study as all samples were collected by the authors during routine diagnostic examinations or necropsies with the consent of the owners. Trachea swabs were washed in 2 ml modified Frey's broth medium [18] and incubated at 37 °C with 5% CO_2 atmosphere. The broth medium consisted of 0.225 g/ml Frey Mycoplasma broth base, 20% porcine serum, 0.01% NAD, 0.01% cysteine, 200 IU/ml penicillin G, 0.5% glucose, 0.5% pyruvate and 0.005% phenol red in distilled water; all products originated from Sigma-Aldrich, Germany. Strains were gained after one-time filter cloning, minimizing the in vitro mutations of the isolates. The QIAamp DNA Mini Kit (Qiagen Inc., Hilden, Germany) was used for DNA extraction according to the manufacturers' instructions for Gram-negative bacteria. The purity of the cultures was confirmed by a universal *Mycoplasma* PCR system targeting the 16S/23S rRNA intergenic spacer region in *Mycoplasmatales* [19] followed by sequencing on an ABI Prism 3100 automated DNA sequencer (Applied Biosystems, Foster City, CA), sequence analysis and BLAST search. Out of a total of 41 *M. synoviae* strains tested in the study 26 strains originated from Hungary, three strains each from Austria, the Czech Republic and from Ukraine, two strains from Russia and one from Serbia (Table 1). Also, three strains isolated in Slovenia between 2002 and 2008 were included in the study. The number of colour changing units (CCU) was calculated by microbroth dilution method, from the highest dilution showing colour change (red to yellow shift) after two weeks of incubation [20].

The following antimicrobial agents were examined during the microbroth dilution tests: the fluoroquinolones: enrofloxacin and difloxacin; the aminocyclitol: spectinomycin; the aminoglycoside: neomycin; the lincosamide: lincomycin; the tetracyclines: doxycycline, oxytetracycline and chlortetracycline; the macrolides: tylosin and tilmicosin; the pleuromutilins: tiamulin and valnemulin; and the amphenicol: florfenicol; all products originated from VETRANAL, Sigma-Aldrich, Germany. Lincomycin and spectinomycin were applied in combination as well, in a ratio of 1:2. The macrolide tylvalosin (Aivlosin, ECO Animal Health Ltd., UK) was also included in the examinations. The antibiotics were diluted and stored according to the recommendations of Hannan [20]. Stock solutions of 1 mg/ml fluoroquinolones were prepared in 0.1 M NaOH; stock solution of 1 mg/ml florfenicol was prepared in 96% ethanol and in sterile distilled water; and the rest of the stock solutions of 1 mg/ml were prepared in sterile distilled water and stored at −70 °C. Freshly prepared two-fold dilutions were used in each microtest after checking the thawed antibiotic solutions for any visible changes in their consistency. The concentration range of the antibiotics was selected to cover values previously suggested to reflect susceptibility, intermediate susceptibility or resistance to the tested agents or which were used in previous publications (Table 2), in details: 0.039–10 μg/ml for fluoroquinolones, doxycycline and pleuromutilins, 0.25–64 μg/ml for neomycin, spectinomycin, lincomycin, oxytetracycline, chlortetracycline and macrolides, 0.125–32 μg/ml for florfenicol and 0.25–64 μg/ml (0.083/0.167–21.333/42.666 μg/ml) for the combination of lincomycin and spectinomycin.

Microbroth dilution examinations were performed according to Hannan [20] on 10^4–10^5 CCU/ml of the strains. In brief, the tests were performed in 96-well microtiter plates containing modified Frey's broth

Table 1 Background data and initial MIC values of the isolated *Mycoplasma synoviae* strains

Strain data							MIC values (μg/ml)														
Strain ID	Host[a]	Production phase	Farm	Region	Country	Year	EFX	DIF	CTC	DX	OTC	TYL	TIL	TVN	N	SPC	LCM	LCM-SPC	TIA	VAL	FFC
MYCAV 31	ch	layer	1	Nógrád	Hungary	2014	0.625	5	0.5	0.078	1	≤0.25	≤0.25	≤0.25	32	1	1	2 (0.666/1.334)	≤0.039	≤0.039	2
MYCAV 79	t	broiler	2	Győr-Moson-Sopron	Hungary	2014	0.312	1.25	≤0.25	0.078	0.5	≤0.25	≤0.25	≤0.25	32	1	1	2 (0.666/1.334)	0.078	≤0.039	2
MYCAV 102	t	broiler	3	Vas	Hungary	2014	1.25	1.25	0.5	0.078	0.5	≤0.25	≤0.25	≤0.25	32	1	1	1 (0.333/0.667)	0.078	≤0.039	2
MYCAV 119	t	broiler	4	Komárom-Esztergom	Hungary	2014	0.312	1.25	≤0.25	0.078	≤0.25	≤0.25	≤0.25	≤0.25	32	2	1	2 (0.666/1.334)	0.078	≤0.039	2
MYCAV 130	t	broiler	5	Győr-Moson-Sopron	Hungary	2014	10	5	0.5	0.078	0.5	≤0.25	≤0.25	≤0.25	32	2	1	2 (0.666/1.334)	0.156	≤0.039	4
MYCAV 167	ch	breeder	6	Jász-Nagykun-Szolnok	Hungary	2015	0.625	0.625	0.5	≤0.039	≤0.25	≤0.25	≤0.25	≤0.25	8	1	≤0.25	0.5 (0.167/0.333)	≤0.039	≤0.039	2
MYCAV 168	ch	layer	7	Pardubice	Czech Republic	2015	>10	5	2	0.312	1	≤0.25	0.5	≤0.25	8	2	1	1 (0.333/0.667)	0.156	≤0.039	8
MYCAV 170	ch	breeder	8	Győr-Moson-Sopron	Hungary	2015	2.5	2.5	0.5	0.078	0.5	≤0.25	≤0.25	≤0.25	16	2	0.5	0.5 (0.167/0.333)	0.156	≤0.039	8
MYCAV 173	ch	layer	9	Oryol	Russia	2015	10	2.5	1	0.156	0.5	≤0.25	1	≤0.25	4	1	0.5	0.5 (0.167/0.333)	≤0.039	≤0.039	2
MYCAV 174	ch	layer	10	Oryol	Russia	2015	>10	10	4	0.312	1	≤0.25	4	≤0.25	32	2	1	2 (0.666/1.334)	0.078	≤0.039	8
MYCAV 183	ch	broiler	11	Komárom-Esztergom	Hungary	2015	1.25	1.25	0.5	0.078	≤0.25	≤0.25	≤0.25	≤0.25	>64	8	0.5	1 (0.333/0.667)	0.078	≤0.039	8
MYCAV 185	ch	breeder	12	Szabolcs-Szatmár-Bereg	Hungary	2015	>10	5	0.5	0.312	0.5	2	64	0.5	16	2	>64	2 (0.666/1.334)	0.156	≤0.039	8
MYCAV 186	ch	layer	13	Borsod-Abaúj-Zemplén	Hungary	2015	>10	2.5	2	0.156	0.5	≤0.25	≤0.25	≤0.25	64	2	0.5	0.5 (0.167/0.333)	0.312	≤0.039	2
MYCAV 188	ch	breeder	14	Zala	Hungary	2015	>10	10	4	0.312	1	≤0.25	≤0.25	≤0.25	32	2	0.5	1 (0.333/0.667)	≤0.039	≤0.039	2
MYCAV 189	ch	layer	15	Cherkasy	Ukraine	2015	10	5	8	0.312	1	≤0.25	2	≤0.25	32	2	1	1 (0.333/0.667)	0.078	≤0.039	8
MYCAV 190	ch	layer	16	Cherkasy	Ukraine	2015	>10	10	4	0.312	0.5	≤0.25	2	≤0.25	32	2	1	0.5 (0.167/0.333)	0.078	≤0.039	8
MYCAV 194[b]	ch	breeder	17	unknown	Slovenia	2002	0.625	1.25	≤0.25	≤0.039	≤0.25	≤0.25	≤0.25	≤0.25	32	4	0.5	0.5 (0.167/0.333)	0.156	≤0.039	4
MYCAV 197[c]	ch	breeder	18	unknown	Slovenia	2002	0.625	10	0.5	≤0.039	≤0.25	≤0.25	≤0.25	≤0.25	32	≤0.25	0.5	2 (0.666/1.334)	0.078	≤0.039	4
MYCAV 198[d]	ch	unknown	19	unknown	Slovenia	2008	0.625	5	≤0.25	0.156	0.5	≤0.25	≤0.25	≤0.25	16	4	0.5	1 (0.333/0.667)	0.312	≤0.039	8
MYCAV 217	t	broiler	20	Békés	Hungary	2015	2.5	10	1	0.078	≤0.25	≤0.25	0.5	≤0.25	64	1	1	1 (0.333/0.667)	0.625	≤0.039	8
MYCAV 236	ch	breeder	21	Veszprém	Hungary	2015	0.312	1.25	1	0.078	≤0.25	≤0.25	≤0.25	≤0.25	16	1	0.5	0.5 (0.167/0.333)	0.078	≤0.039	0.5
MYCAV 249	ch	layer	22	South Moravia	Czech Republic	2016	5	10	≤0.25	0.156	0.5	≤0.25	≤0.25	≤0.25	>64	4	1	1 (0.333/0.667)	0.078	≤0.039	4
MYCAV 256	ch	layer	23	South Moravia	Czech Republic	2016	10	5	1	0.156	0.5	≤0.25	≤0.25	≤0.25	>64	4	1	2 (0.666/1.334)	0.156	≤0.039	4
MYCAV 257	ch	layer	24	Fejér	Hungary	2016	>10	10	2	0.156	1	≤0.25	≤0.25	≤0.25	32	2	1	1 (0.333/0.667)	0.156	≤0.039	4
MYCAV 259	ch	breeder	25	unknown	Serbia	2016	>10	5	0.5	0.078	≤0.25	≤0.25	≤0.25	≤0.25	32	2	≤0.25	0.5 (0.167/0.333)	0.312	≤0.039	2
MYCAV 261	t	broiler	26	Komárom-Esztergom	Hungary	2016	1.25	1.25	0.5	0.078	≤0.25	≤0.25	≤0.25	≤0.25	16	2	≤0.25	0.5 (0.167/0.333)	≤0.039	≤0.039	4
MYCAV 262	t	broiler	27	Komárom-Esztergom	Hungary	2016	0.625	1.25	≤0.25	0.078	≤0.25	≤0.25	≤0.25	≤0.25	16	1	0.5	1 (0.333/0.667)	≤0.039	≤0.039	8
MYCAV 263	t	broiler	28	Győr-Moson-Sopron	Hungary	2016	1.25	1.25	0.5	0.078	≤0.25	≤0.25	≤0.25	≤0.25	8	1	≤0.25	0.5 (0.167/0.333)	≤0.039	≤0.039	2
MYCAV 268	t	broiler	29	Tolna	Hungary	2016	1.25	2.5	0.5	0.078	≤0.25	≤0.25	≤0.25	≤0.25	64	2	0.5	1 (0.333/0.667)	0.156	≤0.039	8
MYCAV 272	ch	layer	30	Ternopil	Ukraine	2016	0.625	1.25	≤0.25	0.078	≤0.25	≤0.25	≤0.25	≤0.25	>64	4	2	1 (0.333/0.667)	0.625	≤0.039	4
MYCAV 274	ch	broiler	31	Vas	Hungary	2016	2.5	2.5	≤0.25	0.078	≤0.25	≤0.25	≤0.25	≤0.25	64	4	1	2 (0.666/1.334)	0.312	≤0.039	8
MYCAV 277	t	broiler	32	Veszprém	Hungary	2016	1.25	1.25	≤0.25	0.078	≤0.25	≤0.25	≤0.25	≤0.25	32	2	0.5	1 (0.333/0.667)	0.078	≤0.039	4
MYCAV 278	t	broiler	33	Veszprém	Hungary	2016	1.25	1.25	≤0.25	0.156	≤0.25	≤0.25	≤0.25	≤0.25	16	2	0.5	1 (0.333/0.667)	≤0.039	≤0.039	2
MYCAV 281	t	broiler	34	Somogy	Hungary	2016	0.312	0.625	≤0.25	0.156	≤0.25	≤0.25	≤0.25	≤0.25	32	2	1	1 (0.333/0.667)	0.156	≤0.039	8
MYCAV 282	ch	layer	13	Borsod-Abaúj-Zemplén	Hungary	2016	10	5	0.5	0.156	0.5	≤0.25	≤0.25	≤0.25	>64	4	1	2 (0.666/1.334)	≤0.039	≤0.039	0.5
MYCAV 284	t	broiler	35	Burgenland	Austria	2016	1.25	2.5	≤0.25	0.078	≤0.25	≤0.25	≤0.25	≤0.25	32	2	0.5	1 (0.333/0.667)	0.156	≤0.039	4

Table 1 Background data and initial MIC values of the isolated *Mycoplasma synoviae* strains *(Continued)*

Strain data							MIC values (µg/ml)															
Strain ID	Host[a]	Production phase	Farm	Region	Country	Year	EFX	DIF	CTC	DX	OTC	TYL	TIL	TVN	N	SPC	LCM	LCM-SPC	TIA	VAL	FFC
MYCAV 285	t	broiler	36	Burgenland	Austria	2016	1.25	2.5	≤0.25	0.078	≤0.25	≤0.25	≤0.25	≤0.25	32	2	≤0.25	0.5 (0.167/0.333)	0.078	≤0.039	4
MYCAV 288	t	broiler	37	Burgenland	Austria	2016	1.25	2.5	≤0.25	0.078	≤0.25	≤0.25	≤0.25	≤0.25	>64	1	0.5	1 (0.333/0.667)	0.078	≤0.039	4
MYCAV 291	t	broiler	38	Győr-Moson-Sopron	Hungary	2016	0.625	2.5	0.5	0.156	0.5	≤0.25	≤0.25	≤0.25	32	1	≤0.25	0.5 (0.167/0.333)	0.078	≤0.039	4
MYCAV 300	ch	breeder	14	Zala	Hungary	2016	>10	10	1	0.312	1	≤0.25	1	≤0.25	64	2	1	1 (0.333/0.667)	0.078	≤0.039	4
MYCAV 306	t	broiler	4	Komárom-Esztergom	Hungary	2016	1.25	2.5	≤0.25	0.078	≤0.25	≤0.25	≤0.25	≤0.25	16	1	1	1 (0.333/0.667)	0.078	≤0.039	4

Abbreviations of antibiotics: *EFX* enrofloxacin, *DIF* difloxacin, *DX* doxycycline, *OTC* oxytetracycline, *CTC* chlortetracycline, *TYL* tylosin, *TIL* tilmicosin, *TVN* tylvalosin, *N* neomycin, *SPC* spectinomycin, *LCM* lincomycin, *TIA* tiamulin, *VAL* valnemulin, *FFC* florfenicol

[a]All strains were isolated from the trachea of the animals, abbreviations stand for: *ch* chicken, *t* turkey

[b]MYCAV194 is sub-clone of strain ULB02/T6 [41]

[c]MYCAV197 is sub-clone of strain IT2/A [41]

[d]MYCAV198 is sub-clone of strain ULB08/T3 [42]

Table 2 Summary of MIC range, MIC$_{50}$ and MIC$_{90}$ values (µg/ml) of the isolated *Mycoplasma synoviae* strains with the suggested non-official breakpoints (in µg/ml; S: susceptible, R: resistant) and MIC values for the type strain WVU1853

	Non-official breakpoints	WVU1853 initial	WVU1853 final	Range initial	Range final	MIC$_{50}$ initial	MIC$_{50}$ final	MIC$_{90}$ initial	MIC$_{90}$ final
Fluoroquinolones									
Enrofloxacin	S ≤ 0.5; *R* ≥ 2 [5]	0.312	1.25	0.312 – >10	0.312 – >10	1.25	1.25	>10	>10
Difloxacin	S ≤ 0.5; *R* ≥ 4 [5]	1.25–2.5	1.25–2.5	0.625 – >10	0.625 – >10	2.5	2.5	10	>10
Aminocyclitol									
Spectinomycin	S ≤ 2; *R* > 4 [28]	2	8	≤0.25–8	1–16	2	2	4	8
Aminoglycoside									
Neomycin	S ≤ 4; R > 4 [25]	64 – >64	>64	4 – >64	8 – >64	32	>64	>64	>64
Lincosamide									
Lincomycin	S ≤ 2; *R* ≥ 8 [43]	0.5	0.5	≤0.25 – >64	≤0.25 – >64	0.5	1	1	4
Tetracyclines									
Doxycycline	S ≤ 4; *R* ≥ 16 [25]	≤0.039	0.156	≤0.039–0.312	0.078–1.25	0.078	0.156	0.312	0.625
Oxytetracycline	S ≤ 4; R ≥ 16 [5]	≤0.25	0.5	≤0.25–1	≤0.25–8	≤0.25	1	1	4
Chlortetracycline	S ≤ 4; R ≥ 16 [25]	0.5	1	≤0.25–8	≤0.25–16	0.5	2	2	8
Macrolides									
Tylosin	S ≤ 1; R ≥ 4 [5]	≤0.25	≤0.25	≤0.25–2	≤0.25–8	≤0.25	≤0.25	≤0.25	≤0.25
Tilmicosin	S ≤ 8; *R* ≥ 32 [5]	≤0.25	≤0.25	≤0.25–64	≤0.25 – >64	≤0.25	≤0.25	1	2
Tylvalosin	S ≤ 0.5; *R* > 2 [28]	≤0.25	≤0.25	≤0.25–0.5	≤0.25–1	≤0.25	≤0.25	≤0.25	≤0.25
Pleuromutilins									
Tiamulin	S ≤ 8; R ≥ 16 [7]	0.078	0.078	≤0.039–0.625	0.078–1.25	0.078	0.156	0.312	0.312
Valnemulin	S ≤ 0.125; *R* > 0.125 [25]	≤0.039	≤0.039	≤0.039	≤0.039	≤0.039	≤0.039	≤0.039	≤0.039
Amphenicol									
Florfenicol	S ≤ 2; R ≥ 8 [25]	1–2	1–4	0.5–8	1–16	4	8	8	8
Combination									
Lincomycin: Spectinomycin	S ≤ 2(0.666/1.334); R > 4(1.332/2.668) [25]	1 (0.333/0.667)	1–2 (0.333/0.667–0.666/1.334)	0.5–2 (0.167/0.333–0.666/1.334)	0.5–4 (0.167/0.333–1.332/2.668)	1 (0.333/0.667)	1 (0.333/0.667)	2 (0.666/1.334)	2 (0.666/1.334)

medium, using growth controls (broth medium without antibiotic), sterility controls (broth medium without antibiotic and *Mycoplasma* inoculum), pH controls (broth medium adjusted to pH 6.8) and quality controls (the duplicate of the *M. synoviae* type strain WVU 1853, NCTC 10124). All strains were tested in duplicates.

The minimum inhibitory concentrations (MIC) were determined from the lowest concentration of the antibiotics where no pH and colour change of the broth was detected, meaning that the growth of the bacteria was completely inhibited in the broth. Initial MIC values were determined when the growth controls showed colour change. Final MIC values were determined when no further growth was detected, generally after two weeks of incubation. MIC$_{50}$ and MIC$_{90}$ values were defined as the lowest concentrations that inhibited the growth of 50% or 90% of the strains [20].

Results

The quality control type strain (WVU 1853, NCTC 10124) showed consistent results throughout the study and the data (Table 2) were in accordance with previously recorded MIC values gained by microbroth dilution method: ranges of initial MIC values were 0.125–0.5 µg/ml for enrofloxacin and difloxacin, 0.1–0.125 µg/ml for oxytetracycline, ≤0.015 µg/ml for doxycycline, 0.025–0.06 µg/ml for tylosin, 0.015–0.06 µg/ml for tilmicosin, and ≤0.03–0.1 µg/ml for tiamulin before [5, 7, 13, 17]. Currently, there are no comparable MIC values available in the case of the *M. synoviae* type strain (WVU 1853, NCTC 10124) for the rest of the antibiotics tested in the present study. The ranges of the initial and final MIC values, MIC$_{50}$ and MIC$_{90}$ values for each antibiotic and for the combination are included in Table 2. In the cases of four antibiotics (oxytetracycline, chlortetracycline, neomycin and lincomycin) at least four-fold difference was observed in the MIC_{50} or MIC_{90} values when initial and final MIC values were compared (Tables 1 and 2 and Additional file 1). The initial MIC values are evaluated and discussed throughout the study [20]. The MIC_{50} values of the strains originating from different countries of the Central and Eastern European region showed high similarity, thus if otherwise not indicated the MIC values of all examined strains are evaluated together.

The distribution of the MIC values for enrofloxacin showed two main peaks (Fig. 1a1), while predominantly even distribution of the MIC values for difloxacin was observed (Fig. 1a2). Among the Hungarian strains the MIC_{50} values for enrofloxacin of the isolates originating from chickens (10 μg/ml, $n = 11$) was notably higher than of the strains originating from turkeys (1.25 μg/ml, $n = 15$), which corresponds to the observed two-peaked distribution (Fig. 1a2). In this comparison, four-fold difference was detected between the MIC_{50} values for difloxacin (with MIC_{50} 1.25 μg/ml and 5 μg/ml of strains from turkeys and chickens, respectively) and the distribution of the MIC values for this agent differed remarkably according to the isolates' host of origin (Fig. 1b2). No outlier strains with high MIC values were observed for the tetracyclines doxycycline, oxytetracycline and chlortetracycline (Fig. 1c, d and e). The strains generally showed low MIC values for the three examined macrolides (Fig. 1f, g and h), with the exception of one strain (MYCAV 185), especially in the case of tilmicosin (MIC 64 μg/ml). Strain MYCAV 185 was isolated from a backyard flock, where excess antibiotic usage was documented, and it showed elevated MIC values for most antibiotics tested. High MIC values were detected for neomycin in most strains (Fig. 1i), especially after two weeks of incubation (final $MIC_{50} > 64$ μg/ml, Table 2 and Additional file 1). The majority of the strains' MIC values for spectinomycin and for lincomycin distributed around the MIC_{50} values (Fig. 1j and k). Outlier strains were detected for both antibiotics; one strain with low MIC value in the case of spectinomycin (MYCAV 197), and one with high MIC value in the case of lincomycin (MYCAV 185). When lincomycin and spectinomycin were applied in combination, the range of the MIC values slightly tightened, no outlier strains were detected and lower concentration of the individual antibiotics was sufficient in the combination to inhibit the growth of 50% of the strains (Fig. 1j, k and l). Pleuromutilins showed high efficacy against the *M. synoviae* strains (Fig. 1m and n). No growth was observed in the presence of valnemulin and most strains were inhibited at the MIC_{50} concentration of tiamulin. The MIC values of the majority of the strains grouped around the MIC_{50} value (4 μg/ml) in the case of florfenicol also (Fig. 1o).

Discussion

Conventional methods for the determination of antibiotic susceptibility of mycoplasmas is time-consuming, laborious and requires special techniques, thus it is not performed routinely [20]. Moreover, the interpretation of the results is hampered by the lack of official standards. In the case of human pathogen mycoplasmas the Clinical and Laboratory Standards Institute (CLSI) has provided official breakpoints for certain antibiotics [21]. However, given the fastidious nature and inherent differences in the cultivation of these pathogens, procedures and media vary according to each of the examined species [22]. Initiations to establish standard CLSI protocols for mycoplasmas with veterinary relevance have been made, but for the time being the recommendations of Hannan [20] are supposed to be applied in these cases [23]. In the lack of official breakpoints, the data of the present study are interpreted according to values previously used in other publications [5, 7, 13, 20, 24] or to breakpoints of other avian pathogens determined by the CLSI [25] (Table 2).

Susceptibility (MIC ≤0.5 μg/ml according to Landman et al. [5]) and also resistance (MICs ≥2 or 4 μg/ml for enrofloxacin or difloxacin, respectively) [5] to fluoroquinolones have been described in *M. synoviae* strains before [5, 12, 16, 17, 24]. Differences in the antibiotic usage and density of poultry flocks were assumed to be responsible for the observed variations [17] and resistance to fluoroquinolones was described in Europe [5]. In the present study, elevated MIC values of fluoroquinolones were observed regardless of the strains' geographical origin. On the other hand, MIC values showed correlation with the host of origin, most probably in connection with the length of the hosts' production cycle. In the interpretation of Landman et al. [5], more than half of the Hungarian strains isolated from chickens (mainly breeders and layers) were regarded resistant to enrofloxacin (MIC ≥2 μg/ml) and difloxacin (MIC ≥4 μg/ml), while most of the strains from meat-type turkeys (short life production cycle) were considered susceptible or intermediately susceptible to these antibiotics.

The MIC values of tetracyclines also varied in previous works according to the strains' country of origin, with most European strains showing susceptibility (MIC ≤4 μg/ml) [20] to these agents [5, 12, 13, 16]. In accordance with previous studies, all strains included in the current study showed high susceptibility to doxycycline and oxytetracycline, and chlortetracycline proved to be highly efficient at least against 90% of the strains.

The 16-membered ring macrolides showed good in vitro activity against *M. synoviae* strains all over the world previously [5, 12, 14, 16, 26–30], but field strains

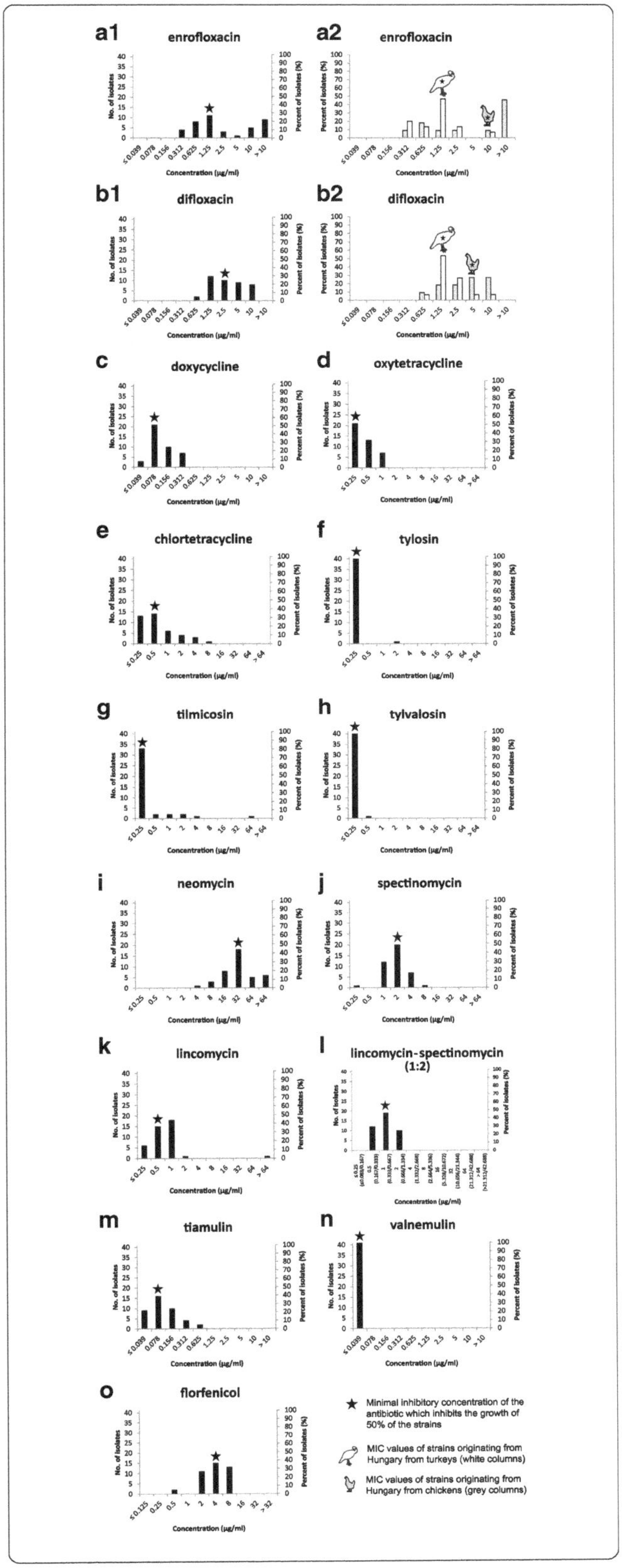

Fig. 1 MIC50 values are marked with asterisks. MIC values of 41 *M. synoviae* strains are demonstrated to enrofloxacin (**a1**), difloxacin (**b1**), doxycycline (**c**), oxytetracycline (**d**), chlortetracycline (**e**), tylosin (**f**), tilmicosin (**g**), tylvalosin (**h**), neomycin (**i**), spectinomycin (**j**), lincomycin (**k**), the combination of lincomycin and spectinomycin (**l**), tiamulin (**m**), valnemulin (**n**) and florfenicol (**o**). The MIC values for enrofloxacin (**a2**) and difloxacin (**b2**) of isolates originating from Hungary from meat-type turkeys (white columns; n = 15) and mostly breeder and layer chickens (grey columns; n = 11) are presented in individual diagrams also

showing intermediate susceptibility or resistance (MIC >1 µg/ml according to Hannan [20]) have been isolated also, even from Europe [13]. In avian *Mycoplasma* strains resistance to tilmicosin developed more readily and quicker than to tylosin under laboratory conditions [31]. Several previous studies reported the slow increase of resistance to tylosin in *M. synoviae* and *M. gallisepticum* in vitro also [7, 32, 33]. In the current examination, the majority of the strains were inhibited by low concentrations of tylvalosin and tylosin, and 90% of the strains were susceptible to tilmicosin (≤1 µg/ml) [5], confirming the high in vitro efficiency of these macrolides against *M. synoviae*. Elevated MIC values were detected primarily in the case of tilmicosin (with four strains reaching MIC >1 µg/ml), which is concordant with previous observations in vitro [31], and assumes the more rapid development of resistance against this agent.

Lincosamides have similar protein synthesis inhibitory mechanism on the 50S subunit of the bacterial ribosome as macrolides [34], and lincomycin was found to be efficacious against avian mycoplasmas before [3, 16]. Cross-resistance was described between macrolides and lincosamides and it was associated with mutations in the 23S ribosomal RNA of *M. synoviae* [35]. In the current study, all isolates showed susceptibility (≤2 µg/ml) [20] to lincomycin except for one outlier strain (MYCAV 185; MIC >64 µg/ml), which showed elevated MIC values to macrolides as well.

Aminoglycosides and aminocyclitols are most commonly administered for the treatment of bacterial enteritis in poultry [36, 37], and by the oral application these compounds absorb poorly from the gastrointestinal tract [38]. Previous in vitro examinations on the efficacy of neomycin against *M. synoviae* revealed that high concentrations of the antibiotic were needed for the inhibition of the pathogen (MICs 32–128 µg/ml) [30]. On the other hand, spectinomycin proved to be effective against the French and Iranian *M. synoviae* strains in vitro with MIC values below the susceptibility breakpoint of 4 µg/ml (according to CLSI [25]) [16, 28]. Potentially lower concentrations of spectinomycin were sufficient for the inhibition of the growth of *M. synoviae* when it was applied in combination with lincomycin [28], and this combination successfully controlled experimental *M. synoviae* infection in vivo before [9]. In the present study, the majority of the strains showed resistance to neomycin (MIC >4 µg/ml according to CLSI [25]) but were inhibited by spectinomycin at concentrations below the assumed breakpoint (MIC ≤4 µg/ml [25]). The combination of lincomycin with spectinomycin improved the efficacy of both antibiotics against most *M. synoviae* strains (Tables 1 and 2 and Additional file 1); therefore the use of their combination is supposed to be preferable in the therapy.

Pleuromutilins showed high in vitro effect against avian mycoplasmas before [7, 13] and have been used in the treatment of mycoplasmosis in poultry [39]. Resistance against these substances in *M. gallisepticum* and *M. synoviae* develops gradually [7], as only one mutation is enough for the elevation of MIC values, but to achieve high level resistance the combination of multiple mutations is required [39]. The *M. synoviae* strains examined in this study showed high susceptibility to tiamulin and valnemulin, assuming their potential in the therapy.

Phenicols are broad-spectrum antibiotics and showed in vitro activity against certain mycoplasmas before [23, 30, 38, 40]. In the present study, although two strains were inhibited by lower concentrations of florfenicol (MIC 0.5 µg/ml), narrow range of MICs was observed among the rest of the strains (MICs between 2 and 8 µg/ml), showing lower effectiveness of florfenicol against *M. synoviae* than reported in other studies or in *M. gallisepticum* [30, 40].

The observed differences between the initial and final MIC values of the mycoplasmastatic antibiotics chlortetracycline and lincomycin [34] lead to the recategorization of certain strains from susceptible to resistant during the interpretation of the results, while in other cases no difference was detected at all. Also, remarkable deviation of the MIC values for neomycin (which has concentration-dependent mycoplasmacidal effect [34]) was observed when initial and final readings were compared, although it did not alter significantly the interpretation of the data. Many factors may influence the growth of the bacteria in the in vitro tests; the discrepancies may indicate the inactivation of the used antibiotics during incubation, or the presence of a slower growing minor population which may have significance in the determination of official breakpoints in the future and in the estimation of the in vivo efficacy of the antibiotics [20, 24, 26]. The combined examination of the in vitro tests with pharmacokinetics/pharmacodynamics studies and in vivo experiments would probably enable the better understanding of the importance of the initial and final MIC values, and the differences in between. Nevertheless, freshly prepared antibiotic solutions are administered during treatment, which minimize the possibility of antibiotic inactivation and initial MIC values are evaluated in the standardized methods for human pathogen mycoplasmas as well [22]; therefore the initial MIC values are advised to be taken into account in the interpretation of the results in mycoplasmas with veterinary relevance.

Strains originating from the same farm but from different years possessed similar MIC values (e.g. strains from farms 4, 13 and 14; Table 1). However, apart from oxytetracycline, doxycycline, tylvalosin, valnemulin and the combination of lincomycin and spectinomycin, strains with elevated MIC values were detected in the cases of all antibiotics tested. Even more, as an alarming example for irresponsible antibiotic usage, one strain (MYCAV 185) showed high MIC values to several antibiotics, especially to fluoroquinolones, macrolides and to lincomycin. It is noteworthy, that the combined application of lincomycin with spectinomycin remarkably reduced the inhibitory antibiotic concentration against this strain (from $MIC_{lincomycin}$ > 64 µg/ml to $MIC_{lincomycin:spectinomycin}$ 2 µg/ml (0.666/1.334 µg/ml)). All of these observations highlight the importance of testing the antibiotic susceptibility of *M. synoviae* before treatment. On the other hand, in clinical cases when rapid intervention is needed (e.g. mortality or high morbidity with severe clinical signs) and the treatment cannot wait for the results of the time-consuming and laborious in vitro tests, the presented data may serve as a guide in the choice of the appropriate antibiotic therapy in the Central and Eastern European region.

Conclusions

Antibiotic susceptibility testing of *M. synoviae* is laborious and time-consuming, and is not performed in routine diagnostics, thus empirical antibiotic treatment is usually applied by the clinicians. The MIC values of the 41 *M. synoviae* strains provided in the present study revealed the in vitro effectiveness of tetracyclines, macrolides and pleuromutilins, and assume the potential usefulness of these agents in the therapy of mycoplasmosis in poultry in Central and Eastern Europe. However, elevated MIC values were observed in several cases during the examinations, which concerns antibiotics with importance in human medicine as well (e.g. fluoroquinolones). In order to preserve these critical antimicrobials for the therapy of humans, prudent antibiotic usage is recommended based on preliminary in vitro antibiotic susceptibility tests and on the careful evaluation of these data by considering the difficulties in the interpretation of the results and the factors influencing antibiotic effectiveness in vivo.

Abbreviation
MIC: Minimal inhibitory concentrations

Acknowledgements
Not applicable

Funding
This work was funded by the National Research, Development and Innovation Office (K119594), by the Lendület (Momentum) program (LP2012–22) of the Hungarian Academy of Sciences and by the MycoPath 2 pan-European antimicrobial susceptibility monitoring programme. MG was supported by the Bolyai János Research Fellowship of the Hungarian Academy of Sciences. The funders had no role in study design, data collection, analysis and interpretation, decision to publish, or preparation of the manuscript.

Authors' contributions
All authors read and approved the final version of this manuscript. ZK, DG, KMS, KN, DB collected the samples, analysed the data and wrote the manuscript. VH performed the examinations. MG designed the study, analysed the data and edited the manuscript.

Consent for publication
Not applicable

Competing interests
The authors declare that they have no competing interests.

Author details
[1]Institute for Veterinary Medical Research, Centre for Agricultural Research, Hungarian Academy of Sciences, Hungária körút 21, Budapest 1143, Hungary. [2]Biotechnical Faculty, University of Ljubljana, Groblje 3, SI-1230 Domžale, Slovenia.

References
1. Kleven SH. Control of avian mycoplasma infections in commercial poultry. Avian Dis. 2008;52:367–74.
2. Feberwee A, de Wit JJ, Landman WJ. Induction of eggshell apex abnormalities by *Mycoplasma synoviae*: field and experimental studies. Avian Pathol. 2009;38:77–85.
3. Stipkovits L, Kempf I. Mycoplasmoses in poultry. Rev Sci Tech. 1996;15: 1495–525.
4. Landman WJM. Is *Mycoplasma synoviae* outrunning *Mycoplasma gallisepticum*? A viewpoint from the Netherlands. Avian Pathol. 2014;43:2–8. doi: 10.1080/03079457.2014.881049.
5. Landman WJ, Mevius DJ, Veldman KT, Feberwee A. In vitro antibiotic susceptibility of Dutch *Mycoplasma synoviae* field isolates originating from joint lesions and the respiratory tract of commercial poultry. Avian Pathol. 2008;37:415–20.
6. McCormack WM. Susceptibility of mycoplasmas to antimicrobial agents: clinical implications. Clin Infect Dis. 1993;17(Suppl 1):200–1.
7. Gautier-Bouchardon AV, Reinhardt AK, Kobisch M, Kempf I. In vitro development of resistance to enrofloxacin, erythromycin, tylosin, tiamulin and oxytetracycline in *Mycoplasma gallisepticum*, *Mycoplasma iowae* and *Mycoplasma synoviae*. Vet Microbiol. 2002;88:47–58.
8. Kleven SH, Anderson DP. In vitro activity of various antibiotics against *Mycoplasma synoviae*. Avian Dis. 1971;15:551–7.
9. Hamdy AH, Kleven SH, McCune EL. Efficacy of Linco-Spectin water medication on *Mycoplasma synoviae* airsacculitis in broilers. Avian Dis. 1976;20:118–25.
10. Olson NO, Sahu SP. Efficacy of chlortetracycline against *Mycoplasma synoviae* isolated in two periods. Avian Dis. 1976;20:221–9.
11. Baughn CO, Alpaugh WC, Linkenheimer WH, Maplesden DC. Effect of tiamulin in chickens and turkeys infected experimentally with avian *Mycoplasma*. Avian Dis. 1978;22:620–6.
12. Bradbury JM, Yavari CA, Giles CJ. In Vitro evaluation of various antimicrobials against *Mycoplasma gallisepticum* and *Mycoplasma synoviae* by the micro-broth method, and comparison with a commercially prepared test system. Avian Pathol. 1994;23:105 15.
13. Hannan PCT, Windsor GD, de Jong A, Schmeer N, Stegeman M. Comparative susceptibilities of various animal-pathogenic mycoplasmas to fluoroquinolones. Antimicrob Agents Chemother. 1997;41:2037–40.
14. Wang C, Ewing M, Aarabi SY. In vitro susceptibility of avian mycoplasmas to enrofloxacin, sarafloxacin, tylosin, and oxytetracycline. Avian Dis. 2001;45: 456–60.
15. McAuliffe L, Ellis RJ, Miles K, Ayling RD, Nicholas RA. Biofilm formation by mycoplasma species and its role in environmental persistence and survival. Microbiol. 2006;152:913–22.
16. Dufour-Gesbert F, Dheilly A, Marois C, Kempf I. Epidemiological study on *Mycoplasma synoviae* infection in layers. Vet Microbiol. 2006;114:148–54.
17. Lysnyansky I, Gerchman I, Mikula I, Gobbo F, Catania S, Levisohn S. Molecular characterization of acquired enrofloxacin resistance in *Mycoplasma synoviae* field isolates. Antimicrob Agents Chemother. 2013;57:3072–7.
18. Frey ML, Hanson RP, Anderson DP. A Medium for the isolation of avian mycoplasmas. Am J Vet Res. 1968;29:2163–71.
19. Lauerman LH, Chilina AR, Closser JA, Johansen D. Avian *Mycoplasma* identification using polymerase chain reaction amplicon and restriction fragment length polymorphism analysis. Avian Dis. 1995;39:804–11.
20. Hannan PCT. Guidelines and recommendations for antimicrobial minimum inhibitory concentration (MIC) testing against veterinary mycoplasma species. Vet Res. 2000;31:373–95.
21. Clinical and Laboratory Standards Institute (CLSI). Methods for antimicrobial susceptibility testing for human mycoplasmas; Approved guideline. CLSI document M43-A. Wayne PA: Clinical and Laboratory Standards Institute; 2011.
22. Waites KB, Duffy LB, Bébéar CM, Matlow A, Talkington DF, Kenny GE, Totten PA, Bade DJ, Zheng X, Davidson MK, Shortridge VD, Watts JL, Brown SD. Standardized methods and quality control limits for agar and broth microdilution susceptibility testing of *Mycoplasma pneumoniae*, *Mycoplasma hominis*, and *Ureaplasma urealyticum*. J Clin Microbiol. 2012;50:3542–7. doi: 10.1128/JCM.01439-12.
23. Waites KB, Lysnyansky I, Bébéar CM. Emerging antimicrobial resistance in mycoplasmas of humans and animals. In: Browning G, Citti C, editors. Mollicutes: molecular biology and pathogenesis. Norfolk: Caister academic press; 2014. p. 289–322.
24. Gerchman I, Lysnyansky I, Perk S, Levisohn S. In vitro susceptibilities to fluoroquinolones in current and archived *Mycoplasma gallisepticum* and *Mycoplasma synoviae* isolates from meat-type turkeys. Vet Microbiol. 2008; 131:266–76. doi: 10.1016/j.vetmic.2008.04.006.
25. Clinical and Laboratory Standards Institute (CLSI). Performance standards for antimicrobial disk and dilution susceptibility tests for bacteria isolated from animals. Wayne, PA. Approved standard (fourth edition) and second informational supplement. CLSI document VET01-A4 and VET01-S2. In: CLSI 2013; 2013.
26. Cooper AC, Fuller JR, Fuller MK, Whittlestone P, Wise DR. In vitro activity of danofloxacin, tylosin and oxytetracycline against mycoplasmas of veterinary importance. Res Vet Sci. 1993;54:329–34.
27. Cerda RO, Giacoboni GI, Xavier JA, Sansalone PL, Landoni MF. In vitro antibiotic susceptibility of field isolates of *Mycoplasma synoviae* in Argentina. Avian Dis. 2002;46:215–8.
28. Behbahan NGG, Asasi K, Afsharifar AR, Pourbakhsh SA. Susceptibilities of *Mycoplasma gallispeticum* and *Mycoplasma synoviae* isolates to antimicrobial agents *in vitro*. Int J Poult Sci. 2008;7:1058–64.
29. Islam KMS, Klein U, Burch DGS. The activity and compatibility of the antibiotic tiamulin with other drugs in poultry medicine—a review. Poult Sci. 2009;88:2353–9.
30. Kibeida, OAI. A comparison of methods used to measure the *in vitro* antimicrobial susceptibilities of *Mycoplasma* species of animal origin. 2010; MSc dissertation, University of Pretoria, Pretoria. http://repository.up.ac.za/handle/2263/26686?show=full Accessed 13 Nov 2017.
31. Wu CM, Wu H, Ning Y, Wang J, Du X, Shen J. Induction of macrolide resistance in *Mycoplasma gallisepticum in vitro* and its resistance-related mutations within domain V of 23S rRNA. FEMS Microbiol Letters. 2005;247:199–205.
32. Zanella A, Martino PA, Pratelli A, Stonfer M. Development of antibiotic resistance in *Mycoplasma gallisepticum in vitro*. Avian Pathol. 1998;27:591–6.
33. Takahashi I, Yoshida T, Higashide Y, Sawada T. Vitro resistance acquisition in *Mycoplasma gallisepticum* against ofloxacin, tylosin and spectinomycin. Jpn J Antibiot. 2002;55:291 301.

34. Lysnyansky I, Ayling RD. *Mycoplasma bovis*: mechanisms of resistance and trends in antimicrobial susceptibility. Front Microbiol. 2016;7:595. doi: 10.3389/fmicb.2016.00595.
35. Lysnyansky I, Gerchman I, Flaminio B, Catania S. Decreased susceptibility to macrolide–lincosamide in *Mycoplasma synoviae* is associated with mutations in 23S ribosomal RNA. Microbial Drug Resist. 2015;21:581–9. doi: 10.1089/mdr.2014.0290.
36. Marrett LE, Robb EJ, Frank RK. Efficacy of neomycin sulfate water medication on the control of mortality associated with colibacillosis in growing turkeys. Poult Sci. 2000;79:12–7.
37. Agunos A, Carson C, Léger D. Antimicrobial therapy of selected diseases in turkeys, laying hens, and minor poultry species in Canada. Can Vet J. 2013; 54:1041–52.
38. Goetting V, Lee KA, Tell LA. Pharmacokinetics of veterinary drugs in laying hens and residues in eggs: a review of the literature. J Vet Pharmacol Therap. 2011;34:521–56. doi: 10.1111/j.1365-2885.2011.01287.x.
39. Li BB, Shen JZ, Cao XY, Wang Y, Dai L, Huang SY, Wu CM. Mutations in 23S rRNA gene associated with decreased susceptibility to tiamulin and valnemulin in *Mycoplasma gallisepticum*. FEMS Microbiol Letters. 2010;308:144–9.
40. Gharaibeh S, Al-Rashdan M. Change in antimicrobial susceptibility of *Mycoplasma gallisepticum* field isolates. Vet Microbiol. 2011;150:379–83.
41. Slavec B, Berčič RL, Cizelj I, Narat M, Zorman-Rojs O, Dovč P, Benčina D. Variation of *vlhA* gene in *Mycoplasma synoviae* clones isolated from chickens. Avian Path. 2011;40:481–9.
42. Dušanić D, Berčič RL, Cizelj I, Salmič S, Narat M, Benčina D. *Mycoplasma synoviae* invades non-phagocytic chicken cells *in vitro*. Vet Microbiol. 2009; 138:114–9.
43. Kempf I, Ollivier C, L'Hospitalier R, Guittet M, Bennejean G. Concentrations minimales inhibitrices de 13 antibiotiques vis-à-vis de 21 souches de mycoplasmes de volailles. Le Point Vétérinaire. 1989;20:935–40.

18

Pathology of carbon monoxide poisoning in two cats

Arya Sobhakumari[1], Robert H. Poppenga[1], J. Brad Pesavento[1] and Francisco A. Uzal[2*]

Abstract

Background: Carbon monoxide (CO), a common cause of poisoning in human beings has also been implicated in the death of animals. Though there are multiple studies on CO poisoning and relevant lethal blood COHb concentrations in humans, there are no reliable reports of diagnostic lethal carboxyhemoglobin percentage of saturation (COHb%) in cats. Additionally, due to shared housing environments, exposures to companion animals can be a surrogate for lethal exposures in human beings and provide valuable information in concurrent forensic investigations.

Case presentation: Two adult Singapura brown ticked cats were submitted to the California Animal Health and Food Safety Laboratory (CAHFS) for necropsy and diagnostic work-up. These animals were found dead along with their two deceased owners. Similar lesions were observed in both cats. At necropsy, gross lesions consisted of multifocal, large, irregular, bright red spots on the skin of the abdomen and the inner surface of ear pinnae, bright red muscles and blood. The carcasses, and tissues fixed in formalin retained the bright red discoloration for up to two weeks. Microscopic lesions included diffuse pulmonary congestion and edema, and multifocal intense basophilia of cardiomyocytes mostly affecting whole fibers or occasionally a portion of the fiber. Based on the clinical history,gross and microscopic changes, cyanide or carbon monoxide poisoning was suspected. Blood samples analyzed for carbon monoxide showed 57 and 41% carboxyhemoglobin COHb%. Muscle samples were negative for cyanide.

Conclusion: There are no established reference values for lethal COHb concentration in cats. The COHb % values detected in this case which fell within the lethal range reported for other species, along with the gross lesions and unique histological findings in the heart suggest a helpful criteria for diagnosis of CO intoxication associated death in cats. This case demonstrates that since pets share the same environment as human beings and often are a part of their activities, they can be useful adjuncts in potential forensic investigations to help solve human cases.

Keywords: Carbon monoxide, Cats, COHb %, Forensic investigation

Background

Carbon monoxide (CO) poisoning has been frequently described in human beings. However, information about CO poisoning and associated lesions in animals is scant to non-existent, especially in cats. In particular, there are no reports of diagnostic lethal carboxyhemoglobin percentage of saturation (COHb%) in cats and the threshold for toxicity in this species has not been established. It is possible that animal cases remain undiagnosed due to lack of adequate testing opportunities in veterinary diagnostic laboratories. The main reason for CO poisoning in human beings is incomplete combustion of hydrocarbons in non-ventilated buildings, associated with faulty furnaces and house fires. This seems to be the same mechanism for CO poisoning in companion animals such as dogs and cats, because of their shared environment with humans.

CO has more than 210 times greater affinity for hemoglobin than oxygen (O_2) [1], readily forming carboxyhemoglobin (COHb), thus reducing the oxygen carrying capacity of red blood cells and leading to hypoxemia and tissue hypoxia. Formation of COHb not only displaces oxygen but CO causes a conformational change in hemoglobin after the binding, resulting in greater affinity for oxygen in the remaining heme moieties. This leads to a shift to left of the O_2 dissociation curve and reduced delivery of O_2 to tissues [2, 3]. CO

* Correspondence: fuzal@cahfs.ucdavis.edu
[2]California Animal Health and Food Safety Laboratory System, San Bernardino branch, School of Veterinary Medicine, University of California Davis, 105 W Central Ave, San Bernardino, CA 92408, USA
Full list of author information is available at the end of the article

has high affinity for myoglobin and binding to cardiac myoglobin can cause myocardial depression, hypotension and arrhythmias. Cardiac decompensation results in further tissue hypoxia which is the ultimate cause of death [4].

Current scientific literature on spontaneous CO intoxication in small animals is limited. While a few papers have been published describing spontaneous CO intoxication in dogs [3, 5, 6], there are no reports that covered gross and histological lesions in various organs in cats. There is only one report on respiratory distress upon CO poisoning in cats, although pathology of the intoxication was not described in that report [7].

This case describes for the first time in detail the gross, microscopic and toxicological findings, specifically the lethal blood COHb concentration, in two cats that died following CO intoxication. This report also indicates the utility of postmortem blood as a feasible sample for diagnostic confirmation. Additionally, it emphasizes the significance of testing animals as a useful adjunct to concurrent human forensic investigations since pets share the same environment as owners and face similar risks with respect to exposure to various chemicals, including CO.

Case presentation

Two adult Singapura brown ticked cats (a spayed female and a neutered male) were submitted to the San Bernardino branch of CAHFS for necropsy and diagnostic work up. The cats had been found dead in a household together with their two deceased owners. The exact date of death was unknown.

Grossly, both cat carcasses were in good nutritional condition and moderate state of postmortem decomposition. The stomach of cat A was almost empty except for ~ 2 mls of mucous fluid and the stomach of cat B had a ~ 50 mls of semi digested kibble. Both cats presented the following gross abnormalities: bright pink-red discoloration of the aqueous fluid (this change was most marked in Cat A), multifocally bright red discoloration on the skin of the abdomen (Fig. 1) and inner surface of the ear pinnae (Fig. 2), bright red skeletal muscles, congestion and bright red discoloration of the abdominal serosa, congested and edematous lungs, mild hydrothorax and hydropericardium. No other significant gross abnormalities were observed in either carcasses. In particular, no gross abnormalities were observed in the brain of either cat.

After necropsy, the carcasses were stored refrigerated for two weeks before they were submitted for cremation, and they retained the bright red discoloration for the whole period (Fig. 3). Formalin fixed tissues and the formalin in which tissues were immersed, retained similar discoloration for the first two weeks after collection; this discoloration faded progressively after that.

Tissue samples from most organs of both cats, including representative areas of the brain (cortex, corpus striatum, thalamus, midbrain, cerebellum and medulla), were routinely processed for the production of HE stained sections. Selected sections of heart from both animals were also stained with Von Kossa to investigate possible calcium deposits and Phosphotungstic acid hematoxylin (PTHA) to highlight the structure of myocardiocytes.

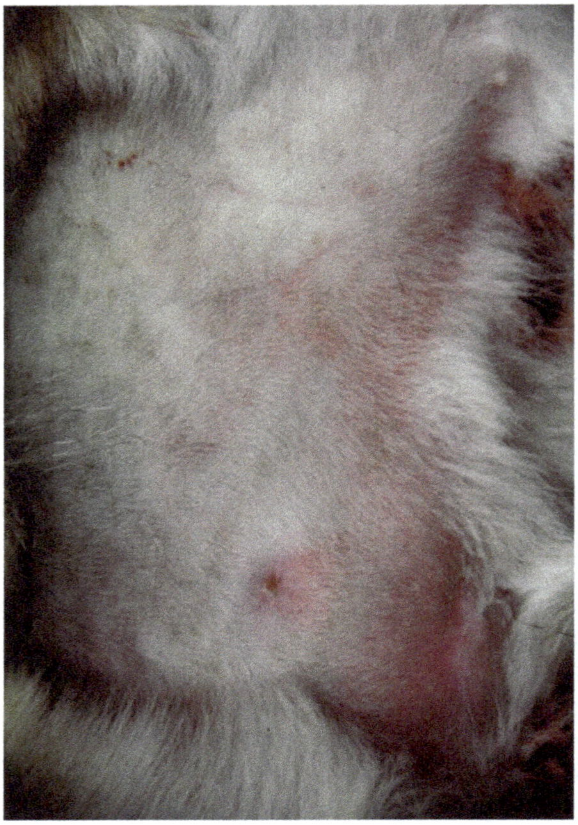

Fig. 1 Gross findings in a cat with carbon monoxide intoxication. Bright red discoloration on the skin of the abdomen

Microscopic lesions were similar in both cats and included diffuse pulmonary congestion, interstitial and alveolar edema, and multifocal intense basophilia of cardiomyocytes (Fig. 4). The latter mostly affected whole fibers but occasionally only a portion of the fiber, with a clear transverse line of demarcation from the rest of the fiber. Rarely, discrete areas of hypercontraction bands were seen in individual cardiomyocytes; these lesions were visible on HE sections but were highlighted on PTHH stained sections. Examination of Von Kossa stained sections of the heart was unremarkable. No other significant microscopic abnormalities were observed in any of these cats. Transmission electron microscopy of formalin fixed heart from both cats was performed but was unrewarding.

Based on the clinical history, gross and microscopic changes, cyanide or carbon monoxide poisoning was suspected. Skeletal muscle from both cats was analyzed

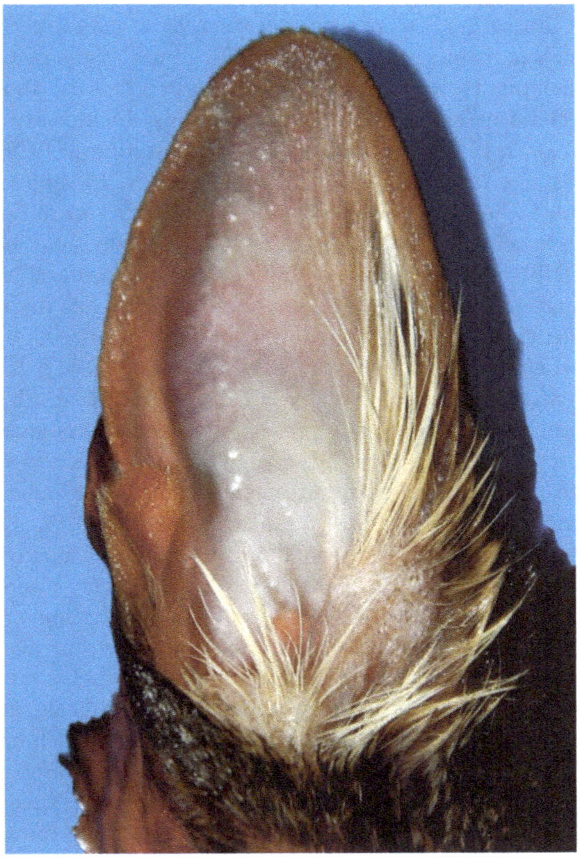

Fig. 2 Gross findings in a cat with carbon monoxide intoxication. Bright red discoloration on the inner surface of the ear pinna

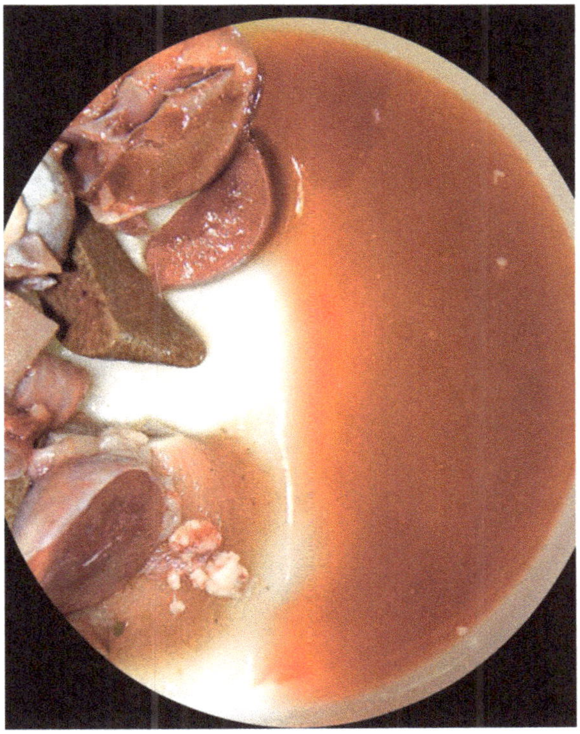

Fig. 3 Gross findings in a cat with carbon monoxide intoxication. Bright red discolored formalin where tissues were immersed for 2 weeks

for cyanide by a distillation method as previously described [8]. Briefly, cyanide in the tissues was converted to hydrogen cyanide gas which was chlorinated and converted to a colored dye. The absorbance was then measured spectrophotometrically at 578 nm and cyanide quantitated from a standard curve. Cyanide was not detected in the muscle of either cat at or above a reporting limit of 1 ppm.

Since the cyanide test was negative, postmortem blood samples were analyzed for CO by a modification of the Comopac® electrochemical gas meter as previously described [9]. Briefly, blood was mixed with saturated sodium chloride in a screw top glass vial adapted to fit onto a Genesis® portable CO monitor (Thermo Scientific) and CO, liberated in a closed headspace, was measured for 5 min. The Hb was measured by an azidemethemoglobin method using HemoCue® Hb 201 System. The blood COHb was reported as % saturation of Hb with CO. COHb saturation was 57% and 41% for cats A and B, respectively.

Discussion and conclusions

In this case, a presumptive diagnosis of CO intoxication was established based on the clinical history, gross and microscopic findings. Gross and microscopic changes have not been described before in cats intoxicated with carbon dioxide. In humans and other animals intoxicated with CO bright red discoloration of skin, mucosas and muscle, cherry red color of the blood and brain changes related to anoxia, including necrosis in the cortex and white matter of cerebral hemispheres, globus pallidus and brainstem have been described and are suggestive, but non-specific for this intoxication [3, 5, 6]. These changes are not, however, considered pathognomonic and confirmation of the diagnosis should be based on detection of toxic levels of COHb in the blood of cadavers, which is standard practice in human forensic medicine.

In this case, both cats had gross findings considered compatible with carbon monoxide intoxication in humans and dogs [3, 5, 6]. In addition, bot animals had blood values of COHb which are considered toxic for humans and, in absence of reference values for cats, this finding was used to confirm the diagnosis of CO intoxication.

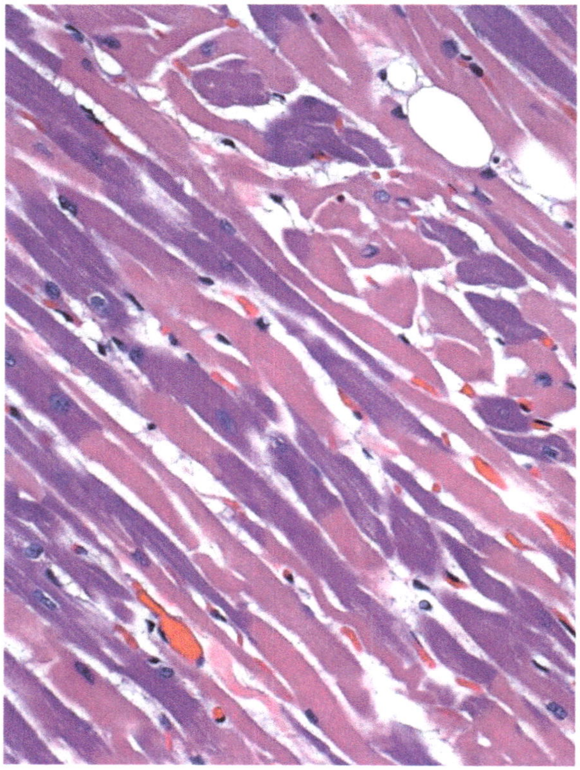

Fig. 4 Microscopic findings in a cat with carbon monoxide intoxication. Multifocal basophilia in cardyomyocytes. HE, 250X

Brain changes have been described in human beings and dogs intoxicated with carbon monoxide before. In the cats presented here, no gross or microscopic lesions were observed in the brain. This might be related to a very acute clinical course with no time for central nervous system lesion development. This is, however, only speculation, as clinical information was not available on these cats which were found dead.

The microscopic discoloration of cardiomyocytes of these two cats is an unusual lesion that has not been described before in humans or animals intoxicated with CO. Because no ultrastructural lesions were observed in the heart of either cat, the pathogenesis of this discoloration could not be determined; it is possible that biochemical alterations not accompanied by morphological (microscopic or ultrastructural) changes occurred associated with CO intoxication.

CO is a colorless, odorless, non-irritant gas produced by incomplete combustion of fuels and is a leading cause of human poisoning and mortality in the US [10]. Two mechanisms of action (acute and delayed) exist for CO intoxication. The formation of COHb in intoxicated individuals decreases the oxygen carrying capacity of hemoglobin and shifts the O_2 dissociation curve to the left impairing O_2 release resulting in tissue hypoxia, which is mainly responsible for the clinical signs of CO poisoning. However, it has been suggested that the above mechanism alone does not account for the toxicity of CO since in many instances the concentration of COHb does not correlate with the clinical signs. In an early study, when dogs were exposed to 13% CO in atmospheric air, the animals died within one hour and had COHb concentrations of 54-90% [5]. However, the transfusion of 80% COHb saturated blood to healthy recipient dogs which resulted in a similar 57 – 64% COHb in their blood did not cause intoxication [5, 11]. It is suggested that acute toxicity of CO may be the result of binding of CO to heme proteins other than hemoglobin such as cytochromes and myoglobin, which interferes with cellular respiration and generation of free radicals through disruption of oxidative metabolism [12, 13]. Additionally, CO has been found to stimulate guanylyl cyclase resulting in relaxation of vascular smooth muscles, cerebral vasodilation and loss of consciousness [6, 14]. CO also displaces nitric oxide (NO) from platelets leading to peroxynitrite formation, endothelial damage, leukocyte adhesion, formation of free radicals, and lipid peroxidation in the brain microvasculature which may be a mechanism for delayed neurological sequelae [15].

Levels of COHb have been measured in many species both at baseline and associated with lethality. In human beings, clinical signs of CO toxicity start at 20% COHb and death occurs between 50 and 80% COHb [16]. In dogs mortality was reported to occur within one hour when exposed to 13% CO in atmospheric air with subsequent COHb concentrations of 54-90% [5]. Ashbaugh measured COHb in healthy, clinically normal dogs and fire victim dogs, and found that the values ranged between 5.6 - 6.4% and 8.3 - 37%, respectively [17]. COHb concentration has been reported in two cats that became ataxic and tachypneic following exposure to generator fumes in a closed warehouse for 8 h [7]. These animals had COHb concentrations of 5 and 9% which declined to baselines levels of 0-4% after oxygen therapy and supportive treatment. However, there are no guidelines to interpret lethal COHb concentrations in blood of cats intoxicated with CO. In the present case, the concentration of COHb in both the cats fell within the lethal ranges reported for dogs and humans. Since no previous data was available to compare, we concluded that the detected concentrations are lethal for cats in the context of the characteristic lesions.

Although measurement of blood COHb is used as a diagnostic tool for CO poisoning, it may not fully correlate with the severity of the symptoms. The COHb in blood is not an absolute index of compromised oxygen delivery at the tissue level. Additionally, unmeasured CO uptake in tissues, which is hypothesized to increase during hypoxia because of the competition of CO and O2 on the binding site of hemoproteins also contributes to the clinical signs. Therefore, the limitation of COHb levels is that it can be used to guide therapeutic strategies but not predict treatment outcomes [7, 18].

The incidence of CO intoxication in pets is unknown. The Pet Poison Helpline (St. Paul, Minnesota) receives an average of 3 – 4 suspected or confirmed cases of CO poisoning every year, with a potential for many suspicious cases unconfirmed due to lack of adequate diagnostic facilities.

Because of the proximity of pets to human beings, investigation of morbidity or mortality can be valuable in concurrent human forensic investigations. The use of dog and cat hair DNA, tissues, saliva and pet food remnants have become more common in criminal investigations helping solve numerous cases [19, 20]. An unusual case of apparent suicide/homicide involving two human beings and a dog was described where the cause of death was identified to be diazepam overdose which was later detected in the liver tissue and dog food remnants [21]. In the present case, the presumed sudden death of both human beings and the cats in the same environment bolsters the argument that a multidisciplinary approach involving pets would be more likely to yield successful investigational outcomes since both species were likely exposed to the same toxicant.

Abbreviations

CAHFS: California Animal Health and Food Safety Laboratory; CO: Carbon monoxide; COHb: Carboxyhemoglobin; COHb%: Carboxyhemoglobin percentage of saturation; HB: Hemoglobin; mls: Milliliters; O_2: Oxygen; ppm: Parts per million; PTAH: Phosphotungstic acid hematoxylin

Acknowledgements

The authors thank Sabine Hargrave and Bill Torres for the chemical analysis.

Funding

CAHFS provided financial support for publication of this article.

Authors' contributions

FAU performed necropsy, described the histopathological findings, wrote part of the manuscript and edited several versions of it including the final version. JBP performed the electron microscopy. AS facilitated the toxicology analysis, interpreted the results and wrote the manuscript. RHP provided helpful discussions, critically reviewed the manuscript and added final corrections. All authors approved the final manuscript.

Ethics approval

Post-mortem samples were collected in accordance with institutional guidelines. The two cats included in this study were submitted to our laboratory (the California Animal health and Food Safety Lab –CAHFS-) by the legal owner of these animals, a state government agency for necropsy and diagnostic work up to establish cause of death. Per UCDavis and CAHFS regulations, neither ethics approval nor consent to use diagnostic material submitted to our lab for publication is required. The submitter signed the following statement in the submission form which accompanied the bodies of these two cats: "I understand that spec mens submitted are the property of CAHFS".

Consent for publication

Not applicable. Please see above.

Competing interests

The authors declare that they have no competing interests.

Author details

[1]California Animal Health and Food Safety Laboratory System, Davis branch, School of Veterinary Medicine, University of California Davis, Davis, USA. [2]California Animal Health and Food Safety Laboratory System, San Bernardino branch, School of Veterinary Medicine, University of California Davis, 105 W Central Ave, San Bernardino, CA 92408, USA.

References

1. Rodkey FL, O'Neal JD, Collison HA, Uddin DE. Relative affinity of hemoglobin S and hemoglobin a for carbon monoxide and oxygen. Clin Chem. 1974;20:83–4.
2. Roughton F, Darling F. The effect of carbon monoxide on oxy-hemoglobin dissociation curve. Am J Phys. 1944;141 17–31.
3. Kent M, Creevy KE, Delahunta A. Clinical and neuropathological findings of acute carbon monoxide toxicity in chihuahuas following smoke inhalation. J Am Anim Hosp Assoc. 2010;46:259–64.
4. Blumenthal I. Carbon monoxide poison ng. J R Soc Med. 2001;94:270–2.
5. Varma D, Chemtob S. Carbonmonoxide: from public health risk to painless killer. In: Gupta RC, editor. Handbook of toxicology of chemical warfare agents. Amsterdam: Academic Press; 2009. p. 267–81.
6. Ashbaugh EA, Mazzaferro EM, McKierman BC, Drobatz KJ. The association of physical examination abnormalities and carboxyhemoglobin concentrations in 21 dogs trapped in a kennel fire. J Vet Emerg Crit Care (San Antonio). 2012;22:361–7.
7. Berent A, Todd J, Sergeeff J, Powell LL. Carbon monoxide toxicity: a case series. J Vet Emerg Crit Care. 2005;15:123–35.
8. APHA. Method 4500-CN. In: Standard methods for examination of water and waste water: American Public Health Association; 1985. https://archive.org/stream/gov.law.apha.method.4500-cn.1992/apha.method.4500-cn.1992_djvu.txt. Accessed 20 Oct 2017.
9. Bogusz M, Aderjan R, Bosche J. The determination of carbon monoxide in blood by means of electrochemical pocket gas meter. J Anal Toxicol. 1988; 12:225–8.
10. American Association of Poison Control Centers provides safety recommendations to avoid poison hazards this holiday season. In: American association of poison control Centres. Alexandria, Virginia; 2016. http://www.aapcc.org/press/52/. Accessed 20 Oct 2017.
11. Goldbaum LR, Ramirez RG, Absalon KB. What is the mechanism of carbon monoxide toxicity? Aviat Space Environ Med. 1975;46:1289–91.
12. Ball EG, Strittmatter CF, Cooper O. The reaction of cytochrome oxidase with carbon monoxide. J Biol Chem. 1951;193:635–47.
13. Cooper CE, Brown GC. The inhibition of mitochondrial cytochrome oxidase by the gases carbon monoxide, nitric oxide, hydrogen cyanide and hydrogen sulfide: chemical mechanism and physiological significance. J Bioenerg Biomembr. 2008;40:533–9.
14. Verma A, Hirsch DJ, Glatt CE, Ronnett GV, Snyder SH. Carbon monoxide: a putative neural messenger. Science. 1993;259:381–4.
15. Utz J, Ullrich V. Carbon monoxide relaxes ileal smooth muscle through activation of guanylate cyclase. Biochem Pharmacol. 1991;41:1195–201.
16. Thom SR. Carbon monoxide-mediated brain lipid peroxidation in the rat. J Appl Physiol. 1990;68:997–1003.
17. Ryter SW, Otterbein LW. Carbon monox de in biology and medicine. BioEssays. 2004;26:270–80.

18. Abelsohn A, Sanborn MD, Jessiman BJ, Weir E. Identifying and managing adverse environmental health effects: carbon monoxide poisoning. CMAJ. 2002;166:1685–90.
19. Menotti-Raymond MA, David VA, O'Brien OJ. Pet cat hair implicates murder suspect. Nature. 1997;386:774.
20. Halverson J. Pet forensics. In: Joy of DNA Sherlock's DNA case files. http://joyofdna.com/dr-joys-story-2/. Accessed 21 Oct 2017.
21. Harding BE, Sullivan LM, Adams S, Middleberg RA, Wolf BC. Multidisciplinary investigation of an unusual apparent homicide/suicide. Am J Forensic Med Pathol. 2011;32:208–12.

19

Trypsin-independent porcine epidemic diarrhea virus US strain with altered virus entry mechanism

Yunjeong Kim, Changin Oh, Vinay Shivanna, Richard A. Hesse and Kyeong-Ok Chang*

Abstract

Background: Porcine Epidemic Diarrhea Virus (PEDV) is a coronavirus that infects the intestinal tract and causes diarrhea and vomiting in older pigs or extreme dehydration and death that could reach 100% mortality in neonatal piglets. In the US, the first PEDV outbreaks occurred in 2013 and since then US PEDV strains have quickly spread throughout the US and worldwide, causing significant economic and public health concerns. Currently two conditionally approved vaccines exist in the US, but there is no live attenuated vaccine, which is considered the best option in controlling PEDV by inducing transferrable mucosal immunity to susceptible neonatal piglets. In this study, we passaged an US PEDV isolate under various conditions to generate three strains and characterized their growth and antigenicity in cell culture using various assays including Western blot analysis, serum neutralization assay, sequencing analysis and confocal microscopy. Finally, these strains were evaluated for pathogenicity in nursing piglets (1–4 days old).

Results: One of the PEDV strains generated in this study (designated as PEDV 8aa) is able to replicate in cells without any protease and grows to a high titer of >8 $\log_{10}$ $TCID_{50}$/ml in cell culture. Interestingly, replication of PEDV 8aa was severely reduced by trypsin and this correlated with the inhibition of virus attachment and entry into the cells. In neonatal nursing piglets, PEDV 8aa (passage number 70 or 105) was found to be fully attenuated with limited virus shedding.

Conclusions: These results suggest that applying selective pressure during viral passages can facilitate attainment of viral attenuation and that PEDV 8aa warrants further investigation as an attenuated vaccine.

Keywords: Porcine epidemic diarrhea virus, Coronavirus, Virus entry, Attenuation, Live attenuated vaccine, trypsin independent, entry

Background

Porcine epidemic diarrhea virus (PEDV) is a coronavirus that can cause diarrhea and vomiting in the affected pigs with high mortality of up to 100% in neonatal piglets. Since the first report of PEDV case in the UK in 1971 [1], PEDV has spread throughout the EU during the 1970s and 1980s [2, 3]. While PEDV strains are classified into two distinct genogroups (1 and 2) and subgroups within the genogroups (a and b) [4, 5], recent reports suggest more than 2 genogroups may exist in the field [6]. In the last 30 years or so, PEDV genogroup 1 (and more recently genogroup 2) caused outbreaks with extensive economic losses in some Asian countries with up to 80% to 100% morbidity and 50% to 90% fatality in suckling piglets [7–9]. In the US, the first PEDV outbreaks occurred in 2013 [10]. Since then the US PEDV strains that belong to subgroup 2a have quickly spread to the most states as well as Canada and Mexico [4, 11–13]. The US PEDV strains were also reported to have caused outbreaks in Asian and European countries [14–23], raising significant economic and public health concerns worldwide [24, 25]. Modified live attenuated vaccines (MLVs) for PEDV genogroup 1 are available in Asian countries, and they have been the major means to control PEDV [26–29]. However, the genogroup 1 MLVs may not provide effective protective immunity to the circulating subgroup 2a PEDV strains due to the genetic diversity of about 10% in the S1 gene between the genogroups [4, 11, 30]. Currently two conditionally approved vaccines exist in the US: alphavirus-based vaccine (Harrisvacccines) and an inactivated vaccine

* Correspondence: kchang@vet.ksu.edu
Diagnostic Medicine and pathobiology, College of Veterinary Medicine, Kansas State University, 1800 Denison Avenue, Manhattan, KS 66506, USA

(Zoetis) [31]. However, MLVs are not yet available for US PEDV strains.

Administration of an MLV, followed by a booster dose of an inactivated vaccine or an MLV in pregnant sows is generally considered an effective measure for controlling PEDV; MLV would effectively prime the immune system of the pregnant sows, especially PEDV naïve sows, for the production of antibodies, which are transferred to neonatal piglets and protect them from viral infections during the most susceptible period (< 2 weeks of age) [26, 32]. In this study, to develop an MLV for US PEDV strains, we isolated an US PEDVstrain and serially passaged the virus under various culture conditions, using trypsin, elastase and glychenodeoxycholic acid (GCDCA), for up to 120 passages in Vero cells. The resulting virus strains, designated as PEDV KD (grown in trypsin), PEDV AA (in elastase) and PEDV 8aa (in GCDCA), were characterized for their growth in cell culture and/or evaluated for attenuation in piglets. After serial passages, PEDV 8aa gained the ability to replicate in cells without any protease, and grew to a high titer of >8 $\log_{10}$ tissue culture infectious dose 50 ($TCID_{50}$)/ml in cell culture. Interestingly, the replication of PEDV 8aa was severely reduced by trypsin and this correlated with the inhibition of virus attachment and entry into the cells. While PEDV KD or PEDV AA retained virulence even after passage number 100, PEDV 8aa showed complete attenuation in neonatal piglets after passage number 70. These results warrant further investigation of PEDV 8aa as an MLV candidiate.

Methods

Ethics statement

All animal studies were conducted at Life Science Annex, University of Nebraska, Lincoln, in strict compliance with the Animal Welfare Act, PHS Policy and other federal statutes and regulations relating to animals and approved by the Institutional Animal Care and Use Committee at University of Nebraska at Lincoln (Protocol Number:1006). Animals were monitored twice daily for illness such as weight loss, dehydration or loss of mobility and all efforts were made to minize suffering. Animals that show clincal signs were assessed by an attending veterinarian and euthanized using euthanasia solution after being anesthetized in accordance with the regulations.

Cells, viruses, and reagents

Vero (ATCC®-CCL-81™) cells were obtained from ATCC (Manassas, VA). Cells were maintained in Dulbecco's minimal essential medium (DMEM) containing 5% fetal bovine serum (FBS) and antibiotics (chlortetracycline [25 μg/ml], penicillin [250 U/ml], and streptomycin [250 μg/ml]). L-1-tosylamide-2-phenylethyl chloromethyl ketone (TPCK)-treated trypsin and GCDCA were purchased from Sigma-Aldrich (St Louis, MO) and elastase from porcine pancreas was obtained from Promega (Madison, WI). For the isolation of an US PEDV strain, the day 4 intestinal contents from a pig inoculated with a stool sample from an Indiana farm with a PEDV outbreak in 2013 [33] were diluted in minimum essential medium (MEM) for 1:10 and filtrated using a 0.2 μm membrane filter. The prepared sample was inoculated to confluent Vero cells grown in the 6-well plates. The cells were then incubated at 37 °C in the presence of trypsin (1–2 μg/ml) in MEM. After 2 or 3 blind passages, apparent cytopathic effects (CPEs) were observed in Vero cells. Viruses were further cloned with the limited dilution method and the cloned virus (P0) was confirmed as PEDV by IFA with an anti-PEDV antibody and the sequencing of spike (S) gene. The individual or pooled convalescent pig serum collected at 43 days after the virus inoculation from the previous pig challenge study [33] were used as the source of anti-PEDV antibody. The pooled sera collected prior to the virus inoculation were used as the negative control.

Virus passages

The isolated PEDV (P0) was passaged in the presence of trypsin (1 μg/ml), elastase (1 μg/ml) or GCDCA (100 μM) in the media to generate PEDV KD, PEDV AA or PEDV 8aa, respectively. Viruses were further passaged in each condition for up to 120 passages. Every 3–5 passages, the titers of PEDV KD, PEDV AA or PEDV 8aa were determined by the $TCID_{50}$ method (Reed-Muench method) in the presence of trypsin (1 μg/ml), elastase (1 μg/ml) or GCDCA (100 μM), respectively. These viruses were characterized using various experiments, including real time reverse transcription-quantitative polymerase chain reaction (RT-qPCR), immunofluorescent assay (IFA), Western blot analysis and inoculation to neonatal piglets. The PEDV N gene from PEDV P0 was amplified with primers of forward primer (aattCTCGAG atggcttctgtcagttttcagg) and reverse primer (aattGCGGC CGCttaatttcctgtgtcgaag) and amplied product was cloned in to the pSI vector (Promega, Madison, WI) using XhoI and NotI enzymes resulted in pSI-PEDV-N. The recombinant plasmid was transfected to Vero cells to express PEDV N to confirm the reactivity of antisera agaisnt the protein. Cell lysates were prepared at 24 h afte the tranfection for the Western blot analysis.

Real-time RT-qPCR

PEDV RNA was extracted from the stool samples or cell culture following repeated freezing and thrawing using the RNeasy Kit (Qiagen, Valencia, CA) according to the manufacturer's protocol. Real-time RT-qPCR was performed by using One-Step Platinum RT-qPCR kit (Invitrogen, Carlsbad, CA) using forward primer- 5′-GCTATGCTCA-GATCGCCAGT-3′, reverse primer- 5′- TCTCGTAA

GAGTCCGCTAGCTC-3′, and Probe- 5′–/56-FAM/TGCTCTTTG/ZEN/GTGGTAATGTGGC/3IABkFQ/–3′ targeting the N gene. The RT-qPCR amplification was performed in a Rotor-Gene Q (Qiagen) with the following conditions: 50 °C for 30 min and 95 °C for 5 min, then 40 cycles of denaturation at 95 °C for 15 s, annealing at 60 °C for 60 s and elongation at 72 °C for 30 s. The Ct values were converted to $TCID_{50}$ equivalent/ml based on the equation derived from the standard curve generated with the serial dilution of cell culture-grown PEDV. The detection limit for this RT-qPCR was approximately 0.1 $TCID_{50}$/ml.

IFA

Confluent Vero cells grown in 96 well plates were infected with PEDV KD, PEDV AA or PEDV 8aa at a various MOI in the presence of trypsin, elastase or GCDCA, respectively. After 24 h of infection, cells were fixed with cold methanol. For IFA, the positive (against WT PEDV) or negative sera were added to each well, followed by the incubation with FITC-conjugated goat anti-swine IgG. The plates were then washed with PBS and visualized for fluorescence under a fluorescence microscope.

Western blot analysis

Confluent Vero cells grown in 6 well plates were infected with PEDV KD, PEDV AA or PEDV 8aa in the presence of trypsin, elastase or GCDCA, respectively. Similarly, growth of PEDV 8aa with trypsin, elastase, GCDCA or without any addition were also monitored by Western blot analysis. Since PEDV 8aa grew to similar titers with or without FBS in the media, FBS was not added to the media. After 24 h post virus infection, cell lysates were prepared for SDS-PAGE (12% Tris-glycine gel), and proteins were transferred to nitrocellulose membranes. Membranes were probed with the positive (against WT PEDV) or negative pig sera followed by horseradish peroxidase-conjugated goat swine IgG. Proteins were visualized by chemiluminescence (Thermo Scientific). Concentrated (×100) PEDV KD, PEDV AA or PEDV 8aa were prepared by ultracentrifugation (100,000×g for 2 h in 30% sucrose cushion) and the concentrated viruses were serially diluted (1:5, 1:50 or 1:500) with PBS for the Western blot analysis.

Determination of antibody titers by SN assay

The SN titers of the sera from pigs infected with WT PEDV [33] or of the serum samples from our pig studies were determined against PEDV KD, PEDV AA or PEDV 8aa P70. Each serum was serially diluted by 2-fold in MEM, and the diluted serum (50 µl each) was mixed with the same volume of media containing 200 $TCID_{50}$ PEDV KD, PEDV AA or PEDV 8aa. The mixture was incubated in 37 °C for 30 min, then transferred to fresh Vero cells. The cells were further incubated in the presence of trypsin (1 µg/ml) for PEDV KD and PEDV AA or GCDCA (100 µM) for PEDV 8aa. Serum neutralization titers were determined by observing the appearance of CPE during the 3 days of incubation. Titers were determined as the reciprocal serum dilution of complete CPE inhibition.

Immunization of inactivated PEDV 8aa in 4 weeks old pigs

To determine immunogenicity, BEI inactivated PEDV 8aa (P75) was inoculated to 4 week old pigs with an adjuvant. BEI was prepared by dissolving BEA in 0.175 M NaOH at 37 C for 1 h. The freshly prepared BEI was added to clarified virus culture (PEDV 8aa, P75, 7.5 log_{10} TCID50/ml) at final BEI concentrations of 1.0 mM. The mixture was incubated at 37 °C with continuous stirring for 24 h. The BEI was inactivated by adding 10% volume of 1 M sodium thio-sulphate in PBS. The inactivation of PEDV was confirmed by inoculating the samples to Vero cells. Approximately 4 week old pigs ($N = 5$) were immunized with intramuscularly (IM) in the neck with 2 ml of inactivated virus containing 20% adjuvant (Emulsigen®, MVP laboratories, Omaha, NE) with additional immunization at 3 weeks later. Final bleeding was done at 2 weeks after the last immunization. Control pigs ($N = 3$) were immunized with MEM and 20% adjuvant. Each serum sample was tested for SN titers against PEDV KD (P80), PEDV AA (P80) or PEDV 8aa (P75) as described above. The fluorescent foci neutralization assay (FFN) was also performed for each sample using a National Veterinary Services Laboratory (NVSL) reference isolate, USA/Colorado/2013 (CO/13) at the SDSU diagnostic laboratory to confirm the immunogenicity.

Sequencing analysis of PEDV 8aa S gene

To investigate the potential underlying mechanism for enzyme-independent growth and/or reduced replication by trypsin of PEDV 8aa, the S gene of PEDV 8aa P0 (the early isolated US PEDV strain with trypsin in the media and P1 is the first virus passage number that was grown in GCDCA, Fig. 1), P70 and P105 were sequenced and compared to among them as well as those of the PEDV strains available in the GenBank (> 100 strains). The GenBank accession numbers for the S gene of PEDV 8aa P0 and P70 are KX834130 and KX834131, respectively. Because the S genes of PEDV P70 and P105 were identical, P70 S gene was deposited in GenBank.

Trypsin pretreatment and time-of-addition assays

Trypsin pretreatment of viruses or cells and time-of-addition assays were performed to study the potential mechanism for the inhibition of PEDV 8aa (P70) replication by trypsin. PEDV KD (P70) was also included in this

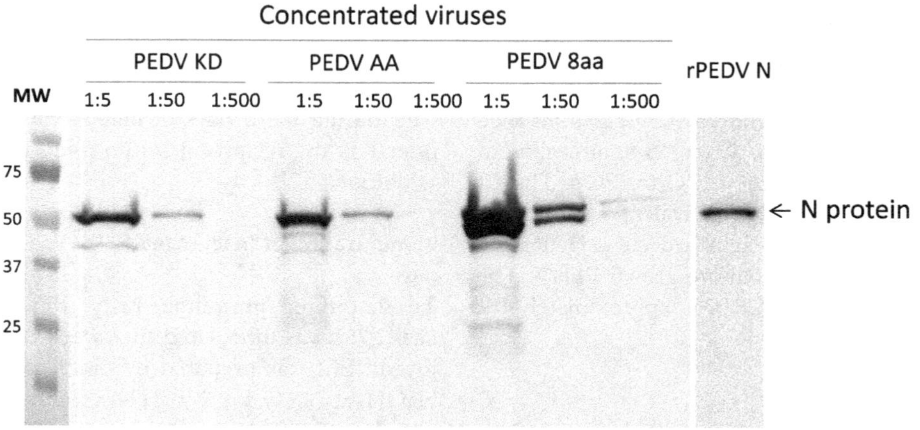

Fig. 1 Western Blot analysis on the serial dilutions of the concentrated PEDV strains obtained in this study. PEDV KD (P120), PEDV AA (P103) or PEDV 8aa (P70) were concentrated by 100-fold with ultracentrifugation, and the concentrated viruses were diluted at 1:5, 1:50 or 1:500 for Western blot analysis. The pooled convalescent sera from US PEDV-infected pigs were used for the analysis. The PEDV N protein expressed in Vero cells (rPEDV N) by transfecting pCI-PEDV-N was included in the figure to confirm the reactivity to the protein by the pooled antisera

study as a control. For trypsin pretreatment of viruses, concentrated (10×) or un-concentrated PEDV 8aa or PEDV KD was incubated with mock-medium or trypsin (5 μg/ml) at 37 °C for 1 h. The mock- or trypsin-treated virus was then added to Vero cells in 6 well plates that were previously washed with cold PBS and the cells were then incubated at 4 °C for 1 h. After the incubation, cells were washed with cold PBS for 3 times, and cell lysates were prepared for real time RT-qPCR or Western blot analysis. The ct values from the real time RT-qPCR were converted to $TCID_{50}$ values, as described below, and the $TCID_{50}$ values were compared between the mock- or trypsin-treated PEDV 8aa or PEDV KD. In a separate experiment, PEDV 8aa pre-treated with mock-medium or trypsin was allowed to enter the Vero cells and replicate for 24 h. PEDV 8aa was incubated with trypsin (1 or 5 μg/ml) at 37 °C for 1 h and then fetal bovine serum (FBS) was added at 1% final concentrations to the mixture to neutralize trypsin. The virus was then inoculated to confluent Vero cells at an MOI of 10. The viral replication was monitored by virus titration or IFA staining at 24 h post inoculation. To determine if pre-treatment of cells by trypsin affects viral replication, confluent Vero cells were incubated with trypsin (5 μg/ml) at 37 ° C for 1 h. After the incubation, the cells were washed 3 times with PBS, and PEDV 8aa or PEDV KD was added to the cell at an MOI of 10. The viral replication was determined by virus titration or IFA staining at 24 h post inoculation. The time-of-addition assay was also performed to determine which replication step of PEDV 8aa is inhibited by trypsin. Confluent Vero cells in 6 or 12-well plates were washed with PBS for 3 times and inoculated with PEDV 8aa (10 MOI). Mock-medium or trypsin (1 μg/ml) was then added at different time points: 0, 30 min, 1, 2, 4, 12 h after virus inoculation. Virus infected cells were further incubated for 24 h, and viral replication was assessed by viral titrations, IFA and Western blot analysis.

Confocal microscopy

Using confocal studies for virus trafficking during entry, we demonstrated the endosomal escape of caliciviruses is critical for virus replication [34–36]. Because the addition of trypsin during up to 2 h post inoculation markedly inhibited virus replication, we examined the cellular trafficking of PEDV 8aa with or without trypsin using the same techniques. Vero cells were seeded onto Lab-Tek II CC2 chamber slide (Fisher Scientific, Pittsburgh, PA), treated with FBS and grown to 90% confluency. Confluent cells on the chamber slides were inoculated with mock-medium or PEDV 8aa (P70) at an MOI of 50 at 4 °C for 1 h. After mock-medium or trypsin (1 μg/ml) was added to the medium, the virus infected cells were further incubated in 37 °C for 30 min or 3 h before fixed for confocal microscopy. Cells were fixed in 4% paraformaldehyde (Sigma-Aldrich) in PBS (pH 7.4) at room temperature for 15 min, permeabilized with 0.1% Triton ×100 in PBS for 10 min at room temperature, washed three times with PBS, and incubated in blocking buffer (PBS containing 0.5% bovine serum albumin) for 15 min. Also fixed cells without permeabilization were prepared as a control. The cells were then incubated with the PEDV antibody (1:200) or Rab7 antibody (1:200) at 37 °C to probe PEDV or endosomes, respectively. After 2 h incubation at 37 °C, cells were washed three times with PBS and further incubated at 37 °C for 2 h with appropriate secondary antibodies. Cell nucleus was stained with sytox orange (0.5 μM in

0.9% NaCl). Coverslips were mounted in Prolong Gold antifade reagent (Molecular Probes), and the cells were scanned with a confocal microscope LSM 510 (Zeiss, Oberkochen, Germany) using a 100× oil-immersion objective. The images were analyzed by Image J software 1.47 (http://imagej.nih.gov/ij/) and merged images were prepared. The colocalization analysis of PEDV and Rab7 was performed using JACoP and colocalization-MBF plugins for ImageJ software. Single channel images were thresholded by Costes' auto threshold method and the Manders split correlation coefficient for colocalization was then determined for each image.

Determination of the level of attenuation of serially passaged PEDV in neonatal piglets

To determine the level of attenuation of serially passaged PEDV in neonatal piglets, we purchased PEDV-negative pregnant sows and their negative status with known enteric pathogens were confirmed with RT-qPCR. After farrowing of the sows, piglets were nursed by the sows in the farrowing crates for the duration of the virus attenuatioin study. The 1–4 day old piglets were orally inoculated with PEDV KD (P120), PEDV AA (P103), or PEDV 8aa (P40, P70 and P105). The virus inoculum was 1×10^6 $TCID_{50}$ per animal. After inoculation, clinical symptoms, survival and virus shedding (daily rectal swabs) were examined for up to 14 days. Stool samples were assessed by visual observation of rectal swabs and described as normal, loose stool or diarrhea (liquid with or without some solid content). Virus shedding was determined by real time RT-qPCR as described above. Serum samples were collected from each piglet weekly and tested for SN titers against PEDV 8aa.

Results

Cell culture adaptation of an US PEDV strain

Initial attempt to isolate the US PEDV strain required 2 or 3 blind passages with trypsin (1–2 μg/ml) until apparent CPE appeared in Vero cells. Virus growth in cell culture was confirmed by IFA using the PEDV antisera generated from the previous pig challenge study with a PEDV US strain [33]. The S gene of this PEDV isolate (designated as P0) showed a high sequence identity with those of other US PEDV strains (less than 10 amino acid residue differences from most of US PEDV strains detected or isolated during 2013–2014). To generate the PEDV KD, P0 was serially passaged in the presence of trypsin (1–2 μg/ml). After about 20 passages of PEDV, PEDV KD began to grow faster based on the apparent CPE appearance at 24 h post inoculation, leading to complete cell lysis by 48 h post inoculation. Syncytia formation was also observed in the cell monolayers. After passage number 20, PEDV KD titers consistently reached to 6.2–6.5 log_{10} $TCID_{50}$/ml (Table 1).

For PEDV AA, P0 was serially passaged in the presence of elastase (1–2 μg/ml). Apparent CPE began to appear after 2–3 passages of PEDV and PEDV AA titers gradually increased during the first 20 passages with syncytia formation. Interestingly, PEDV AA grew well with trypsin or elastase, which allowed virus titration to be performed using trypsin or elastase (Table 1). The titers of PEDV AA grown with elastase reached to 6.8 log_{10} $TCID_{50}$/ml when titration was done with trypsin, which is slighly higher than those of PEDV KD (Table 1). However, when PEDV AA grown with elastase was titrated with elastase, the titers were approximately 10-fold lower than those determined with trypsin (Table 1). Nonetheless, antigenic masses of PEDV KD and PEDV AA strains were similar to each other when they were assessed with Western blot analysis after each virus was concentrated at the same ratio (Fig. 1).

To generate PEDV 8aa, P0 was serially passaged with GCDCA (100 μM), but without adding any enzyme. PEDV 8aa began to efficiently grow after about 10 passages. Interestingly, syncytia formation was not observed in the cells infected with PEDV 8aa. Instead, extensive cell death (lysis) of cell monolayers occurred at approximately 40–48 h following virus infection. The virus titers of PEDV 8aa reached higher than 8.0 log_{10} $TCID_{50}$/ml after passage number 20, which is substantially higher than those of PEDV KD or PEDV AA (Table 1). It is of note that, after 10 passages of initial adaptation to GCDCA, PEDV 8aa no longer required GCDCA for replication (Fig. 2a, Panels 2 and 3) and was able to grow in the presence or absence of FBS. The CPE progress or titers of PEDV 8aa grown in the presence with GCDCA were slightly faster or higher than those grown in mock (media only) or 2% FBS, respectively. It is noteworthy that the replication of PEDV 8aa became greatly inhibited by trypsin once viruses were completely adapted to grow with GCDCA after passage number 20 (Fig. 2a, Panel 4 and Table 1). The majority of the cells infected with PEDV 8aa with GCDCA or mock-medium were positively stained for PEDV (Fig. 2a, Panels 2 and 3). On the contrary, only few positive cells were observed by IFA staining when PEDV 8aa was grown with trypsin (1 μg /ml) (Fig. 2a, Panel 4). The inhibitory effects of trypsin on the replication of 8aa PEDV (passage number 21) was also confirmed by Western blot analysis in which the reduction of PEDV N protein levels was commensurate with trypsin concentrations in cell culture (Fig. 2b). On the contrary, PEDV KD (P70) efficiently replicated only in the presence of trypsin (Fig. 2a, Panels 5 and 6).

Replication of PEDV KD, PEDV AA or PEDV 8aa in cell culture was also determined by Western blot analysis, IFA and SN assay using the PEDV antisera. Figure 1 shows that the antisera from the pigs infected with a

Table 1 The adapted US PEDV strains passaged in three different culture conditions (trypsin, elastase and GCDCA) were designated as PEDV KD, AA or 8aa, respectively

PEDV KD		PEDV AA			PEDV 8aa		
Passage No	Titration with	Passage No	Titration with		Passage No	Titration with	
	Trypsin		Trypsin	Elastase		GCDCA	Trypsin
P4	5.1	P4	3.8	2.5	P4	2.5	3.1
P10	5.8	P10	5.2	4.1	P14	6.6	5.1
P20	6.3	P20	6.7	5.3	P17	7.5	2.2
P30	6.2	P30	6.5	5.1	P21	8.1	< 2
P40	6.5	P40	6.7	5.5	P40	8.1	< 2
P60	6.2	P60	6.8	5.3	P70	8.2	< 2
P120	6.3	P120	6.7	5.2	P120	8.1	< 2

The table shows PEDV titers (log_{10} $TCID_{50}$/ml) which were determined in the presence of trypsin, elastase or GCDCA, as indicated

WT PEDV reacted to the tissue culture adapted viruses in Western blot analysis. The detection of N protein by the sera was confirmed with the recombinant PEDV N protein expressed from the plasmid (pCMV-PEDV N) carrying PEDV N gene under the CMV promoter. The N protein of PEDV 8aa appeared as two fragments in the Western blot analysis (Fig. 1) and this may be due to further modification (cleavage) of the N protein during replication as noted by Jaru-Ampornpan et al. [37]. When we determined the IFA and SN titers of the convalescent antisera against PEDV KD, PEDV AA or PEDV 8aa P70, the IFA titers against PEDV KD, PEDV AA or PEDV 8aa were 1255 ± 23, 1195 ± 41 or 1243 ± 31, respectively, and SN titers against PEDV KD, PEDV AA or PEDV 8aa were 48 ± 16, 43 ± 8.3, or 52 ± 4.7, respectively. The average SN titers of antisera immunized with the inactivated PEDV 8aa (with adjuvant) in 4 weeks old pigs against PEDV KD, PEDV AA or PEDV 8aa were 54.5 ± 8.0, 51.3 ± 6.9 or 57.6 ± 17, respectively. The average SN titers of the antisera (from the inactivated PEDV 8aa) against USA/Colorado/2013 (CO/13) was 52.8 ± 12.3 determined at the SDSU diagnostic laboratory. However, the sera from the control pigs immunized with MEM and 20% adjuvant did not show SN activity (<10) against these PEDV strains. These results indicate that PEDV AA, PEDV KD and PEDV 8aa retained comparable immunogenicity to wild type PEDV after cell-culture adaptation.

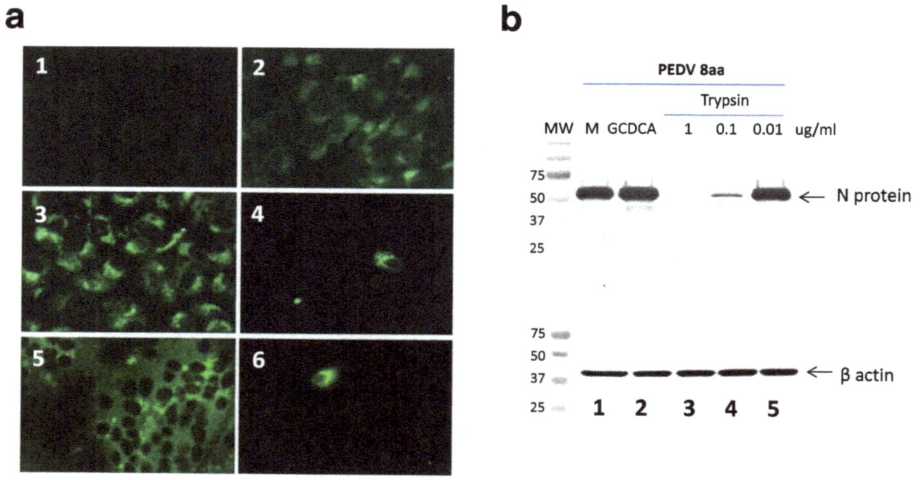

Fig. 2 IFA and Western blot analysis of PEDV 8aa (P70) and PEDV KD grown in various culture conditions. **a** IFA: Vero cells were inoculated with mock-medium (Mock) (Panel 1), PEDV 8aa (P70) (Panels 2–4) or PEDV KD (P70) (Panels 5 and 6). PEDV 8aa-infected cells were further incubated in MEM containing mock (Panel 2), GCDCA (100 μM) (Panel 3) or trypsin (1 μg/ml) (Panel 4). Vero cells inoculated with PEDV KD (P70) (Panels 5 and 6) were further incubated in MEM containing trypsin (1 μg/ml) (Panel 5) or mock (Panel 6). At 24 h post virus infection, cells were fixed for IFA. **b** Western blot analysis: Vero cells were inoculated with PEDV 8aa (P70) at an MOI of 1, and virus infected cells were incubated with MEM only (M), GCDCA (100 uM) or various concentrations of trypsin (0.01 to 1 μg/ml) for 24 h. After 24 h of incubation, cell lysates were prepared for Western blot analysis for PEDV or β-actin

Sequencing analysis of PEDV 8aa S gene

The amino acid sequences of the S gene of PEDV 8aa P70 or P105 were identical. However, PEDV 8aa P70 (or P105) had 6 amino acid residue changes in the S gene when compared to P0 (Fig. 3a). Interestingly, the mutated 6 amino acids found in PEDV 8aa P70 or P105 are conserved in US PEDV strains (over 100 strains) whose sequences are available in the PubMed. Those conserved and mutated 6 amino acids, aa 214, 457, 777, 825, 958 and 976, are shown in Fig. 3a.

Trypsin pretreatment and time-of-addition assays

Pretreament of cells with trypsin (5 μg/ml) did not affect the replication of PEDV 8aa or PEDV KD. However, pretreatment of PEDV 8aa with trypsin (5 μg/ml) led to a marked reduction (> 90%) in virus binding to the cells determined by real time RT-qPCR (Fig. 3b) or Western blot analysis (Fig. 3c) compared to the mock-medium treatment. In contrast, pretreatment of PEDV KD with trypsin (5 μg/ml) had little effect on the binding of PEDV KD to the cells (Fig. 3b and c). When PEDV 8aa pretreated with trypsin (1 or 5 μg/ml) for 30 min or 1 h was allowed to replicate in the cells for 24 h, viral replication was significantly reduced determined by viral titration (Table 2) or IFA staining compared to mock-medium treatment (Fig. 3d, Panels 3 and 4). Pretreatment of PEDV 8aa with trypsin (5 μg/ml) for 1 h resulted in over 10-fold reduction in viral titers compared to mock-medium treatment (Table 2).

The time-of-addition assay showed that the addition of trypsin during 0 to 2 h post inoculation markedly inhibited PEDV 8aa replication determined at 24 h (Fig. 4a and b and Table 2). When trypsin was added at the same time of PEDV 8aa inoculation (0 h) or 1 h post

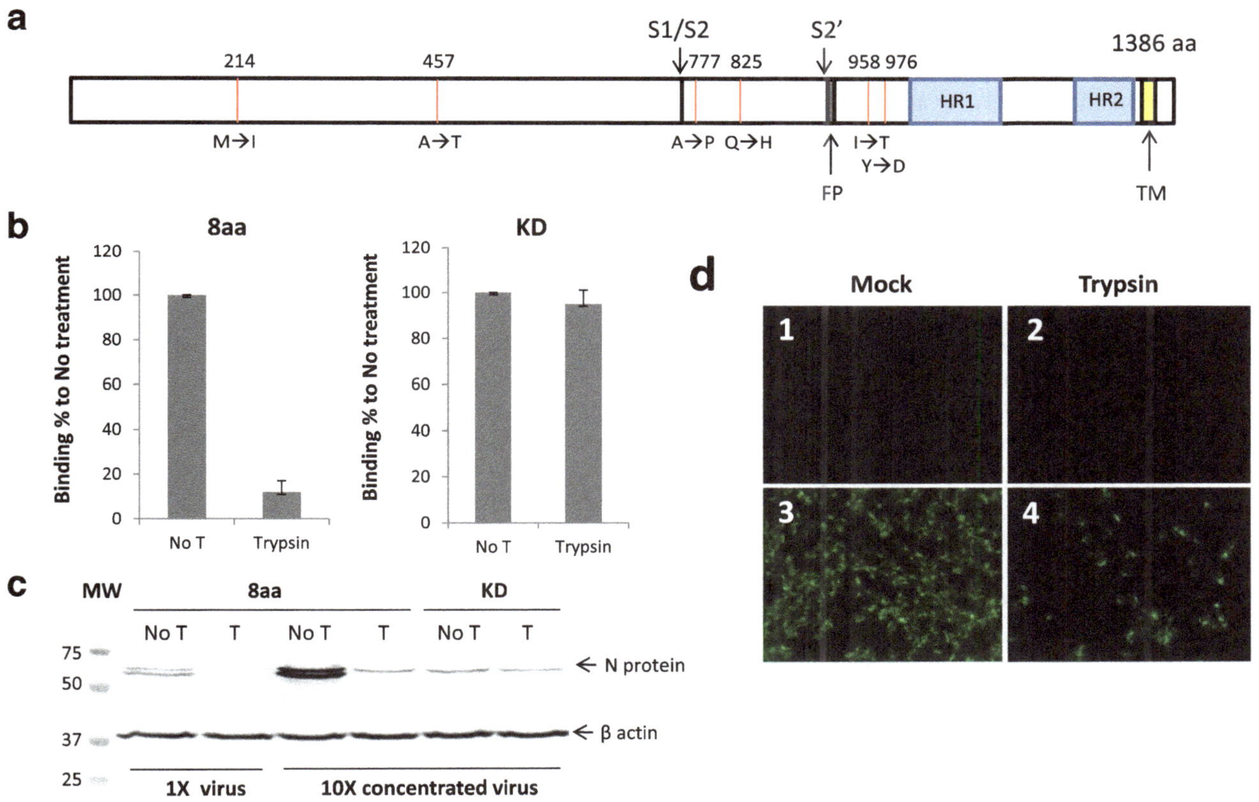

Fig. 3 Mutations identified in the PEDV 8aa S gene and the effects of trypsin treatment on PEDV 8aa on virus binding or viral replication. **a** Amino acid changes in PEDV 8aa P70 or P105 from multiple sequence alignments with the parental PEDV 8aa P0 and >100 US PEDV strains. The S1/S2 junction (758/579), HR1 (aa 979–1088) and HR2 (aa 1239–1277) are indicated based on the literature [44, 45]. Fusion peptide (FP, aa 895–912) and transmembrane (TM) region are also shown in the schematic drawing. **b** and **c** Effects of trypsin treatment on PEDV 8aa or PEDV KD on virus binding. Unconcentrated or concentrated (10 ×) PEDV 8aa (P70) or PEDV KD (P70) was treated with trypsin (5 μg/ml) or mock-medium at 37 °C for 1 h and the treated virus was added to confluent Vero cells. The cells were then incubated in a cold room (4 °C) for 1 h and cell lysates were prepared for real time RT-qPCR (**b**) or Western blot analysis (**c**). The percentage of trypsin-treated viruses bound to the cells were compared to mock-medium treatment (No T, no treatment). **d** Effects of trypsin pre-treatment on PEDV 8aa on virus replication. Concentrated (10 ×) PEDV 8aa was pre-treated with trypsin (5 μg/ml) or mock-medium at 37 °C for 1 h, and added to confluent Vero cells. After incubation of the virus infected cells at 37 °C for 24 h, they were fixed for IFA staining for PEDV. Panels 1 and 2 show the cells incubated with trypsin or with mock-medium without virus infection, respectively. Panels 3 and 4 show PEDV 8aa grown in the cells with mock medium or trypsin respectively

inoculation, greater than 10^5- or 10^3-fold reduction in viral titers was observed compared to mock-medium treatment, respectively (Table 2). Both Western blot analysis and IFA results correlated with the reduced viral titration (Fig. 4a and b). However, there was no significant difference in viral replication when trypsin was added at 4 h post inoculation (Fig. 4a and Fig. 4b, Panel 4).

Confocal studies

Confocal studies for virus trafficking during the virus entry demonstrated that PEDV 8aa was not able to escape from endosomes in the presence of trypsin. At 30 min post inoculation of PEDV 8aa, there was no noticeable difference in the fluorescence signals for virus (green) in the cells with or without trypsin (Fig. 5a, panels 6 and 8). At 3 h post inoculation, fluorescence signals for virus disappeared in the cells without trypsin, (Fig. 5b, Panel 6), suggesting successful PEDV release to the cytoplasm at the time point. However, in the presence of trypsin, fluorescence signals still remained (and increased) in the cells (Fig. 5b, Panel 10). The increased signals in Fig. 6b, Panel 10 suggest accumulation of PEDV in the compartments without releasing to cytoplasm at that time point. Fluorescence signals remained in the cells even at 24 h post inoculation in the presence of trypsin (data not shown). Fluorescence signals for virus (green) co-localized (white) with the endosomal marker Rab7 (red) with Manders split colocalization coefficient of >0.90 (Fig. 5a, Panels 8 and 12 and Fig. 5b, Panels 8 and 12). These results suggest that PEDV 8aa failed to escape from the endosomal compartments in the presence of trypsin, while viruses in the trypsin-free media were able to exit the endosomal compartments to the cytoplasm and to initiate virus replication.

Pathogenicity of serially passaged PEDVs in neonatal piglets

The results of the animal studies to determine the level of attenuation of PEDV KD, PEDV AA, and PEDV 8aa (P40, P70 and P105) in neonatal piglets are summarized in Table 3. Fatality varied among groups from 0 to 100% (Table 3, Fig. 6a). The onset and duration of symptom (diarrhea) and virus shedding also differed among groups (Table 3, Fig. 6b and c).

In PEDV KD P120 group, 2-day old piglets were inoculated with the strain, and three out of five piglets died during 6 to 8 days post-infection (DPI) (60% fatality) (Table 3, Fig. 6a). Virus shedding and diarrhea started at 2 and 3 DPI, respectively. Fecal viral titers reached to 4.5 $\log_{10}$ $TCID_{50}$ equivalent/ml at 4 DPI and remained above 3–4 $\log_{10}$ $TCID_{50}$ equivalent/ml until 11 DPI (end of observation)(Fig. 6b). In PEDV AA P103 group, 2-day old piglets were inoculated with PEDV AA P103. During 5 to 8 DPI, 7 out of 14 piglets died (50% fatality) (Table 3 and Fig. 6a). Virus shedding and diarrhea started at 1 and 2 DPI, respectively. Fecal viral titers reached to 5.2 and 5.5 $\log_{10}$ $TCID_{50}$ equivalent/ml at 1 and 2 DPI, respectively, and remained higher than 4–5 $\log_{10}$ $TCID_{50}$ equivalent/ml until 6 DPI. Fecal virus titers gradually reduced to lower than 1 $\log_{10}$ $TCID_{50}$ equivalent/ml after 9 DPI (Fig. 6b).

Three groups were inoculated with three different passage numbers (P40, P70 and P105) of PEDV 8aa. They were comprised of piglets of 1 day-old (P70), 1–2 day old (P105) or 2 or 4 day old (P40) at the time of virus inoculation (Table 3). The piglets infected with PEDV 8aa P40 sustained high fatality during 1–6 DPI (83.3% fatality) with high viral shedding and diarrhea starting at 2 and 3 DPI, respectively (Fig. 6a and c). In this group, the average fecal viral titers reached to 5.7 $\log_{10}$ $TCID_{50}$ equivalent/ml at 6 DPI (Fig. 6c). However, inoculation of piglets with PEDV 8aa P70 or P105 led to only one (6.7% fatality) or no death, respectively (Table 3, Fig. 6a). One piglet died after inoculation of PEDV 8aa P70 does not seem to be related to PEDV as there was no clinical symptom or virus shedding. In some animals infected with PEDV 8aa P70, loose stool was observed at 1 and 2 DPI, which resolved after 2 DPI, and limited virus shedding (< 1 $\log_{10}$ $TCID_{50}$ equivalent/ml) was observed (Fig. 6c). In the PEDV 8aa P105 group, there was no loose stool or diarrhea with limited virus shedding with <1 $\log_{10}$ $TCID_{50}$ equivalent/ml (Fig. 6c). The survival rates of the piglets and viral shedding/diarrhea indicate that PEDV 8aa became greatly attenuated after passage number 70.

Discussion

Until recently, most PEDV strains circulating in the Asia belonged to the genogroup 1 and, in those countries,

Table 2 The effect of trypsin pretreatment of PEDV 8aa and time-of-addition assay with trypsin. Concentrated PEDV 8aa was used for this study

	Pre-treatment of virus with trypsin					Time-of-addition assay (post-inoculation)				
	Mock	1 μg/ml		5 μg/ml		Mock	1 μg/ml			
		30 min	1 h	30 min	1 h		0 h	2 h	4 h	12 h
$\log_{10}$, $TCID_{50}$/ml	7.23	6.59*	6.26*	6.34*	5.37*	7.10	1.60*	3.50*	6.00*	6.80

For trypsin pretreatment study, virus was incubated with trypsin at 1 or 5 μg/ml for 1 h at 37 °C and added to Vero cells. For time-of-addition assay, trypsin at 1 μg/ml was added to Vero cells infected with PEDV 8aa at the designated time points post infection. Viral titration was done at 24 h post infection for both pre-treatment and time-of-addition assay. Mock indicates treatment with mock-medium. * $P < 0.05$ compared to the control (Mock)

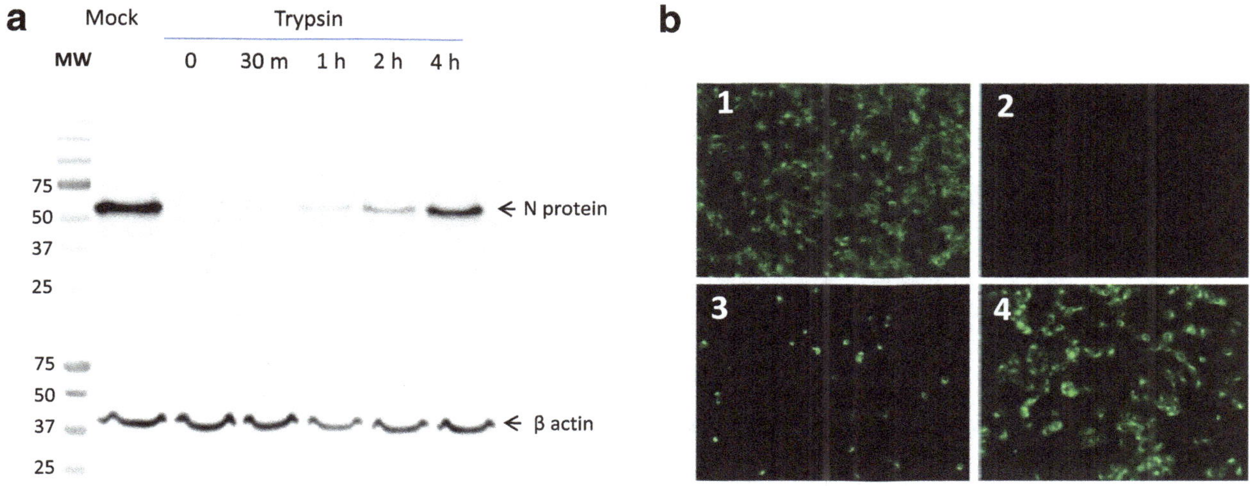

Fig. 4 Replication of PEDV 8aa (P70) by the addition of trypsin at various time points determined by Western blot analysis or IFA. Confluent Vero cells were inoculated with PEDV 8aa (10 MOI) and mock-medium or trypsin (1 μg/ml) was added at different time points of 0, 30 min, 1, 2, or 4 h after virus inoculation. **a** Cell lysates were prepared at 24 h post inoculation for Western blot analysis with antibody against PEDV or β-actin. **b** Cells were fixed at 24 h post inoculation for IFA staining. Panel 1 shows the cells with mock-medium treatment. Panels 2–4 show the virus-infected cells where trypsin was added at 0, 1 or 4 h post virus inoculation, respectively

genogroup 1 PEDV MLVs have been used for the control of PEDV [26–29]. The MLVs (including 83P-5 and DR13 strain) were generated by continuous passages of wild-type viruses in Vero cells (> 100 times) and their attenuation in piglets and sows and induction of a robust immune response in sows were previously demonstrated [38]. The US PEDV strains have approximately 10% genetic diversity in the S1 gene compared to that of the genogroup 1 and the US PEDV strains are phylogenetically grouped in subgroup 2a [4, 11, 30]. Although there is a varying degree of cross-reactivity and cross-neutralization among some US PEDV strains and the genogroup 1 PEDV prototype strain CV777 in in vitro assays [39], the protective efficacy of the genogroup 1 PEDV MLV against the genogroup 2 PEDV strains has not been reported. Considering the genetic and antigenic differences in S1 between the genogroups, effective control of US PEDV outbreaks is expected to require both genogroups 1 and 2 PEDV vaccines. For both killed vaccines or MLV production, generation of high-titered PEDV in cell culture is important for vaccine production [40]. However, propagation of PEDV to high titers (>8 $\log_{10}$ $TCID_{50}$/ml) is not easily achieved. In this study, to generate US PEDV strains with properties suitable for vaccine production, we investigated the effects of various selective pressures on viral growth characteristics by serially-passaging an US PEDV isolate in cell culture. Since trypsin is typically required for isolation and propagation of PEDV in cell culture, we first passaged PEDV in the presence of trypsin to generate PEDV KD. Although PEDV can be ultimately adapted to grow in cell culture without trypsin, exemplified by DR13 or PEDV 8aa, PEDV is the only known coronavirus which requires trypsin in the medium for isolation and replication in cell culture. Using trypsin during viral passages, we generated PEDV KD that induces typical extensive cell fusion with syncytium formation and its titers are similar to those reported by other groups [11, 12, 40]. In addition to PEDV KD adapted to grow in the presence of trypsin, we generated PEDV AA and 8aa that do not require trypsin for viral propagation. PEDV AA was obtained by passaging the WT US strain with elastase in cell culture. Elastase is a proteolytic enzyme produced by pancreas or neutrophils and involved in nutrient digestion in the intestines or catalyzing the breakdown of elastin or bacteria during inflammation in the lung. Elastase recognizes the carboxyl groups of small hydrophobic amino acid such as glycine, alanine and valine for proteolytic activity, while trypsin recognizes basic amino acids such as arginine or lysine. Interestingly, the resulting PEDV AA retains the ability to grow either in the presence of elastase or trypsin and induces extensive cell fusion similar to that by PEDV KD. PEDV 8aa was generated by serially passageing the WT PEDV in the presence of bile acid. We and other groups have previously shown that bile acids influence the replication of various viruses that propagate in the bile-rich organs such as liver and intestines, which include porcine enteric calicivirus, hepatitis B and C viruses and rotaviruses [41–43]. Bile acids are synthesized in the liver, stored in the gallbladder and released into the duodenum, where they play important roles in absorption of nutrients, lipid and cholesterol metabolism and also imunomodulation [44]. Interestingly, PEDV 8aa gradually lost its ability to grow in the presence of trypsin during adaptation to bile acid (Table 1 and Fig. 2). The other change observed

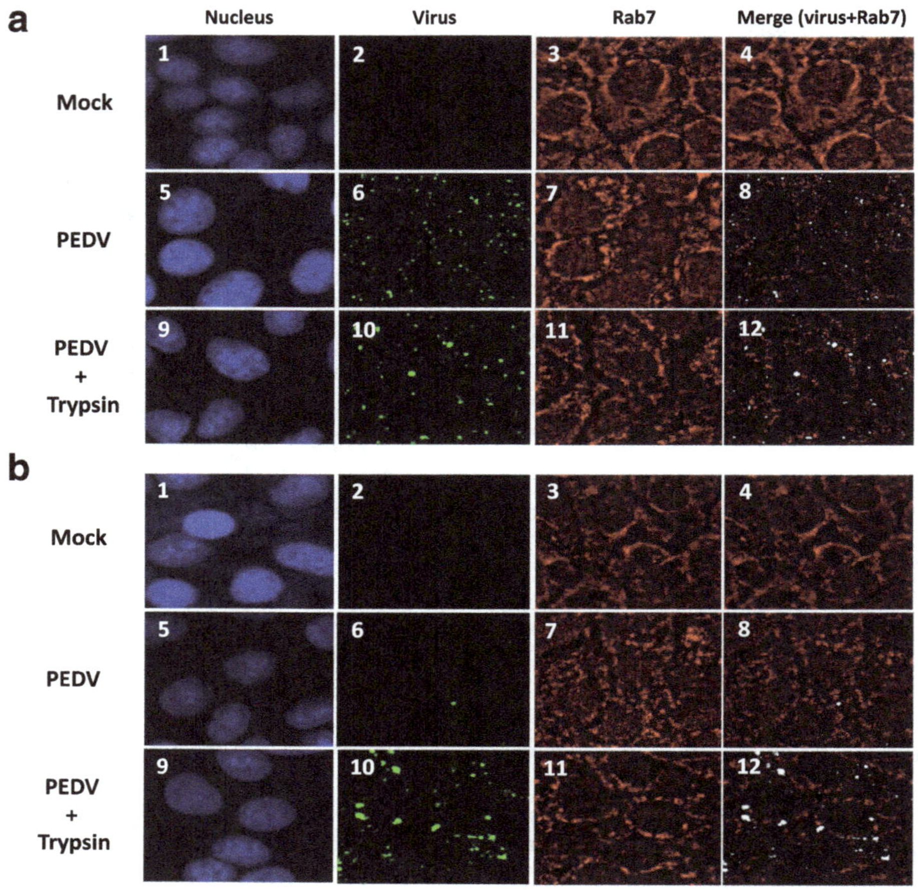

Fig. 5 Confocal microscopic study on the effects of trypsin on the entry of PEDV 8aa (P70) into the cells. (a and b) Vero cells were inoculated with mock-medium (Panel 1 to 4) or PEDV 8aa (50 MOI) and incubated at 4 °C for 1 h, then mock-medium (Panels 5 to 8) or trypsin (Panels 9 to 12) were added to the cells. The cells were further incubated at 37 °C for 30 min (**a**) or 3 h (**b**) and then fixed for confocal microscopy. Fixed cells were probed with sytox orange (blue) for nucleus, anti-Rab7 antibody (red) for the endosomes or anti-PEDV antibody (green). Merged images of viruses and the endosomes (white) were prepared (Panel 4, 8, 12 in **a** and **b**)

concurrently is that PEDV 8aa induced extensive cell death (lysis) without cell fusion. The role of GCDCA in the replication of PEDV is unknown, however, it was previously reported that serial passages of PEDV in cell culture (> 100 passages) led to generation of viruses that grow in trypsin-free media (DR13 vaccine strain). Therefore, it can be speculated that GCDCA may facilitate the adaptation of the virus to trypsin-free growth during the early phases of adaptation. However, once PEDV are fully adapted to the absence of these extraneous supplement in media, GCDCA does not substantially promote or reduce viral replication in cell culture. Importantly, PEDV KD, AA and 8aa retained immonogenicity (IFA and SN) to the pooled sera generated against the WT PEDV. Since PEDV 8aa consistently grows to high titers in FBS or enzyme-free media, this adapted virus would offer advantages in cell-culture based production of viruses for vaccines.

The sequence analysis of the S gene of PEDV 8aa P70 and P105 revealed that they have six unique mutations compared to the parental P0 virus and other reported US PEDV strains. Four out of six mutations are located near the S1/S2 junction and the fusion peptide (Fig. 3a). Recently, Wicht et al. [45] demonstrated that the S protein determines trypsin-dependency of PEDV replication and that trypsin-enhanced PEDV entry was mapped to the region from S1/S2 junction to HR1 by using a recombinant PEDV carrying the S protein of CV777 (trypsin-dependent strain) or DR13 (trypsin-independent strain). In this study, trypsin pretreatment and the time-of-addition assays using PEDV 8aa showed that trypsin prevents viral attachment to the host cells and inhibits the early phase of virus replication, including virus entry (Figs. 3 and 4, Table 2). The confocal microscopy study demonstrated that PEDV 8aa failed to exit the endosomal compartments for viral replication in the presence of trypsin (Fig. 5). The PEDV 8aa was detected in the endosomal compartments even after 24 h post inoculation in the presence of trypsin (data not shown). We

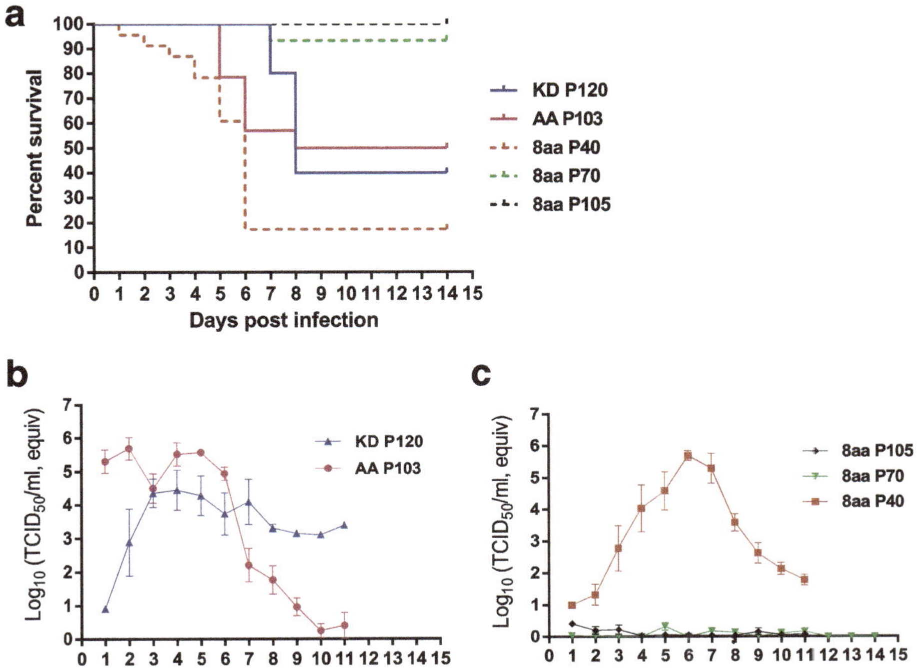

Fig. 6 Survival curves and virus shedding of nursing piglets inoculated with PEDV KD, AA, or 8aa at various passage numbers. **a** Survival curves of 1–4 day old piglets inoculated with PEDV KD P120 (KD P120), PEDV AA P103 (AA P103), PEDV 8aa P40 (8aa P40), PEDV 8aa P70 (8aa P70) or PEDV 8aa P105 (8aa P105). **b** and **c** Virus shedding of piglets inoculated with each strain. Daily rectal swabs were collected and virus shedding was determined by real-time RT-qPCR. The Ct values were converted to $TCID_{50}$/ml equivalent values (log_{10}). The mean and the standard errors are shown

have previously reported that endosomal uptake and subsequent endosomal escape of caliciviruses (porcine enteric calicivirus and murine norovirus) is critical for virus replication by showing that virus replication was completely or significantly reduced when the endosomal escape event was blocked [34–36]. Based on our results, it can be speculated that those mutations found in the S protein of PEDV 8aa may be associated with trypsin-independent viral growth as well as trypsin-mediated inhibition of virus entry to the host cells. Currently, we are investigating the roles of the mutations in both trypsin independent growth and viral entry inhibition.

In the neonatal piglets, PEDV KD and PEDV AA at the passage number over 100 still retained virulence (Fig. 6), and further passages may be required for attenuation of these strains. It was previously shown that about 100 passages of genogroup 1 PEDV in Vero cells resulted in attenuation in piglets, which are 83P-5 and DR13 MLVs [26, 29]. It is possible that genogroup 2 PEDV may require more serial passages in cell culture to become attenuated in piglets, as shown in a recent report where attenuation of a US PEDV was achieved with at least 160 passages in cell culture [46]. In this study, PEDV 8aa P70 and P105 were found to be fully attenuated in the neonatal piglets (Fig. 6) and substantial attenuation seems to have occurred between P40 and P70 (Fig. 6a and c). These results suggest that growth inhibition of PEDV 8aa by trypsin or elastase may be the key

Table 3 Summary of pathogenicity (attenuation) studies of PEDV KD (P120), PEDV AA (P103) or PEDV 8aa (P40, P70 or P105) in 1–4 day old piglets

Group	Inoculum	Age at inoculation (numbers)	No. of death (fatality %)	Clinical symptoms	Virus shedding
1	PEDV KD P120	2-day old (N = 5)	3/5 (60%)	Diarrhea: 3–9 DPI	Started at 2 DPI
2	PEDV AA P103	2-day-old (*N* = 14)	7/14 (50%)	Diarrhea: 2–9 DPI	Started at 1 DPI
3	PEDV 8aa P40	2 or 4-day old (*N* = 24)	20/24 (83.3%)	Diarrhea: 3–8 DPI	Started at 2 DPI
4	PEDV 8aa P70	1-day-old (*N* = 15)	1/15 (6.7%) 1 died (non-PEDV related)	Loose stool at 1–2 DPI	Limited virus shedding
5	PEDV 8aa P105	1- or 2-day old (*N* = 16)	0/16 (0%)	No diarrhea	Limited virus shedding

After virus inoculation, piglets were observed daily for clinical signs and rectal swabs were collected daily for the determination of virus shedding for up to 14 days post inoculation. DPI, days post infection for the fully attenuated phenomenon of PEDV 8aa in piglets. Of note, it was previously suggested that ORF3 protein is also involved in the PEDV attenuation [47] but the sequencing results of ORF3 gene from PEDV 8aa P70 or P105 showed no mutation in the ORF3 in these strains compared to the earlier passage numbers. We plan to investigate the mechanism of attenuation of PEDV 8aa P70 and P105 by conducting various experiments.

Conclusions

We showed that US PEDV strains (genogroup 2) adapted to various culture conditions have different growth characteristics. One (PEDV 8aa) of the generated strains is able to replicate in cells without any protease. Interestingly, replication of PEDV 8aa is severely reduced by the presence of trypsin and this correlates with impaired virus entry into the cells. Because PEDV 8aa P70 (and P105) was significantly attenuated in neonatal piglets, this strain may warrant further investigation as a candidate for MLV for the control of emerging US PEDV. Further investigation would include vaccination and passive protection study using PEDV 8aa in pregnant sows and neonatal piglets.

Abbreviations

BEA: Bromoethylamine hydrobromide; BEI: Binary ethyleneimine; CPE: Cytopathic effect; DMEN: Dulbecco's minimal essential medium; FBS: Fetal bovine serum; GCDCA: Glychenodeoxycholic acid; IFA: Immunofluorescent assay; MEM: Minimum essential medium; MLV: Modified live attenuated vaccine; PEDV: Porcine epidemic diarrhea virus; RT-qPCR: Real time-quantitative polymerase chain reaction; S: Spike; SN: Serum neutralization; TCID50: Tissue culture infectious dose 50; TPCK: L-1-tosylamide-2-phenylethyl chloromethyl ketone

Acknowledgements

We thank Drs Erin Strait and Pravina Kitikoon at Merck Animal Health for helpful discussion, David George and Amanda Schlagel for technical assistance in the virus and serum analysis, Dr. Jianfa Bai for providing primers and probe for PEDV real time RT-qPCR, and Vicky Samek, Bayliegh Murphy and Brittany Smola at UNL Life Sciences Annex for animal cares.

Funding

This work was supported by the National Institutes of Health (R01AI109039) for the overall design and in vitro studies, and Merck Animal Health Fund (Memorandum of Agreement, BG4117) for in vivo studies with data collection, analysis and interpretation for the manuscript.

Authors' contributions

Conceived and designed the experiments: YK, RH and KOC. Performed the experiments and analyzed data: YK, CO, VS, RH and KOC. Wrote the paper: YK and KOC. All authors have read and approved the final version of this manuscript.

Consent for publication

Not applicable.

Competing interests

YK, RH and KOC declare patent application (PCT application No: WO 2016/126853 or PCT/US2016/016417).

References

1. Oldham J. Letter to the editor. Pig Farming. 1972;10:72–3.
2. Pensaert MB, de Bouck P. A new coronavirus-like particle associated with diarrhea in swine. Arch Virol. 1978;58(3):243–7.
3. Lee C. Porcine epidemic diarrhea virus: an emerging and re-emerging epizootic swine virus. Virol J. 2015;12(1):193.
4. Huang YW, Dickerman AW, Pineyro P, Li L, Fang L, Kiehne R, Opriessnig T, Meng XJ. Origin, evolution, and genotyping of emergent porcine epidemic diarrhea virus strains in the United States. MBio. 2013;4(5):e00737–13.
5. Jung K, Saif LJ. Porcine epidemic diarrhea virus infection: etiology, epidemiology, pathogenesis and immunoprophylaxis. Vet J. 2015;204(2): 134–43.
6. Choudhury B, Dastjerdi A, Doyle N, Frossard JP, Steinbach F. From the field to the lab - an European view on the global spread of PEDV. Virus Res. 2016;226:40–9.
7. Sun RQ, Cai RJ, Chen YQ, Liang PS, Chen DK, Song CX. Outbreak of porcine epidemic diarrhea in suckling piglets, China. Emerg Infect Dis. 2012;18(1):161–3.
8. Song D, Park B. Porcine epidemic diarrhoea virus: a comprehensive review of molecular epidemiology, diagnosis, and vaccines. Virus Genes. 2012;44(2): 167–75.
9. Sun D, Wang X, Wei S, Chen J, Feng L. Epidemiology and vaccine of porcine epidemic diarrhea virus in China: a mini-review. J Vet Med Sci. 2016; 78(3):355-63.
10. Stevenson GW, Hoang H, Schwartz KJ, Burrough ER, Sun D, Madson D, Cooper VL, Pillatzki A, Gauger P, Schmitt BJ, et al. Emergence of porcine epidemic diarrhea virus in the United States: clinical signs, lesions, and viral genomic sequences. J Vet Diagn Investig. 2013;25(5):649–54.
11. Chen Q, Li G, Stasko J, Thomas JT, Stensland WR, Pillatzki AE, Gauger PC, Schwartz KJ, Madson D, Yoon KJ, et al. Isolation and characterization of porcine epidemic diarrhea viruses associated with the 2013 disease outbreak among swine in the United States. J Clin Microbiol. 2014;52(1):234–43.
12. Vlasova AN, Marthaler D, Wang Q, Culhane MR, Rossow KD, Rovira A, Collins J, Saif LJ. Distinct characteristics and complex evolution of PEDV strains, North America, may 2013-February 2014. Emerg Infect Dis. 2014;20(10): 1620–8.
13. Pasma T, Furness MC, Alves D, Aubry P. Outbreak investigation of porcine epidemic diarrhea in swine in Ontario. Can Vet J. 2016;57(1):84–9.
14. Stadler J, Zoels S, Fux R, Hanke D, Pohlmann A, Blome S, Weissenbock H, Weissenbacher-Lang C, Ritzmann M, Ladinig A. Emergence of porcine epidemic diarrhea virus in southern Germany. BMC Vet Res. 2015;11:142.
15. Boniotti MB, Papetti A, Lavazza A, Alborali G, Sozzi E, Chiapponi C, Faccini S, Bonilauri P, Cordioli P, Marthaler D. Porcine epidemic diarrhea virus and discovery of a recombinant swine enteric coronavirus, Italy. Emerg Infect Dis. 2016;22(1):83–7.
16. Zhao PD, Tan C, Dong Y, Li Y, Shi X, Bai J, Jiang P. Genetic variation analyses of porcine epidemic diarrhea virus isolated in mid-eastern China from 2011 to 2013. Can J Vet Res. 2015;79(1):8–15.
17. Van Diep N, Norimine J, Sueyoshi M, Lan NT, Hirai T, Yamaguchi R. US-like isolates of porcine epidemic diarrhea virus from Japanese outbreaks between 2013 and 2014. Spring. 2015;4:756.
18. Suzuki T, Murakami S, Takahashi O, Kodera A, Masuda T, Itoh S, Miyazaki A, Ohashi S, Tsutsui T. Molecular characterization of pig epidemic diarrhoea viruses isolated in Japan from 2013 to 2014. Infect Genet Evol. 2015;36:363–8.
19. Steinrigl A, Revilla Fernandez S, Stoiber F, Pikalo J, Sattler T, Schmoll F. First detection, clinical presentation and phylogenetic characterization of porcine epidemic diarrhea virus in Austria. BMC Vet Res. 2015;11(1):310.
20. Ojkic D, Hazlett M, Fairles J, Marom A, Slavic D, Maxie G, Alexandersen S, Pasick J, Alsop J, Burlatschenko S. The first case of porcine epidemic diarrhea in Canada. Can Vet J. 2015;56(2):149–52.
21. Mesquita JR, Hakze-van der Honing R, Almeida A, Lourenco M, van der Poel WH, Nascimento MS. Outbreak of porcine epidemic diarrhea virus in Portugal, 2015. Transbound Emerg Dis. 2015;62(6):586–8.
22. Kim SH, Lee JM, Jung J, Kim IJ, Hyun BH, Kim HI, Park CK, Oem JK, Kim YH, Lee MH, et al. Genetic characterization of porcine epidemic diarrhea virus in Korea from 1998 to 2013. Arch Virol. 2015;160(4):1055–64.
23. Dastjerdi A, Carr J, Ellis RJ, Steinbach F, Williamson S. Porcine epidemic diarrhea virus among farmed pigs, Ukraine. Emerg Infect Dis. 2015; 21(12):2235–7.
24. Schulz LL, Tonsor GT. Assessment of the economic impacts of porcine epidemic diarrhea virus in the United States. J Anim Sci. 2015;93(11):5111–8.

25. Opriessnig T. Re-emergence of porcine epidemic diarrhea virus in the global pig population. Vet J. 2015;204(2):131.
26. Song D, Moon H, Kang B. Porcine epidemic diarrhea: a review of current epidemiology and available vaccines. Clin Exp Vaccine Res. 2015;4(2):166–76.
27. Kweon CH, Kwon BJ, Lee JG, Kwon GO, Kang YB. Derivation of attenuated porcine epidemic diarrhea virus (PEDV) as vaccine candidate. Vaccine. 1999; 17(20–21):2546–53.
28. Sato T, Takeyama N, Katsumata A, Tuchiya K, Kodama T, Kusanagi K. Mutations in the spike gene of porcine epidemic diarrhea virus associated with growth adaptation in vitro and attenuation of virulence in vivo. Virus Genes. 2011;43(1):72–8.
29. Song DS, JS O, Kang BK, Yang JS, Moon HJ, Yoo HS, Jang YS, Park BK. Oral efficacy of Vero cell attenuated porcine epidemic diarrhea virus DR13 strain. Res Vet Sci. 2007;82(1):134–40.
30. Meng F, Ren Y, Suo S, Sun X, Li X, Li P, Yang W, Li G, Li L, Schwegmann-Wessels C, et al. Evaluation on the efficacy and immunogenicity of recombinant DNA plasmids expressing spike genes from porcine transmissible gastroenteritis virus and porcine epidemic diarrhea virus. PLoS One. 2013;8(3):e57468.
31. JAVMA. news: PED vaccine gains conditional approval. J Am Vet Med Assoc. 2014;245(3):267.
32. Chattha KS, Roth JA, Saif LJ. Strategies for design and application of enteric viral vaccines. Annu Rev Anim Biosci. 2015;3:375–95.
33. Niederwerdera MC, Nietfelda JC, Jianfa B, Peddireddia L, Breazealeb B, Andersonb J, Kerrigana MA, Anb B, Oberst RD, Crawford K, et al. Tissue localization, shedding, virus carriage, antibody response, and aerosol transmission of porcine epidemic diarrhea virus (PEDV) following inoculation of 4-week-old feeder pigs. J Vet Diagn Investig. 2016;6:671–8.
34. Shivanna V, Kim Y, Chang KO. The crucial role of bile acids in the entry of porcine enteric calicivirus. Virology. 2014;456-457:268–78.
35. Shivanna V, Kim Y, Chang KO. Endosomal acidification and cathepsin L activity is required for calicivirus replication. Virology. 2014;464-465:287–95.
36. Shivanna V, Kim Y, Chang KO. Ceramide formation mediated by acid sphingomyelinase facilitates endosomal escape of caliciviruses. Virology. 2015;483:218–28.
37. Jaru-Ampornpan P, Jengarn J, Wanitchang A, Jongkaewwattana A. Porcine Epidemic Diarrhea Virus 3C-Like Protease-Mediated Nucleocapsid Processing: Possible Link to Viral Cell Culture Adaptability. J Virol. 2017;91(2):201660-16.
38. Song DS, Yang JS, JS O, Han JH, Park BK. Differentiation of a Vero cell adapted porcine epidemic diarrhea virus from Korean field strains by restriction fragment length polymorphism analysis of ORF 3. Vaccine. 2003; 21(17–18):1833–42.
39. Lin CM, Gao X, Oka T, Vlasova AN, Esseili MA, Wang QH, Saif LJ. Antigenic relationships among porcine epidemic diarrhea virus and transmissible gastroenteritis virus strains. J Virol. 2015;89(6):3332–42.
40. Collin EA, Anbalagan S, Okda F, Batman R, Nelson E, Hause BM. An inactivated vaccine made from a U.S. field isolate of porcine epidemic disease virus is immunogenic in pigs as demonstrated by a dose-titration. BMC Vet Res. 2015;11:62.
41. Chang KO, George DW. Bile acids promote the expression of hepatitis C virus in replicon-harboring cells. J Virol. 2007;81(18):9633–40.
42. Chang KO, Sosnovtsev SV, Belliot G, Kim Y, Saif LJ, Green KY. Bile acids are essential for porcine enteric calicivirus replication in association with down-regulation of signal transducer and activator of transcription 1. Proc Natl Acad Sci U S A. 2004;101(23):8733–8.
43. Kim Y, Chang KO. Inhibitory effects of bile acids and synthetic farnesoid X receptor agonists on rotavirus replication. J Virol. 2011;85(23):12570–7.
44. Trauner M, Boyer JL. Bile salt transporters: molecular characterization, function, and regulation. Physiol Rev. 2003;83(2):633–71.
45. Wicht O, Li W, Willems L, Meuleman TJ, Wubbolts RW, van Kuppeveld FJ, Rottier PJ, Bosch BJ. Proteolytic activation of the porcine epidemic diarrhea coronavirus spike fusion protein by trypsin in cell culture. J Virol. 2014; 88(14):7952–61.
46. Lin CM, Hou Y, Marthaler DG, Gao X, Liu X, Zheng L, Saif LJ, Wang Q. Attenuation of an original US porcine epidemic diarrhea virus strain PC22A via serial cell culture passage. Vet Microbiol. 2017;201:62–71.
47. Park SJ, Moon HJ, Luo Y, Kim HK, Kim EM, Yang JS, Song DS, Kang BK, Lee CS, Park BK. Cloning and further sequence analysis of the ORF3 gene of wild- and attenuated-type porcine epidemic diarrhea viruses. Virus Genes. 2008;36(1):95–104.

20

Domestic feline contribution in the transmission of *Sporothrix* in Rio de Janeiro State, Brazil: a comparison between infected and non-infected populations

Pãmella A. Macêdo-Sales[1], Simone R. L. S. Souto[2], Carolina A. Destefani[3], Ricardo P. Lucena[3], Ricardo Luiz D. Machado[3], Marcia R. Pinto[3], Anderson M. Rodrigues[4], Leila M. Lopes-Bezerra[5], Elisabeth M. S. Rocha[3] and Andréa Regina S. Baptista[3*]

Abstract

Background: Sporotrichosis is a neglected zoonosis caused by pathogenic fungi belonging to the *Sporothrix schenckii* complex. In Rio de Janeiro state, this disease reached an epidemic status with over 4700 domestic felines and around 4000 humans affected since the mid-90s. The present study evaluated clinical and epidemiological aspects and also the frequency of colonization and infection by these fungi in healthy cats and among those with suspicious cutaneous lesions, inhabiting four Rio de Janeiro state distinct areas.

Results: Three hundred and seventy-one cats were included in two groups: 175 healthy cats [CRG] and 196 cats showing lesions suggesting sporotrichosis [SSG]. Mycological diagnosis allowed SSG animals to be divided in positive [104 cats; +SG] and negative [92 cats; -SG] groups. Nails, oral mucosa and lesions swabs were submitted to culture and potential colonies were subculture for micromorphologycal analysis, dimorphism and molecular tests. In the CRG, only one cat was colonized in the oral cavity [0.57%]; in the -SG group, four animals showed colonization of the nail and/or oral cavity [4.3%]; while the highest frequency of colonization [39.4%] was observed in the +SG. All molecularly typed isolates were identified as *S. brasiliensis*.

Conclusion: The results obtained here indicate that healthy cats have a minor role in sporotrichosis transmission within the state of Rio de Janeiro. Conversely, a higher participation of diseased feline in sporotrichosis transmission was evidenced, especially by the colonization of their oral cavity. *Sporothrix brasiliensis* equally affects and colonizes animals from distinct Rio de Janeiro state areas. Thus, we hypothesize that sporotrichosis is a uniform endemic throughout the state, whose transmission depends mainly on the contact with cats with sporotrichosis. Since Rio de Janeiro displays a world unique epidemic model of the disease, not fully understood, data on the infected and non-infected animals can be of major importance for future strategies of sporotrichosis prevention and control. Finally, considering the importance of the current concept of "one health", the experience here observed can be helpful for distinct epizootias and/or zoonosis.

Keywords: Sporotrichosis, Subcutaneous infection, Zoonosis, Cat (*Felis catus*), Neglected diseases

* Correspondence: andrearegina@id.uff.br
[3]Medical and Molecular Mycology Laboratory, Microbiology and Parasitology Department, Biomedical Institute, Fluminense Federal University (UFF), Rua Prof. Hernani Melo, 101 São Domingos, Niterói, RJ CEP: 24210-130, Brazil
Full list of author information is available at the end of the article

Background

Sporotrichosis is a subcutaneous mycosis caused by pathogenic dimorphic fungi belonging to the recently described *Sporothrix schenckii* complex, associated with plant organic matter and/or decaying matter in hot and humid climate regions and usually [1–3]. The disease was formerly known as Rose gardener's disease because of its acquisition through traumatic inoculation of plant organic matter, but it is currently considered a zoonosis because of its transmittance through scratches or bites of cats. In fact, the feline particular behavior exposes them to possible environmental niches of the fungi in its saprophytic phase since scratching tree trunks and other surfaces, burying their feces and licking their bodies, facilitates nails and nasopharynx/oral cavity to carry particles of these fungi [4, 5]. Therefore, these animals are at higher risk for *Sporothrix* spp. conidia colonization and subsequent infection, playing a key role in the transmission of this zoonosis because they promote the traumatic implantation of the fungi in the subcutaneous tissue of humans and of other animals and also because they have an exuberant clinical presentation of sporotrichosis with intense proliferation of the parasitic form of the fungus [4–6].

In feline sporotrichosis, the spectrum of lesions ranges from self-limiting forms with the presence of a single lesion that may regress spontaneously to fatal systemic clinical cases. The difficulties regarding the treatment of feline sporotrichosis, such as prolonged treatment time, high cost, drug dosage forms and isolation of affected animals, often contribute to their abandonment, which eventually die [7–12]. Currently, soil contamination by infected carcasses represents a major environmental concern because it can greatly increase the spread of fungi and hold back the control of this mycosis, closing the cat-environment-man cycle [10, 13].

Sporotrichosis has been described in the last decades as one of the most important zoonosis and also as a neglected disease, having reached an epidemic status in the state of Rio de Janeiro [7, 9, 13] with over 4700 domestic felines [14] and around 4000 humans [13] affected since the mid-90s. Until 2009, approximately 3244 cats, 2200 humans and 120 dogs presenting this subcutaneous mycosis were reported by the most important sporotrichosis reference center in Rio de Janeiro, the National Institute of Infectious Diseases of the Oswaldo Cruz Foundation (IPEC-FIOCRUZ) [10]. Still, all these cases were reported from a single reference center/institution [14]. Therefore, there is a pressing need for larger investigations in order to provide a broader view of sporotrichosis in its different aspects such as epidemiology, fungal biology and environmental particularities of transmission within this state. Thus, it is clear that sporotrichosis has reached an epidemic magnitude in the only Brazilian state wherein notification is compulsory and the disease is considered an important zoonosis [8, 13, 15]. Additionally, although in reduced numbers compared to Rio de Janeiro, sporotrichosis zoonotic transmission by domestic felines have been reported in other Brazilian states [16]. Given its relevance, routine laboratory procedures for investigating its etiological agent are well established and include the in vitro isolation of *Sporothrix* spp., identification of these fungi based on their macro and microscopic features, and in vitro thermal conversion techniques. Nevertheless, the epidemiological data show that the disease still affects humans and domestic felines with growing frequencies, especially for this state.

Several authors have investigated the clinical-epidemiological, immunological and molecular aspects of sporotrichosis, and they have primarily focused on the metropolitan region of Rio de Janeiro [2, 4, 8, 11, 15, 17, 18]. Despite these studies, data on the presence of the fungi on the nails and in the oral cavity of cats that do not carry the disease as well as of those infected are inconclusive. Indeed, the few studies that have addressed this issue in Brazil have been restricted to the states of Rio Grande do Sul and São Paulo and also the metropolitan region of Rio de Janeiro [4–6, 9, 16, 19, 20]. None of these studies included domestic felines inhabiting areas other than the metropolitan region of the state of Rio de Janeiro.

The aim of the present study was to compare the potential role of *Sporothrix* infected and non-infected domestic feline in the transmission of sporotrichosis by investigating colonization and infection by these fungi in cat populations from different regions of Rio de Janeiro state, Brazil.

Methods

The inclusion of animals was performed regardless of breed, age or gender, and the study was conducted over a period of 12 months (August 2012–2013). Similarly, the owners were informed of the objectives and methodology of the study and were asked to sign an informed consent form and answer questions related to epidemiological variables. Animals from the distinct location covered by the studied area were included. Likewise, cat populations from west, central-south and north regions of the municipality of Rio de Janeiro (Capital), Baixada Fluminense (Metropolitan region I, including Duque de Caxias, Nilópolis, São João do Meriti and Magé cities), Grande Niterói (Metropolitan region II – including Niterói, São Gonçalo and Itaboraí cities), Mountain (including Teresópolis and Petrópolis cities), Baixada Litorânea (Cabo Frio, Araruama, Arraial do Cabo, Búzios, São Pedro da Aldeia and Saquarema cities) and central-south Fluminense (Areal city) regions, as described by the Health State Secretary of Rio de Janeiro (SES/RJ), were investigated in the present study.

All animals were submitted to clinical evaluation by the veterinarians of this study, and clinical and epidemiological factors, such as gender, age, castration and contact with soil/plants and other domestic animals, were evaluated. All data were registered on a standardized data collection form. A total of 371 animals were included and divided into groups according to the presence/absence of skin lesions indicative of sporotrichosis as follows: 196 cats with clinical suspicion of sporotrichosis (Suspicious Sporotrichosis Group – SSG) and 175 apparently healthy cats (Colonization Research Group - CRG).

The following biological samples were collected based on clinical conditions, type of lesion and availability at the time of the study: swab from the lesion exudate; swab of the oral cavity; and nail tip fragments from both thoracic members. For diagnostic purposes, cytopathology analysis was conducted by impression smears of the skin lesion prepared on clean and dry glass slides, subsequently stained by the quick panoptic method (Laborclin, Pinhais, PR, Brazil), a Romanowsky-type stain. The slides were analyzed by light microscopy using 40× and 100× objective lenses for the identification of *Sporothrix* yeast-like suggestive structures. All the clinical specimens were immediately transported to the Medical and Molecular Mycology Laboratory, Biomedical Institute of the Fluminense Federal University (LMMI-UFF). Samples that were collected with a swab (lesion exudate and oral cavity) were submitted to routine mycological examination as follows: seeding onto Sabouraud agar 2% dextrose (BD, Franklin Lakes, NJ, USA) and Mycosel® (BD, Franklin Lakes, NJ, USA). The nail tip fragments were processed according to the method developed by the LMMI-UFF staff. Briefly, 5 × 7 mm plastic Ziploc bags containing 5–10 nail tips were used for storage, and the tips were subsequently transferred to 2.0 ml Eppendorf tubes containing 500 µl of 0.9% sterile saline solution. These tubes were submitted to vortexing for 15 s to dislodge possible adhered particles and then centrifuged at 1677 *xg* (Hettich Zentrifugen, Tuttlingen, Germany) for 15 min. Thirty microliters of the obtained pellet were then transferred and streaked on two 90 × 15 mm Petri dishes containing Sabouraud agar 2% dextrose (BD, Franklin Lakes, NJ, USA) and Mycosel® (BD, Franklin Lakes, NJ, USA). All media were incubated at room temperature (25–28 °C) and observed over four weeks for fungal growth. As previously described [3], colonies showing features suggestive of the *Sporothrix* genus were subcultivated on Sabouraud agar 2% dextrose (BD, Franklin Lakes, NJ, USA) at room temperature for colony isolation. The fungi were initially identified based on macro- and microscopic characteristics. Later, potential colonies were subcultured in brain–heart infusion agar (BHI; BD, Franklin Lakes, NJ, USA) at 37 °C for conversion to the yeast stage of *Sporothrix*. A random sampling subset on each study group/area, comprising approximately half of all studied isolates ($n = 51$), was submitted to molecular identification according to a species-specific PCR targeting the calmodulin gene (*CAL*), as previously described [21]. Briefly, fungal cells were recovered from 10-day-old colonies grown on Sabouraud dextrose agar, further used for genomic DNA extraction with the Fast DNA kit (MP Biomedicals, Vista, CA, USA), according to the manufacturer's protocol. DNA extracts concentrations were estimated with a NanoDrop 2000 spectrophotometer (Thermo Fisher Scientific, USA) and stored at − 20 °C until use. We performed a 25 µL reaction as a final volume for the PCR experiments, conducted as follows: 12.5 µL PCR Master Mix buffer (2×), which consisted of 3 mM $MgCl^2$, 400 mM each dNTPs, and 50 U/mL Taq Polymerase (Promega Corporation, Madison, WI, USA); 9.5 µL water, 1 µL each of forward and reverse primers (10 pmol/µL; Integrated DNA Technologies, USA), and 1 µL of target DNA [100 ng/µL], using the touchdown PCR method on a Eppendorf Mastercycler Pro machine (Eppendorf, Hamburg, Germany). The resulting PCR amplicons were separated and visualized on 1.2% agarose gel electrophoresis for 1 h at 100 V in the presence of GelRed (Biotium, Hayward, CA, USA). The L-Pix Touch (Loccus Biotecnologia, São Paulo, Brazil) imaging system was used to visualize the stained bands under UV light.

The data were processed and analyzed with the aid of statistical software BioEstat 5.3 (Belém, PA, Brazil). To analyze the results, the chi-square test and risk estimate test were used, and the nature of the variables was considered. For all tests, the level of significance was set at $p < 0.05$.

Results

Epidemiological and clinical evaluation

Of the 371 animals included in the present study, most inhabited the northern region of the capital (Metropolitan region I; 37%; 138/371), with the remaining cats distributed as follows: Grande Niterói (Metropolitan region II; 19%; 70/371), western region of the capital (Metropolitan region I; 18%; 66/371), Baixada Litorânea (15%; 56/371), Mountain region (6%; 24/371), Baixada Fluminense (Metropolitan region I; 2%; 8/371), Central-south Fluminense region (2%; 6/371) and Central-south capital region (1%; 3/371; Fig. 1). Table 1 shows the distribution of clinical-epidemiological data of the cat populations according to the study group, Colonization Research Group (CRG; $n = 175$) or Suspicious Sporotrichosis Group (SSG; $n = 196$), with the latter group divided into

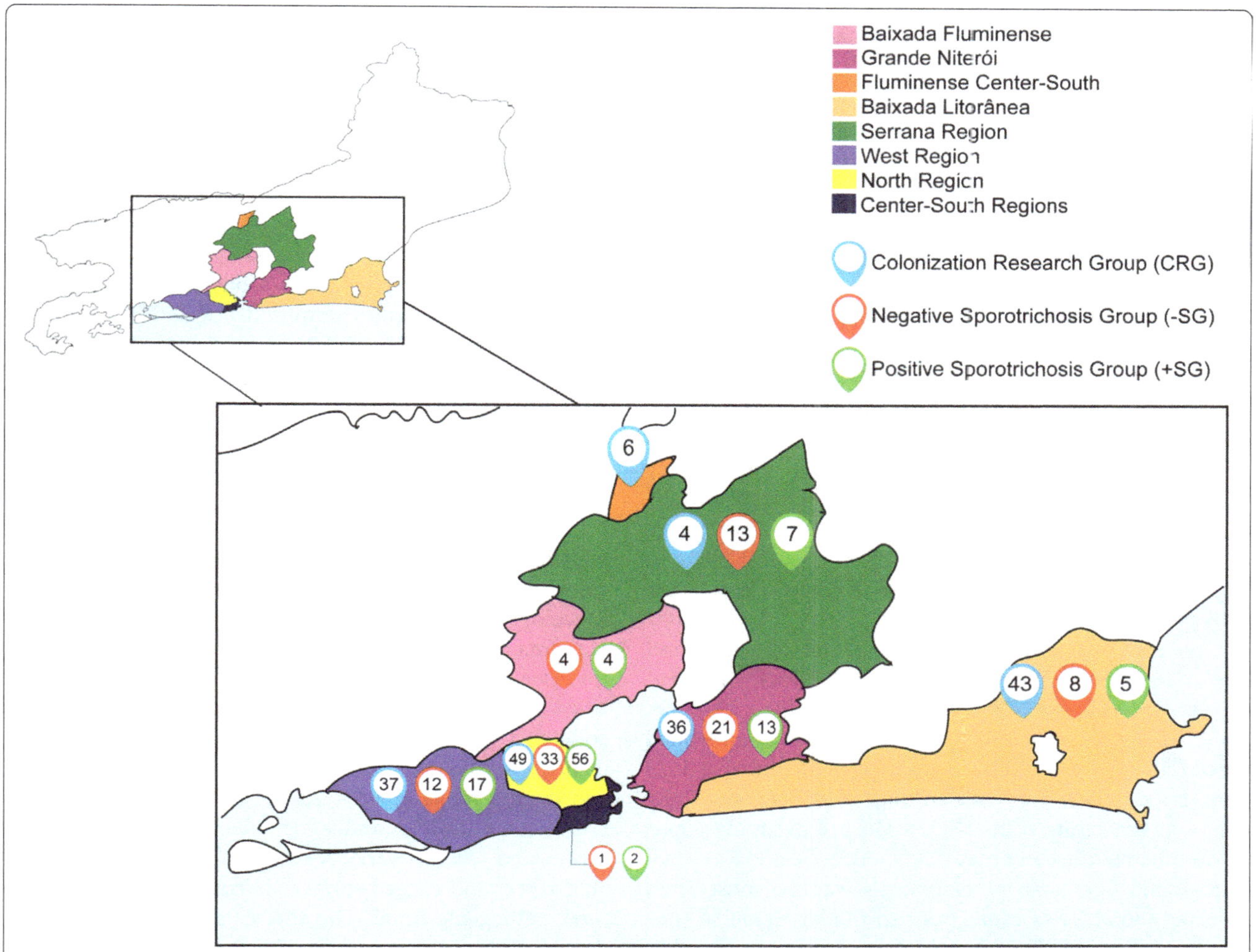

Fig. 1 Map of the state of Rio de Janeiro highlighting the regions inhabited by the cats included in the present study. In each region, the absolute number of cats and groups to which they belong are depicted: CRG (Colonization Research Group), Negative Sporotrichosis Group (-SG) and Positive Sporotrichosis Group (+SG)

Table 1 Absolute number and percentage (%) distribution of cats according to group and clinical-epidemiological variables

Study populations Clinical-epidemiological variables	CRG n (%)	SSG -SG n (%)	 +SG n (%)	TOTAL n (%)	p-value
	175	92	104	371	
Age (mean in years)	2.85 ± 2.8	4.45 ± 3.9	3.75 ± 3.1	3,51 ± 3,2	
Male	88 (50.3)	41 (44.6)	62 (59.6)	191 (51,5)	0,035†
Neutering	100 (57.1)	52 (56.5)	47 (45.2)	199 (53,6)	0,037*
Undefined Breed (UDB)	129 (92.1)	82 (95.3)	92 (94.8)	303 (93,8)	
Urban Area	133 (76.0)	78 (84.8)	82 (78.8)	293 (79,0)	
Contact with Soil/Plants	145 (82.9)	68 (73.9)	75 (72.1)	288 (77,6)	0,034*
Contact with Animals	164 (93.7)	80 (87.0)	76 (73.1)	215 (57,9)	0,0004*
Contact with Cats with Sporotrichosis	59 (33.7)	24 (26.1)	40 (38.5)	123 (33,2)	
Risk Event Prior to Lesion	n.a.	28 (30.4)	43 (41.3)	71 (36,2)	

CRG Colonization Research Group, *SSG* Sporotrichosis Suspicion Group, *-SG* Negative Sporotrichosis Group, *+SG* Positive Sporotrichosis Group
*$p < 0.05$ between CRG and +SG; Chi-square Test
†$p < 0.05$ between -SG and +SG; Chi-square Test
n.a.: not analyzed

two subgroups after laboratory diagnosis by culture (gold-standard): +SG, Positive Sporotrichosis Group ($n = 104$); and -SG, Negative Sporotrichosis Group ($n = 92$; other skin pathologies). A comparison of cat populations of the different geographical areas showed they were similar in all investigated clinical-epidemiological parameters ($p > 0.05$).

The mean age of the studied domestic feline population was 42 months ($\sigma \pm 39$ months), ranging from 2 months to 22 years. There was no significant difference in the mean age of the animals among the three groups studied, even when age was stratified in different groups (< 24 months, 24 to 60 months and > 60 months; $p > 0.05$; data not shown). Approximately half of the cats were male (51.5%), and 58.4% of the population was neutered. No differences were observed in the number of females and males between the +SG and CRG groups ($p = 0.124$). However, the +SG group had more males (59.6%) than the -SG group (44.6%; $p = 0.035$) and a higher number of unneutered animals (54.8%) compared with CRG (42.9%; $p = 0.037$).

A comparison of the cat breed, nutritional status, and area of origin (urban or rural) among the +SG, CRG and -SG groups did not present significant differences ($p > 0.05$). Most of the animals were identified as undefined breed (UDB; 93.8%; 303/323), some were identified as Persian (1.5%; 5/323) and Siamese (4.2%; 14/323), and only one was Himalayan (0.3%; 1/323). Most of the study population inhabited urban areas (CRG: 76%; -SG: 84.8%; +SG: 78.8%), and fight with other animals was the most often reported (36.2%) risk event prior to the suspicion of sporotrichosis lesion (SSG), followed by contact with other animals with sporotrichosis without any record of fight (25%). The majority (83%) of the CRG animals had contact with soil or plants in the house where they lived, and this potential exposure to the fungi was higher than in the +SG animals (72.1%; $p = 0.034$; Table 1). In the CRG, over half of the population was free-roaming (60%), and owners reported that the majority (93.7%) of cats shared their home environment with other animals. In turn, animals with sporotrichosis had less contact with other animals in their own houses (+SG: 73.1%; $p = 0.0004$) compared with the healthy group (CRG).

Crust, ulceration and blood and pus represented the most frequent macroscopic aspects of lesions in infected cats (Fig. 2; Table 2). In many animals, pruritus in varying degrees was reported (69.6%) as a clinical symptom concomitant with lesions; however, this clinical sign was not preferentially observed in cats with sporotrichosis (+SG versus -SG; $p = 0.299$; Table 2). Sneezing and weight loss were more commonly found among +SG cats (sneezing: 62.5%, 65/104; weight loss: 26%, 27/104; Table 2) when compared with -SG animals (sneezing: 39.1%, 36/92; weight loss: 13%, 12/92). Sneezing in cats with suspicious skin lesions was associated with a greater probability of positive sporotrichosis diagnosis (38.6%; $p = 0.001$; OR: 0.386; 95% CI: 0.217 to 0.687).

Infection with pathogenic fungi of the *S. schenckii* complex

Mycological examinations revealed colonies that showed both macro- and micro-morphological characteristics of the *Sporothrix* genus. The macromorphological characteristics of the colonies included an initially cream brown color that turned to a dark brown color after 5–7 days of incubation and a dark brown color with velvety aspect and rugged topography at 25 °C. The colonies showed a cream color at 37 °C, and some colonies showed a creamy aspect and smooth surface, whereas others showed a friable aspect and rugged surface, all compatible with *Sporothrix* pathogenic fungi. The species-specific PCR showed that all 51 isolates correspond to *S. brasiliensis*: 25 from sporotrichosis lesions (+SG = northern region: 8; Grande Niterói: 4; western region: 5; Baixada Litorânea: 2; Mountain region: 3; Baixada Fluminense: 2; Central-south capital region: 1), 12 from nails (+SG = northern region: 4; Grande Niterói: 3; western region: 2; Baixada Litorânea: 2; Baixada Fluminense: 1), 13 from oral mucosa (+SG = northern region: 4; Grande Niterói: 4; western region: 2; Baixada Litorânea: 2; Baixada Fluminense: 1), plus one

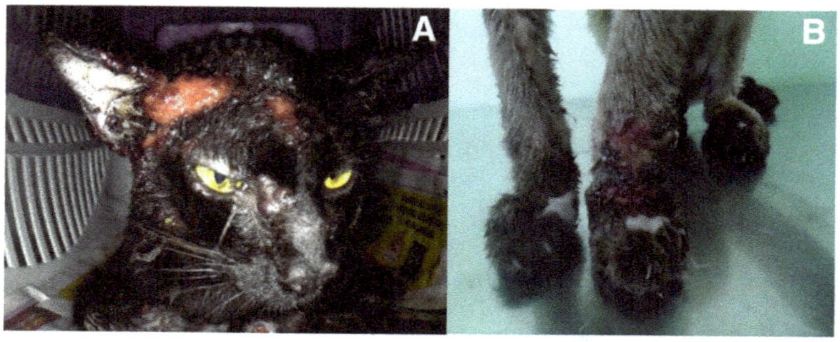

Fig. 2 Most commonly observed sporotrichosis cutaneous lesions in two infected domestic feline showing crust, ulceration, blood and pus in the cephalic region (**a**) and thoracic member (**b**)

Table 2 Absolute number and percentage (%) of cats according to group and clinical variables

Populations	+SG *n* = 104 (%)	−SG *n* = 92 (%)	*p*-value	OR (IC95%)
Clinical Signs				
Respiratory Distress	37 (35.6)	24 (26.1)		
Nasal Secretion	51(49.0)	33(35.9)		
Sneezing	65(62.5)	36 (39.1)	0.001	0.386 (0.217–0.687)
Lack of Appetite	2 (1.9)	3 (3.3)		
Weight Loss	27 (26.0)	12 (13.0)	0.024	0.428 (0.202–0.904)
Apathy	20 (19.2)	18 (19.6)		
Ocular Secretion	3 (2.9)	2 (2.2)		
Epistaxis	5 (4.8)	1 (1.1)		
Macroscopic Aspect of Lesions				
Crust	61 (58.7)	41 (44.6)	0.049	0.567 (0.321–0.999)
Peeling	5 (4.8)	8 (8.7)		
Erythema	31 (29.8)	20 (21.7)		
Ulceration	77 (74.0)	45 (48.9)	< 0.001	0.336 (0.184–0.611)
Presence of Pus	31 (29.8)	13 (14.1)	0.009	0.388 (0.188–0.797)
Presence of Blood	71 (68.3)	39 (42.4)	< 0.001	0.342 (0.191–0.614)
Nodule	38 (36.5)	23 (25.0)		
Depigmentation	5 (4.8)	1 (1.1)		
Vesicle	7 (6.7)	2 (2.2)		
Degree of Pruritus				
Absent	29 (27.9)	26 (28.3)		
Mild	24 (23.1)	22 (23.9)		
Moderate	22 (21.2)	11 (12.0)		
Severe	24 (23.1)	23 (25.0)		

+SG Positive Sporotrichosis Group, *-SG* Negative Sporotrichosis Group
OR odds ratio

from the oral mucosa in the CRG group; all obtained from different domestic feline, as detailed below.

Swab samples from the exudate of lesions suggestive of sporotrichosis and at least one slide obtained via imprint were obtained from 196 animals (SSG), and 53% (104/196; +SG) showed a positive diagnosis, with no confirmed diagnosis in the remaining cats with suspicious skin lesions (-SG).

There was no difference in the frequency of infected animals among the surveyed geographic regions ($\chi^2 = 3.878$; $p = 0.6932$), distributed as follows: central-south region, north and west regions of the capital (67–59%), Baixada Fluminense (50%) and, finally, Grande Niterói, Baixada Litorânea and Mountain region (38–35%).

Colonization versus studied groups

CRG (colonization) and –SG (Sporotrichosis negative diagnosis)

Table 3 summarizes the frequency of colonization by fungi of the *Sporothrix* genus in animals of the three groups according to anatomical site (nails and/or oral mucosa). *Sporothrix brasiliensis* was isolated by culture in a single case of the "healthy" group (CRG; 0.57%, 1/175) from an animal inhabiting the northern region of the municipality of Rio de Janeiro. As for the -SG animals, the same agent was isolated from four cats (4.3%) of the Baixada Fluminense, Mountain region, Grande Niterói and northern region, and one of these animals was colonized both in the nai_ and in the oral mucosa.

Table 3 Frequency of colonization by *Sporothrix* in the three groups according to anatomical site

	Nail Fragments	Oral Cavity	Both Sites	Total *n* = 371 (%)
CRG n = 175 (%)	0	1 (0.57%)	0	1 (057%)
-SG n = 92 (%)	1(1.1%)	2(2.1%)	1(1.1%)	4(4.3%)
+SG n = 104 (%)	11(10.6%)	12(11.5%)	18(17.3%)	41 (39.4%)

CRG Colonization Research Group, *+SG* Positive Sporotrichosis Group, *-SG* Negative Sporotrichosis Group

+SG (Sporotrichosis positive diagnosis)
The highest frequency of colonization was observed in the population with sporotrichosis at 39.4% (41/104; $p < 0.0001$). The northern region of the capital and Grande Niterói showed a similar frequency of colonized animals (47.6 and 50%, respectively). In these regions, cats with colonized nails represented 33.3 and 25% of the population, whereas those with colonized oral mucosa were 19 and 25%, respectively. Among the diseased and colonized animals living in the western region of the capital, half were colonized in the oral mucosa and the other half at both anatomical sites. The same percentage was observed in the population of Baixada Fluminense. In Baixada Litorânea, half of the cats with sporotrichosis carried the fungi in the nails, while the other half had this agent in the oral cavity.

Nail fragments and oral mucosa colonization
A total of 340 nail fragments and 190 swabs of the oral cavity mucosa were obtained from the 371 evaluated cats (Table 4). Overall, 31 nail fragments were colonized (9.18%; 31/340), whereas 34 swabs of the oral mucosa (17.9%; 34/190) were positive.

In the CRG, the prevalence of fungal isolation in the oral cavity was 1.49% (1/66); however, none of the nail fragments were colonized (0/174). As for the -SG, the fungi were isolated from two nail fragments (2.5%; 2/80) and three swabs of the oral cavity (5.3%; 3/57).

The highest frequency of colonized clinical specimens was observed in animals with sporotrichosis (+SG) with 33% of nails (29/86) and 54% of the oral mucosa swabs (36/66) testing positive; significant differences were not observed between these sites ($\chi^2 = 2.158$; $p = 0.1418$).

Discussion
Since the first report of sporotrichosis zoonotic transmission in 1998, the disease has shown a progressive increase in the number of human and animal cases, most of them admitted at the National Institute of Infectious Diseases of the Oswaldo Cruz Foundation (IPEC-FIOCRUZ), which is the reference center for diagnosis and treatment of the disease [2, 4, 7, 9, 17, 18, 20]. Thus, the available literature on clinical-epidemiological data of sporotrichosis in the state of Rio de Janeiro is limited to these populations. The present study investigated infection and colonization by pathogenic fungi of the *S. schenckii* complex in domestic feline populations with or without sporotrichosis from different regions of the state of Rio de Janeiro.

One of the postulated hypotheses was that specific clinical-epidemiological features of cat populations inhabiting different geographic regions would be observed because of the remarkable climatic and demographic differences between these regions, especially the Mountain region and Baixada Litorânea versus the metropolitan areas (Capital, Grande Niterói and Baixada Fluminense). Such a result would be expected because both the Mountain and Baixada Litorânea regions have milder climate and lower population density and are geographically distant from the Baixada Fluminense, which represents the initial epicenter the epidemic. However, the groups of domestic cats surveyed were similar in age, sex, breed, nutritional status, environmental exposure to the fungi, origin (rural or urban) and neutered status, regardless of the region studied. One possible explanation is the fact that both the Mountain region and Baixada Litorânea represent popular tourist regions, which increases the movement of people and subsequently favors the displacement of their animals to these regions [22].

The mean age of the different domestic feline populations of the +SG was homogeneous among the groups, as reported by Madrid et al. [5]. At approximately 3 years of age, cats have reached sexual maturity and come into heat, increasing the chance of fighting for females and subsequent exposure to infected animals. This hypothesis is corroborated by the fact that the studied cats with suspicious lesions (SSG) were involved in fights prior to the onset of the wounds. Despite the predominance of males, this difference was significant only when +SG was compared with the group with other skin pathologies (-SG). The higher number of females in the (-SG) group is noteworthy because females could have been affected by dermatophytosis or parasite infections such as scabies, which are acquired independent of trauma [23]. As expected, a higher number of unneutered animals was observed in the infected population, signaling an increased risk of exposure to the etiological agent of sporotrichosis because of fights over territory and females [4, 9, 15]. Interestingly, cats here defined as "healthy" (CRG) had greater contact with environmental niches compared to animals with sporotrichosis (+SG). Taken together, these results reinforce that feline sporotrichosis in Rio de Janeiro is acquired from other cats affected by this mycosis rather than by direct contact with environmental sources.

Cutaneous lesions in cats with sporotrichosis were compatible with previously described wounds in different cat populations including crust, ulceration and presence of

Table 4 *Sporothrix* isolation within different biological samples

	CRG (p/n)	+SG (p/n)	-SG (p/n)	Total (p/n)
Nail Fragments	0/174	29/86*	2/80	31/340
Oral Cavity	1/66	30/66*	3/57	34/190

CRG Colonization Research Group, *+SG* Positive Sporotrichosis Group, *-SG* Negative Sporotrichosis Group; p = positive
*Differences were not observed in colonization between oral cavity and nail fragments ($\chi^2 = 2.158$; p = 0.1418)

pus and blood [4, 5, 20, 24], as well as respiratory signs and weight loss [20, 24] with the sneezing being the most frequent. Weight loss could be a result of respiratory distress, which may lead to eating difficulties. Data on clinical manifestations of feline sporotrichosis point toward a closer attention by veterinary medicine professionals to respiratory symptoms, especially sneezing, associated with weight loss, crusted lesions, and blood and pus as frequent symptoms of this disease.

Different authors reported the isolation of *Sporothrix* from environmental sources [1, 16, 25]. Surprisingly, nearly all of the 175 healthy cats inhabiting Rio de Janeiro endemic areas did not harbor the fungus either in their oral cavity or their nails, although the great majority of them had prior contact with soil or plants [1, 25, 26]. The single oral cavity colonized cat within this group lived in a cattery and shared the same feeder and drinker with other cats with diagnosed sporotrichosis. Therefore, we postulate that this animal's colonization began by sharing such fomites.

In Table 5 we summarize published data on *Sporothrix* spp. colonization in different Brazilian domestic feline populations. The low frequency of colonization in the healthy cat population from distinct Rio de Janeiro state regions (0.57%) detected is consistent with those reported for cats living in its capital [4] (Table 5; 3.57%) and in the city of São Paulo [19] (SP; Southeast Brazil; 0.7%, 1/120). The authors attributed the low percentage of isolation to the fact that São Paulo is not an endemic area for sporotrichosis. In contrast, a study performed in Rio Grande [27] (RS; South Brazil) in a shelter with 90 animals with or without sporotrichosis, reported fungal isolation from the nails of seven healthy cats (29.1%) amongst all 24 healthy ones as detected by direct claw impressions in a culture medium. This finding may be associated with the presence of *Sporothrix* conidia in the paws or in soil fragments attached to them and not necessarily to the nail exclusive colonization. Considering these results, we conclude that environmental exposure may not be a determining factor for colonization in cats of the surveyed areas. Therefore, nails of non-infected cats are not important as a fungal inoculum reservoir, greatly diminishing the importance of trauma caused by healthy animals in this zoonosis transmission.

Four animals with suspicious of sporotrichosis and negative mycological culture (-SG) were colonized by *S. brasiliensis* in their nails and/or oral mucosa (Tables 3 and 5). These four animals lived with other cats diagnosed with sporotrichosis, except by one of them. Noteworthy, this last domestic feline had been under treatment with itraconazole for 23 months and was persistently colonized in the oral mucosa. Therefore, the present study stands out, for the first time, the potential for sporotrichosis transmission even by cats undergoing antifungal therapy for a long period and with negative mycological results.

Among cats with sporotrichosis here investigated, over half (54%) were colonized in the oral cavity, while approximately one-third were colonized in the nails (33%; Table 3). As summarized in Table 5, these results are similar to previous studies performed in cat

Table 5 Scientific articles on *Sporothrix* colonization in cats from different Brazilian regions, including the present study

Author/Year	Location	CRG (n)	+SG (n)	-SG (n)	Technique used to investigate the nails	Frequency of isolation in the nails (%)			Frequency of isolation in the oral cavity (%)			Frequency of isolation in the nasal cavity (%)		
						CRG	+SG	-SG	CRG	+SG	-SG	CRG	+SG	-SG
Schubach et al. [4][c]	Rio de Janeiro/RJ	84	148	–	Seeding of the *pool* of nail fragments	–	39.5	–	3.57	41.8	–	–	66.2	–
Schubach et al. [15][c]	Rio de Janeiro/RJ	10	347	–	–	–	–	–	–	49,1	–	0	70,5	–
Souza et al. [27][d]	Rio Grande/RS	24	–	–	Paw impressions in culture medium	29.1	–	–	–	–	–	–	–	–
Leme et al., [d] [20]	Rio de Janeiro/RJ	12	11	–	–	–	–	–	16.7	45.5	–	25	72.7	–
Madrid et al. [5][c]	Rio Grande do Sul/ Brasil[a]	–	92	–	–	–	–	–	–	45.2	–	–	–	–
Borges et al. [19][d]	São Paulo/SP	119	1	–	Paw impressions in culture medium	0	0.7	–	–	–	–	–	–	–
Present study[c]	Rio de Janeiro/ Brasil[b]	175	104	92	Seeding of the pool of nail fragments	0	33	2.5	1.49	54	5.3	–	–	–

CRG Colonization Research Group, *+SG* Positive Sporotrichosis Group, *-SG* Negative Sporotrichosis Group

[a]Study performed in eight municipalities of Rio Grande do Sul (Rio Grande, Pelotas, Capão do Leão, Pedro Osório, Morro Redondo, Canguçu, São Lourenço and Bento Gonçalves)

[b]Animals in this study inhabited the following areas of the state of Rio de Janeiro: west, central-south and north regions of the city of Rio de Janeiro, Baixada Fluminense, Grande Niterói, Serrana and dos Lagos Regions and central-south Fluminense

[c] Data referring to clinical specimens

[d] Data referring to domestic cats surveyed

populations from Rio de Janeiro capital [4, 15] as well as from Rio Grande do Sul [5]. As expected, the highest frequency of colonization occurred among domestic feline with sporotrichosis since the these animals have the habit of cleaning themselves by licking and also licking the wound itself where this yeast is abundant [4, 5]. In addition, as pruritus was repeatedly noted in the lesions of several animals here included (approximately 70%), it may have served as stimulus for increasing licking, thus favoring the maintenance of these fungi in the oral cavity. Nasal and oral cavities were more often colonized compared with the nails (present study, [4, 5, 20]), indicating that bites would be the traumatic event with the greatest potential for sporotrichosis transmission rather than scratching.

Conclusions

Because of distinct urbanization, socioeconomic level, climate and demographic aspects of each surveyed area in the present study, which could affect fungal environmental distribution, differences in the sporotrichosis Rio de Janeiro endemics were expected. Nevertheless, in addition to the city of Rio de Janeiro and Baixada Fluminense region, *Sporothrix* equally affects and colonizes animals from other areas, including Grande Niterói, Baixada Litorânea and the Mountain region. Furthermore, our data confirm *S. brasiliensis* as the most prevalent species in the Brazilian feline sporotrichosis epidemics. Thus, we hypothesize that sporotrichosis is a uniform epidemic throughout the state, whose transmission depends mainly on the contact with cats with sporotrichosis.

Colonized feline populations with or without sporotrichosis are concentrated in Rio de Janeiro, São Paulo and Rio Grande do Sul states, and despite their marked geoclimatic differences uniform results are observed. The healthy cat population is of limited importance in the maintenance of epizootic and epidemic sporotrichosis in Rio de Janeiro, whereas cats with confirmed clinical and mycological diagnosis are those with a greater chance of acting as sources of transmission since these animals often carry *Sporothrix* in skin lesions, nails and oral mucosa.

We believe that since Rio de Janeiro displays a world unique epidemic model of the disease, not fully understood, data on the infected and non-infected animals can be of major importance for future strategies of sporotrichosis prevention and control. Finally, considering the importance of the current concept of "one health", the experience here observed can be helpful for distinct epizootias and/or zoonosis.

Acknowledgements
The authors would like to thank the veterinarian collaborators and cat owners for allowing their animals to be part of this study. We also thank Karen Rafaella Silva Diniz for her technical support on laboratorial diagnosis.

Funding
The authors would like to thank the National Council for Scientific and Technological Development (Conselho Nacional de Desenvolvimento Científico e Tecnológico – CNPq) for granting fellowships (PIBIC-CNPq-UFF and Master's) and the Rio de Janeiro Research Foundation (Fundação de Amparo à Pesquisa do Estado do Rio de Janeiro - FAPERJ; E-26/103.198/2011) for funding this study and for granting the IC-FAPERJ fellowship.

Authors' contributions
ARSB and EMSR conceived the study and participated in its design and coordination. PAMS, EMSR, LMLB and ARSB wrote the final version of the manuscript. SRLSS, RPL and EMSR collected and evaluated the clinical and epidemiological data. PAMS, RLDM and CAD performed phenotypic laboratorial diagnosis while AMR conducted molecular analysis. ARSB, LMLB and MRP conducted statistical analysis and interpreted the data obtained. RLDM revised the manuscript critically on its intellectual content and English language adequacy. All authors have read and approved the final manuscript.

Consent for publication
Not applicable.

Competing interests
The authors declare that they have no competing interests.

Author details
[1]Applied Microbiology e Parasitology Postgraduation Program, Fluminense Federal University (UFF), Niterói, RJ, Brazil. [2]Veterinary Medicine Postgraduation Program, Fluminense Federal University (UFF), Niterói, RJ, Brazil. [3]Medical and Molecular Mycology Laboratory, Microbiology and Parasitology Department, Biomedical Institute, Fluminense Federal University (UFF), Rua Prof. Hernani Melo, 101 São Domingos, Niterói, RJ CEP: 24210-130, Brazil. [4]Microbiology, Immunology and Parasitology Department, São Paulo Federal University (UNIFESP), São Paulo, SP, Brazil. [5]Cellular Mycology and Fungal Proteomics Laboratory, Rio de Janeiro State University (UERJ), Rio de Janeiro, RJ, Brazil.

References

1. Marimon R, Cano J, Gené J, Sutton DA, Kawasaki M, Guarro J. *Sporothrix brasiliensis*, *S. globosa*, and *S. mexicana*, three new *Sporothrix* species of clinical interest. J Clin Microbiol. 2007;45:3198–206.
2. Barros MBL, Schubach TMP, Galhardo MCG, Schubach AO, Monteiro PCF, Reis RS, Zancopé-Oliveira RM, Lazéra MS, Cuzzi-Maya T, Blanco TCM, Marzochi KBF, Wanke B, Valle ACF. Sporotrichosis: an emergent Zoonosis in Rio de Janeiro. Mem Inst Oswaldo Cruz. 2001;96(6):777–9.
3. Rippon JW. Sporotrichosis. In: Medical mycology: the pathogenic fungi and the pathogenic Actinomycetes. Philadelphia: W.B. Saunders Co.; 1988. p. 325–52.
4. Schubach TMP, Schubach AO, Reis RS, Cuzzi-Maya T, Blanco TCM, Monteiro DF, Barros MBL, Brustein R, Zancopé-Oliveira RM, Monteiro PCF, Wanke B. *Sporothrix schenckii* isolated from domestic cats with and without sporotrichosis in Rio de Janeiro, Brazil. Mycopathologia. 2001;153:83–6.
5. Madrid IM, Mattei AS, Fernandes CG, Nobre MO, Meireles MCA. Epidemiological findings and laboratory evaluation of Sporotrichosis: a description of 103 cases in cats and dogs in southern Brazil. Mycopathologia. 2012;173:265–73.
6. Schubach AO, Barros MBL, Wanke B. Epidemic sporotrichosis. Curr Opin Infect Dis. 2008;21:129–33.
7. Barros MBL, Paes RA, Schubach AO. *Sporothrix schenckii* and Sporotrichosis. Clin Microbiol Rev. 2011;24:633–54.
8. Barros MBL, Schubach AO, Schubach TMP, Wanke B, Lambert-Passos SR. An epidemic of sporotrichosis in Rio de Janeiro, Brazil: epidemiological aspects of a series of cases. Epidemiol Infect. 2008;136:1192–6.
9. Pereira SA, Gremião IDF, Kitada AAB, Boechat JS, Viana PG, Schubach TMP. The epidemiological scenario of feline sporotrichosis in Rio de Janeiro, state of Rio de Janeiro, Brazil. Rev Soc Bras Med Trop. 2014;47:392–3.

10. Barros MBL, Schubach TP, Coll JO, Gremião ID, Wanke B, Schubach A. Esporotricose: a evolução e os desafios de uma epidemia. Rev Panam Salud Publica. 2010;27(6):455–60.
11. Pereira SA, Schubach TMP, Gremião IDF, Silva DT, Figueiredo FB, Assis NV, Passos SRL. Aspectos terapêuticos da esporotricose felina. Acta Sci Vet. 2009; 37(4):311–21.
12. Gremião IDF, Menezes RC, Schubach TMP, Figueiredo ABF, Cavalcanti MCH, Pereira SA. Feline sporotrichosis: epidemiological and clinical aspects. Med Mycol. 2015;53(1):15–21.
13. Silva MB, Costa MM, Torres CC, Galhardo MC, Valle AC, Magalhães Mde A, Sabroza PC, Oliveira RM. Urban sporotrichosis: a neglected epidemic in Rio de Janeiro, Brazil. Cad Saude Publica. 2012;28(10):1867–80.
14. Gremião IDF, Miranda LHM, Reis EG, Rodrigues AM, Pereira AS. Zoonotic epidemic of Sporotrichosis: cat to human transmission. PLoS Pathog. 2017; https://doi.org/10.1371/journal.ppat.1006077.
15 Schubach TMP, Schubach AO, Okamoto T, Barros MBL, Figueiredo FB, Cuzzi T, Fialho-Monteiro PC, Reis RS, Perez M, Wanke B. Evaluation of an epidemic of sporotrichosis in cats: 347 cases (1998-2001). J Am Vet Med Assoc. 2004; 224(10):1623–9.
16 Sanchotene KO, Madrid IM, Klafke GB, Bergamashi M, Della Terra PP, Rodrigues AM, de Camargo ZP, Xavier MO. *Sporothrix brasiliensis* outbreaks and the rapid emergence of feline sporotrichosis. Mycoses. 2015;58(11):652–8.
17 Reis RS, Almeida-Paes R, Muniz MDM, Tavares PMES, Monteiro PCF, Schubach TMP, Gutierrez-Galhardo MC, Zancopé-Oliveira RM. Molecular characterisation of *Sporothrix schenckii* isolates from humans and cats involved in the sporotrichosis epidemic in Rio de Janeiro, Brazil. Mem Inst Oswaldo Cruz. 2009;104(5):769–74.
18 Schubach AO, Schubach TMP, de Lima Barros MB, Wanke B. Cat-transmitted Sporotrichosis, Rio de Janeiro, Brazil. Emerg Infect Dis. 2005;11(12):1952–4.
19 Borges TS, Rossi CN, Fedullo JDL, Taborda JP, Larsson CE. Isolation of *Sporothrix schenckii* from the claws of domestic cats (indoor and outdoor) and in captivity in São Paulo (Brazil). Mycopathologia. 2013;176(1–2):129–37.
20 Leme LRP, Schubach TMP, Santos IB, Figueiredo FB, Pereira SA, Reis RS, Mello MFV, Ferreira AMR, Quintella LP, Schubach AO. Mycological evaluation of bronchoalveolar lavage in cats with respiratory signs from Rio de Janeiro, Brazil. Mycoses. 2007;50(3):210–4.
21 Rodrigues AM, Hoog GS, De Camargo ZP. Molecular diagnosis of pathogenic *Sporothrix* species. PLoS Negl Trop Dis. 2015;9(12):1–22.
22 IBGE census 2010. Brazil, Instituto Brasileiro de Geografia e Estatística (updated 1st December 2010). Available at: http://censo2010.ibge.gov.br/ Accessed on 9 Jan 2017.
23 Neves RDDM, Cruz FACS, Lima SR, Torres MM, Dutra V, Sousa VRF. Retrospectiva das dermatofitoses em cães e gatos atendidos no Hospital Veterinário da Universidade Federal de Mato Grosso, nos anos de 2006 a 2008. Cienc Rural. 2011;41(8):1405–10.
24 Madrid IM, Mattei AS, Martins A, Nobre M, Meireles M. Feline sporotrichosis in the southern region of Rio Grande Do Sul, Brazil: clinical, zoonotic and therapeutic aspects. Zoonoses Public Health. 2010;57(2):151–4.
25 Fernandes GF, Santos PO, do Amaral CC, Sasaki AA, Godoy-Martinez P, Camargo ZP. Characteristics of 151 Brazilian *Sporothrix schenckii* isolates from 5 different geographic regions of Brazil: a forgotten and re-emergent pathogen. Open Mycol J. 2009;3:48–58.
26 Rodrigues AM, Bagagli E, Camargo ZP, Bosco SMG. *Sporothrix schenckii* Sensu stricto isolated from soil in an armadillo's burrow. Mycopathologia. 2014; https://doi.org/10.1007/s11046-014-9734-8.
27 Souza LL, Nascente PDS, Nobre MDO, Meinerz ARM, Meireles MCA. Isolation of *Sporothrix schenckii* from the nails of healthy cats. Brazilian J Microbiol. 2006;37:372–4.

21

Inflammatory markers before and after farrowing in healthy sows and in sows affected with postpartum dysgalactia syndrome

Marianne Kaiser[1*], Magdalena Jacobson[2], Pia Haubro Andersen[2], Poul Bækbo[3], José Joaquin Cerón[4], Jan Dahl[5], Damián Escribano[4] and Stine Jacobsen[1]

Abstract

Background: The pathogenesis of postpartum dysgalactia syndrome (PDS) in sows is not fully elucidated and affected sows often present vague clinical signs. Accurate and timely diagnosis is difficult, and PDS is often recognized with a delay once piglets begin to starve. Increased rectal temperature of the sow is an important diagnostic parameter, but it may also be influenced by a number of other parameters and is thus difficult to interpret. Inflammatory markers may be important adjuncts to the clinical assessment of sows with PDS, but such markers have only been studied to a limited extent. The objective was to characterize the inflammatory response in healthy sows and in sows suffering from PDS, and to identify biomarkers that may assist in early identification of PDS-affected sows.

Results: Thirty-eight PDS-affected (PDS+) and 38 healthy (PDS-) sows underwent clinical examination and blood sampling every 24 h, from 60 h before the first piglet was born to 36 h after parturition. In both groups, inflammatory markers changed in relation to parturition. Most inflammatory markers changed 12-36 h after parturition [white blood cell counts (WBC), neutrophil counts, lymphocyte counts, tumor necrosis factor alpha (TNF-α), interleukin 6 (IL-6), serum amyloid A (SAA), C-reactive protein (CRP), haptoglobin (Hp), iron (Fe) and albumin (ALB)]. Changes in neutrophil counts, lymphocyte counts, CRP, Fe and ALB were observed -12 to 0 h before parturition. WBC, neutrophil and lymphocyte counts, serum concentrations of TNF-α, IL-6, Hp and Fe differed between PDS+ and PDS- sows. These differences were mainly apparent 12 to 36 h after parturition, but already at 12 h before parturition, PDS+ sows had lower lymphocyte counts than PDS- sows.

Conclusions: Parturition itself caused significant inflammatory changes, but PDS+ sows showed a more severe response than PDS- sows. WBC, neutrophil and lymphocyte counts, and concentrations of TNF-α, IL-6, Hp and Fe can be potential biomarkers for PDS. Lymphocyte counts may be used to detect PDS at pre-partum. To assess their diagnostic potential, these markers must be investigated further and most likely combined with assessment of clinical parameters and other biomarkers for improved identification of sows at risk of developing PDS.

Keywords: PDS, Inflammatory markers, Postpartum, Dysgalactia, Sow

* Correspondence: kaiser@sund.ku.dk
[1]Department of Veterinary Clinical Sciences, Faculty of Health and Medical Sciences, Copenhagen University, Højbakkegård Alle 5, 2630 Taastrup, Denmark
Full list of author information is available at the end of the article

Background

Postpartum dysgalactia syndrome (PDS) is a common disease in sows with recently reported prevalences varying from 6.0 to 48.2% [1–4]. The pathogenesis of PDS is complex and not fully elucidated. Mastitis, metritis and agalactia syndrome (MMA) and coliform mastitis may all cause dysgalactia, but these disease complexes are considered to be the more readily observable components of the PDS complex [5, 6]. Therefore, a subgroup of sub-clinically affected sows, which are difficult to detect in the early stages of the disease, seems to occur. These cases of PDS may only be discovered once piglets start to lose weight and display milk-searching behaviour. Mortality increases when colostrum intake during the first 24 h of life is less than 200 g per piglet [7], and increased piglet mortality among MMA-affected litters has been reported [8]. Furthermore, increased prevalence of stillborn piglets has been found in litters from sows with fever or elevated rectal temperature before [9] and after farrowing [10]. The impact of PDS on the welfare of sows and piglets is thus substantial.

Currently, elevated rectal temperature seems to be one of the more reliable indicators of PDS [4, 11, 12], but as rectal temperature is influenced by metabolic status, parity, circadian rhythm and days postpartum (p.p.), interpretation of the measured rectal temperature is not straight forward [4]. A threshold temperature of 39.5°C is most often applied as a cut-off value when used for detection of PDS [11, 13–20]. Other clinical signs, e.g. anorexia, inflamed udder, decreased demeanor, and milk-searching behavior among piglets, have been used in conjunction with rectal temperatures in an attempt to identify sows with PDS [13, 18, 19, 21, 22].

Systemic inflammation in sows with PDS has only been investigated to a limited degree. Increased blood levels of haptoglobin (Hp) [8, 23], tumor necrosis factor alpha (TNF-α) and interleukin-6 (IL-6) [24] have been found in sows diagnosed with MMA, and a decrease in white blood cell counts (WBC) and neutropenia was observed in sows developing agalactia after experimental intramammary infusion of *Escherichia (E.) coli* [25]. Furthermore, increases in concentrations of cytokines and acute phase proteins (APPs) have been demonstrated in sows with experimental mastitis elicited by intramammary infusion of *E. coli* [26] or lipopolysaccharide (LPS) [27].

Detection of PDS remains elusive, and it is thus possible that the prevalence of sub-clinically affected sows is significant. Consequently, the diagnosis may be delayed until the piglets start expressing hunger, at which time the disease has severe consequences on animal welfare and production. Early detection of the disease (most preferably before or during parturition, or at least before piglets show signs of starvation) is thus desirable and may be aided by assessment of biomarkers in blood. The objective of our study was to characterize the periparturient inflammatory response in healthy sows and in sows suffering from PDS with the goal of identifying biomarkers that may assist in identification of affected animals early in the course of disease.

Methods

Herd and animals

A case-cohort study was performed from March 2014 to November 2014, including 38 PDS affected (PDS+) and 38 healthy (PDS-) multiparous sows. Samples were collected from a Danish sow herd within the Danish Specific Pathogen-Free (SPF) system. The farm was chosen based on a treatment rate of at least 20% of all farrowing sows. Usually, 20–30% of the sows would receive medical treatment in the periparturient period. The sows were housed in confined crates from 1 week before farrowing until 3 weeks after farrowing. Between each batch of sows, the farrowing units were cleaned and disinfected. The farrowing pens had partly slatted floors with 2/3 solid concrete and 1/3 iron bars measuring 1.6 × 2.6 m^2. The sows were fed 4 times per day with liquid feed and assigned straw according to the Danish law of animal welfare. All sows were of the Danish cross-breed (Landrace/Yorkshire).

Experimental design

According to the following and assumptions of the syndrome [28], a broad clinical definition of PDS was adopted. PDS+ sows would have at least two of the following clinically visible characteristics: 1. anorexia, defined as "trough not empty 30 minutes after feeding", 2. inflammation of the udder, characterized by redness, swelling and increased skin temperature, 3. rectal temperature ≥ 39.5°C.

From each of 9 batches, approximately 12 sows were randomly selected and monitored when they entered the farrowing unit. All sows (n = 109) were sampled every 24 h from 60 h before expected parturition and to a maximum of 36 h p.p. or until PDS occurred. For ethical reasons, sows were treated as described below and precluded from further sampling as soon as PDS was detected. In the following order, monitoring prior to parturition included: 1. samplings of saliva and ear venous blood before morning feeding (these data were used for other research purposes and are not shown), 2. veterinary clinical assessment after feeding with recording of the general demeanor, appetite, rectal temperature, respiration frequency, capillary re-filling time, skin color, eye mucosa color, vaginal mucosa color, vaginal discharges, fecal consistency, and signs of inflammation (subjective assessment of skin temperature by palpation, capillary refill time, and hyperemia) of the mammary glands, 3. blood sampling from *v. jugularis* as described below, and 4. blood sampling from *v. epigastrica caudalis superficialis* [*v. mammaria cranialis*] (these data were used for other research purposes and are not shown). After parturition, a morning and an afternoon milking was included in the procedure for other research purposes.

Sows categorized as PDS+ were administered medical treatment by the farmer immediately after the clinical examination and sample collection. The medical treatment consisted of systemic antibiotics, either 10.000 IU/kg bw of benzyl procaine penicillin (Noropen® vet., ScanVet, Denmark) or 16 mg/kg bw of trimethoprim-sulfadiazin (Norodine® vet., ScanVet, Denmark), and 0.4 mg/kg bw of meloxicam (Loxicom®, ScanVet, Denmark). Sows that farrowed prematurely and sows treated for reasons other than PDS were excluded from the study.

Eventually, 38 sows were defined as PDS+ sows, and these were retrospectively matched with 38 PDS- sows. The match was done in the following descending order of importance: 1. batch, 2. parity, and 3. date of parturition. Data from the remaining 33 sows were not included in the study.

Sampling

Blood samples were collected from *v. jugularis* in tubes with no additive for preparation of serum (BD, New Jersey, US) and with EDTA for haematological analyses (BD, New Jersey, US). To reduce stress and build up confidence, the sows were fed small sugar cubes after handling. All blood samples were kept at room temperature for a maximum of 30 minutes before being processed. The additive-free tubes were centrifuged for 10 min. at 3,000 × g and the serum was separated and stored at − 80°C until analysis, which was performed within 15 months from first sampling date. The EDTA tubes were carefully mixed and blood smears prepared within 2 h. Blood smears underwent cytological examination. Blood samples were stored at 5°C for a maximum of 48 hours before they were shipped to the Veterinary Diagnostic Laboratory at University of Copenhagen for determination of WBC count, hematocrit (Ht), hemoglobin (Hb), iron (Fe), Albumin (ALB) and total protein (TP), which were performed by the Hematology System Complete Blood Count method using an automated biochemistry analyzer (ADIVA 2120/2120i, Siemens Healthcare A/S, Denmark). Blood smears were stained with modified Wright stain (Siemens AG, Germany), and differential count of WBC was performed as described [29]. Concentrations of the cytokines interleukin-1 (IL-1), IL-6 and TNF-α in serum were determined by commercially available pig-specific ELISAs (Porcine IL-1 beta/IL-1F2 Quantikine ELISA Kit, Porcine IL-6 Quantikine ELISA Kit, and Porcine TNF-alpha Quantikine ELISA Kit, all from R&D Systems, Minneapolis, USA) as described previously [30]. The absorbance was read at 450 nm using a microtiter plate reader (Multiskan EX, Thermo LabSystems, Massachusetts, USA). Concentrations below the detection limit of the assay were set at the detection limit for the assay in question in the calculations (TNF-α = 23.40 pg/mL, IL-1 = 39.10 pg/mL, IL-6 = 18.80 pg/mL). Concentrations in serum of the acute phase protein serum amyloid A (SAA) was determined by a previously described commercial multispecies SAA ELISA kit (Tridelta Development Ltd., Ireland) according to the manufacturer's instructions [31]. The absorbance was read at 450 nm using a microtiter plate reader (BIO-TEK, Vermont, US). Hp and C-reactive protein (CRP) levels were measured in serum using an automated biochemistry analyzer (Olympus AU600 Automatic Chemistry Analyzer, Olympus Europe GmbH, Germany) with commercial quantitative turbidimetric tests produced by SPINREACT, S.A.U (Spain) and Beckman Coulter® (California, USA), respectively. Assays for Hp and CRP were performed as reported before [32]. The APP assays all had intra-run and inter-run coefficients of variation < 10%, and the limits of detection were 10 mg/L for Hp, 0.6 mg/L for CRP and 3.06 mg/L for SAA. Where concentrations were higher than the upper limit of the assay, concentrations were set at the concentrations of the highest calibrator (SAA, 500 mg/L, n = 7 samples).

Statistical analyses

Retrospectively, the exact sampling times (date:hour:-min.) were determined relative to the exact time of farrowing of the first piglet (date:hour:min.) which was recorded by videos. Sampling times were grouped into time intervals where 0 h was the parturition time of the first piglet: A. -60 to -36 h; B. -36 to -24 h; C. -24 to -12 h; D. -12 to 0 h; E. 0 to 12 h; F. 12 to 24 h, and G. 24 to 36 h. The number of observations (n) within each interval varied because of variation in the individual sampling times relative to parturition (0 h) [For illustrative explanation, see Additional file 1].

For statistic evaluation, two autoregressive linear regression models (A and B) were performed in the PROC MIXED procedure of Statistic Analytical Software, Enterprise Guide 7.1 (SAS® Institute, Cary, North Carolina, USA). Least-squares means (LSMEANS) and standard deviation (SD) were included in the statistic model A. Model A was $\text{OUTCOME PARAMETER}_{ij} = \mu + \text{TIME}_i + \text{GROUP}_j + \text{TIME*GROUP}_{ij} + \varepsilon$ where $\text{OUTCOME PARAMETER}_{ij}$ was the measured value of the inflammatory parameter, μ was the observations value at time 0, TIME_i was explanatory variable "time intervals A-G", GROUP_j the explanatory variable "PDS+/PDS-", TIME*GROUP_{ij} the interaction between the two groups and change over time and ε was the random residual error term. When significant interaction was identified using model A, differences between the relevant groups and time intervals were accepted. In case of non-significant interaction, model A were replaced with model B which was OUTCOME $PARAMETER_{ij} = \mu + TIME_i + GROUP_j + \varepsilon$. If a non-significant change in $TIME_i$ occur in model B, the OUTCOME $PARAMETER_{ij}$ was considered non-significant. For significant $TIME_i$ value, differences in the relevant groups were still accepted and recorded from the model A output. In case of a significant effect of $GROUP_j$, an overall effect of group was accepted. Significance was considered if $p<0.05$. Parity and body condition score were included as explanatory variables. By preliminary analyses, obstetric aid and farrowing length were found not to be associated with any of the outcome variables. Natural logarithm was performed for lymphocytes, IL-6, TNF-α, CRP, SAA and TP because assumptions concerning residual plots and test for normality were unlikely.

Results

Clinical findings

The 38 sows categorized as PDS+ constituted 34.9% of the farrowings in the randomly selected 109 sows. PDS+ sows were on average treated 18.6 h (range 6-26.9 h) after the first piglet was born. Obstetric aid was performed in 18 PDS+ sows and 11 PDS- sows. Reduced appetite was observed in 10 PDS+ sows and 5 PDS- sows at 0-12 h, while 12 PDS+ sows and 12 PDS- showed reduced appetite at 12-24 h (with 1 sow having complete anorexia). Mean parity, relevant production results, and clinical findings are shown in Table 1.

Inflammatory markers

Change in level of inflammatory markers in relation to parturition

In both PDS+ and PDS- sows, inflammatory markers changed in relation to parturition. Developments over time for both groups are illustrated by raw data for WBC, neutrophils, lymphocytes, TNF-α, IL-6, SAA, CRP, Hp, Fe and ALB (Figs. 1, 2, 3, 4, 5, 6, 7, 8, 9 and 10). Some markers (IL-1, TP, Hb, and Ht) did not change significantly over time in any group [See Additional file 2, Additional file 3, Additional file 4 and Additional file 5]. A leukocyte left shift was detected in one time interval in 5 PDS+ sows and 1 PDS- sow. Mild neutrophilic toxic changes were observed in one time interval in 5 PDS+ sows and 7 PDS- sows. Reactive lymphocytes in low numbers were observed in 2 PDS+ sows and in 7 PDS- sows.

Table 1 Parity and productions results for 38 sows with postpartum dysgalactia syndrome (PDS+) and 38 healthy sows (PDS-) together with key clinical parameters in time interval A, E and F. The number of observations (*n*) in each interval varies because of variation in individual sampling times relative to parturition (0 h) [For further explanation see Additional file 1]

Sow related observations	PDS+				PDS-			
	n	Mean	Min	Max	*n*	Mean	Min	Max
Parity and production								
Parity, no.	38	4.26	2	7	38	4.12	2	7
Liveborn, no.	37	16.9	10	23	38	17.3	6	24
Stillborn, no.	38	0.18	0	3	38	0.32	0	3
Clinical findings time point A (-60 to -36 h p.p.)								
Rectal temp, °C	18	38.1	37.4	38.7	22	38.2	37.6	38.8
Increased mammary skin temperature, no. of glands/sow	18	0.1	0	1	22	0.9	0	14
Heart rate, beats/min.	18	122	96	152	22	112	82	160
Respiratory rate, breaths/min.	18	46	22	86	22	45	22	88
Clinical findings time point E (0 to12 h p.p.)								
Rectal temp, °C	15	38.9	38.0	40.1	10	38.6	37.3	39.3
Increased mammary skin temperature, no. of glands/sow	14	4.4	0	16	10	1.5	0	15
Heart rate, beats/min.	14	112	68	144	10	117	92	144
Respiratory rate, breaths/min.	15	31	13	112	10	37	12	84
Clinical findings time point F (12 to 24 h p.p.)								
Rectal temp., °C	23	39.5	38.1	40.5	25	39.0	38.1	39.3
Increased mammary skin temperature, no. of glands/sow	23	10.4	0	17	24	6.0	0	16
Heart rate, beats/min.	23	117	84	158	25	101	74	144
Respiratory rate, breaths/min.	23	25	12	38	24	27	12	66

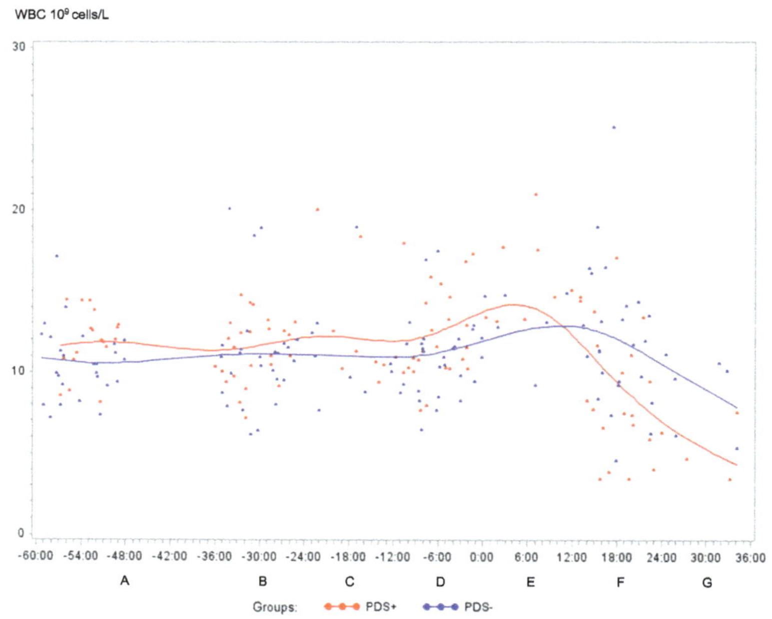

Fig. 1 White blood cell (WBC) counts (10^9 cells/L) in sows with postpartum dysgalactia syndrome (PDS+, red) and healthy sows (PDS-, blue) sampled from 60 h before until 36 h after parturition (time interval A-G). Each dot represents the exact sample time of each observation relative to the exact birth of the first piglet (0 h). The lines show the mean value (Normal range; 11.3-22.8 × 10^9 cells/L)

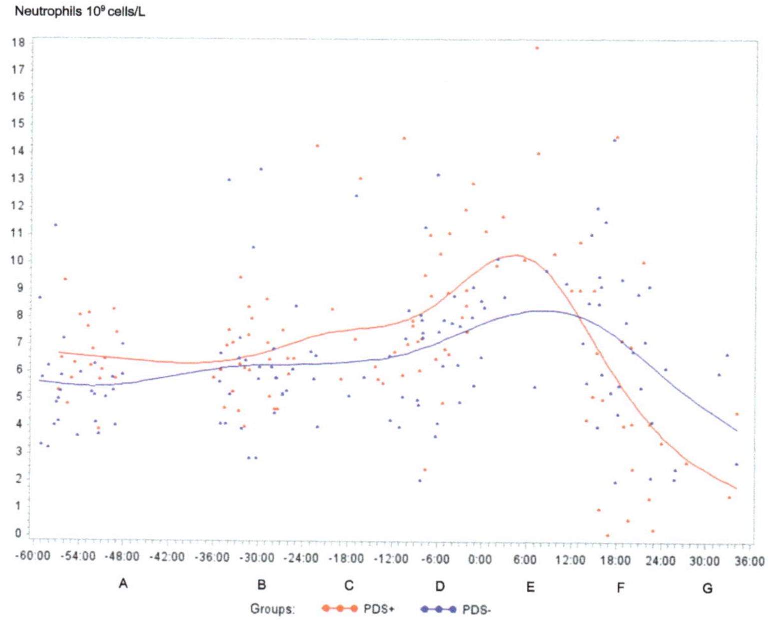

Fig. 2 Neutrophils counts (10^9 cells/L) in sows with postpartum dysgalactia syndrome (PDS+, red) and healthy sows (PDS-, blue) sampled from 60 h before until 36 h after parturition (time interval A-G). Each dot represents the exact sample time of each observation relative to the exact birth of the first piglet (0 h). The lines show the mean value (Normal range; 3.1-9.6 × 10^9 cells/L)

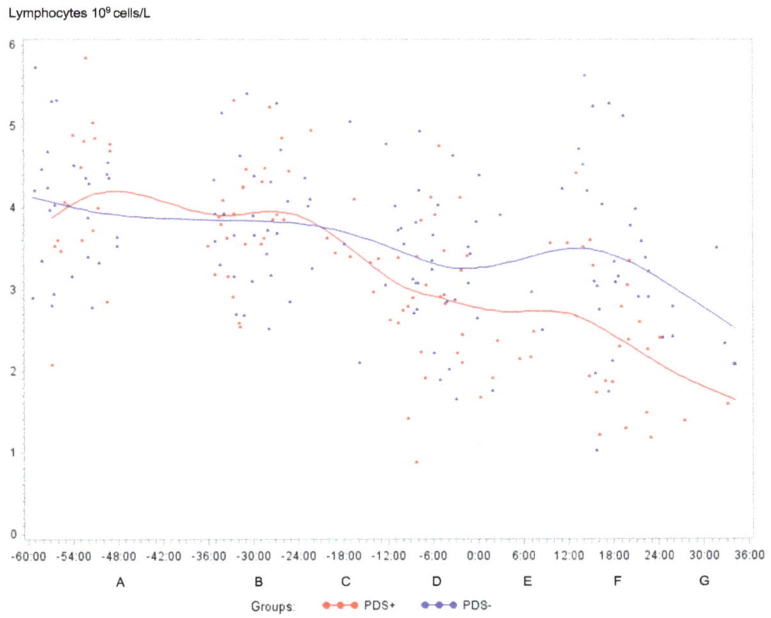

Fig. 3 Lymphocyte counts (10^9 cells/L) in sows with postpartum dysgalactia syndrome (PDS+, red) and healthy sows (PDS-, blue) sampled from 60 h before until 36 h after parturition (time interval A-G). Each dot represents the exact sample time of each observation relative to the exact birth of the first piglet (0 h). The lines show the mean value (Normal range; 4.6 – 10.0 × 10^9 cells/L)

Statistically significant changes of the inflammatory markers in relation to parturition for both PDS- and PDS+ sows are summarized in Fig. 11. Most inflammatory markers were changed relative to baseline (time interval A) between 12 and 36 h p.p. [WBC (Fig. 1), neutrophil counts (Fig. 2), lymphocyte counts (Fig. 3), TNF-α (Fig. 4), IL-6 (Fig. 5), SAA (Fig. 6), CRP (Fig. 7), Hp (Fig. 8), Fe (Fig. 9) and ALB (Fig. 10)], while changes in neutrophil counts (Fig. 2), lymphocyte counts (Fig. 3), CRP (Fig. 7), Fe (PDS+ sows only, Fig. 9), ALB (PDS-

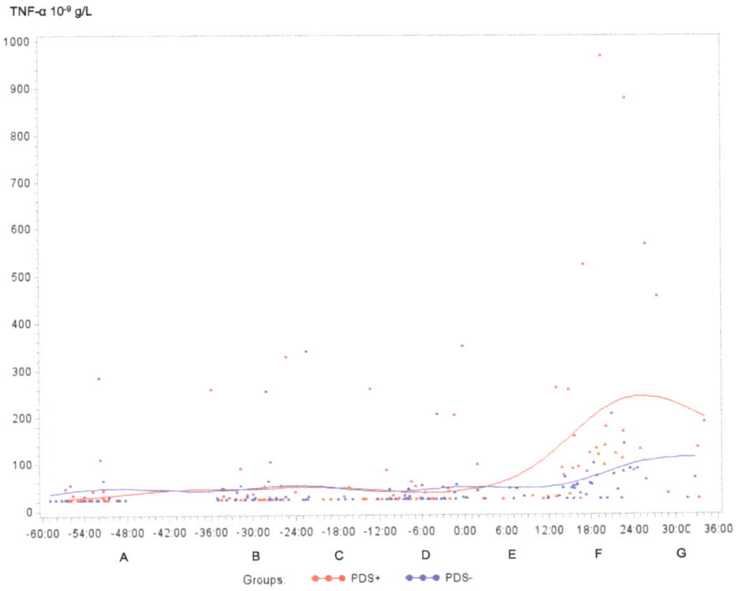

Fig. 4 Tumor necrosis factor alpha (TNF-α) concentration (10^{-9}g/L) in sows with postpartum dysgalactia syndrome (PDS+, red) and healthy sows (PDS-, blue) sampled from 60 h before until 36 h after parturition (time interval A-G). Each dot represents the exact sample time of each observation relative to the exact birth of the first piglet (0 h). The lines show the mean value

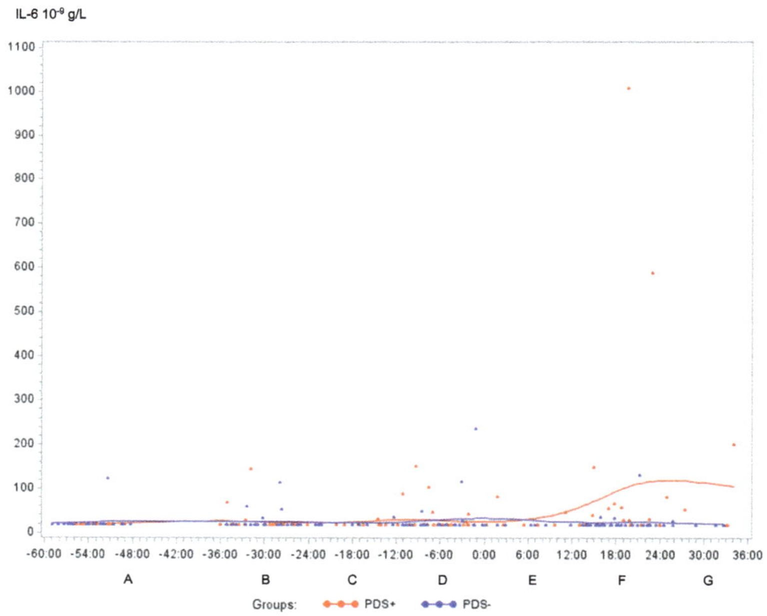

Fig. 5 Interleukin 6 (IL-6) concentration (10^{-9} g/L) in sows with postpartum dysgalactia syndrome (PDS+, red) and healthy sows (PDS-, blue) sampled from 60 h before until 36 h after parturition (time interval A-G). Each dot represents the exact sample time of each observation relative to the exact birth of the first piglet (0 h). The lines show the mean value

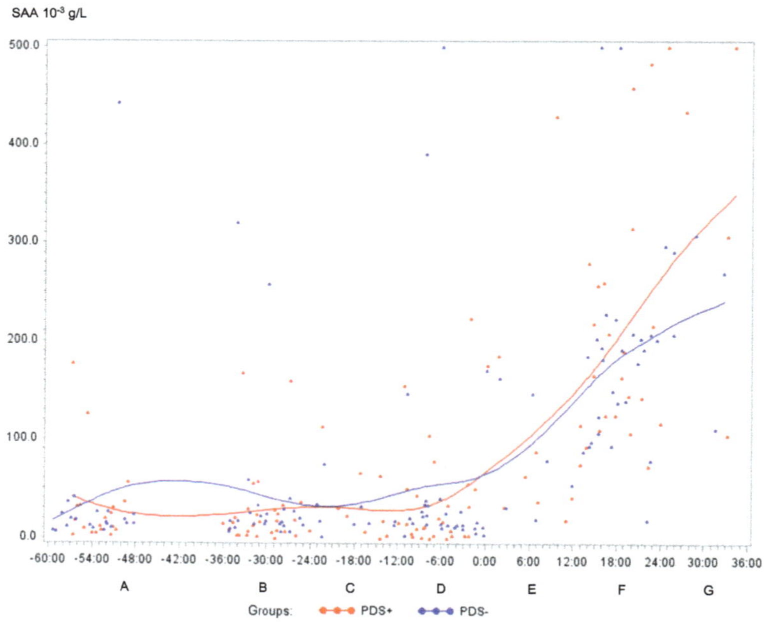

Fig. 6 Serum amyloid A (SAA) (10^{-3} g/L) in sows with postpartum dysgalactia syndrome (PDS+, red) and healthy sows (PDS-, blue) sampled from 60 h before until 36 h after parturition (time interval A-G). Each dot represents the exact sample time of each observation relative to the exact birth of the first piglet (0 h). The lines show the mean value

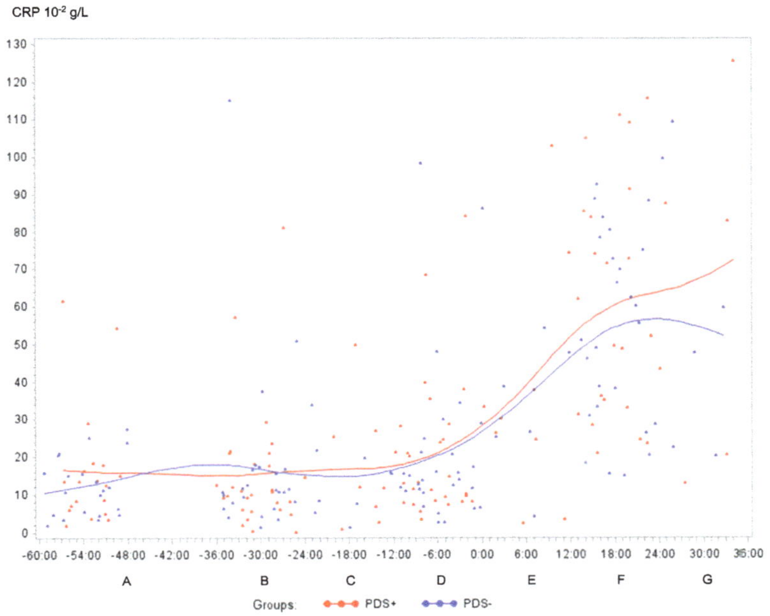

Fig. 7 C-reactive protein (CRP) concentration (10^{-2} g/L) in sows with postpartum dysgalactia syndrome (PDS+, red) and healthy sows (PDS-, blue) sampled from 60 h before until 36 h after parturition (time interval A-G). Each dot represents the exact sample time of each observation relative to the exact birth of the first piglet (0 h). The lines show the mean value

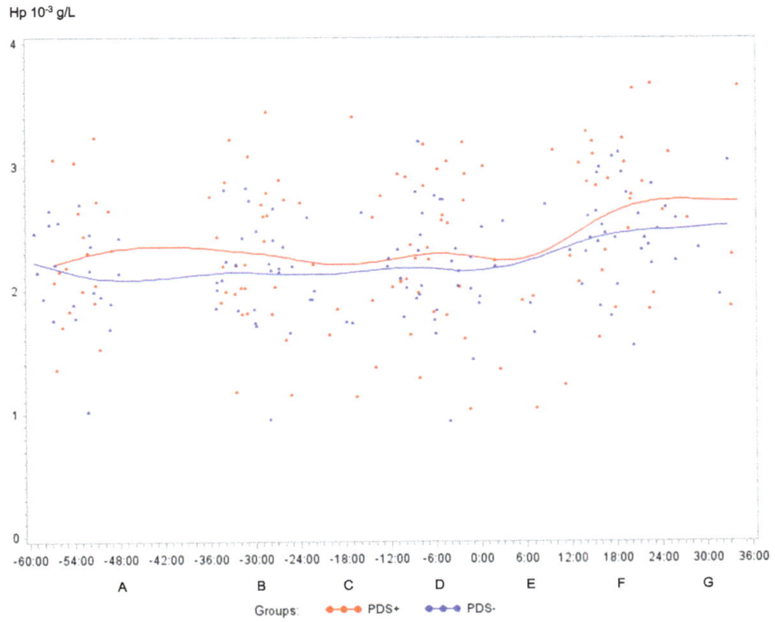

Fig. 8 Haptoglobin (Hp) concentration (10^{-3} g/L) in sows with postpartum dysgalactia syndrome (PDS+, red) and healthy sows (PDS-, blue) sampled from 60 h before until 36 h after parturition (time interval A-G). Each dot represents the exact sample time of each observation relative to the exact birth of the first piglet (0 h). The lines show the mean value

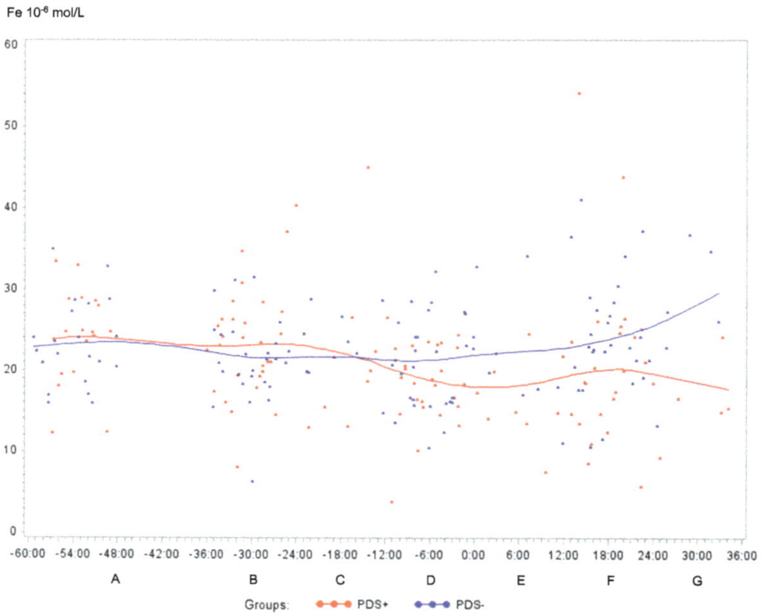

Fig. 9 Iron (Fe) concentration (10^{-6} mol/L) in sows with postpartum dysgalactia syndrome (PDS+, red) and healthy sows (PDS-, blue) sampled from 60 h before until 36 h after parturition (time interval A-G). Each dot represents the exact sample time of each observation relative to the exact birth of the first piglet (0 h). The lines show the mean value (Normal range is 9.0 – 30.4 10^{-6} mol/L)

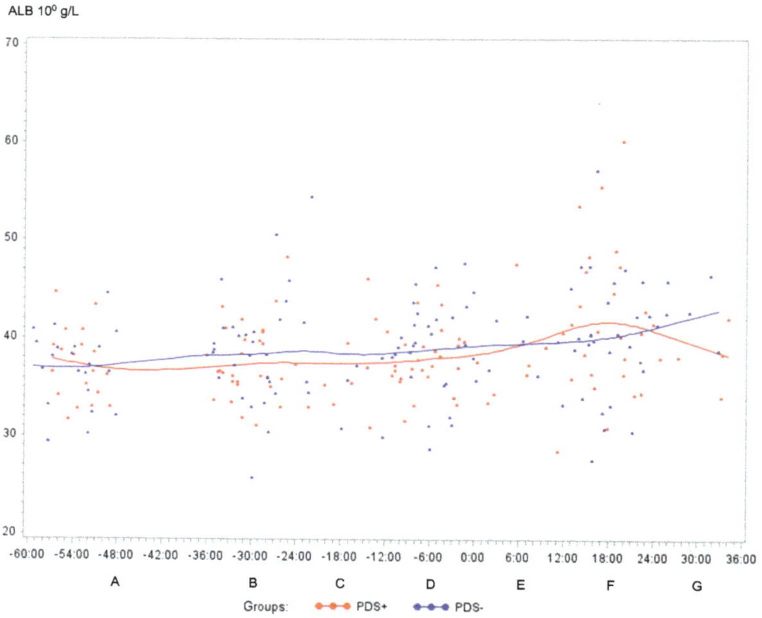

Fig. 10 Albumin (ALB) concentration (10^{0} g/L) in sows with postpartum dysgalactia syndrome (PDS+, red) and healthy sows (PDS-, blue) sampled from 60 h before until 36 h after parturition (time interval A-G). Each dot represents the exact sample time of each observation relative to the exact birth of the first piglet (0 h). The lines show the mean value (Normal range is 32 – 48 10^{0} g/L)

	A. -60 to -36 h	B. -36 to -24 h	C. -24 to -12 h	D. -12 to 0 h	E. 0 to 12 h	F. 12 to 24 h	G. 24 to 36 h
PDS+				↑Neutrophil ** ↓Lymphocyte **** ↑CRP * ↓Fe **	↑WBC ** ↑Neutrophil **** ↓Lymphocyte **** ↑SAA ** ↑CRP *** ↓Fe **	↓WBC ** ↓Lymphocyte **** ↑TNF-α **** ↑IL-6 **** ↑SAA **** ↑CRP **** ↑Hp **** ↑ALB **	↓WBC ** ↓Neutrophil * ↓Lymphocyte **** ↑TNF-α **** ↑IL-6 * ↑SAA **** ↑CRP **** ↑Hp **** ↓Fe *
PDS-				↑Neutrophil * ↓Lymphocyte ** ↑CRP ** ↑ALB *	↑WBC * ↑Neutrophil ** ↑SAA ** ↑CRP ****	↑Neutrophil ** ↓Lymphocyte * ↑TNF-α *** ↑SAA **** ↑CRP **** ↑Hp **** ↑ALB *	↓Lymphocyte ** ↑TNF-α * ↑SAA **** ↑CRP **** ↑Hp **** ↑ALB **

Asterisk symbols indicate differences between time interval A and each of the time intervals B, C, D, E, F or G: **** $p<0.0001$, *** $p<0.001$, ** $p<0.01$, * $p<0.05$

Fig. 11 Changes in levels of inflammatory markers over time in 38 sows with postpartum dysgalactia syndrome (PDS+) and 38 healthy (PDS-) sows, with asterisk symbols indicating significant differences between time interval A and the subsequent time intervals (D to G). Upward pointing arrows indicate increasing concentrations. Downward pointing arrows indicate decreasing concentrations

sows only and Fig. 10) were observed also before parturition (Fig. 11).

Differences between PDS+ and PDS- sows

WBC, neutrophil counts, lymphocyte counts, TNF-α, IL-6, Hp and Fe differed between PDS+ and PDS- sows (Table 2). Lymphocyte counts differed between PDS- and PDS+ sows pre-partum, with lymphocyte counts being lower in PDS+ than in PDS- sows from -12 h to 36 h. While WBC and neutrophil counts tended to be higher in PDS+ than in PDS- sows immediately around parturition (-12 to 12 h p.p.), WBC and neutrophil counts dropped in PDS+ sows and were significantly lower than in PDS- sows 12-24 h p.p. After parturition, concentrations of TNF-α, IL-6 and Hp were significantly higher in PDS+ than in PDS- sows at 12-36 h. Concentrations of Fe were significantly lower in PDS+ than in PDS- sows 24-36 h p.p. Concentrations of SAA, CRP, ALB, TP, Hb and Ht did not differ between PDS+ and PDS- sows.

Discussion

Periparturient inflammation

In the present study, hematological and blood biochemical changes indicate the presence of systemic inflammation in both healthy and PDS-affected sows. Periparturient inflammation in healthy individuals has previously been described in other species [33, 34] as well as in sows [35]. In horses, WBC [34] and SAA concentrations [36] were increased within 2 and 36 h, respectively, after foaling. In healthy primiparous sows, blood neutrophil counts increased significantly between day 3 before parturition and day 1 p.p. [37, 38], followed by a decrease back towards antepartum levels on day 3 p.p. [38]. In healthy sows, SAA and Hp concentrations were increased relative to antepartum levels 48-72 h and 24-96 h p.p., respectively [26]. Several factors may cause periparturient changes in inflammatory markers. Hormonal changes with fast antepartum cortisol increase have been suggested to be the cause of periparturient leukocytosis and neutrophilia [34]. Release of cytokines and APPs after parturition could be caused by tissue trauma to the birth canal, elicited by the foetus as well as by obstetric interventions. Understanding periparturient inflammation in otherwise healthy sows is important for differentiating physiology from pathology when using inflammatory markers for assessing periparturient disease, as inflammatory markers are non-specific in nature and will be released in infectious as well as non-infectious inflammation. Limiting periparturient inflammation may be beneficial to avoid inflammatory-induced physiological and behavioural changes such as malaise, pain, fatigue and anorexia, which may affect the sow's ability to provide for the piglets and thus impact welfare of both sow and piglets. PDS+ as well as PDS- sows had increased serum concentrations of TNF-α and IL-6 12-36 h p.p., and these two cytokines have been shown to cause a wide range of clinical signs [39, 40]. The link between parturition-induced inflammation and disease is unexplored, but sows with larger litters and sows receiving birth interventions, and thus potentially more trauma to the birth canal, were more likely to develop coliform mastitis [14]. Pre-existing inflammation may also be a problem if animals are subsequently affected by an infectious agent. It has been shown that exposure to exogenous LPS exacerbates tissue injury and mortality in experimentally induced ischemia and reperfusion lesions [41, 42].

In sow mammary tissue, lymphocytes are located in the interalveolar tissue, in the epithelium and, during lactation within the alveolar lumen [43, 44]. At the end

Table 2 Least-squares means (LSMEANS) and standard deviation (SD) for white blood cell counts (WBC), neutrophil counts, lymphocyte counts, tumor necrosis factor alpha (TNF-α), interleukin 6 (IL-6), serum amyloid A (SAA), C-reactive protein (CRP), haptoglobin (Hp), iron (Fe) and albumin (ALB) in 38 sows with postpartum dysgalactia syndrome (PDS+) and 38 healthy sows (PDS-)

			A. (-60 to -36 h)		B. (-36 to -24 h)		C. (-24 to -12 h)		D. (-12 to 0 h)		E. (0 to 12 h)		F. (12 to 24 h)		G. (24 to 36 h)	
Parameter	Group	*n*	LSMEANS	±SD	LSMEANS	±SD	LSMEANS	±SD	LSMEANS	±SD	LSMEANS	±SD	LSMEANS	±SD	LSMEANS	±SD
White blood cells	PDS+	110	11.46	0.69	11.29	0.58	12.62	1.04	12.14	0.58	15.45	1.04	8.74****	0.66	6.15	1.45
	PDS-	126	10.77	0.58	11.22	0.57	11.68	0.97	11.09	0.55	13.94	1.16	12.20****	0.60	9.24	1.18
Neutrophils	PDS+	110	6.35	0.59	6.36	0.49	7.93	0.90	8.34	0.49	11.53	0.89	5.22**	0.56	3.35	1.25
	PDS-	126	5.57	0.49	6.39	0.49	6.43	0.83	7.09	0.48	8.9	1.00	7.46**	0.51	4.35	1.01
Lymphocytes	PDS+	110	3.96	1.07	3.81	1.05	3.69	1.10	2.74*	1.05	2.43	1.10	2.22****	1.06	1.90*	1.14
	PDS-	126	3.95	1.05	3.75	1.05	3.83	1.01	3.20*	1.05	3.23	1.12	3.30****	1.06	2.69*	1.12
Tumor necrosis factor-α	PDS+	121	30.04	1.15	31.81	1.13	32.27	1.21	31.02	1.13	34.35	1.21	130.43****	1.14	130.36*	1.26
	PDS-	119	31.53	1.15	32.80	1.13	29.87	1.20	31.71	1.13	34.23	1.22	55.21****	1.14	58.99*	1.25
Interleukin 6	PDS+	121	19.10	1.13	22.28	1.11	19.94	1.20	24.61	3.03	24.76	1.20	39.20***	1.13	39.54	1.25
	PDS-	119	20.50	1.13	22.23	1.12	21.15	1.20	22.81	1.11	20.70	1.22	22.06***	1.12	21.47	1.24
Serum amyloid A	PDS+	120	15.01	1.27	12.81	1.22	13.33	1.42	14.84	1.23	54.20	1.42	187.41	1.26	234.58	1.53
	PDS-	122	18.45	1.26	20.63	1.24	19.81	1.41	21.36	1.23	69.06	1.46	145.13	1.24	292.72	1.52
C-reactive protein	PDS+	122	10.03	1.18	8.71	1.13	13.72	1.26	14.86	1.16	24.60	1.26	56.30	1.17	71.52	1.32
	PDS-	122	9.23	1.18	11.80	1.16	11.05	1.25	14.65	1.16	29.14	1.27	48.52	1.17	53.02	1.31
Haptoglobin	PDS+	122	2.24	0.08	2.26	0.08	2.35	0.10	2.30	0.08	2.31	0.10	2.73*	0.08	2.92*	0.12
	PDS-	122	2.11	0.08	2.15	0.08	2.16	0.10	2.15	0.08	2.23	0.10	2.46*	0.08	2.56*	0.11
Iron	PDS+	122	24.36	1.51	23.40	1.23	22.16	2.23	18.30	1.27	16.75	2.22	20.86	1.38	17.97*	2.73
	PDS-	125	23.30	1.44	21.22	1.30	23.42	2.20	21.12	1.25	21.28	2.32	24.08	1.30	26.40*	2.68
Albumin	PDS+	122	37.31	1.09	37.38	0.90	37.82	1.60	37.74	0.93	38.38	1.59	41.99	1.00	40.15	1.95
	PDS-	125	36.67	1.04	38.52	0.94	37.17	1.57	39.73	0.91	37.79	1.66	39.88	0.95	42.83	1.91
Total protein	PDS+	122	72.29	1.03	71.20	1.02	72.76	1.04	70.74	1.02	70.73	1.04	76.14	1.03	76.50	1.05
	PDS-	125	69.30	1.03	72.54	1.02	68.87	1.04	73.29	1.02	68.92	1.04	72.93	1.02	77.71	1.05
Hemoglobin	PDS+	110	6.51	0.12	6.32	0.10	6.31	0.17	6.31	0.10	6.02	0.17	6.41	0.11	6.50	0.23
	PDS-	126	6.44	0.10	6.34	0.10	6.38	0.16	6.29	0.10	6.46	0.18	6.22	0.10	6.39	0.19
Hematocrit	PDS+	110	0.35	0.01	0.34	0.01	0.34	0.01	0.34	0.01	0.32	0.01	0.34	0.01	0.34	0.01
	PDS-	126	0.34	0.01	0.34	0.01	0.35	0.01	0.33	0.01	0.35	0.01	0.33	0.01	0.34	0.01

Asterisk symbols indicating significant differences between PDS+ and PDS- sows: **** $p<0.0001$, *** $p<0.001$, ** $p<0.01$, * $p<0.05$

of gestation, the total number of lymphocytes in the mammary tissue increases but at parturition the amount decreases temporarily, followed by a second increase from the day of parturition [43, 44]. Moreover, increased opsonic activity in mammary secretion are found p.p. [38]. The observed decrease in lymphocyte counts observed between -12 and 36 h in PDS+ sows, and to some extent in PDS- sows, could therefore be explained by recruitment of lymphocytes into the mammary tissue for colostrum production. Further, Salmon [43] demonstrated a temporal association between lymphocyte accumulation and expression of prolactin-receptors on the epithelial cells which indicate that prolactin plays a role directing lymphocytes to the mammary tissue. Though, lymphocytopenia also occur in response to glucocorticoid administration in humans [44–46] and an association between increased serum cortisol and decreased numbers of mononuclear cells are found in healthy sows during parturition [37, 38]. Magnusson and Fossum [37] therefore concluded that variations in numbers of mononuclear cells could be influenced by cortisol. This could also be the case in the present study.

Inflammatory changes in sows with PDS

The prevalence of PDS+ sows (34.9 %) in the herd indicates that high herd health and SPF status did not protect the sows from developing PDS.

Leukocyte counts (WBC, neutrophil and lymphocyte counts), serum concentrations of the proinflammatory cytokines (TNF-α and IL-6) and acute phase reactants (Hp and Fe) differed between healthy and PDS affected sows. These changes suggest that PDS+ sows suffered from more severe systemic inflammation than did the PDS- sows. The cause of this inflammation was not determined. A previous study in gilts demonstrated a decrease in WBC and neutrophils 12-36 h after LPS infusion at parturition [25] and a non-significant decrease of WBC and neutrophils was found among sows with clinical signs of agalactia day 1 and 2 p.p. [35]. The leukopenia and low neutrophil counts that developed in PDS+ sows 12-36 h p.p. could be related to overwhelming infection or exposure to LPS, as LPS may cause profound leukopenia in several species including pigs [47]. *E. coli* has been found in larger amount among agalactic sows [17], which indicate that LPS could be involved in the pathogenesis of PDS. Leukocyte left shift has been demonstrated among sows affected with porcine agalactia [48] after exposure to LPS [49] and E. coli [50], so release of this substance from the mammary gland or intestine may have resulted in the cytological changes observed in the PDS+ sows.

There was a tendency ($p<0.1$) for transient elevated neutrophil counts in PDS+ sows from -12 to 12 h compared to PDS- sows (Fig. 2). This could reflect an endocrine stress response with increased blood cortisol, as cortisol causes leukocytosis and neutrophilia by preventing migration of leukocytes to the extracellular space [51].

Concentrations of the pro-inflammatory cytokines TNF-α and IL-6 were higher in PDS+ than in PDS- sows. A previous study demonstrated higher serum TNF-α and IL-6 concentrations in sows affected with MMA compared to healthy sows for up to 72 h p.p. [24]. Experimental induction of udder inflammation by intra-mammary infusion of LPS [27] or *E. coli* inoculation [26] has been shown to cause increased blood concentrations of TNF-α and IL-6. Based on these findings, previous studies have suggested that TNF-α and IL-6 could be potential biomarkers for detection of sows with coliform mastitis or MMA [24, 26], thus corroborating the results of the present study.

Proinflammatory cytokines are responsible for the induction of hepatic synthesis of APPs. Concentrations of the three measured APPs, CRP, SAA and Hp, increased significantly peripartum in both groups of sows, but only Hp concentrations differed in PDS- and PDS+ sows. While p.p. concentrations of Hp were similar in healthy sows and sows receiving intramammary administration of *E. coli* in one study [26], another study detected higher Hp concentrations in sows with MMA than in healthy sows 1-10 days p.p. [8]. Based on our results, Hp seems to be the most useful of the three APPs measured. Considering the modest difference in Hp concentrations in PDS+ and PDS- sows (peak Hp concentration was 14 % higher in PDS+ sows than in PDS- sows), the diagnostic potential of Hp may be limited. It is not clear why concentrations of SAA, which is considered to be a very sensitive marker of inflammation [52], did not differ between the groups. In a previous study, higher blood concentrations of SAA were detected in sows undergoing intra-mammary inoculation with *E. coli* as compared to healthy controls [26]. The discrepancy between studies may be related to the timing of sampling, as different APPs have different response patterns, with some increasing more slowly than others. In the study by Zhu et al. [26] sows were sampled until 96 h p.p., and the study showed that SAA concentrations peaked at 48 h p.p. following intramammary infusion of *E. coli*, whereas concentrations of proinflammatory cytokines peaked at 24 h. To the authors knowledge, CRP has not been investigated in sows at parturition. However, CRP has well described APP properties in the porcine species, as increased concentrations have been found in pigs with clinical signs of disease [53], pigs with lesions at slaughter [54] and after experimental injection of LPS [55] or turpentine [56]. Similar to SAA, CRP could not distinguish PDS+ from PDS- sows.

Iron is a so-called negative acute phase reactant, as its concentration decreases during inflammation. In accordance with this, PDS+ sows had lower serum Fe concentrations than PDS- sows. A decrease in Fe and an increase in Hp has been shown previously in pigs following experimental inoculation with Actinobacillus [57]. Odink et al. [58] found lower serum Fe concentrations in slaughter pigs with abscesses and other inflammatory processes than in pigs with no postmortem findings. In ruminants and horses, Fe have been shown to be a fast reacting marker, with concentrations decreasing within few hours following an inflammatory stimulus, and returning to normal values within 48 h [59, 60]. In horses, assessment of serum Fe was more useful for detection of acute inflammation than was the assessment of fibrinogen [61]. The results of the present study indicate that Fe may be used for distinguishing PDS+ and PDS- sows 12-36 h p.p.

Conclusions

This study suggests that inflammation is part of the pathogenesis in PDS. WBC, neutrophil and lymphocyte counts, and serum concentrations of TNF-α, IL6, Hp and Fe differed between PDS+ and PDS- sows and may potentially serve as diagnostic adjuncts for detection of PDS. However, considering the inflammatory changes found also in PDS- sows, the diagnostic value of measuring inflammatory markers needs further investigation in larger study populations, where diagnostic capacity (positive and negative predictive value) of the investigated markers may be fully assessed. Combining measurements of inflammatory markers with assessment of clinical and behavioral parameters may improve identification of sows at risk of developing PDS. Development of assay systems that allow farmers and veterinarians to measure relevant inflammatory markers sow-side may enhance future use of clinical-chemical parameters in porcine herd health medicine markedly. Early (antepartum) detection of sows at risk of developing PDS is desirable, but only lymphocyte counts were different in PDS+ and PDS- sows before parturition.

Additional files

Additional file 1: Three fictive examples of sampling points. The figure illustrates how the number of observations (*n*) in each time interval differ between variables because of individual sampling times relative to parturition (0 h).

Additional file 2: Interleukin 1 (IL-1). IL-1 concentration (10^{-9} g/L) in sows with postpartum dysgalactia syndrome (PDS+, red) and healthy sows (PDS-, blue) sampled from 60 h before until 36 h after parturition (time interval A-G). Each dot represents the exact sample time of each observation relative to the exact birth of the first piglet (0 h). The lines show the mean value.

Additional file 3: Total protein (TP). TP concentration (10^{0} g/L) in sows with postpartum dysgalactia syndrome (PDS+, red) and healthy sows (PDS-, blue) sampled from 60 h before until 36 h after parturition (time interval A-G). Each dot represents the exact sample time of each observation relative to the exact birth of the first piglet (0 h). The lines show the mean value.

Additional file 4: Hemoglobin (Hb). Hb concentration (10^{-3} mol/L) in sows with postpartum dysgalactia syndrome (PDS+, red) and healthy sows (PDS-, blue) sampled from 60 h before until 36 h after parturition (time interval A-G). Each dot represents the exact sample time of each observation relative to the exact birth of the first piglet (0 h). The lines show the mean value. Normal range is $6.2 - 9.4 \times 10^{-3}$ mol/L.

Additional file 5: Hematocrit (Ht). Ht (L/L) in sows with postpartum dysgalactia syndrome (PDS+, red) and healthy sows (PDS-, blue) sampled from 60 h before until 36 h after parturition (time interval A-G). Each dot represents the exact sample time of each observation relative to the exact birth of the first piglet (0 h). The lines show the mean value. Normal range is 0.31 – 0.46 L/L.

Abbreviations

ALB: Albumin; APP's: Acute phase proteins; CRP: C-reactive protein; *E. coli*: *Escherichia coli*; Fe: Iron; Hb: Hemoglobin; Hp: Haptoglobin; Ht: Hematocrit; IL-1: Interleukin 1; IL-6: Interleukin 6; LPS: Lipopolysaccharide; LSMEANS: Least-squares means; MMA: Mastitis, metritis and agalactia syndrome; p.p. : Postpartum; PDS: Postpartum dysgalactia syndrome (PDS+ is cases and PDS- is healthy sows); SAA: Serum amyloid A; SD: Standard deviation; SPF: Specific pathogen-free; TNF-α: Tumor necrosis factor alpha; TP: Total protein; WBC: White blood cell counts

Acknowledgements

The authors thank the staff and the vet at the farm Jørn Skov Jensen, Anna Bech and Christian Pårup Nielsen for getting assess to the barn and helping with practical work; Karen Bach-Mose, Hanne Præstgaard, Jens-Ove Hansen, Peter Nøddebo Hansen, Kristina Nøddebo Balle, Sarah Mortensen, Peter Hansen, Hanne Nissen, are thanked for technical work collecting our data; Estrid Hasager, Susana Ros, Josefa Hernandez, Isabel Rodriguez, Annlouise Jansson, Anna Svensson, Claus Sivertsen Stjernegaard, Anne Kristine Havnsøe Krogh, Birgitta Svensmark, for helping with the laboratory work; Ken Steen Pedersen for professional sparring; and Henrik Thoning for parts of the statistical analysis.

Funding

This work is partly funded by the Innovation Fund Denmark (IFD) under File No. 1355-00121 and SEGES, Danish Pig Research Center. The study design was approved by SEGES and IFD. SEGES contributed with technical support during data collection and statistical analysis.

Authors' contributions

The study was designed by MK, MJ, PHA, PB and SJ. Data and samples were collected by MK and MJ. JC, DE and MK performed laboratory analyses. MK, JD and SJ performed statistical analyses. MK and SJ drafted the manuscript. All authors interpreted, read, revised, and approved the final manuscript.

Consent for publication

Not applicable.

Competing interests

The authors declare that they have no competing interests.

Author details

[1]Department of Veterinary Clinical Sciences, Faculty of Health and Medical Sciences, Copenhagen University, Højbakkegård Alle 5, 2630 Taastrup, Denmark. [2]Department of Clinical Sciences, Faculty of Veterinary Medicine and Animal Science, Swedish University of Agricultural Sciences, p.o. Box 7054, SE-750 07 Uppsala, Sweden. [3]SEGES, Danish Pig Research Center, Danish Agriculture & Food Council, Agro Food Park 15, 8200 Aarhus N, Denmark. [4]Department of Animal Medicine and Surgery, Regional "Campus of Excellence Mare Nostrum", University of Murcia, 30100 Espinardo, Murcia, Spain. [5]Danish Agriculture and Food Council, Axelborg, Axeltorv 3, 1709 Copenhagen V, Denmark.

References

1. Kemper N, Gerjets I. Bacteria in milk from anterior and posterior mammary glands in sows affected and unaffected by postpartum dysgalactia syndrome (PPDS). Acta Vet Scand. 2009;51:26.
2. Papadopoulos GA, Vanderhaeghe C, Janssens GPJ, Dewulf J, Maes DGD. Risk factors associated with postpartum dysgalactia syndrome in sows. Vet J. 2010;184:167–71.
3. Preissler R, Hinrichs D, Reiners K, Looft H, Kemper N. Estimation of variance components for postpartum dysgalactia syndrome in sows. J Anim Breed Genet. 2012;129:98–102.
4. Stiehler T, Heuwieser W, Pfuetzner A, Burfeind O. The course of rectal and vaginal temperature in early postpartum sows. J Swine Health Prod. 2015; 23:72–83.
5. Maes D, Papadopoulos G, Cools A, Janssens GPJ. Postpartum dysgalactia in sows: pathophysiology and risk factors. Tierärztl Prax. 2010;38(Suppl 1):15–20.
6. Martineau GP, Le Treut Y, Guillou D, Waret-Szkuta A. Postpartum dysgalactia syndrome: a simple change in homeorhesis? J Swine Health Prod. 2013;21: 85–93.
7. Quesnel H, Farmer C, Devillers N. Colostrum intake. Influence on piglet performance and factors of variation. Livest Sci. 2012;146:105–14.
8. Mirko CP, Bilkei G. Acute phase proteins, serum cortisol and prewearing litter performance in sows suffering from periparturient disease. Acta Vet (Beograd). 2004;54:153–61.
9. Persson A. Mastitis in Sows. Clinical, bacteriological and cytological examinations in assessing udder health during early lactation and at weaning. Doctoral thesis. Acta Universitatis Agriculturae Sueciae. Veterinaria 10. Uppsala: Swedish University of Agricultural Sciences; 1997.
10. Hales J, Moustsen VA, Nielsen MBF, Hansen CF. Individual physical characteristics of neonatal piglets affect preweaning survival of piglets born in a noncrated system1. J Anim Sci. 2013;91:4991–5003.
11. Furniss SJ. Measurement of rectal temperature to predict 'mastitis, metritis and alagactia' (MMA) in Sows after farrowing. Prev Vet Med. 1987;5:133–9.
12. Hoy S. The impact of puerperal diseases in sows on their fertility and health up to next farrowing. Anim Sci. 2006;82:701–4.
13. Backstrom L, Morkoc AC, Connor J, Larson R, Price W. Clinical study of mastitis-metritis-agalactia in sows in Illinois. J Am Vet Med Assoc. 1984;185:70–3.
14. Gerjets I, Traulsen I, Reiners K, Kemper N. Assessing individual sow risk factors for coliform mastitis: a case-control study. Prev Vet Med. 2011;100: 248–51.

15. Göransson L. The effect of dietary crude fibre content on the frequency of post partum agalactia in the sow. J Vet Med. 1989;36:474–9.
16. Göransson L. The effect of feed allowance in late pregnancy on the occurrence of agalactia post partum in the sow. J Vet Med. 1989;36:505–13.
17. Persson A, Pedersen Mörner A, Kuhl W. A long-term study on the health status and performance of sows on different feed allowances during late pregnancy. III. Escherichia coli and other bacteria, total cell content, polymorphonuclear leucocytes and pH in colostrum and milk during the first 3 weeks of lactation. Acta Vet Scand. 1996;37:293–313.
18. Preissler R, Gerjets I, Reiners K, Looft H, Kemper N. Prevalence of postpartun dysgalactia syndrome in sows. Vienna: International Society for Animal Hygiene (ISAH); 2011. p. 63–5.
19. Preissler R, Tetens J, Reiners K, Looft H, Kemper N. Biological pathway analysis of postpartum dysgalactia syndrome in sows via a genome-wide association study. Vienna: International Society for Animal Hygiene (ISAH); 2011. p. 67–9.
20. Osterlundh I, Hulten F, Johannisson A, Magnusson U. Sows intramammarily inoculated with Escherichia coli at parturition: I. Functional capacity of granulocytes in sows affected or non-affected by clinical mastitis. Vet Immunol Immunopathol. 2002;90:35–44.
21. Gerjets I, Traulsen I, Reiners K, Kemper N. Comparison of virulence gene profiles of Escherichia coli isolates from sows with coliform mastitis and healthy sows. Vet Microbiol. 2011;152:361–7.
22. Hirsch AC, Philipp H, Kleemann R. Investigation on the efficacy of meloxicam in sows with mastitis-metritis-agalactia syndrome. J Vet Pharmacol Ther. 2003;26:355–60.
23. van Gelder KN, Bilkei G. The course of acute-phase proteins and serum cortisol in mastitis metritis agalactia (MMA) of the sow and sow performance. Tijdschr Diergeneeskd. 2005;130:38–41.
24. Szczubial M, Urban-Chmiel R. Tumor Necrosis Factor-α and Interleukin-6 contentration in the serum of sows with the MMA syndrome. Bull Vet Inst Pulawy. 2008;52:267–70.
25. Nachreiner RF, Ginther OJ. Induction of agalactia by administration of endotoxin (Escherichia coli) in swine. Am J Vet Res. 1974;35:619–22.
26. Zhu Y, Osterlundh I, Hulten F, Magnusson U. Tumor necrosis factor-alpha, interleukin-6, serum amyloid A, haptoglobin, and cortisol concentrations in sows following intramammary inoculation of Escherichia coli. Am J Vet Res. 2004;65:1434–9.
27. Wang JF, Wang M, Ma JL, Jiao LG, Zhou XY, Lindberg JE. The influence of intramammary lipopolysaccharide infusion on serum Ca, P, vitamin D, cytokines and cortisol concentrations in lactating sows. J Vet Med A Physiol Pathol Clin Med. 2006;53:113–8.
28. Martineau GP, Farmer C, Peltoniemi O. Mammary system. In: Zimmerman JJ, Karriker LA, Ramirez A, Schwartz KJ, Stevenson GW. Diseases of swine. 10 ed. Chichester: Wiley. 2012. p. 270–93.
29. Wright JH. A rapid method for the differential staining of blood films and malarial parasites. J Med Res. 1902;7:138–44.
30. Kruse R, Essen-Gustavsson B, Fossum C, Jensen-Waern M. Blood concentrations of the cytokines IL-1beta, IL-6, IL-10, TNF-alpha and IFN-gamma during experimentally induced swine dysentery. Acta Vet Scand. 2008;50:32.
31. Tecles F, Fuentes P, Martinez Subiela S, Parra MD, Munoz A, Ceron JJ. Analytical validation of commercially available methods for acute phase proteins quantification in pigs. Res Vet Sci. 2007;83:133–9.
32. Hernandez-Caravaca I, Gourgues SF, Rodriguez V, Estrada ED, Ceron JJ, Escribano D. Serum acute phase response induced by different vaccination protocols against circovirus type 2 and Mycoplasma hyopneumoniae in piglets. Res Vet Sci. 2017;114:69–73.
33. Hebisch G, Neumaier-Wagner PM, Huch R, von Mandach U. Maternal serum interleukin-1 beta, -6 and -8 levels and potential determinants in pregnancy and peripartum. J Perinat Med. 2004;32:475–80.
34. Nagel C, Trenk L, Aurich J, Wulf M, Aurich C. Changes in blood pressure, heart rate, and blood profile in mares during the last 3 months of gestation and the peripartum period. Theriogenology. 2016;86:1856–64.
35. Hermansson I, Einarsson S, Ekman L, Larsson K. On the agalactia post partum in the sow. A hematological and blood chemical study in affected and healthy sows. Nordisk veterinaermedicin. 1978;30:474–81.
36. Coutinho da Silva MA, Canisso IF, ML MP, Johnson AE, Divers TJ. Serum amyloid A concentration in healthy periparturient mares and mares with ascending placentitis. EVJ. 2013;45:619–24.
37. Magnusson U, Fossum C. Numerical Variations among Blood Mononuclear Cells during the Peripartal Period in the Gilt. J Vet Med Ser B. 1990;37:459–67.
38. Osterlundh I, Holst H, Magnusson U. Hormonal and immunological changes in blood and mammary secretion in the sow at parturition. Theriogenology. 1998;50:465–77.
39. Bluthe RM, Laye S, Michaud B, Combe C, Dantzer R, Parnet P. Role of interleukin-1beta and tumour necrosis factor-alpha in lipopolysaccharide-induced sickness behaviour: a study with interleukin-1 type I receptor-deficient mice. Eur J Neurosci. 2000;12:4447–56.
40. Harden LM, du Plessis I, Poole S, Laburn HP. Interleukin (IL)-6 and IL-1 beta act synergistically within the brain to induce sickness behavior and fever in rats. Brain Behav Immun. 2008;22:838–49.
41. Colletti LM, Green M. Lung and liver injury following hepatic ischemia/reperfusion in the rat is increased by exogenous lipopolysaccharide which also increases hepatic TNF production in vivo and in vitro. Shock. 2001;16:312–9.
42. Koike K, Moore FA, Moore EE, Poggetti RS, Tuder RM, Banerjee A. Endotoxin after gut ischemia/reperfusion causes irreversible lung injury. J Surg Res. 1992;52:656–62.
43. Salmon H. The intestinal and mammary immune system in pigs. Vet Immunol Immunopathol. 1987;17:367–88.
44. Slade JD, Hepburn B. Prednisone-induced alterations of circulating human lymphocyte subsets. J Lab Clin Med. 1983;101:479–87.
45. Fukuda R, Ichikawa Y, Takaya M, Ogawa Y, Masumoto A. Circadian variations and prednisolone-induced alterations of circulating lymphocyte subsets in man. Intern Med. 1994;33:733–8.
46. Fauci AS, Dale DC. The effect of Hydrocortisone on the kinetics of normal human lymphocytes. Blood. 1975;46:235–43.
47. Borissov I, Andonova M. Escherichia coli lipopolysaccharide-induced experimental infection in piglets: clinical and laboratory findings. Revue Méd. Vét. 2000;151:931–6.
48. Nachreiner RF, Ginther OJ. Porcine Agalactia: Hematologic, Serum Chemical, and Clinical Changes during the Preceding Gestation. Am J Vet Res. 1972;33:799–8.
49. Cort N. A clinical study on the effect of a gram-negative bacterial endotoxin and cloprostenol in non-pregnant and 60-day-pregnant gilts. Anim Reprod Sci. 1986;10:133–45.
50. Nachreiner RF, Garcia MC, Ginther OJ. Clinical, Hematologic, and Blood Chemical Changes in Swine Given Endotoxin (Escherichia coli) During the Immediate Postpartum Period. Am J Vet Res. 1972;33:2489–99.
51. Elenkov IJ, Webster EL, Torpy DJ, Chrousos GP. Stress, corticotropin-releasing hormone, glucocorticoids, and the immune/inflammatory response: acute and chronic effects. Ann N Y Acad Sci. 1999;876:1–11.
52. Jacobsen S, Andersen PH. The acute phase protein serum amyloid A (SAA) as a marker of inflammation in horses. Equine Vet Educ. 2007;19:38–46.
53. Pallares FJ, Martinez-Subiela S, Seva J, Ramis G, Fuentes P, Bernabe A, Munoz A, Ceron JJ. Relationship between serum acute phase protein concentrations and lesions in finishing pigs. Vet J. 2008;177:369–73.
54. Gutierrez AM, Martinez-Subiela S, Ceron JJ. Diagnostic accuracy of porcine acute phase proteins in meat juice for detecting disease at abattoir. Vet Rec. 2015;177:15.
55. Escribano D, Campos PH, Gutierrez AM, Le Floc'h N, Ceron JJ, Merlot E. Effect of repeated administration of lipopolysaccharide on inflammatory and stress markers in saliva of growing pigs. Vet J. 2014;200:393–7.
56. Escribano D, Tvarijonaviciute A, Tecles F, Ceron JJ. Serum paraoxonase type-1 activity in pigs: assay validation and evolution after an induced experimental inflammation. Vet Immunol Immunopathol. 2015;163:210–5.
57. Baarsch MJ, Foss DL, Murtaugh MP. Pathophysiologic correlates of acute porcine pleuropneumonia. AVMA. 2000;61:684–90.
58. Odink J, Smeets JF, Visser IJ, Sandman H, Snijders JM. Hematological and clinicochemical profiles of healthy swine and swine with inflammatory processes. J Anim Sci. 1990;68:163–70.

59. Jacobsen S, Nielsen JV, Kjelgaard-Hansen M, Toelboell T, Fjeldborg J, Halling-Thomsen M, Martinussen T, Thoefner MB. Acute phase response to surgery of varying intensity in horses: a preliminary study. Vet surg. 2009;38: 762–9.
60. Jacobsen S, Toelboell T, Andersen PH. Dose dependency and individual variability in selected clinical, haematological and blood biochemical responses after systemic lipopolysaccharide challenge in cattle. Vet Res. 2005;36:167–78.
61. Borges AS, Divers TJ, Stokol T, Mohammed OH. Serum iron and plasma fibrinogen concentrations as indicators of systemic inflammatory diseases in horses. J Vet Intern Med. 2007;21:489–94.

Prevalence and molecular characterization of *Staphylococcus aureus* isolated from goats in Chongqing, China

Zuoyong Zhou[1,2*†], Mengsi Zhang[1,2,3†], Hexian Li[1,2], Haoyue Yang[1,2], Xiaoxia Li[1,2], Xinyue Song[1,2] and Zhiying Wang[1,2]

Abstract

Background: *Staphylococcus aureus* is an important zoonotic pathogen which not only causes significant economic loss in livestock production but also poses a potential threat to public health. Compared with bovine and swine, the information on the colonization of *S. aureus* in goats is very limited. To understand the prevalence and characteristics of *S. aureus* in goats, we used the nasal swabs collected from apparently healthy goats to isolate *S. aureus*, and tested their antimicrobial susceptibility, virulence gene carrying levels, and multilocus sequence typing (MLST).

Results: In 74 nasal swabs of apparently healthy goats, 32 (43.24%) *S. aureus* strains were isolated and identified, most of which were susceptible to many antibiotics, except for trimethoprim, furazolidone, amoxicillin, lincomycin and roxithromycin, and the resistance incidence of which were 50%, 40.63%, 37.5%, 28.13%, and 21.88% respectively. All the isolates were methicillin-susceptible *S. aureus* (MSSA) and *mecA*-negative. Enterotoxin genes were found in 53.13% of the strains. Of which, *sej* was the most prevalent (21.88%), followed by *seb*, *sec*, and *see* with the same level (18.75%). The most prevalent combination were *seb* + *see* and *seb* + *tst*. None of the *S. aureus* isolates harbored *sea, sed, seh, eta* and *etb*. Multilocus sequence typing (MLST) revealed 6 new alleles (*aroe*-552, *aroe*-553, *glpf*-500, *pta*-440, *yqil*-482 and *yqil*-496) and 5 new sequence types (STs) (3431,3440,3444,3445 and 3461). Using eBURST, the 5 STs were assigned to clonal complex 522 (CC522) and a further CC with no predicted ancestor. Phylogenetic analysis of seven concatenated MLST alleles revealed that the 5 STs were grouped into cluster I composed of *S. aureus* mainly from goats and sheep.

Conclusion: We provide the data for prevalence of *S. aureus* in goats in Chongqing municipality and their characterization which will help in tracking evolution of epidemic strains and their control methods.

Keywords: *Staphylococcus aureus*, Goats, Antimicrobial resistance, Virulence genes, MLST

Background

Staphylococcus aureus is an important opportunistic pathogen and the cause of infection among human, domestic and wild animals [1–3]. Due to its broad spectrum of inherent virulence factors, the infection of *S. aureus* usually plays an important role for the causing of abscesses, mastitis, pneumonia and meningitis in mammals [4–6]. The invasion of *S. aureus* in domestic animals not only causes significant economic loss in livestock production but also poses a potential threat to public health since these animals can act as the reservoir of methicillin-resistant *S. aureus* (MRSA) [7, 8]. The livestock-associated methicillin-resistant *S. aureus* (LA-MRSA) represented by clonal complex 398 (CC 398) have been shown to be able to colonize and cause serious infections in people having close contact with animals such as veterinarians, farmers and their family members [9–11]. In addition, both handling and consumption of products of these animals colonized by MRSA may provide a potential transmission to humans

* Correspondence: zzyxnny@163.com
†Equal contributors
[1]College of Animal Science, Rongchang Campus of Southwest University, No. 160 Xueyuan Road, Rongchang District, Chongqing 402460, China
[2]Veterinary Science Engineering Research Center of Chongqing, No. 160 Xueyuan Road, Rongchang District, Chongqing 402460, China
Full list of author information is available at the end of the article

Table 1 Primers used for *nuc*, *mecA* and virulence genes amplification

Gene Primer	Primer sequence (5'to 3')	Amplification size (bp)	Reference
nuc	SF:GCGATTGATGGTGATACGGTT	279	[13]
	SR:AGCCAAGCCTTGACGAACTAAAGC		
mecA	SF: AAAATCGATGGTAAAGGTTGGC	533	[15]
	SR: AGTTCTGCAGTACCGGATTTGC		
sea	SF: GGTTATCAATGTGCGGGTGG	102	[16]
	SR: CGGCACTTTTTTCTCTTCGG		
seb	SF: GTATGGTGGTGTAACTGAGC	164	[16]
	SR: CCAAATAGTGACGAGTTAGG		
sec	SF: AGATGAAGTAGTTGATGTGTATGG	451	[16]
	SR: CACACTTTTAGAATCAACCG		
sed	SF:CCAATAATAGGAGAAAATAAAAG	278	[16]
	SR: ATTGGTATTTTTTTTCGTTC		
see	SF:AGGTTTTTTCACAGGTCATCC	209	[16]
	SR: CTTTTTTTTCTTCGGTCAATC		
seg	SF: TGCTATCGACACACTACAACC	704	[17]
	SR:CCAGATTCAAATGCAGAACC		
seh	SF:CGAAAGCAGAAGATTTACACG	495	[17]
	SR: GACCTTTACTTATTTCGCTGTC		
sei	SF:GACAACAAAACTGTCGAAACTG	630	[17]
	SR: CCATATTCTTTGCCTTTACCAG		
sej	SF: CATCAGAACTGTTGTTCCGCTAG	142	[18]
	SR: CTGAATTTTACCATCAAAGGTAC		
tst	SF: ACCCCTGTTCCCTTATCATC	326	[16]
	SR: TTTTCAGTATTTGTAACGCC		
eta	SF: ATATCAACGTGAGGGCTCTAGTAC	1155	[20]
	SR: ATGCAGTCAGCTTCTTACTGCTA		
etb	SF: CACACATTACGGATAATGCAAG	604	[20]
	SR: TCAACCGAATAGAGTGAACTTATCT		
pvl	SF: GTGCCAGACAATGAATTACCC	255	[19]
	SR: TTCATGAGTTTTCCAGTTCACTTC		

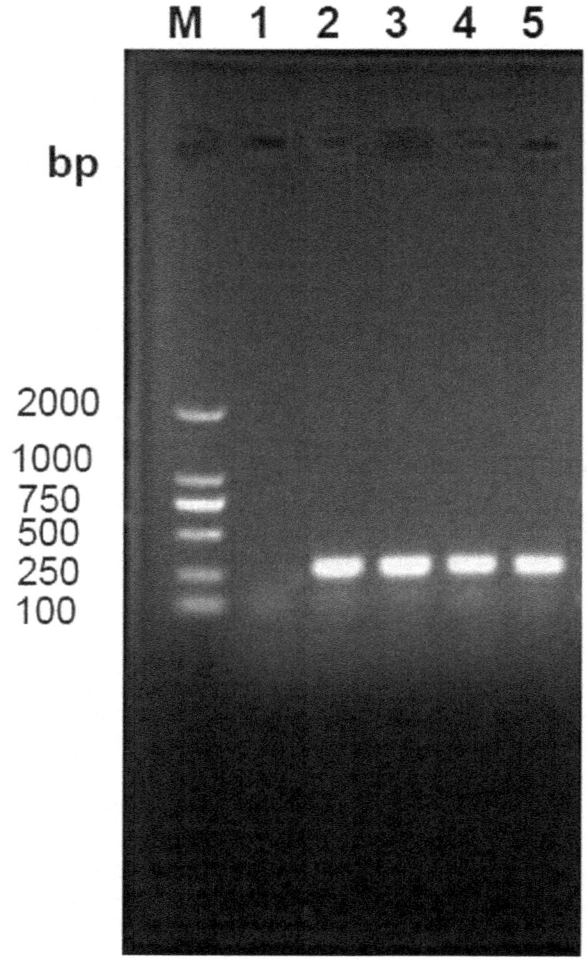

Fig. 1 Gel electrophoresis of amplified *nuc* in *S. aureus* isolated from goats in Chongqing. M: DL-2000 DNA marker; 1: *Staphylococcus sciuri*; 2–5: the *nuc* gene of some *S. aureus* isolates by amplified at 297 bp

[12]. Thus, it is of importance to understand the prevalence and characterization of *S. aureus* colonizing the livestock.

In contrast to the studies of *S. aureus* infections in bovine and human, less is known on these bacteria in goats or their relevant products. In 2008, Chongqing municipality was incorporated into the national "Advantage of agricultural products regional planning" in China and recognized as the key areas for beef cattle and goats breeding. The number of live sheep and goats in Chongqing was about 2.26 million and 2.74 million slaughtered was provided by the end of 2015 (Chongqing Statistical Yearbook, 2016). However, there is no investigation on the incidences of colonization in goats by *S. aureus* in Chongqing. To understand the prevalence and characteristics of *S. aureus* in goats, we used the nasal swabs from apparently healthy goats to isolate *S. aureus*, tested their antimicrobial susceptibility and virulence gene carrying levels, and defined multilocus sequence typing (MLST).

Methods

Sample collection and *S. aureus* isolation

The nasal swabs were collected from 74 apparently healthy goats from 10 herds in 4 counties (Rongchang, Jiangjing, Zhongxian and Dazu) of Chongqing municipality, transported to the laboratory and stored at 4 °C prior to isolation. The bacteria were enriched in a common broth at 37 °C for 18 h, and then inoculated on 7.5% NaCl agar plates for cultivation at 37 °C for 24 h. The colonies suspected to be *S. aureus* were identified by Gram staining, colony morphology, and coagulase

Table 2 Results of drug sensitivity test for *S. aureus* ($n = 32$)

Antibiotics	No. of *S. aureus*			Percentage of resistance or sensitive	
	R	I	S	Resistance rate (%)	Sensitive rate (%)
Macrodantin	2	4	26	6.25	81.25
Streptomycin	2	2	28	6.25	87.50
Gentamicin	1	1	30	3.13	93.75
Norfloxacin	4	0	28	12.50	87.50
Kanamycin	2	4	26	6.25	81.25
Vancomycin	3	1	28	9.38	87.50
Ceftriaxone	3	17	12	9.38	37.50
Tetracycline	2	8	22	6.25	68.75
Cefotaxime	1	5	26	3.13	81.25
Chloramphenicol	5	6	21	15.63	65.63
Trimethoprim	16	5	11	50.00	34.38
Cefepime	1	1	30	3.13	93.75
Roxithromycin	7	14	11	21.88	34.38
Levofloxacin	5	0	27	15.63	84.38
Lincomycin	9	10	13	28.13	40.63
Minocyline	0	4	28	0	87.50
Cefoxitin	0	1	31	0	96.88
Clarithromycin	5	2	25	15.63	78.13
Amoxicillin	12	4	16	37.50	50.00
Furazolidone	13	8	11	40.63	34.38

"R" represents resistance; "I" represents intermediate; "S" represents susceptible

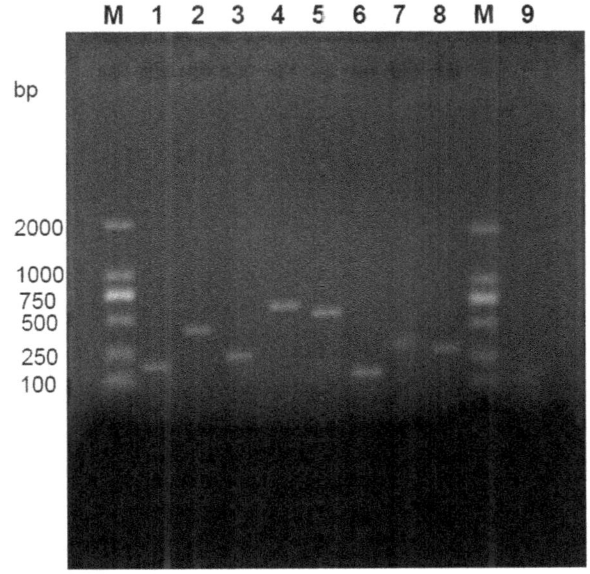

Fig. 2 Gel electrophoresis of amplified virulence gene products of *S. aureus* isolates from goats in Chongqing. M: DL-2000 DNA marker; 1: *seb* (164 bp); 2: *sec* (451 bp); 3: *see* (209 bp); 4: *seg* (704 bp); 5: *sei* (630 bp); 6: *sej* (142 bp); 7: *tst* (326 bp); 8: *pvl* (255 bp); 9: amplification of *seb* in *Staphylococcus sciuri*

testing. All the presumptive *S. aureus* colonies were then subcultured and confirmed by the PCR amplification of *nuc* (a thermonuclease gene characteristic of *S. aureus*) [13] (Table 1) with the following conditions: denaturation for 4 min at 94 °C, followed by 30 cycles for 1 min at 94 °C, 30 s at 58 °C and 90 s at 72 °C, and a final extension at 72 °C for 3.5 min. *S. sciuri* was used as *nuc*-negative control strain.

Antimicrobial resistance profile

The *S. aureus* isolates were used for antimicrobial susceptibility test using disk diffusion method according to Clinical and Laboratory Standards Institute (CLSI) guidelines [14]. Following antibiotics with stated concentrations (μg/disc) were used: cefotaxime (30), ceftriaxone (30), streptomycin (10),kanamycin (30), gentamicin (10),tetracycline (30), chloramphenicol (30),lincomycin (2), macrodantin (300),furazolidone (300), vancomycin (30), norfloxacin (10),minocyline (30), amoxicillin (10), cefoxitin (30),clarithromycin (15), levofloxacin (5),roxithromycin (15),trimethoprim (5) and cefepime (30). The presence of *mecA* (staphylococci methicillin resistance gene) [15] (Table 1) was analyzed by PCR method under the same amplification conditions as stated earlier for *nuc*, ATCC 43300 (*mecA* positive) and ATCC 29213 (*mecA* negative) were used as control strains.

Detection of virulence genes

DNA extraction was done using a commercial DNA extraction kit (Dalian TaKaRa Biotechnology Co.,Ltd.) following the manufacturer's instructions. Thirteen *S. aureus* virulence genes including enterotoxins (SEs), *sea, seb, sec, sed, see, seg, seh, sei, sej* [16–18]; cytotoxin *pvl* [19]; exfoliative toxins (ETs), *eta, etb* [20]; and a toxic shock syndrome toxin 1(*tst*) [16] (Table 1) were selected

Table 3 Distribution of virulence genes among *S. aureus* isolates from goats ($n = 32$)

Gene	Number of isolates	Detection rate(%)	Genes	Number of isolates	Detection rate(%)
seb	6	18.75	*seb + see + pvl*	2	6.25
sec	6	18.75	*seb + tst + pvl*	2	6.25
see	6	18.75	*seb + see + sej*	2	6.25
seg	1	3.13	*seb + see*	4	12.50
sei	3	9.38	*see + sej*	3	9.38
sej	7	21.88	*seb + tst*	4	12.50
tst	6	18.75	*seb + pvl*	3	9.38
pvl	6	18.75	*sec + pvl*	2	6.25
			sec + tst	2	6.25

Table 4 The alleles and STs of *S. aureus* isolates from goats in Chongqing

Isolates	MLST allelic profile							ST
	arcc	*aroe*	*glpf*	*gmk*	*pta*	*tpi*	*yqil*	
1	8	***552***	135	2	***440***	127	***482***	***3431***
2	18	***552***	***500***	2	7	15	5	***3440***
3	8	***552***	135	2	***440***	127	***496***	***3444***
4	8	***552***	135	2	***440***	127	***496***	***3444***
5	8	***552***	135	2	***440***	127	***496***	***3444***
6	18	***552***	45	2	7	15	5	***3445***
7	8	***552***	135	2	***440***	127	***496***	***3444***
8	8	***552***	135	2	***440***	127	***496***	***3444***
9	8	***552***	135	2	***440***	127	***496***	***3444***
10	8	***552***	135	2	***440***	127	***496***	***3444***
11	18	***552***	45	2	7	15	5	***3445***
12	8	***552***	135	2	***440***	127	***496***	***3444***
13	8	***553***	45	2	7	15	5	***3461***

The bold-italic numbers indicate new alleles or STs

for PCR with the following amplification conditions: initial denaturation for 5 min at 94 °C, followed by 30 cycles of 94 °C for 1 min, 50 °C for 1 min (55 °C for *seg* and *pvl*), and 72 °C for 1 min, with a final elongation of 72 °C for 10 min. *S. aureus* reference strains including ATCC 25923 (*pvl* positive) and ATCC 29213 (*sea, sec, see* and *tst* positive).

Multilocus sequence typing (MLST) of *S. aureus*

A random selection of 13 *S. aureus* isolates were analyzed by MLST. The 7 housekeeping genes, carbamate kinase (*arcc*), shikimate dehydrogenase (*aroe*), glycerol kinase (*glpf*), guanylate kinase (*gmk*), phosphate acetyltransferase (*pta*), triosephosphate isomerase (*tpi*), and acetyl coenzyme A acetyltransferase (*yqil*) (http://saureus.mlst.net/misc/info.asp), were amplified by PCR method consisting of initial denaturation at 95 °C for 5 min, followed by a total of 35 cycles of 30 s denaturation at 94 °C, 30 s annealing at 55 °C, and 1 min elongation at 72 °C, with a final elongation step of 10 min at 72 °C. PCR products were sequenced both in forward and reverse directions by Shanghai Invitrogen Biotechnology Co., Ltd. The sequences for each locus were compared to the allele sequences through the MLST website (http://www.mlst.net). Isolates were defined by their alleles at the seven loci (allelic profile), and each allelic profile was submitted to the database to obtain a sequence type (ST) number.

Clonal complexes (CCs) clustering and phylogenetic analysis of *S. aureus* STs

The clustering of STs was performed using eBURST algorithm (http://eburst.mlst.net/) [21] by comparing the present dataset to that of the MLST database of 4066 STs by the end of May 2017, and ran with the default settings. Clonal complexes (CCs) were composed of STs that shared at least six alleles in common and a predicted ancestral ST and its associated single locus variants (SLVs: the variants differ at one of the seven MLST alleles from the ancestor) and double locus variants (DLVs: the variants differ at two of the seven MLST alleles from the ancestor) [3]. Along with the STs obtained in this research, 23 STs from human (ST7, 12,13, 15, 27, 88, 101 and 240), goats and sheep (ST130, 133, 398, 425, 522, 1595, 1740, 1742, 1743, 1758, 1780, 1781, 2011, 2305, 2328) [2, 9, 22, 23] were collected for phylogenetic analyses. The concatenated sequences of all seven MLST alleles for each ST were aligned using the CLUSTAL X program with default parameters followed by manual inspection. MEGA 4.0 was used to construct neighbour-

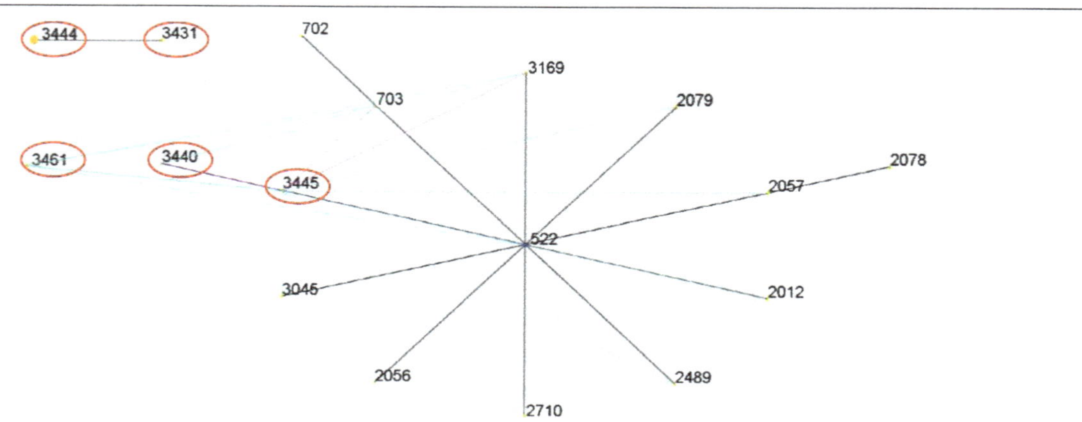

Fig. 3 eBURST-generated CC522 containing the major ST522 comprising 14 STs. The primary founder (ST522) is colored blue and positioned centrally in the cluster, and subgroup founders are colored yellow; the SLVs were connected by red lines, and the DVLs were connected by blue lines; the areas of each of the circles indicate the prevalence of the ST in the input data. The novel STs in this study were marked by red oval circle

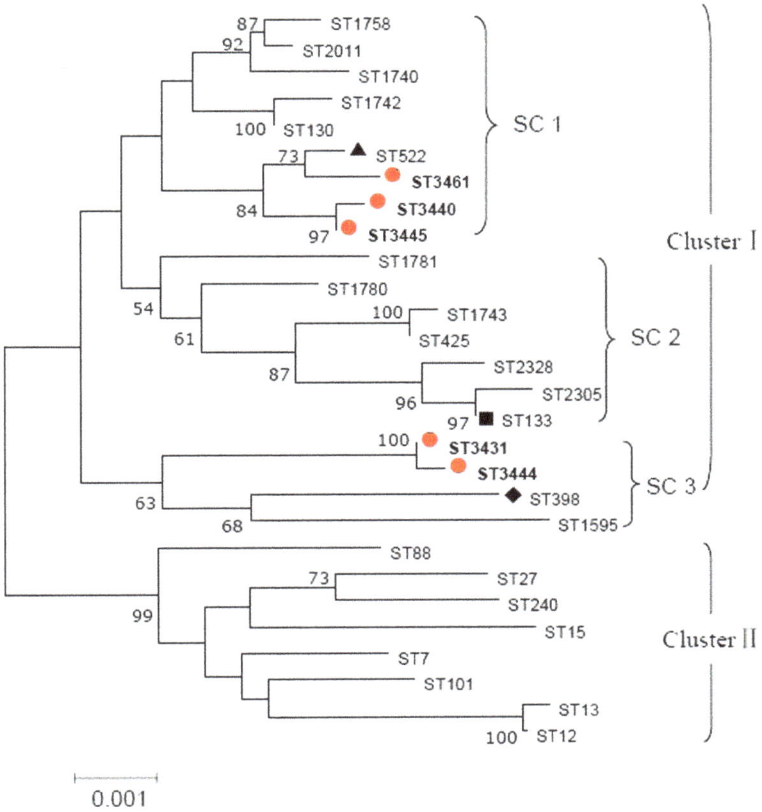

Fig. 4 Phylogenetic tree of *S. aureus* STs using the concatenated sequences of the seven MLST genes mainly from human, goats and sheep. ClusterI: mainly from goats and sheep; Cluster II: mainly from human. In clusterI, the STs divided into three sub-clusters (SCs), and the new STs (marked by red filled circles) obtained in this study were clustered in SC1 and SC3. ST398 (marked by black filled diamond), is associated with animals infection [9]; ST522 (marked by black filled triangle) is associated with goats and sheep [2]; ST133 (marked by black filled square) appears to be an ungulate-animal-specific genotype [3]

joining trees [24]. Bootstrapping was performed with 1000 replicates.

Results

Isolation and identification of *S. aureus*

Of 74 nasal swabs of goats collected from 10 herds, 32 (43.24%) were identified as *S. aureus* through *nuc* amplification (Fig. 1), and all the *S. aureus* isolates were found to be coagulase positive.

Antimicrobial resistance profile

The antimicrobial susceptibility test showed most of the *S. aureus* isolates susceptible to a majority of antibiotics and the resistance rates below 20%, with the exceptions of following: trimethoprim (50% resistant), furazolidone (40.63%), amoxicillin (37.5%), lincomycin (28.13%), and roxithromycin (21.88%) (Table 2). All the isolates (n = 32) were methicillin-susceptible *S. aureus* (MSSA) and cefoxitin-susceptible.

Distribution of virulence genes among *S. aureus* isolates

Since every *S. aureus* carries several virulence genes, but here 19/32 strains carried at least one of the small chosen set of virulence genes (Fig. 2). Enterotoxin genes were detected in majority (53.13%) of the strains, and *sej* gene was found in 7 (21.88%), followed by *seb*, *sec* and *see* in 18.75% isolates each, *sei* (9.38%), *seg* (3.13%). In addition, both *tst* gene and *pvl* gene were detected in 6 (18.75%) isolates. The most prevalent combination was determined to be *seb* + *see* and *seb* + *tst* in 12.5% of all isolates (Table 3). There were 8 isolates which only encode a virulence gene.

MLST analysis

After MLST analysis, 6 new alleles (*aroe*-552, *aroe*-553, *glpf*-500, *pta*-440,*yqil*-482 and *yqil*-496) and 5 new STs (ST 3431,ST 3440,ST 3444,ST 3445 and ST 3461) were identified and added to the *S. aureus* MLST database (Table 4). The dominant type of *aroE* was *aroE*-552, which was present in 92.31% (12/13) of *S. aureus* isolates, followed by *pta*-440 and *yqiL*-496, which accounted for 69.23% (9/13) and 61.54% (8/13) respectively. The ST3444 was the most common ST type which accounted for 61.54% (8/13) of the *S. aureus* isolates, followed by ST3445 (2 strains), and ST 3431, ST 3440, ST 3461 which just had one strain.

Clonal complexes (CCs) clustering and phylogenetic analysis of *S. aureus* STs

eBURST generated 103 groups and 483 singletons. The *S. aureus* isolates tested in this study were clustered into CC522 containing ST3440 and ST3445, and a further CC with no predicted ancestor containing ST3431 and ST3444, while ST3461 was a singleton (Fig. 3). The phylogenetic relationship of 28 STs, based on concatenated sequences of seven MLST alleles, resulted in two main clusters: clusterI(mainly from goats and sheep) and cluster II (from humans). In clusterI, there were three sub-clusters (SCs) (SC1 containing ST130, 522, 1740, 1742, 1758, 2011, 3440, 3445 and 3461; SC2 containing ST133, 425, 1743, 1780, 1781, 2305 and 2328; SC3 containing ST 398, 1595, 3431 and 3444) (Fig. 4).

Discussion

This is the first study of the prevalence of *S. aureus* from the nose swabs of apparently healthy goats in Chongqing. Our results were comparable to the carriage frequency of *S. aureus* in healthy sheep in Tunisia [25] approaching to ~ 45% level, which were higher than reported by other investigators in dairy sheep and goats [26–28], but lower than that in goats in Norway and Denmark [22, 29].

It is interesting that all the *S. aureus* isolates in this study were methicillin-susceptible *S. aureus* (MSSA) since they were sensitive or medium sensitivity to cefoxitin and *mecA* tested negative. The majority of *S. aureus* showed relatively low resistance to vancomycin, ceftriaxone, macrodantin, streptomycin, kanamycin, tetracycline, gentamicin, cefotaxime and cefepime, which is similar to the resistance of *S. aureus* isolated from sheep and goat in Spain [23], but lower than the resistance of *S. aureus* from goats in Taiwan [26]. The relatively high sensitivity spectrum of *S. aureus* from Chongqing is likely due to a limited use of antimicrobials for goats [28].

The infections caused by *S. aureus* is associated with its virulence factors which allow it to adhere to surface, invade or avoid the immune system, and cause harmful toxic effects to the host [30, 31]. More than half of isolates in this study were tested positive for SE genes, which is similar to other reports in *S. aureus* from dairy goats [29] and their milk products [32], and higher than the result in goats and cows affected with mastitis [33]. Of the SE genes tested, *sej* was the most predominantly occurring gene which is different from the detection rates in goats from Taiwan or sheep in Tunisia where there were no *sej* occurrence [25, 26]. Except for *sej*, the *seb*, *sec*, *see*, *tst* and *pvl* carriage rate of 18.75% is similar to the other reports in *S. aureus* from goats and their milk products [26, 32, 34, 35] but lower than *sec* and *tst* found in *S. aureus* from dairy goats [29], or in MSSA from sheep [25]. In contrast to the other report [29], although *sec* and *tst* showed the same detection rates, they were not always co-detected. In the previous study, *see* was identified only in *S. aureus* associated with mastitis in goat [26], the carry level of *seb* and *see* in this study are inconsistent with other reports [32, 35] where there were no *S. aureus* strain harboured *seb* and *see*. *Pvl* is associated with *S. aureus* causing goat subclinical mastitis [36]. Different from the previous report [25], we found 18.75% isolates *pvl*-positive.

To understand the molecular characteristics of *S. aureus* isolates from Chongqing goats, we used MLST typing and found 6 new alleles (*aroe*-552, *aroe*-553, *glpf*-500, *pta*-440,*yqil*-482 and *yqil*-496) and 5 new STs (3431,3440,3444,3445 and 3461). The dominant alleles belonged to *aroE* was *aroE*-552, which occurred in most of *S. aureus* strains, followed by *pta*-440 and *yqiL*-496. In the newly found STs, ST3444 was the most common, which occurred in approximately 60% of the *S. aureus* isolates. It is relatively normal for *S. aureus* from goats to possess novel alleles or STs in contrast to human or bovine strains, which may be simply due to the investigation of a new population, since most reports have focused on human clinical isolates or bovine mastitis [37].

The eBURST analyses assigned *S. aureus* isolates to CC522 containing ST3440 and ST3445, and a further CC with no predicted ancestor. The results from phylogenetic analyses showed that STs from goats and sheep were separated from that of human, thus formed two main clusters. Three new STs (ST3440, 3445 and 3461) were sub-grouped in the branch of SC1 containing ST522, the primary founder ST of CC522, which was reported previously from cases of goat mastitis or goat's milk samples [2, 3, 23]. ST3444, the predominate ST in this study, and ST3431 were sub-clustered into the branch SC3 containing ST398, which is associated with animals infection [9]. In SC2, ST133 was found in variety of animals including cows, goats and sheep [2, 3, 22, 23], and was found to be the most common animal-associated MLST type [3]. Our results confirmed the relative close relationship of ST 3440, ST3445 and ST3461 with ST522, and ST3444, ST3431 with ST398.

Conclusion

This is the first study to report the prevalence rate, antimicrobial resistance profile, virulence genes association and MLST characteristics of *S. aureus* from goats in Chongqing municipality. This study will help in tracking evolution of *S. aureus* epidemic strains and proving the methods to control *S. aureus* in goats in China.

Abbreviations

CC: Clonal complex; DLVs: Double locus variants; ETs: Exfoliative toxins; LA-MRSA: Livestock-associated methicillin-resistant *S. aureus*; MLST: Multilocus sequence typing; MSSA: Methicillin-susceptible *S. aureus*; PCR: Polymerase chain reaction; SEs: Enterotoxins; SLVs: Single locus variants; STs: Sequence types

Acknowledgements

We really appreciate Dr. Shijun Hu, Fangjun Cheng and Cailiang Fan for their practical support, Mr. Youdong Gong and Peng Chen for their assistant in sample collection. We also thank Dr. Narayan C. Rath and Yang Zhou for English-language editing of this manuscript.

Funding

This research is funded by the the Social Undertakings and Livelihood Security Technology Innovation Projects of Chongqing (CSTC2015SHMSZX80020), the Project of Youth Fund of Southwest University (No. 20700926) and Fundamental Research Funds for the Central Universities (XDJK2017D078). The funding bodies had no role in study design, data collection or analysis, decision to publish or preparation of the manuscript.

Authors' contributions

ZYZ and MSZ designed the study and wrote the manuscript. MSZ, HXL, HYY, XXL, XYS, and ZYW performed the experiments, analyzed the data, and drafted the manuscript. All authors read and approved the final manuscript.

Consent for publication

Not applicable.

Competing interests

The authors declare that they have no competing interests.

Author details

[1]College of Animal Science, Rongchang Campus of Southwest University, No. 160 Xueyuan Road, Rongchang District, Chongqing 402460, China. [2]Veterinary Science Engineering Research Center of Chongqing, No. 160 Xueyuan Road, Rongchang District, Chongqing 402460, China. [3]College of Veterinary Medicine and State Key Laboratory of Agrobiotechnology, China Agricultural University, No. 2 Yuanmingyuan West Road, Haidian District, Beijing 100193, China.

References

1. Monecke S, Gavier-Widen D, Hotzel H, Peters M, Guenther S, Lazaris A, Loncaric I, Muller E, Reissig A, Ruppelt-Lorz A, Shore AC, Walter B, Coleman DC, Ehricht R. Diversity of *Staphylococcus aureus* isolates in European wildlife. PLoS One. 2016;11(12):e168433.
2. Bar-Gal GK, Blum SE, Hadas L, Ehricht R, Monecke S, Leitner G. Host-specificity of *Staphylococcus aureus* causing intramammary infections in dairy animals assessed by genotyping and virulence genes. Vet Microbiol. 2015;176(1–2):143–54.
3. Smyth DS, Feil EJ, Meaney WJ, Hartigan PJ, Tollersrud T, Fitzgerald JR, Enright MC, Smyth CJ. Molecular genetic typing reveals further insights into the diversity of animal-associated *Staphylococcus aureus*. J Med Microbiol. 2009;58(Pt 10):1343–53.
4. Spini RG, Ferraris V, Glasman MP, Orofino G, Casanovas A, Debaisi G. Methicillin resistant *Staphylococcus aureus* community acquired meningitis: a case report. Arch Argent Pediatr. 2014;112(6):e266–8.
5. Song Z, Gu FF, Guo XK, Ni YX, He P, Han LZ. Antimicrobial resistance and molecular characterization of *Staphylococcus aureus* causing childhood pneumonia in shanghai. Front Microbiol. 2017;8:455.
6. El-Ashker M, Gwida M, Tomaso H, Monecke S, Ehricht R, El-Gohary F, Hotzel H. *Staphylococci* in cattle and buffaloes with mastitis in Dakahlia governorate, Egypt. J Dairy Sci. 2015;98(11):7450–9.
7. Petersen A, Stegger M, Heltberg O, Christensen J, Zeuthen A, Knudsen LK, Urth T, Sorum M, Schouls L, Larsen J, Skov R, Larsen AR. Epidemiology of methicillin-resistant *Staphylococcus aureus* carrying the novel mecC gene in Denmark corroborates a zoonotic reservoir with transmission to humans. Clin Microbiol Infect. 2013;19(1):E16–22.
8. Verkade E, Kluytmans J. Livestock-associated *Staphylococcus aureus* CC398: animal reservoirs and human infections. Infect Genet Evol. 2014;21:523–30.
9. Loncaric I, Brunthaler R, Spergser J. Suspected goat-to-human transmission of methicillin-resistant Staphylococcus Aureus sequence type 398. J Clin Microbiol. 2013;51(5):1625–6.
10. De Martino L, Lucido M, Mallardo K, Facello B, Mallardo M, Iovane G, Pagnini U, Tufano MA, Catalanotti P. Methicillin-resistant *staphylococci* isolated from healthy horses and horse personnel in Italy. J Vet Diagn Investig. 2010;22(1):77–82.
11. Lozano C, Aspiroz C, Charlez L, Gomez-Sanz E, Toledo M, Zarazaga M, Torres C. Skin lesion by methicillin-resistant *Staphylococcus aureus* ST398-t1451 in a Spanish pig farmer: possible transmission from animals to humans. Vector Borne Zoonotic Dis. 2011;11(6):605–7.
12. EFSA. Assessment of the public health significance of meticillin resistant *Staphylococcus aureus* (MRSA) in animals and foods. EFSA J. 2009;993:2–3.
13. Brakstad OG, Aasbakk K, Maeland JA. Detection of *Staphylococcus aureus* by polymerase chain reaction amplification of the nuc gene. J Clin Microbiol. 1992;30(7):1654–60.
14. CLSI CALS. Performance standards for antimicrobial SusceptibilityTesting; twenty-second informational supplement; CLSI document M100-S22. Wayne, PA, USA: Clinical and Laboratory Standards Institute; 2013.
15. Murakami K, Minamide W, Wada K, Nakamura E, Teraoka H, Watanabe S. Identification of methicillin-resistant strains of *staphylococci* by polymerase chain reaction. J Clin Microbiol. 1991;29(10):2240–4.
16. Mehrotra M, Wang G, Johnson WM. Multiplex PCR for detection of genes for *Staphylococcus aureus* enterotoxins, exfoliative toxins, toxic shock syndrome toxin 1, and methicillin resistance. J Clin Microbiol. 2000;38(3): 1032–5.
17. McLauchlin J, Narayanan GL, Mithani V, O'Neill G. The detection of enterotoxins and toxic shock syndrome toxin genes in *Staphylococcus aureus* by polymerase chain reaction. J Food Prot. 2000;63(4):479–88.
18. Monday SR, Bohach GA. Use of multiplex PCR to detect classical and newly described pyrogenic toxin genes in *staphylococcal* isolates. J Clin Microbiol. 1999;37(10):3411–4.
19. Wang Q, Yang LM, Luo FJ, F MS: The resistance and mecA, qacA/B, pvl gene detection of *Staphylococcus aureus*. In: *2008 Annual Meeting of Zhejiang Provincial Laboratory Medicine*. Hangzhou Zhejiang, China: China Academic Journal Electronic Publishing House; 2008: 5.
20. Noguchi N, Nakaminami H, Nishijima S, Kurokawa I, So H, Sasatsu M. Antimicrobial agent of susceptibilities and antiseptic resistance gene distribution among methicillin-resistant *Staphylococcus aureus* isolates from patients with impetigo and staphylococcal scalded skin syndrome. J Clin Microbiol. 2006;44(6):2119–25.
21. Feil EJ, Li BC, Aanensen DM, Hanage WP, Spratt BG. eBURST: inferring patterns of evolutionary descent among clusters of related bacterial genotypes from multilocus sequence typing data. J Bacteriol. 2004; 186(5):1518–30.
22. Eriksson J, Espinosa-Gongora C, Stamphoj I, Larsen AR, Guardabassi L. Carriage frequency, diversity and methicillin resistance of *Staphylococcus aureus* in Danish small ruminants. Vet Microbiol. 2013;163(1–2):110–5.
23. Porrero MC, Hasman H, Vela AI, Fernandez-Garayzabal JF, Dominguez L, Aarestrup FM. Clonal diversity of *Staphylococcus aureus* originating from the small ruminants goats and sheep. Vet Microbiol. 2012;156(1–2):157–61.
24. Tamura K, Dudley J, Nei M, Kumar S. MEGA4: molecular evolutionary genetics analysis (MEGA) software version 4.0. Mol Biol Evol. 2007;24(8):1596–9.
25. Gharsa H, Ben SK, Lozano C, Gomez-Sanz E, Klibi N, Ben SR, Gomez P, Zarazaga M, Boudabous A, Torres C. Prevalence, antibiotic resistance,

23

Molecular characterization and expression patterns of a non-mammalian toll-like receptor gene (TLR21) in larvae ontogeny of common carp (*Cyprinus carpio* L.) and upon immune stimulation

Hua Li†, Ting Li†, Yujie Guo, Yujun Li, Yan Zhang, Na Teng, Fumiao Zhang* and Guiwen Yang*

Abstract

Background: In the host innate immune system, various pattern recognition receptors (PRRs) recognize conserved pathogen-associated molecular patterns (PAMPs) and represent an efficient first line of defense against invading pathogens. Toll-like receptors (TLRs) are a major class of PRRs, which are able to recognize a wide range of PAMPs and play a central role in initiating innate immune responses. TLR21 is one of the non-mammalian TLRs identified in some bird and fish species.

Results: In the present study, we reported the cloning and identification of a TLR21 cDNA from the head kidney of common carp (*Cyprinus carpio* L.), named CcTLR21. The full-length CcTLR21 cDNA was 3557 bp long, including an open reading frame (ORF) of 2895 bp, which encoded a putative protein of 964 amino acids. The putative CcTLR21 protein was found to comprise a signal peptide, 14 LRR domains in the extracellular region and a TIR domain in the cytoplasmic region, which fits with the characteristic TLR domain architecture. The phylogenetic analysis showed that CcTLR21 possessed high amino acid identities with the TLR21s in other freshwater teleosts. A Real-time PCR assay showed that CcTLR21 mRNA was expressed in almost all tissues examined in healthy common carp, while the levels obviously varied among different tissues. During the embryonic and early larval developmental stages of common carp, the CcTLR21 showed two peaks of expression, with the first at 1 dpf and the second at 10 dpf. When challenged with poly(I:C) (a viral model) or *Aeromonas hydrophila*, the expression level of CcTLR21 was up-regulated in a variety of common carp tissues.

Conclusions: Our findings indicate that CcTLR21 plays a significant role in innate immune defense during larvae ontogeny and in responses to viral or bacterial pathogens.

Keywords: Common carp (*Cyprinus carpio* L.), TLR21, Evolutionary relationship, Expression pattern, Innate immunity

* Correspondence: zhangfumiao@sdnu.edu.cn; yanggw@sdnu.edu.cn
†Equal contributors
Shandong Provincial Key Laboratory of Animal Resistance Biology, College of Life Sciences, Shandong Normal University, No. 88 East Wenhua Road, Jinan 250014, People's Republic of China

Background

Toll-like receptors (TLRs) are one class of pattern recognition receptors (PRRs), which recognize various pathogens-associated molecular patterns (PAMPs) in the host innate immune system, such as lipopolysaccharide (LPS), peptidoglycan, lipoteichoic acid, non-methylated CpG DNA and so on [1, 2]. To date, 11 kinds of TLRs have been identified in humans, 13 in mice and 17 in fish [3, 4]. Among these, TLR21 is a kind of non-mammalian TLR found in fish, birds and amphibians; some examples are chicken (*Gallus gallus*) [5], south African clawed frog (*Xenopus laevis*) [6], zebrafish (*Danio rerio*) [7], grass carp (*Ctenopharyngodon idella*) [8], orange-spotted grouper (*Epinephelus coioides*) [9], channel catfish (*Ictalurus punctatus*) [10], Atlantic salmon (*Salmo salar*) [11], turbot (*Scophthalmus maximus*) [12], large yellow croaker (*Larimichthys crocea*) [13], yellow catfish (*Pelteobagrus fulvidraco*) [14], rock bream (*Oplegnathus fasciatus*) [15] and yellowtail (*Seriola lalandi*) [16].

TLRs are type-I transmembrane proteins that are composed of three domains: an intracellular Toll/interleukin-1 receptor (TIR) domain, a transmembrane region and an extracellular leucine-rich repeat (LRR) domain. The LRR domain binds to PAMPs, and the TIR domain transmits signals into the cytosol by recruiting Myeloid differentiation factor 88 (MyD88) or TIR-domain-containing adapter-inducing interferon-β (TIRF) [17], which are responsible for the production of pro-inflammatory cytokines or type I interferons [18]. Previous studies reported that fish TLR21 could recognize non-methylated CpG DNA and were considered a functional homologue of mammalian TLR9 [12]. Accordingly, upon stimulation with viral stimulants, such as turbot reddish body iridovirus (TRBIV), infectious salmon anaemia virus (ISAV), rock bream iridovirus (RBIV), polyinosinic: polycytidylic acid [poly(I:C)] or CpG oligodeoxynucleotides (CpG-ODN), the TLR21 mRNA expression was up-regulated in turbot [12], Atlantic salmon [11], large yellow croaker [13], yellow catfish [14] and rock bream [15]. In addition, upon stimulation with bacteria, such as *Aeromonas hydrophila*, *Streptococcus iniae*, *Edwardsiella tarda*, *Vibrio alginolyticus* or *Vibrio parahaemolyticus*, the mRNA expression levels of the TLR21 gene were also up-regulated in grass carp [8], large yellow croaker [13], yellow catfish [14] and rock bream [15]. This suggests that fish TLR21s play key roles in immune defense against both viral and bacterial infections.

Common carp (*Cyprinus carpio* L.) is a freshwater fish widespread in Europe and Asia. To date, TLR1 and TLR2 [19, 20], TLR3 [21], TLR4 [22], TLR9 [23], TLR18 [24], TLR20 [25] and TLR22 [26] were reported in common carp. Since TLRs play an important role in host anti-pathogen responses, the study of TLRs will be beneficial to the disease control of common carp. In this study, we reported the cloning and identification of a TLR21 cDNA from common carp (named CcTLR21). We analysed the gene expression profiles of CcTLR21 in various tissues and during embryonic and early larval developmental stages of common carp. Moreover, the gene expression of CcTLR21 is studied after viral or bacterial stimulation to speculate on the possible role of TLR21 in fish immune response against pathogenic infections.

Methods

Fish rearing and sample collection

Common carp, with an average weight of 75 g, were obtained from the Fresh Water Fishery Research Institute of Shandong Province. Before the start of the experiment, the fish were reared at 20–25 °C in a recirculating freshwater system for at least two weeks, and fed once a day with commercial carp diet. The fish were euthanatized by immersion in a solution of Tricaine Methane Sulfonate (MS222, Sigma Aldrich) at a concentration of 100 mg/l of water, and the tissue samples obtained from three healthy common carp, including liver, spleen, head kidney, foregut, hindgut, gills, skin, brain, gonad, muscle and buccal epithelium, were separately frozen in liquid nitrogen until use for RNA extraction.

To study the gene expression of CcTLR21 during the embryonic and early larval stages, four pairs of parent fish were selected for artificial propagation. Fertilized eggs were incubated in water reservoir at 28–30 °C with enough oxygen. After fertilization, the embryonic stage of common carp is from one to two days, and the hatching was at three days post fertilization (dpf). At 1, 2, 3, 4, 6, 10, 16 and 24 dpf, embryo or larvae samples were sampled randomly for RNA extraction (three repeats for each time piont).

Viral and bacterial challenges in vivo

The fish for the in vivo challenge were divided equally into two independent groups. One group was injected intraperitoneally with formalin-inactivated *A. hydrophila* with 5×10^7 CFU per fish [27–29], and the other group injected intraperitoneally with 500 μl of poly(I:C) (SIGMA) solution per fish at a dose of 1.6 mg/ml [30, 31]. After challenge, the tissues (liver, spleen, head kidney, foregut and hindgut) of fish were sampled at different time points from three fish in each group, and total RNA were extracted (Tiangen) and reverse transcripted to cDNA (Tiangen).

Cloning and analysis of CcTLR21 cDNA

Primers TLR21 F1 and TLR21 R1, which were designed based on the conserved regions of the other species TLR21 sequences, were used to amplify the cDNA fragment of CcTLR21 from the head kidney of common carp. PCR was performed with the following setting: 30 cycles of 94 °C for 30 s, 55 °C for 45 s, and 72 °C for 1 min. The PCR products were ligated into the pMD18-

T vector and transformated into competent *E. coli* DH-5α for sequencing. The full-length of the TLR21 cDNA were obtained by RACE (rapid amplification of the cDNA ends) using the 3′-full and 5′-full RACE core set (TaKaRa). The primers used are shown in Table 1.

The structural domains of CcTLR21 were characterized using the SMART (a simple modular architecture research tool) program (http://smart.embl-heidelberg.de/). The amino acid sequence alignment of TLR21s was performed with MegAlign in DNAstar 7.0 using the method of Clustal W. The phylogenetic tree was generated with MEGA 6.0 using the Neighbour-Joining method.

Real-time PCR

The Real-time PCR analysis of CcTLR21 gene expression was performed with a Rotor-Gene Q PCR instrument (Qiagen) using SYBR Green Real Master Mix (Tiangen). The amplification scheme was: incubated for 1 min at 94 °C, followed by 40 cycles of 20 s at 94 °C, 20 s at 59 °C and 50 s at 70 °C. For each mRNA, gene expression was corrected by the 40S ribosomal protein S11 in each sample. Relative expression of CcTLR21 mRNA was determined using the $2^{(-\Delta\Delta Ct)}$ method. The primers used are shown in Table 1. In all cases, each PCR was performed with triplicate samples.

Statistical analysis

Differences in relative gene expression between the challenged group and the control group were analysed using the Graphpad Prism 6 and were considered significant when $p < 0.05$. A two-way analysis of variance (ANOVA) was performed to test differences in gene expression in each tissue.

Results

cDNA sequence of CcTLR21

The full-length CcTLR21 cDNA (GenBank accession number MF615210) was amplified from the head kidney of common carp, which was 3557 bp long, including a 149 bp 5`-untranslated region (UTR), an open reading frame (ORF) of 2895 bp and a 513 bp 3`-UTR. The ORF of CcTLR21 encoded a putative protein of 964 amino acids. Using the SMART program, the CcTLR21 protein was found to comprise a signal peptide (24 amino acids), 14 LRR domains in the extracellular region and a TIR domain in the cytoplasmic region (Fig. 1).

Homology alignment and phylogenetic analysis of TLR21

Homology alignment analysis showed that the deduced CcTLR21 protein exhibited significant similarity (from 43. 4% to 81.7%) to other known TLR21s (Additional file 1: Table S1). Moreover, the amino acid sequences of CcTLR21 showed a relatively higher degree of similarity with other fish TLR21 than with bird TLR21. The TIR domain of TLR21 presented three conserved regions: box 1 (YDXFXSY), box 2 (LCLHHRDFXPG) and box 3 (FWXXLXXA), which were all found through multiple sequence alignment with the TLR21 family proteins (Additional file 2: Figure S1). To investigate the evolutionary relationships of TLR21 in fish and birds, a phylogenetic tree was constructed. In the tree, all teleost TLR21 members were separated from the TLR21 in birds (Fig. 2).

Constitutive expression of the CcTLR21 gene in common carp

The expression of CcTLR21 mRNA was found in almost all tissues examined, but the levels varied strongly between different tissues. The highest expression level of CcTLR21 mRNA was detected in the spleen, head kidney and gills, with a moderate level of expression observed in the brain, gonad, hindgut and muscle, while very low expression was observed in the foregut, skin, buccal epithelium and liver (Fig. 3).

We analyzed the constitutive expression of the CcTLR21 gene in embryo and early larvae of common carp from 1 to 24 days post fertilization (dpf). The results showed that CcTLR21 have two peaks of expression, with the first at 1 dpf and the second at 10 dpf (Fig. 4).

Expression profiles of CcTLR21 gene in common carp upon poly(I:C) challenge

The expression level of CcTLR21 mRNA in common carp after poly(I:C) stimulation was up-regulated in the spleen, foregut, hindgut and liver (Fig. 5, $p < 0.05$ or

Table 1 The primers and their applications in this study

Primer	Sequence (5` → 3`)	Application
TLR21 F1	CTACAGTTTCAGGAGTTGCA	cDNA amplification
TLR21 R1	TACGATTGTATCGATAGCTCAG	
5′- GSP Outer	TGGCAAGCGAGTTTGGTAGACGGGTGGA	RACE gene specific primers
5′- GSP Inner	TAGACGGGTGGAGTGATGCAGGGTG	
3′- GSP Outer	CCAGCTATCGTCTCTTTCAAGA	
3′- GSP Inner	GCAACYGTCTACTTATCACC	
TLR21 F2	AAGGACCAGGAGGAGAAAT	Real-time PCR
TLR21 R2	AGAGCCGAAATGAAGAACC	
40S F	CCGTGGGTGACATCGTTACA	
40S R	TCAGGACATTGAACCTCACTGTCT	

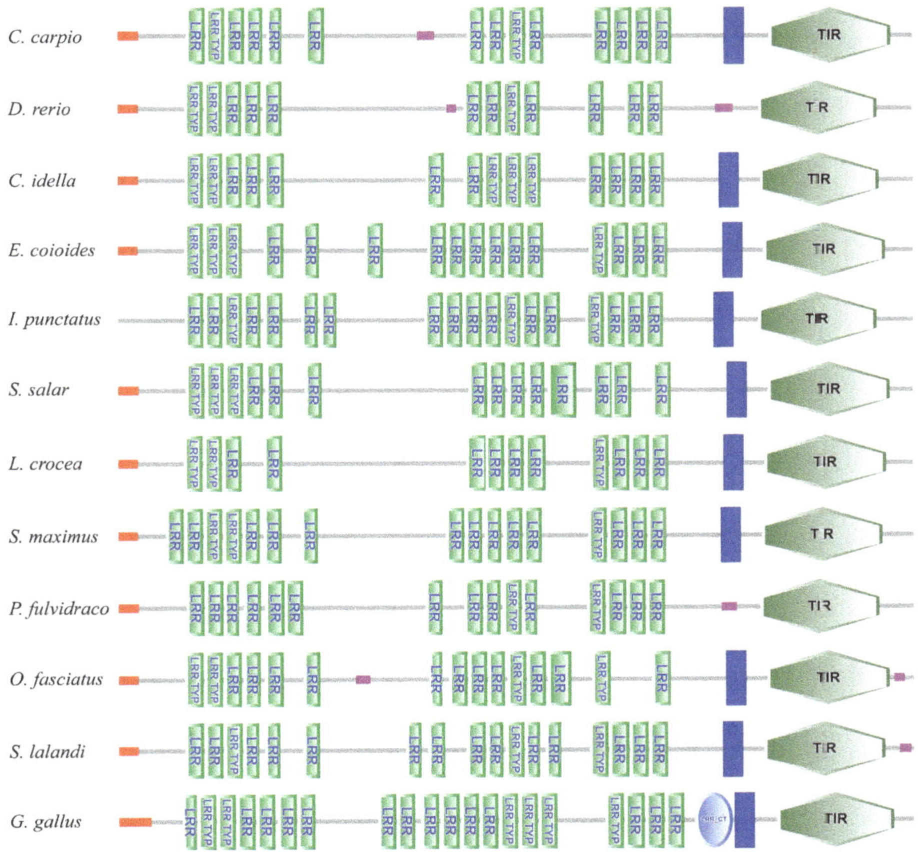

Fig. 1 The domain organizations for TLR21 in various species. Schematic representation of TLR21 domains was predicted by SMART. N-terminal signal peptide (red box), LRRs and LRR-CT domain are denoted at the extracellular region, followed by a transmembrane domain (blue box), and a TIR domain in the cytoplasmic region

$p < 0.01$), with an increase of 5.29-, 2.73-, 6.22-, and 14.44-fold, respectively. The highest induced expression level was found at 3 hpi in the foregut, 12 hpi in the spleen and hindgut, and 24 hpi in the liver. However, CcTLR21 expression was down-regulated in the head kidney at 3 hpi ($p < 0.01$).

Expression profiles of CcTLR21 gene in common carp upon *A. hydrophila* challenge

After i.p. injection with formalin-inactivated *A. hydrophila*, the expression level of CcTLR21 mRNA was up-regulated in the head kidney, foregut, hindgut and liver of common carp (Fig. 6, $p < 0.05$), with an increase of 1. 96-, 6.99-, 8.95-, and 7.30-fold, respectively. The highest induced expression level was found at 3 hpi in the foregut, 6 hpi in the head kidney and hindgut, and 24 hpi in the liver. However, CcTLR21 expression remained unchanged in the spleen after *A. hydrophila* challenge.

Discussion

In the present study, the full-length CcTLR21 cDNA was first amplified from common carp. The ORF of CcTLR21 encoded a putative protein of 964 amino acids, which was found to comprise a signal peptide, 14 LRR domains in the extracellular region and a TIR domain in the cytoplasmic region. This represents the characteristic TLR domain architecture, although the number of LRR domains in different fish TLR21s differs greatly. Like CcTLR21, the TLR21 of *C. idella* and *S. salar* exhibit 14 LRR domains, while the TLR21 of *D. rerio* and *L. crocea* contain 12, *P. fulvidraco* and *O. fasciatus* contain 15, *E. coioides* and *S. maximus* contain 16, *S. lalandi* contains 17, *I. punctatus* contains 18 and *G. gallus* contains 21 LRR domains (Fig. 1). The LRR motif was involved in ligand recognitions that bind to PAMPs for the purpose of subsequent signal transduction [32, 33]. The exact reasons for species-wise variations in number of LRR remain unknown, but the variation in the number of LRR domains suggest that fish TLR21 may exhibit a special mode of ligand binding [34, 35].

The TIR domain of CcTLR21 presented three conserved regions: box 1 (YDXFXSY), box 2 (LCLHHRDFXPG) and box 3 (FWXXLXXA), which were also found in other species TLR21 proteins (Additional file 2: Figure S1). The

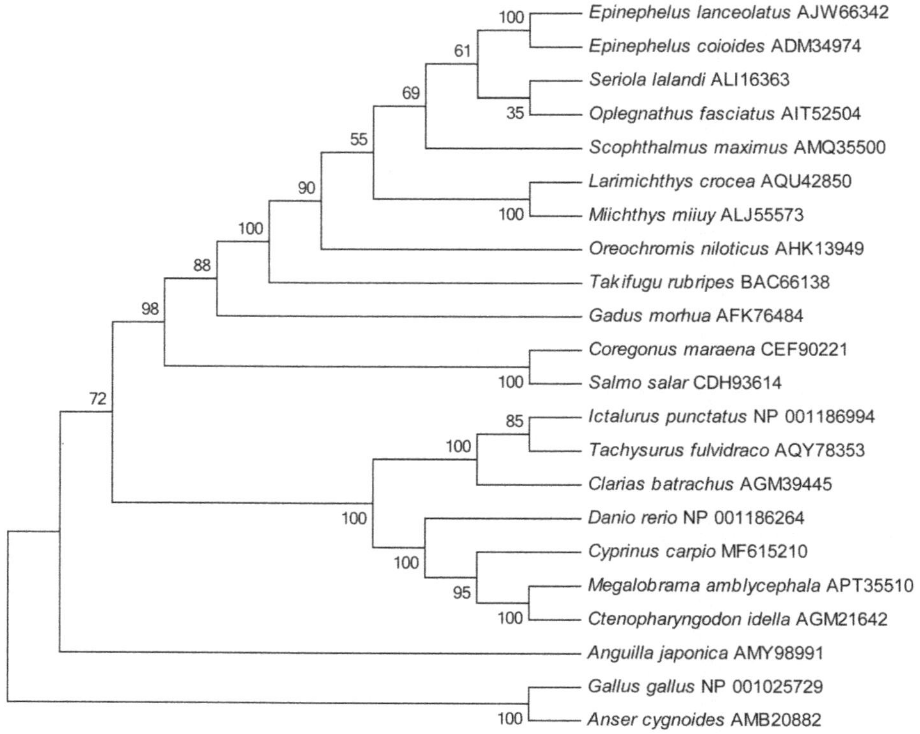

Fig. 2 Phylogenetic analysis of TLR21 amino acid sequences. The evolutionary tree of known TLR21s in fish and birds. These trees are generated using the method of Neighbour-Joining in MEGA 6. The GenBank accession numbers of these sequences are shown in the trees

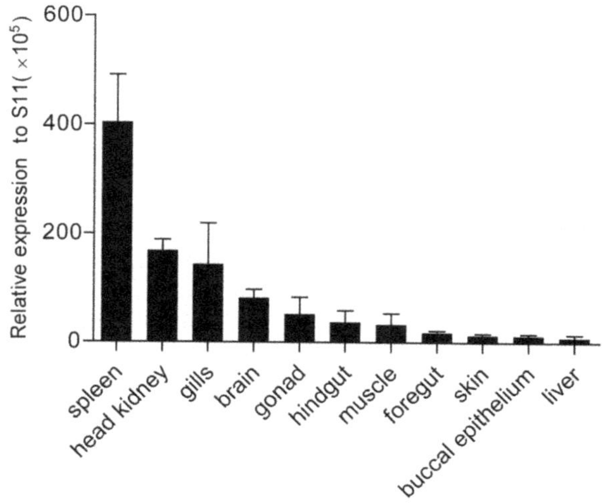

Fig. 3 Tissue expression of CcTLR21 in healthy common carp. CcTLR21 transcripts in the spleen, head kidney, gills, brain, gonad, hindgut, muscle, foregut, skin, buccal epithelial and liver of common carp are detected by Real-time PCR. Amplification of 40S ribosomal protein S11 in each tissue is performed as an internal control. $n = 3$

conserved box 1 and box 2 motifs were known to mediate the coupling of receptor molecules in signal transduction pathways, while the function of box3 region was to control subcellular location of these receptors [12]. Thus, the TIR domain is structurally and functionally conserved

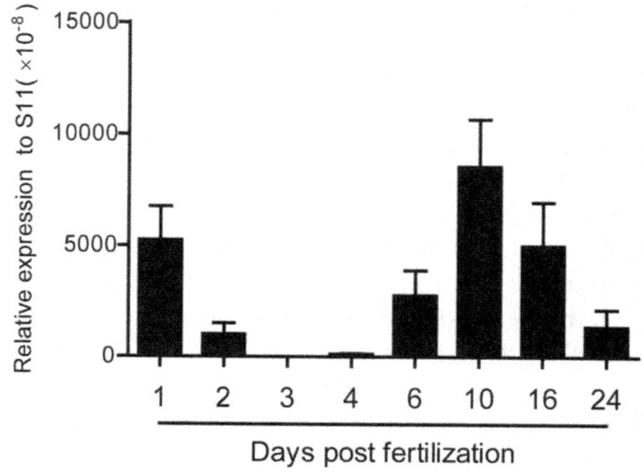

Fig. 4 CcTLR21 gene expression during common carp larvae ontogeny. A normalized expression of CcTLR21 gene during the development of common carp larvae between 1 and 24 days post fertilization. Amplification of 40S ribosomal protein S11 in each tissue is performed as an internal control. $n = 3$

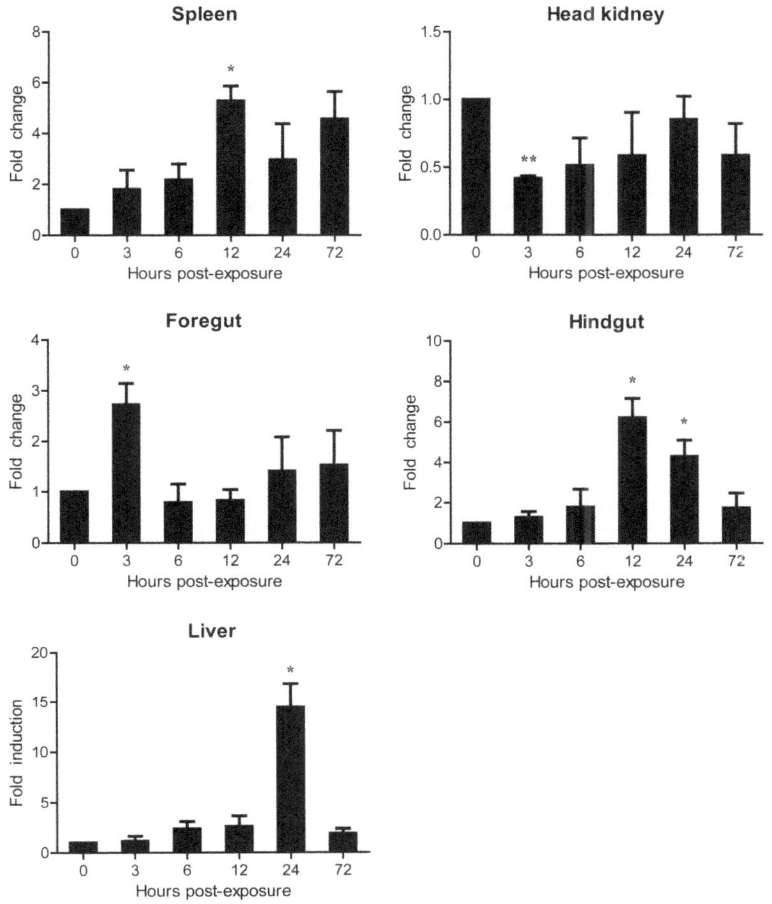

Fig. 5 The relative expression of CcTLR21 in common carp after i.p. injection with poly(I:C). The relative expression of CcTLR21 in the spleen, head kidney, foregut, hindgut and liver of common carp was examined at different time points by Real-time PCR. All these results are corrected by 40S ribosomal protein S11. Data are presented as a fold increase of the challenged group to the un-stimulated control group (denoted by 0 h) and shown as the mean ± SEM ($n = 3$). $^*p < 0.05$ or $^{**}p < 0.01$ versus un-stimulated fish

among different species and seems to trigger similar intracellular signal transduction pathways.

To investigate the evolutionary relationships of TLR21 in fish and birds, a phylogenetic tree was constructed in which all teleost TLR21 members were separated from the TLR21 in birds. As for teleost TLR21, there were two distinct subgroups, one of which consisted of marine teleost TLR21 proteins, including TLR21 of *S. salar, C. maraena, E. coioides, E. lanceolatus, S. lalandi, O. fasciatus, T. rubripes, S. maximus, O. niloticus, M. miiuy, L. crocea* and *G. morhua*; the other was comprised of freshwater teleost TLR21 proteins, including *C. carpio, M. amblycephala, C. idella, D. rerio, I. punctatus, C. batrachus* and *T. fulvidraco*. Interestingly, the TLR21 of *A. japonica* was in a signal branch. The result suggested that TLR21 in marine and freshwater teleosts might undergo different evolutionary processes.

The expression of CcTLR21 mRNA was found in almost all examined tissues of the healthy common carp, but the levels varied strongly among different tissues. In fish, the spleen and head kidney are important systemic lymphoid organs [36], and a high expression of CcTLR21 in these organs suggests an important role of CcTLR21 in the immunity of common carp. Similar high expression of the TLR21 gene in the spleen and head kidney was found in grass carp [8], orange-spotted grouper [9], Atlantic salmon [11], large yellow croaker [13], yellow catfish [14], rock bream [15] and yellowtail [16]. Meanwhile, the gills, hindgut, foregut, buccal epithelium and skin are mucosal immune organs in fish. The high expression level of the CcTLR21 gene in the gills and hindgut suggests that CcTLR21 might play a role in the mucosal defenses of common carp, although there is much lower expression in the foregut, skin and buccal epithelium. Similarly, high expression of the TLR21 gene in gills was found in grass carp [8], orange-spotted grouper [9], Atlantic salmon [11], large yellow croaker [13] and rock bream [15]. In addition, in grass carp [8], large yellow croaker [13] and yellowtail

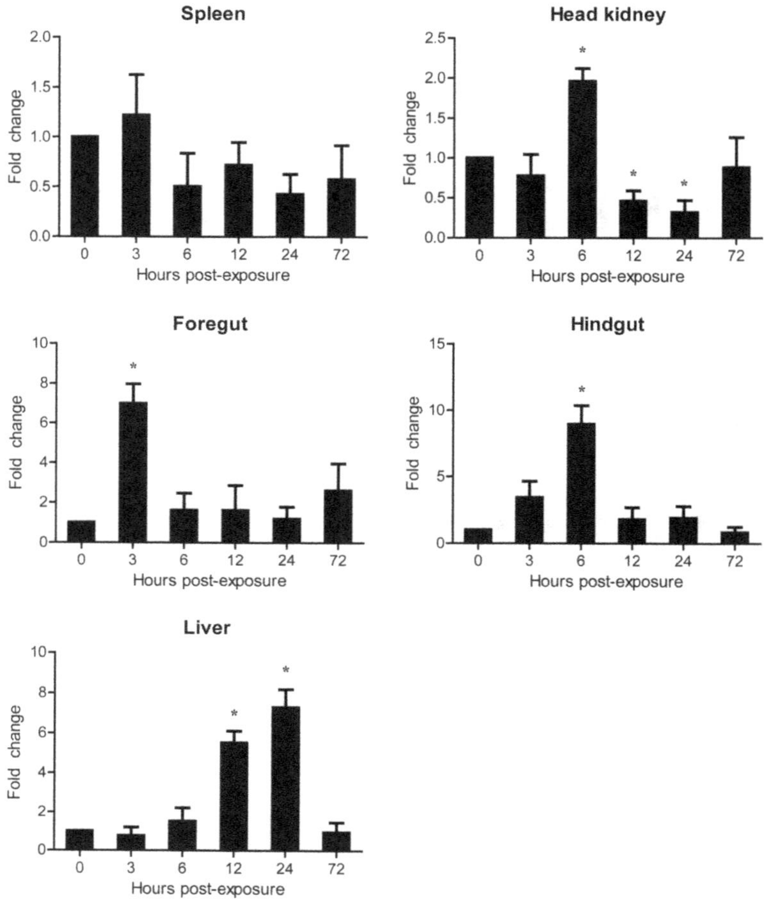

Fig. 6 The relative expression of CcTLR21 in common carp after i.p. injection with *A. hydrophila*. The relative expression of CcTLR21 in the spleen, head kidney, foregut, hindgut and liver of common carp was examined at different time points by Real-time PCR. All these results are corrected by 40S ribosomal protein S11. Data are presented as a fold increase of the challenged group to the un-stimulated control group (denoted by 0 h) and shown as the mean ± SEM ($n = 3$). *$p < 0.05$ or **$p < 0.01$ versus un-stimulated fish

[16], the TLR21 gene also had high expression in the intestine and skin, indicating that the tissue expression pattern of TLR21 varied among different fish species.

We analyzed the constitutive expression of the CcTLR21 gene in embryo and early larvae of common carp post fertilization. The results showed that CcTLR21 had two peaks of expression. Similarly, in yellow catfish, the expression of TLR21 mRNA was at a high level from the fertilized egg stage to the late blastula stage, and subsequently showed an significant up-regulation from 1 to 30 days post hatching (dph) [14]. Additionally, the mRNA expression of other TLRs during embryonic development of fish, such as TLR3, TLR5, TLR18 and TLR19 genes were also reported. The TLR3 mRNA had a higher expression at the fertilized egg stage than at other embryonic developmental stages in rohu [37], and the expression level of TLR5 mRNA was the highest at 5 h post fertilization in mrigal [38]. In yellow catfish, the expressions of TLR18 and TLR19 mRNA were high during the early-stage embryonic development from the fertilized egg to the late blastula [14]. These results suggested that the mRNAs of maternal TLRs might be transferred to the fertilized eggs of fish and will be gradually consumed during the embryonic developmental stage [39]. After hatching, the CcTLR21 mRNA expression levels increased in common carp. In line with this, the mRNA expressions of other TLR genes have also been reported to be up-regulated post hatching of fish, such as rohu, mrigal and yellow catfish [14, 37, 38]. All these results suggest that TLRs may be involved in some immune-related activities, as the larvae will be exposed to the complicated water environment after hatching. Therefore, CcTLR21 might play important immune roles in the embryonic and early larval developmental stages of common carp.

In some reported fish species, significant up-regulation of the TLR21 mRNA was observed after viral or bacterial stimulation, suggesting a possible immune function of fish TLR21. Accordingly, in the present study, we analysed the expression pattern of CcTLR21 mRNA after poly(I:C) and *A. hydrophila* challenges in a variety of immune-related tissues.

Poly(I:C) is used here as a model of double-stranded genome virus infection [40, 41]. After poly(I:C) challenge, the expression level of CcTLR21 mRNA was up-regulated in the spleen, foregut, hindgut and liver. Similarly, upon stimulation with poly(I:C), TRBIV and CpG-ODN, the TLR21 mRNA expression was up-regulated in the gills, head kidney, spleen and muscle of turbot [12]. Additionally, three CpG-ODNs were found to significantly up-regulate the expression of TLR21 in large yellow croaker head kidney cells [13], and TLR21 mRNA levels significantly increased in the spleen tissues of rock bream in response to RBIV infection [15]. The changes of gene expression induced by various infections might be due to the cell migration or proliferation, or actual modulation of gene transcription in resident cells. Although the viral stimulation and subsequent up-regulation of TLR21 gene expression does not claim the recognition of specific ligands by TLR21, induction of TLR21 gene expression is consistent over different studies across different fish species, at least indicating the involvement of fish TLR21 in innate immune defense against viral pathogens [42]. Otherwise, in the head kidney of common carp, the CcTLR21 expression was down-regulated upon poly(I:C). Similarly, the TLR21 expression was down-regulated in the kidneys of Atlantic salmon after ISAV infection [11], and in the liver and spleen of grass carp upon aquareovirus induction [8]. The down-regulation of TLR21 gene expression indicates an altered rate of transcription or a migration of the relevant cell type away from the tissues, implying that TLR21 may have different roles in different tissues of fish.

In the present study, *A. hydrophila*, a Gram-negative bacterium found in fresh or brackish water and associated with some diseases of freshwater fish and amphibians [24, 26, 29, 31], was performed to investigate the possible role of CcTLR21 in the immune defenses against bacterial pathogens in common carp. After i.p. injection with formalin-inactivated *A. hydrophila*, the expression level of CcTLR21 mRNA was up-regulated in the head kidney, foregut, hindgut and liver of common carp. Similar results have been reported in some other fish species. After challenge with *A. hydrophila*, the expression level of the TLR21 gene was up-regulated in the spleen, head kidney, trunk kidney, liver and blood of yellow catfish [14], and in the liver and spleen of grass carp [8]. Post *C. irritans* infection, TLR21 transcript was induced in the skin and gill of orange-spotted grouper [9]. Upon stimulation with *S. iniae* or *E. tarda*, TLR21 mRNA levels was significantly up-regulated in the spleen of rock bream [15]. The expression of TLR21 gene was quickly increased in the spleen and head kidney of large yellow croaker, in response to a trivalent bacterial vaccine consisting of *V. alginolyticus*, *V. parahaemolyticus*, and *A. hydrophila* [13]. Thus, similar to the results of viral stimulation, the induced expression of TLR21 indicates its potential role in the innate immune response of fish against bacterial pathogens.

Conclusions

The structure, evolutionary relationship and expression characteristics of a TLR21 gene in common carp were reported in the present study. CcTLR21 seems to have a closer evolutionary relationship with other freshwater fish TLR21s than those of marine fish species. The constitutive expression of CcTLR21 in various tissues and during early larval ontogeny implies its possible relevance to immune function of common carp. Moreover, the up-regulated expression of CcTLR21 strongly indicates that CcTLR21 plays a significant role in innate immune defense against viral and bacterial pathogenic microbes.

Additional files

Additional file 1: Table S1. Percent identity of CcTLR21 with other species.

Additional file 2: Figure S1. Alignment of CcTLR21 with other species TLR21s. The signal peptide, LRRs domain, transmembrane region and TIR domain were denoted, respectively. The three active motifs in TIR domain are boxed: box 1 (YDXFXSYN), box 2 (LCLHHRDFXXG) and box 3 (FWXXL). X denotes an arbitrary amino acid.

Abbreviations

ANOVA: two-way analysis of variance; CpG-ODN: CpG oligodeoxynucleotides; dpf: days post fertilization; dph: days post hatching; ISAV: infectious salmon anaemia virus; LB: Luriae Bertani; LPS: lipopolysaccharide; LRR: leucine-rich repeat; MyD88: Myeloid differentiation factor 88; ORF: open reading frame; PAMPs: pathogen-associated molecular patterns; poly(I:C): polyinosinic: polycytidylic acid; PRRs: pattern recognition receptors; RACE: rapid amplification of the cDNA ends; RBIV: rock bream iridovirus; SMART: a simple modular architecture research tool; TIR: Toll/interleukin-1 receptor; TIRF: TIR-domain-containing adapter-inducing interferon-β; TLR: toll-like receptor; TRBIV: turbot reddish body iridovirus; UTR: untranslated region

Funding

This work was supported by the National Natural Science Foundation of China (31602186), the Shandong Provincial Natural Science Foundation, China (ZR2014CZ004, ZR2014CQ051) and the University Independent Innovation Project of Jinan, China (200906020).

Authors' contributions

HL and GWY participated in the design of the study, performed the experiments, collected and analysed data, and drafted the manuscript. TL and YJG cloned and sequenced the CcTLR21 gene. YJL and YZ helped with the animal experiments. TL and NT participated in the acquisition of preliminary data and performed the statistical analysis. FMZ conceived the study and participated in its design and coordination. All authors read and approved the final manuscript.

Competing interests

The authors declare that they have no competing interests.

References

1. Belvin MP, Anderson KV. A conserved signaling pathway: the Drosophila toll-dorsal pathway. Annu Rev Cell Dev Biol. 1996;12:393–416.
2. Medzhitov R. Toll-like receptors and innate immunity. Nat Rev Immunol. 2001;1(2):135–45.
3. Beutler BA. TLRs and innate immunity. Blood. 2009;113(7):1399–407.
4. Munoz I, Sepulcre MP, Meseguer J, Mulero V. Toll-like receptor 22 of gilthead seabream, Sparus aurata: molecular cloning, expression profiles and post-transcriptional regulation. Dev Comp Immunol. 2014;44(1):173–9.
5. Temperley ND, Berlin S, Paton IR, Griffin DK, Burt DW. Evolution of the chicken toll-like receptor gene family: a story of gene gain and gene loss. BMC Genomics. 2008;9:62.
6. Ishii A, Kawasaki M, Matsumoto M, Tochinai S, Seya T. Phylogenetic and expression analysis of amphibian Xenopus toll-like receptors. Immunogenetics. 2007;59(4):281–93.
7. Jault C, Pichon L, Chluba J. Toll-like receptor gene family and TIR-domain adapters in Danio rerio. Mol Immunol. 2004;40(11):759–71.
8. Wang W, Shen Y, Pandit NP, Li J. Molecular cloning, characterization and immunological response analysis of toll-like receptor 21 (TLR21) gene in grass carp, Ctenopharyngodon idella. Dev Comp Immunol. 2013;40(3–4):227–31.
9. Li YW, Luo XC, Dan XM, Qiao W, Huang XZ, Li AX. Molecular cloning of orange-spotted grouper (Epinephelus coioides) TLR21 and expression analysis post Cryptocaryon irritans infection. Fish Shellfish Immunol. 2012;32(3):476–81.
10. Baoprasertkul P, Xu P, Peatman E, Kucuktas H, Liu Z. Divergent toll-like receptors in catfish (Ictalurus punctatus): TLR5S, TLR20, TLR21. Fish Shellfish Immunol. 2007;23(6):1218–30.
11. Lee PT, Zou J, Holland JW, Martin SA, Collet B, Kanellos T, Secombes CJ. Identification and characterisation of TLR18-21 genes in Atlantic salmon (Salmo salar). Fish Shellfish Immunol. 2014;41(2):549–59.
12. Li S, Wang G, Liu D, Liu Q, Hu G. Cloning and expression analysis of a toll-like receptor 21 (TLR21) gene from turbot, Scophthalmus maximus. Dev Comp Immunol. 2017;73:163–8.
13. Sun M, Mu Y, Ding Y, Ao J, Chen X. Molecular and functional characterization of Toll-like receptor 21 in large yellow croaker (*Larimichthys crocea*). Fish Shellfish Immunol. 2016;59:179–88.
14. Wang KL, Ji W, Zhang GR, Wei KJ, Shi ZC, Zhang XT, Zheng H, Fan QX. Molecular characterization and expression analysis of three TLR genes in yellow catfish (Pelteobagrus fulvidraco): responses to stimulation of Aeromonas hydrophila and TLR ligands. Fish Shellfish Immunol. 2017;66:466–79.
15. Priyathilaka TT, Elvitigala DA, Whang I, Lim BS, Jeong HB, Yeo SY, Choi CY, Lee J. Molecular characterization and transcriptional analysis of non-mammalian type toll like receptor (TLR21) from rock bream (Oplegnathus fasciatus). Gene. 2014;553(2):105–16.
16. Reyes-Becerril M, Ascencio-Valle F, Hirono I, Kondo H, Jirapongpairoj W, Esteban MA, Alamillo E, Angulo C. TLR21's agonists in combination with Aeromonas antigens synergistically up-regulate functional TLR21 and cytokine gene expression in yellowtail leucocytes. Dev Comp Immunol. 2016;61:107–15.
17. Hacker H, Redecke V, Blagoev B, Kratchmarova I, Hsu LC, Wang GG, Kamps MP, Raz E, Wagner H, Hacker G, et al. Specificity in toll-like receptor signalling through distinct effector functions of TRAF3 and TRAF6. Nature. 2006;439(7073):204–7.
18. Akira S. Pathogen recognition by innate immunity and its signaling. Proc Jpn Acad Ser B Phys Biol Sci. 2009;85(4):143–56.
19. Fink IR, Pietretti D, Voogdt CG, Westphal AH, Savelkoul HF, Forlenza M, Wiegertjes GF. Molecular and functional characterization of toll-like receptor (Tlr)1 and Tlr2 in common carp (Cyprinus carpio). Fish Shellfish Immunol. 2016;56:70–83.
20. Ribeiro CM, Hermsen T, Taverne-Thiele AJ, Savelkoul HF, Wiegertjes GF. Evolution of recognition of ligands from gram-positive bacteria: similarities and differences in the TLR2-mediated response between mammalian vertebrates and teleost fish. J Immunol. 2010;184(5):2355–68.
21. Yang C, Su J. Molecular identification and expression analysis of toll-like receptor 3 in common carp Cyprinus carpio. J Fish Biol. 2010;76(8):1926–39.
22. Pietretti D, Spaink HP, Falco A, Forlenza M, Wiegertjes GF. Accessory molecules for toll-like receptors in teleost fish. Identification of TLR4 interactor with leucine-rich repeats (TRIL). Mol Immunol. 2013;56(4):745 56.
23. Kongchum P, Hallerman EM, Hulata G, David L, Palti Y. Molecular cloning, characterization and expression analysis of TLR9, MyD88 and TRAF6 genes in common carp (Cyprinus carpio). Fish Shellfish Immunol. 2011;30(1):361–71.
24. Shan S, Liu D, Liu R, Zhu Y, Li T, Zhang F, An L, Yang G, Li H. Non-mammalian Toll-like receptor 18 (Tlr18) recognizes bacterial pathogens in common carp (*Cyprinus carpio* L.): Indications for a role of participation in the NF-kappaB signaling pathway. Fish Shellfish Immunol. 2017;72:187–98.
25. Pietretti D, Scheer M, Fink IR, Taverne N, Savelkoul HF, Spaink HP, Forlenza M, Wiegertjes GF. Identification and functional characterization of nonmammalian toll-like receptor 20. Immunogenetics. 2014;66(2):123–41.
26. Li H, Yang G, Ma F, Li T, Yang H, Rombout JH, An L. Molecular characterization of a fish-specific toll-like receptor 22 (TLR22) gene from common carp (Cyprinus carpio L.): evolutionary relationship and induced expression upon immune stimulants. Fish Shellfish Immunol. 2017;63:74–86.
27. Li H, Zhang F, Guo H, Zhu Y, Yuan J, Yang G, An L. Molecular characterization of hepcidin gene in common carp (Cyprinus carpio L.) and its expression pattern responding to bacterial challenge. Fish Shellfish Immunol. 2013;35(3):1030–8.
28. Yang G, Guo H, Li H, Shan S, Zhang X, Rombout JH, An L. Molecular characterization of LEAP-2 cDNA in common carp (Cyprinus carpio L.) and the differential expression upon a Vibrio anguillarum stimulus; indications for a significant immune role in skin. Fish Shellfish Immunol. 2014;37(1):22–9.
29. Zhu YY, Xing WX, Shan SJ, Zhang SQ, Li YQ, Li T, An L, Yang GW. Characterization and immune response expression of the rig-I-like receptor mda5 in common carp Cyprinus carpio. J Fish Biol. 2016;88(6):2188–202.
30. Shan SJ, Liu DZ, Wang L, Zhu YY, Zhang FM, Li T, An LG, Yang GW. Identification and expression analysis of irak1 gene in common carp Cyprinus carpio L.: indications for a role of antibacterial and antiviral immunity. J Fish Biol. 2015;87(2):241–55.
31. Li T, Li H, Peng S, Zhang F, An L, Yang G. Molecular characterization and expression pattern of X box-binding protein-1 (XBP1) in common carp (Cyprinus carpio L.): indications for a role of XBP1 in antibacterial and antiviral immunity. Fish Shellfish Immunol. 2017;67:667–74.
32. Kobe B, Deisenhofer J. Proteins with leucine-rich repeats. Curr Opin Struct Biol. 1995;5(3):409–16.
33. Panda RP, Chakrapani V, Patra SK, Saha JN, Jayasankar P, Kar B, Sahoo PK, Barman HK. First evidence of comparative responses of toll-like receptor 22 (TLR22) to relatively resistant and susceptible Indian farmed carps to Argulus siamensis infection. Dev Comp Immunol. 2014;47(1):25–35.
34. Takeda K, Akira S. TLR signaling pathways. Semin Immunol. 2004;16(1):3–9.
35. Lee MS, Kim YJ. Signaling pathways downstream of pattern-recognition receptors and their cross talk. Annu Rev Biochem. 2007;76:447–80.
36. Rauta PR, Nayak B, Das S. Immune system and immune responses in fish and their role in comparative immunity study: a model for higher organisms. Immunol Lett. 2012;148(1):23–33.
37. Samanta M, Basu M, Swain B, Panda P, Jayasankar P. Molecular cloning and characterization of toll-like receptor 3, and inductive expression analysis of type I IFN, mx and pro-inflammatory cytokines in the Indian carp, rohu (Labeo rohita). Mol Biol Rep. 2013;40(1):225–35.
38. Basu M, Swain B, Maiti NK, Routray P, Samanta M. Inductive expression of toll-like receptor 5 (TLR5) and associated downstream signaling molecules following ligand exposure and bacterial infection in the Indian major carp, mrigal (Cirrhinus mrigala). Fish Shellfish Immunol. 2012;32(1):121–31.
39. Yu Y, Zhong Q, Li C, Jiang L, Yan F, Wang Z, Zhang Q. Isolation and characterization of toll-like receptor 9 in half-smooth tongue sole Cynoglossus semilaevis. Fish Shellfish Immunol. 2009;26(3):492–9.
40. Zhu Y, Qi C, Shan S, Zhang F, Li H, An L, Yang G. Characterization of common carp (Cyprinus carpio L.) interferon regulatory factor 5 (IRF5) and its expression in response to viral and bacterial challenges. BMC Vet Res. 2016;12(1):127.
41. Shan S, Qi C, Zhu Y, Li H, An L, Yang G. Expression profile of carp IFN correlate with the up-regulation of interferon regulatory factor-1 (IRF-1) in vivo and in vitro: the pivotal molecules in antiviral defense. Fish Shellfish Immunol. 2016;52:94–102.
42. Pietretti D, Wiegertjes GF. Ligand specificities of toll-like receptors in fish: indications from infection studies. Dev Comp Immunol. 2014;43(2):205–22.

Randomized clinical trial to evaluate the pathogenicity of *Bibersteinia trehalosi* in respiratory disease among calves

Christy J Hanthorn[1], Reneé D Dewell[1,2], Vickie L Cooper[1], Timothy S Frana[1], Paul J Plummer[1,3], Chong Wang[1,4] and Grant A Dewell[1*]

Abstract

Background: *Bibersteinia trehalosi* causes respiratory disease in ruminants particularly in wild and domestic sheep. Recently, there has been an increased number of *B. trehalosi* isolates obtained from diagnostic samples from bovine respiratory disease cases. This study evaluated the role of *B. trehalosi* in bovine respiratory disease using an intra-tracheal inoculation model in calves. Thirty six cross bred 2–3 month old dairy calves were inoculated intra-tracheally with either leukotoxin negative *B. trehalosi*, leukotoxin positive *B. trehalosi* isolate, *Mannheimia haemolytica*, a combination of leukotoxin negative *B. trehalosi* and *M. haemolytica* or negative control. Calves were euthanized and necropsy performed on day 10 of study.

Results: *B. trehalosi* inoculated calves did not have increased lung involvement compared to control calves. Additionally, *B. trehalosi* was only cultured once from the lungs of inoculated calves at necropsy.

Conclusions: Based on these findings *B. trehalosi* may not be a primary pathogen of respiratory disease in cattle. Culture of *B. trehalosi* from diagnostic submissions should not be immediately identified as a primary cause of respiratory disease.

Keywords: *Bibersteinia trehalosi*, Bovine respiratory disease, Calf, Pneumonia, Pasteurellosis

Background

Bibersteinia trehalosi is a known pathogen of ruminants and has been identified worldwide [1]. *B. trehalosi* was formerly included in a single species *of Pasteurella haemolytica* as biotype T [2]. This pathogen was recently reclassified as *B. trehalosi* on the basis of phylogenetic studies [3]. *B. trehalosi* has been associated with systemic pasteurellosis or septicaemia in lambs [4] and pneumonia in bighorn sheep (Ovis canadensis) [5,6].

Although *B. trehalosi* infections are considered rare in cattle, the agent is occasionally isolated from bovine lungs. Diagnostic reports of severe non-responsive Bovine Respiratory Disease (BRD) outbreaks associated with multi-drug resistant *B. trehalosi* have been documented [7]. Clinical manifestations of these strains are often associated with multi-drug resistance and severe lung pathology. The reasons for development of these potentially highly virulent strains remain unclear. It has been hypothesized that *B. trehalosi* may have acquired increased pathogenicity from other bacteria. Some reports in the literature suggest that *B. trehalosi* and *Mannheimia haemolytica* can share genetic material [8,9]. Earlier work has shown that nucleotide diversity of lktA from *B. trehalosi* is minimal (0.7%) compared to *M. haemolytica* (22.0%) and were genetically different from M. *haemolytica* [10]. However, this report included only *B. trehalosi* isolates from ovine samples. Bovine adapted isolates of *B. trehalosi* may have acquired some genetic material from *M. heamolytica* increasing its ability to infect cattle.

Understanding the role different pathogens play in BRD is critical to understanding and effectively treating clinical cases. The primary objective of this study was to evaluate the pathogenicity of *B. trehalosi* in respiratory disease among calves using field strains of *B. trehalosi.*

* Correspondence: gdewell@iastate.edu
[1]Department of Veterinary and Diagnostic Production Animal Medicine, College of Veterinary Medicine, Iowa State University, 2237 Lloyd Vet Med, Ames, IA 50011, USA
Full list of author information is available at the end of the article

Methods

Two *B. trehalosi* isolates were identified from diagnostic submissions of bovine cases for the challenge study. Isolate identification was confirmed by 16S ribosomal RNA analysis. One isolate was PCR positive for the leukotoxin (lktA) gene [11] and the other isolate was negative. The lktA gene was amplified with a 5′ primer lktA9 (5′-TCAAGAAGAGCTGGCAAC-3′) and the 3′ primer lktA7 (5′-AGTGAGGGCAACTAAACC-3′). Amplification parameters were: denaturation at 94°C for 45 s, annealing at 62°C for 45 s, and extension at 72 C for 2 min. The leukotoxin-PCR-positive *B. trehalosi* isolate was cultured from the lungs, along with a *Pasteurella multocida,* from a feedlot calf that had been treated with antibiotics multiple times for Bovine Respiratory Disease that had fibrinosuppurative bronchopneumonia from a group of 273 kg Southeastern feedlot calves with 16% respiratory morbidity and 10% mortality. The leukotoxin-PCR-negative *B. trehalosi* isolate was cultured from the brain of a bull with multifocal, suppurative meningoencephalitis.

Thirty six 8–12 week old individually housed Holstein cross steer calves were obtained from a private calf raiser. Calves were tested for persistent infection by BVDV by immunohistochemistry prior to purchase and confirmed PI negative. Nasal swab samples were collected from each calf and submitted for bacterial culture to the diagnostic lab prior (Day −1) to inoculation. During the experimental challenge, calves were housed in a Biosecurity Level 2 facility at the ISU Livestock Infectious Disease Isolation Facility. Each calf was confined separately in raised 0.9 × 1.8 meter pens that provided no opportunity for calf-to-calf contact in a room that held 12 calves at a time. Three groups of calves were utilized to accommodate room layout. Calves were provided free choice water and were fed mixed grass hay and a pre-mixed calf starter. Biosecurity procedures such as changing protective gloves and clothing between calves were employed by all research personnel working with calves. Calves were randomly assigned by a random number generator [12] to one of five treatments. Treatments were randomly assigned to 1 of 3 replicates (Table 1). Eight calves were assigned to each bacterial challenge treatment and 4 calves to a negative control treatment.

Table 1 Replicate and treatment group assignments

	Replicate 1	Replicate 2	Replicate 3
Control Calves	1	1	2
Leukotoxin negative *B. trehalosi*	3	3	2
Leukotoxin postive *B. trehalosi*	3	3	2
M. haemolytica	3	2	3
M. haemolytica and leukotoxin negative *B. trehalosi*	2	3	3

Assignment of calves to treatment groups by replicate of study presented in table format.

The 5 treatment groups were:

1) Negative control (Brain Heart Infusion broth),
2) Leukotoxin negative *B. trehalosi,*
3) Leukotoxin positive *B. trehalosi,*
4) *M. haemolytica*
5) Combination of leukotoxin negative *B. trehalosi* and *M. haemolytica*

Prior to inoculation, each isolate was grown overnight on two blood agar plates and then transferred to a Brain Heart Infusion broth immediately prior to inoculation to obtain an estimated 2.5×10^9 CFU of bacteria per ml. Isolates for group 5 had an estimated 2.5×10^9 CFU of bacteria per ml for both leukotoxin negative *B. trehalosi* and *M. haemolytica* for a total of 5×10^9 CFU of bacteria per ml. A small sample of the inoculum was enumerated on blood agar plates to determine exact concentration of the inoculum. Inoculums ranged on average from 1.7×10^9 to 3.3×10^9 CFU of bacteria per ml of broth. A sterile 90 cm number 8 French Foley catheter (MILA International) was used to inoculate each calf. The researcher administering the inoculum was masked to the treatment being administered. For each inoculation, a sterile catheter was passed intranasal to approximately the bifurcation of the trachea and 20 ml of the inoculum was infused. Following inoculation, the calf's head was briefly elevated.

Following inoculation, calves were monitored twice daily by trained personnel masked to treatment on Days 0–9. Measurements recorded included rectal temperature, pulse rate and respiration rate. In addition each calf was clinically assessed and assigned a respiratory and depression score during twice daily monitoring. The following scoring systems were used for the study.

Respiratory scores:

0 – Normal, eyes are clear, nose is clean with no discharge, normal breathing
1 – Mild Respiratory, serous discharge from eyes and\or nose, slight cough
2 – Moderate Respiratory, muco-purulent discharge, cough, increased respiratory rate
3 – Severe Respiratory, excessive muco-purulent discharge, harsh cough, open mouth breathing

Depression scores

0 – Normal, cattle are bright and alert, hold their head up and readily move away from the observer
1 – Mild depression, cattle's attitude is slightly depressed but respond quickly to observer and appear normal

2 – Moderate depression, cattle stand with head down, ears droop, abdomen lack of fill and may appear floppy, cattle move away slowly from observer
3 – Severe depression, cattle stand with head down and very reluctant to move, very noticeable gauntness of abdomen

Any calf that was assigned a respiratory and/or depression score of three was considered a candidate for euthanasia. If calf was determined to be moribund from physical exam, it was humanly euthanized. All surviving calves were euthanized on day 9 of the study by use of captive bolt followed by pithing. All euthanasias followed American Veterinary Medical Association guidelines [13].

Immediately following euthanasia, a necropsy was performed on each calf. The respiratory system was evaluated by a diagnostic pathologist. The percent abnormal lung was visually estimated for each lobe and total lung involvement calculated as a percentage of total lung as described by Jericho and Langford [14]. Samples of representative lung as determined by the pathologist were submitted ISU Veterinary Diagnostic Laboratory for routine culture and histology. For culture, samples were plated on bovine blood agar and incubated aerobically at 35°C, sheep blood agar and incubated anaerobically at 35°C and tergitol-7 agar and incubated aerobically at 35°C. All samples were incubated overnight and suspect hemolytic and non-hemolytic colonies were selected for identification by matrix-assisted laser desorption/ionization–time of flight (MALDI-TOF).

This protocol was approved by the Iowa State University Institutional Animal Care and Use Committee (#5-12-7352-B) and the Institutional Biosafety Committee (#12-I-0017-A). Personnel conducting daily monitoring, the pathologist and the statistician were blinded to calves treatment group.

Statistical analysis

Our goal was to describe the magnitude and variation of our collected measurements and assess the association of these variables with BRD and *B. trehalosi.* The primary outcome of interest included percent lung involvement, temperature, depression score and respiratory score. The percent abnormal lung response was analyzed using mixed effect Analysis of Variance (ANOVA) model, with Treatment as fixed effect and Group as a random effect. The remaining responses (Temperature, Depression score, and Respiratory score) were analyzed using repeated measures ANOVA model, with Treatment, time and their interaction as fixed effects and group as random effect. Comparisons among treatment groups were performed using Tukey's t-tests. SAS® Version 9.2 (SAS® Institute Inc., Cary, NC, USA) was used in analyses. A p-value <0.05 was considered significant.

Results

Thirty five of the thirty six candidates were enrolled in the study. One calf assigned to the *M. haemolytica* group died prior to enrollment in study. *Pasturella multocida* was isolated from nasal swab samples from 34 of 35 calves. *M. haemolytica* was isolated from 3 of 35 calves. *M. haemolytica* positive nasal swab calves were fairly evenly spread across all five treatment groups (1/4 in Control group, 1/8 in Leukotoxin negative *B. trehalosi* group, 2/8 Leukotoxin positive *B. trehalosi* group, 1/7 *M. haemolytica* group, 3/8 leukotoxin negative *B. trehalosi* and *M. haemolytica* combination group). Six of the 35 enrolled calves were euthanized prior to day 9 of the study. Three of the euthanized calves (3/7) in *M. haemolytica* group (days 1, 2 and 2) and three calves (3/8) from the leukotoxin negative *B. trehalosi* and *M. haemolytica* combination treatment (days 2, 4 and 7) were euthanized according to protocol because of a clinical assessment of moribund. Overall, the mean estimated percent lung involvement was highest for the *M. haemolytica* group (49%) followed by the mixed infection of *M. haemolytica* and leukotoxin negative *B. trehalosi* (26%). The leukotoxin postive *B. trehalosi* had a mean 18% estimated lung involvement while the leukotoxin negative *B. trehalosi* mean lung involvement was estimated to be 13%. The control group had a mean lung involvement estimate of 13% (Table 2). Calves with lung involvement had histologic lesions that were consistent with bronchointerstitial pneumonia (26 of 35 calves) and 20 of these calves also had evidence of pyogranulomatus pneumonia.

M. haemolytica was isolated from5 of 7 lungs of the *M. haemolytica* inoculated group and 4 of 8 lungs from the leukotoxin negative *B. trehalosi* and *M. haemolytica* combination group. *B. trehalosi* was isolated from one of 24 lungs that were inoculated with *B. trehalosi.* Calf number 6 in the leukotoxin negative *B. trehalosi* and *M. haemolytica* combination inoculation treatment group was euthanized on day 2 of the study as reported above. The calf had 71.6% lung involvement and both *M. haemolytica* and a *B. trehalosi* were isolated from the lung tissue. *B. trehalosi* was not isolated from the lung tissue of any other calves that were inoculated with a *B. trehalosi* isolate.

Rectal temperature (Figure 1), depression scores (Figure 2) and respiratory scores (Figure 3) followed an expected pattern after inoculation. Overall, rectal temperatures ranged from 35.3-41.3°C. Depression scores ranged from 0–3 and respiratory scores ranged from 0–3.There were occasional time periods when differences in rectal temperatures, depression score or respiratory score between the *M. haemolytica* and the *B. trehalosi* or

Table 2 Percent lung involvement by treatment group

	Control	Leukotoxin negative *B. trehalosi*	Leukotoxin postive *B. trehalosi*	*M. haemolytica*	*M. haemolytica* and leukotoxin negative *B. trehalosi*
Calves	20.4	0	36.55	57.25	71.6
	26.2	24.25	27.1	53.95	61.3
	0	21.7	28.1	26	62.85
	4.4	32.1	27.1	33.15	0
		18.05	14.2	28.6	1.8
		6.15	1.5	63.6	0.6
		3.6	11.35	75.1	4.75
		0	1.45		6.1
Mean*	12.75 a	13.2 a	18.4 a	48.2 b	26.1 a, b
Adj P value**		0.9999	0.9981	0.0715	0.8049

*means with different letters are statistically different ($p < 0.05$).
**Adj p value of treatment from the control group.
Individual and mean lung involved in disease process as a percentage of total lung volume. Treatment group means that were statistically different from other treatment groups are indicated by different letters (a or b) in table. Adjusted p-values of treatment group from control group is reported.

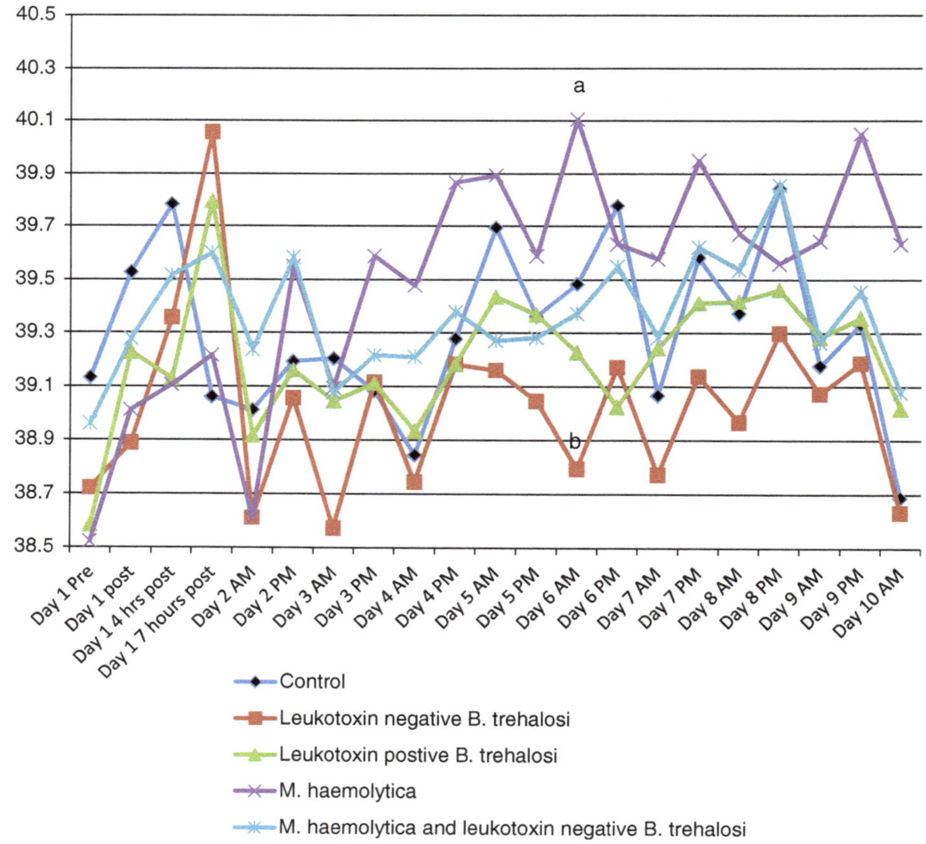

Figure 1 Temperature over time by treatment group. Line graph of rectal temperature by treatment group for each time point when temperature was recorded. Time points that were statistically different are indicated by different letters (a or b).

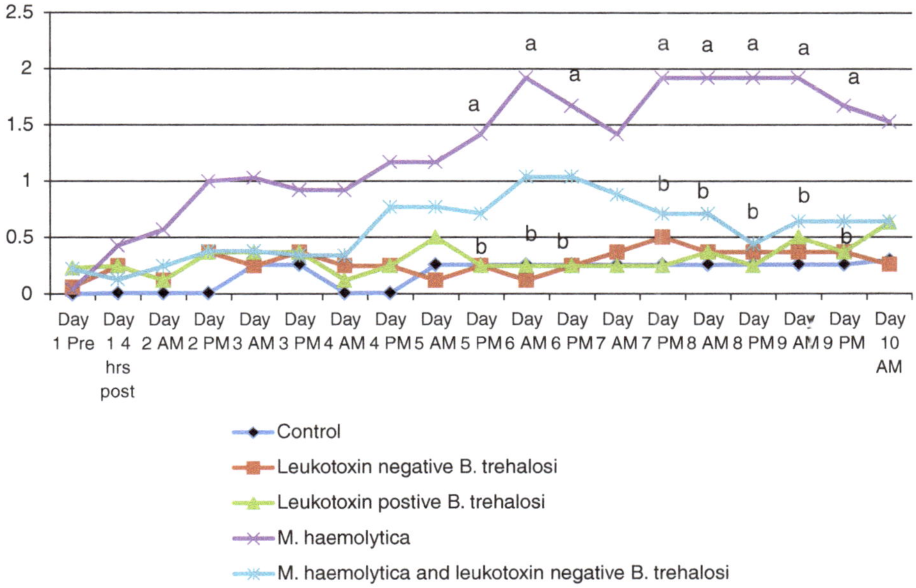

Figure 2 Depression score over time by Treatment group. Line graph of depression score by treatment group for each time point when depression score was recorded. Time points that were statistically different are indicated by different letters (a or b).

control groups were statistically significant (Figures 1, 2 and 3).

The calves from both groups inoculated with *B. trehalosi* demonstrated increased rectal temperature (>39.5°C) at 7 hours after inoculation compared to calves that had been inoculated with *M. haemolytica*. Temperatures for the two *B. trehalosi* only treatment groups returned to normal levels (37.5 – 39.5°C) within 12 hours. Calves in the *M. haemolytica* only inoculation group did not demonstrate increased rectal temperatures (>39.5°C) on average until 24 hours following inoculation and temperatures of these calves remained elevated except for morning

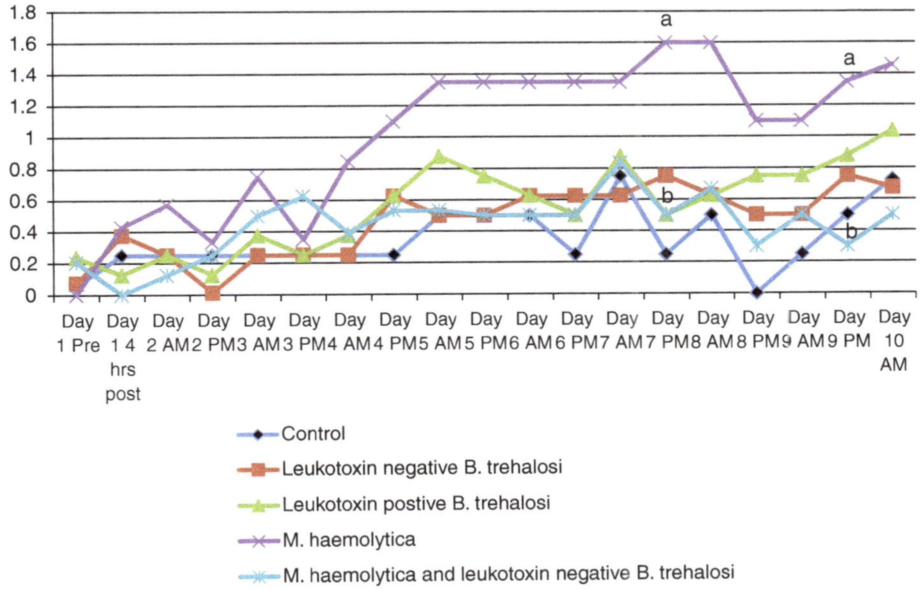

Figure 3 Respiratory score over time by treatment group. Line graph of respiratory score by treatment group for each time point when respiratory score was recorded. Time points that were statistically different are indicated by different letters (a or b).

of day 2. Calves in the combined inoculation group fluctuated above and below 39.5°C throughout the study (Figure 1).

Depression scores (Figure 2) for the *M. haemolytica* inoculation group began to increase 4 hours post inoculation and remained elevated at 1 or greater throughout the study. The combined inoculation group did not have increased depression scores (≥1) until Day 3 of the study and never reached the severity of the *M. haemolytica* only inoculation group. Neither of the *B. trehalosi* inoculation groups had elevated depression scores. The average depression score for the control group was 0.2. Both *B. trehalosi* only inoculation groups had an average depression score of 0.3 while the *M. haemolytica* inoculation group had an average of 1.3. The combined inoculation group had an average depression score of 0.6.Respiratory scores for the *M. haemolytica* inoculation group ranged from 0–3 and were not consistently abnormal (≥1) until Day 3 of the study. None of the other groups had elevated average respiratory scores (Table 3).

Discussion

Results of this study indicate that *B. trehalosi* isolates used in this study are not associated with significant disease in a research setting. Calves inoculated with either a leukotoxin positive (PCR positive for the leukotoxin (lktA) gene) or leukotoxin negative isolate of *B. trehalosi* did not demonstrate increased lung involvement compared to control calves. This finding contradicts some perceptions that *B. trehalosi* is an emerging primary respiratory pathogen of cattle [7]. In contrast, this study's results are more supportive of *B. trehalosi's* role in BRD as secondary and perhaps opportunistic bacteria. Reports of *B. trehalosi* associated pneumonia are from diagnostic submissions, often without access to history of inciting causes of respiratory disease, nutritional health of calves, additional stressors or information on antimicrobial therapies. In this challenge model healthy calves were challenged with field isolates of *B. trehalosi* and extensive lung involvement was not identified post inoculation.

Table 3 Average depression and respiratory score by treatment group

	Average peak depression score (Range)	Average peak respiratory score (Range)
Control	0.25 (0–1)	1 (1–1)
Leukotoxin negative *B. trehalosi*	0.75 (0–2)	1 (0–1)
Leukotoxin postive *B. trehalosi*	1 (0–2)	1.25 (1–2)
M. haemolytica	2 (0–3)	1.7 (1–3)
M. haemolytica and leukotoxin negative *B. trehalosi*	1.25 (0–3)	1.25 (0–3)

Average depression and respiratory scores over the course of the study are reported for each treatment group in table format.

The limitations of this study include the small size of the study, isolate credibility, the inoculation method and the health status of the calves prior to inoculation. The study was designed as a pilot study to evaluate the pathogenicity of *B. trehalosi* in cattle. The number of calves in each group was limited as much as possible to decrease the number of calves sacrificed while still providing important information. The small size of the study decreases the statistical power to identify statically significant differences even though numerically the difference between the negative control group (inoculated with broth only) and the positive control group (*M. haemolytica*) were substantial.

The authors are unaware of any *B. trehalosi* isolates that have demonstrated pathogenicity in a challenge model in cattle. The *B. trehalosi* isolates selected for this study originated from field submissions to a diagnostic laboratory. Our approach was to use leukotoxin positive and negative *B. trehalosi* isolates that had been associated with respiratory disease and could potentially be associated with lung pathology in the study calves.

Though unlikely, it is possible that, during the inoculation procedure, the dose was inadvertently misplaced into the esophagus instead of the lungs. There are multiple bovine respiratory disease challenge models cited in the literature including trans-tracheal injection, trans-thoracic injection, bronchoscope and using a nasal-tracheal approach that this study utilized. Confirmation that the catheter was correctly placed in the trachea as opposed to the esophagus can be difficult. However, the *M. haemolytica* positive control group, had substantial lung involvement and a p-value of 0.07 compared to the negative control group suggesting that the inoculation technique and the challenge model was valid.

Calves in the study were conventionally reared dairy crossbred calves. Calves were purchased from a calf raiser and were considered clinically normal at the time of purchase and did not exhibit signs of respiratory disease at enrollment. However, two calves in the control group had lung lesions (20–26% lung involvement). Thus, this pathology was presumed to have resulted from a previous infection not associated with inoculation. Evidence of lung pathology from prior respiratory disease in some control calves may confound results between treatment groups. Histologic lesions characteristic of a previous BRSV infection was seen in 17 of the calves. Since two control calves demonstrated some lung pathology, the potential difference between treatment groups and the control group was affected.

Pre-study pharyngeal swabs did not identify any calves carrying *B. trehalosi* and the calf farm did not have a history of *B. trehalosi* disease. Despite this, it is still possible that calves could have had exposure to *B. trehalosi* prior to enrollment in the project. Given the age of the calves, it is also possible that passive immunity played a role in immune response. However, there is currently not a validated serologic test for cattle to determine previous exposure to *B. trehalosi*. Therefore, it is possible that calves may have had previous unknown exposure to *B. trehalosi* that enhanced their immunological response.

It was surprising that calves inoculated with a combination of *M. haemolytica* and *B. trehalosi* tended to have numerically less lung involvement than that of *M. haemolytica* inoculation alone (difference was not significant). One would expect that mixed infections would potentiate increased lung involvement and subsequent pathology. Other research has suggested that *B. trehalosi* can inhibit the growth of *M. haemolytica*. Dassanayake et al. [15] reported that *B. trehalosi* inhibited the growth of *M. haemolytica* in co-culture when *B. trehalosi* enters the stationary phase. One possible explanation for this finding is that; when both bacteria are inoculated simultaneously, *B. trehalosi* may inhibit *in vivo* growth of *M. haemolytica* until the immune system removes *B. trehalosi*. This postulated in vivo inhibition may delay the onset of clinical signs of BRD (such as a temperature spike and decrease the subsequent severity of lung involvement.

Our goal was to determine if *B. trehalosi* is really an emerging primary BRD pathogen as has been reported or if infection occurs secondary to some other viral/bacterial insult. Cortese et al. [7] have reported peracute fatal pneumonia in healthy adult cattle attributed to *B. trehalosi*. Other, anecdotal reports concerning *B. trehalosi* and BRD, suggest that *B. trehalosi* is associated with severe fibinous pneumonia with consolidation (especially caudal lobes) and pleuritis that is unresponsive to antimicrobial therapy. The more minor role that *B. trehalosi* may play in BRD is supported by the isolation results described in this study. *B. trehalosi* was isolated from only one set of lungs post inoculation and in that case the sample was obtained only 3 days following inoculation from a calf that had been inoculated with both *B. trehalosi* and *M. haemolytica*. This finding suggests that *B. trehalosi* may not persist long term in bovine lung. The temperature response of calves inoculated with *B. trehalosi* or *M. haemolytica* was different ($p < 0.05$) over time. The early spike and rapid return to normal in rectal temperature from the *B. trehalosi* inoculated calves may indicate that the immune system in the lungs may more rapidly identify and respond to a *B. trehalosi* bacterial insult compared to the *M. haemolytica* inoculated calves. The authors acknowledge that *B. trehalosi* isolates have been obtained from samples submitted from field cases. These "positives" suggest the occurrence of an opportunistic infection and proliferation of *B. trehalosi* after normal lung defenses have been compromised by other primary respiratory pathogens. The plausibility of *B. trehalosi* as a secondary, perhaps even an opportunistic, pathogen is a stronger argument than *B. trehalosi* as an emerging primary BRD pathogen of economic importance.

Conclusion

This pilot study suggests that *B. trehalosi* may not be an important primary pathogen of respiratory disease in cattle. The study's results suggest that *B. trehalosi* is likely a secondary, or perhaps opportunistic, BRD pathogen. Culture of this bacterium from diagnostic submissions should not necessarily be interpreted cited as a primary cause of respiratory disease but may still have a role as a secondary pathogen or an opportunistic invader. Clinicians and diagnosticians should temper a *B. trehalosi* culture in context of the clinical setting. Practically, identification of *B. trehalosi* as the primary isolate from a submitted lung sample may suggest a failure in identification or treatment of a major BRD pathogen such as M. haemolytica. Further challenge studies designed to assess *B.trehalosi's* interaction with other BRD pathogens (IBR, BVDV, *Mycoplasma bovis*, *Histophilus somni*) should be conducted. Additionally, a challenge model designed to evaluate if *B. trehalosi*, inoculated after *M. haemolytica* has already initiated lung damage, can lead to more severe BRD would be beneficial.

Competing interests

The authors declare that they have no competing interests.

Authors' contributions

GD and PP conceived and coordinated the experiment. CH and RD performed the experiment. VC evaluated lungs. CW conducted statistical analysis. TF helped with bacteriology guidance and draft of the manuscript. All authors read and approved the final manuscript.

Acknowledgements

The authors thank Boehringer Ingelheim Vetmedica, Inc. for their support of research through the Iowa State University Foundation. Jessica Ninneman is acknowledged for her excellent laboratory assistance.

Author details

[1]Department of Veterinary and Diagnostic Production Animal Medicine, College of Veterinary Medicine, Iowa State University, 2237 Lloyd Vet Med, Ames, IA 50011, USA. [2]Center for Food Security and Public Health, Department of Veterinary Microbiology and Preventive Medicine, College of Veterinary Medicine, Iowa State University, Ames, IA 50011, USA. [3]Department of Veterinary Microbiology and Preventive Medicine, College of Veterinary Medicine, Iowa State University, Ames, IA 50011, USA. [4]Department of Statistics, College of Liberal Arts and Sciences, Iowa State University, Ames, IA 50011, USA.

References

1. Franck GH: **Pasteurellosis in cattle.** In *Pasteurella and Pasteurellosis*. Edited by Adlam C, Rutter JM. London, UK Academic Press; 1989:197–222.
2. Adlam C: **The structure, function and properties of cellular and extracellular components of *Pasteurella haemolytica*.** In *Pasteurella and Pasteurellosis*. Edited by Adlam C, Rutter JM. London, UK: Academic Press; 1989:75–92.

3. Blackall PJ, Bojesen AM, Christensen H, Bisgaard M: **Reclassification of [*Pasteurella*] *trehalosi* as *Bibersteinia trehalosi* gen. nov., comb. nov.** *Int J Syst Evol Microbiol* 2007, **57:**666–674.
4. Gilmour NJL, Gilmour JS: **Pasteurellosis of sheep.** In *Pasteurella and Pasteurellosis.* Edited by Adlam C, Rutter JM. London, UK: Academic Press; 1989:223–262.
5. Wolfe LL, Diamond B, Spraker TR, Sirochman MA, Walsh DP, Machin CM, Bade DJ, Miller MW: **A bighorn sheep die-off in southern Colorado involving a Pasteurellaceae strain that may have originated from syntopic cattle.** *J Wildl Dis* 2010, **46:**1262–1268.
6. Dassanayake RP, Shanthalingam S, Subramaniam R, Herndon CN, Bavananthasivam J, Haldorson GJ, Foreyt WJ, Evermann JF, Herrmann-Hoesing LM, Knowles DP, Srikumaran S: **Role of *Bibersteinia trehalosi*, respiratory syncytial virus, and parainfluenza-3 virus in bighorn sheep pneumonia.** *Vet Microbiol* 2013, **162:**166–172.
7. Cortese VS, Braun DA, Crouch D, Townsend C, Zukowski B: **Case report – Peracute to acute fatal pneumonia in cattle caused by *Bibersteinia trehalosi*.** *Bov Pract* 2012, **46:**138–142.
8. Kelley ST, Cassirer EF, Weiser GC, Safaee S: **Phylogenetic diversity of Pasteurellaceae and horizontal gene transfer of leukotoxin in wild and domestic sheep.** *Infect Genet Evol* 2007, **7:**13–23.
9. Lee I, Davies RL: **Evidence for a common gene pool and frequent recombinational exchange of the tbpBA operon in *Mannheimia haemolytica*, *Mannheimia glucosida* and *Bibersteinia trehalosi*.** *Microbiology* 2010, **157:**123–135.
10. Davies RL, Campbell S, Whittam TS: **Mosaic structure and molecular evolution of the leukotoxin operon (lktCABD) in Mannheimia (Pasteurella) haemolytica, Mannheimia glucosida, and Pasteurella trehalosi.** *J Bacteriol* 2002, **184:**266–277.
11. Davies RL, Whittam TS, Selander RK: **Sequence diversity and molecular evolution of the leukotoxin (lktA) gene in bovine and ovine strains of Mannheimia (Pasteurella) haemolytica.** *J Bacteriol* 2001, **183:**1394–1404.
12. **RANDOM.ORG** [www.random.org].
13. AVMA: **AVMA guidelines for the euthanasia of Animals: 2013 Edition.** https://www.avma.org/KB/Policies/Documents/euthanasia.pdf.
14. Jericho KW, Langford EV: **Aerosol vaccination of calves with pasteurella haemolytica against experimental respiratory disease.** *Can J Comp Med* 1982, **46:**287–292.
15. Dassanayake RP, Call DR, Sawant AA, Casavant NC, Weiser GC, Knowles DP, Srikumaran S: **Bibersteinia trehalosi inhibits the growth of Mannheimia haemolytica by a proximity-dependent mechanism.** *Appl Environ Microbiol* 2010, **76:**1008–1013.

PERMISSIONS

All chapters in this book were first published in VR, by BioMed Central; hereby published with permission under the Creative Commons Attribution License or equivalent. Every chapter published in this book has been scrutinized by our experts. Their significance has been extensively debated. The topics covered herein carry significant findings which will fuel the growth of the discipline. They may even be implemented as practical applications or may be referred to as a beginning point for another development.

The contributors of this book come from diverse backgrounds, making this book a truly international effort. This book will bring forth new frontiers with its revolutionizing research information and detailed analysis of the nascent developments around the world.

We would like to thank all the contributing authors for lending their expertise to make the book truly unique. They have played a crucial role in the development of this book. Without their invaluable contributions this book wouldn't have been possible. They have made vital efforts to compile up to date information on the varied aspects of this subject to make this book a valuable addition to the collection of many professionals and students.

This book was conceptualized with the vision of imparting up-to-date information and advanced data in this field. To ensure the same, a matchless editorial board was set up. Every individual on the board went through rigorous rounds of assessment to prove their worth. After which they invested a large part of their time researching and compiling the most relevant data for our readers.

The editorial board has been involved in producing this book since its inception. They have spent rigorous hours researching and exploring the diverse topics which have resulted in the successful publishing of this book. They have passed on their knowledge of decades through this book. To expedite this challenging task, the publisher supported the team at every step. A small team of assistant editors was also appointed to further simplify the editing procedure and attain best results for the readers.

Apart from the editorial board, the designing team has also invested a significant amount of their time in understanding the subject and creating the most relevant covers. They scrutinized every image to scout for the most suitable representation of the subject and create an appropriate cover for the book.

The publishing team has been an ardent support to the editorial, designing and production team. Their endless efforts to recruit the best for this project, has resulted in the accomplishment of this book. They are a veteran in the field of academics and their pool of knowledge is as vast as their experience in printing. Their expertise and guidance has proved useful at every step. Their uncompromising quality standards have made this book an exceptional effort. Their encouragement from time to time has been an inspiration for everyone.

The publisher and the editorial board hope that this book will prove to be a valuable piece of knowledge for researchers, students, practitioners and scholars across the globe.

LIST OF CONTRIBUTORS

Nicole Willems, Anna R. Tellegen, Niklas Bergknut, Jeannette Wolfswinkel and Marianna A. Tryfonidou and Björn P. Meij
Department of Clinical Sciences of Companion Animals, Faculty of Veterinary Medicine, 3584 CM Utrecht, The Netherlands

Laura B. Creemers
Department of Orthopaedics, University Medical Center, 3584 CX Utrecht, The Netherlands

Christian Freudigmann and Karin Benz
NMI Natural and Medical Sciences Institute at the University of Tuebingen, Regenerative Medicine II, 72770 Reutlingen, Germany

Guy C. M. Grinwis
Department of Pathobiology, Faculty of Veterinary Medicine, 3508 TD Utrecht, The Netherlands

Yuiko Kato, Kazuhiko Ochiai, Shota Kawakami, Daigo Azakami and Toshinori Omi
School of Veterinary Nursing and Technology, Faculty of Veterinary Science, Nippon Veterinary and Life Science University, Tokyo 180-8602, Japan

Nobuhiro Nakao
Laboratory of Animal Physiology, School of Animal Science, Nippon Veterinary and Life Science University, Tokyo 180-8602, Japan

Makoto Bonkobara
Department of Veterinary Clinical Pathology, Faculty of Veterinary Science, Nippon Veterinary and Life Science University, Tokyo 180-8602, Japan

Masaki Michishita
Department of Veterinary Pathology, Faculty of Veterinary Science, Nippon Veterinary and Life Science University, Tokyo 180-8602, Japan

Masami Morimatsu
Laboratory of Laboratory Animal Science and Medicine, Department of Disease Control, Graduate School of Veterinary Medicine, Hokkaido University, Sapporo 060-0818, Japan

Masami Watanabe
Department of Urology, Graduate School of Medicine, Dentistry and Pharmaceutical Sciences, Okayama University, Okayama 700-8558, Japan

Eun-Sil Park, Michio Suzuki, Masanobu Kimura, Koichi Imaoka and Shigeru Morikawa
Department of Veterinary Science, National Institute of Infectious Diseases, Tokyo 162-8640, Japan

Hiroshi Mizutani, Ryuichi Saito, Nami Kubota, Youko Hasuike, Jungo Okajima, Hidemi Kasai and Keiji Maruyama
Tokyo Metropolitan Animal Care and Consultation Center, Jounanjima Branch Office, Tokyo 143-0002, Japan

Yuko Sato and Noriko Nakajima
Department of Pathology, National Institute of Infectious Diseases, Tokyo 162-8640, Japan

Nitin M. Kamble and John Hwa Lee
College of Veterinary Medicine and Bio-Safety Research Institute, Chonbuk National University, Iksan Campus 570-752, Republic of Korea

Aline S. Hora, Paulo E. Brandão and Hilda F. J. Pena
Department of Preventive Veterinary Medicine and Animal Health, College of Veterinary Medicine, University of São Paulo, São Paulo, SP, Brazil

Samantha I. Miyashiro and Archivaldo Reche-Junior
Department of Veterinary Medicine, College of Veterinary Medicine, University of São Paulo, São Paulo, SP, Brazil

Fabiana C. Cassiano
Veterinary Hospital, College of Veterinary Medicine, University of São Paulo, São Paulo, SP, Brazil

Khadija Khataby
Laboratory of Virology, Microbiology, Quality and Biotechnologies/Ecotoxicology & Biodiversity, Faculty of Sciences and Techniques, University Hassan II of Casablanca, Mohammedia, Morocco
Society Biopharma, Km 2, Route de Casa, B.P. 4569, Rabat, Morocco

Faouzi Kichou
Department of Veterinary Pathology and Public Health, Hassan 2nd Institute of Agronomy and Veterinary Medicine, B.P. 6202, Madinat Al Irfane, Rabat, Morocco

Chafiqa Loutfi
Society Biopharma, Km 2, Route de Casa, B.P. 4569, Rabat, Morocco

My Mustapha Ennaji
Laboratory of Virology, Microbiology, Quality and Biotechnologies/Ecotoxicology & Biodiversity, Faculty of Sciences and Techniques, University Hassan II of Casablanca, Mohammedia, Morocco

Qing Lin Zeng, Xian Mei, Jia Su and Xiao Hong Li
National Laboratory of Safety Evaluation of veterinary Drugs, College of Veterinary Medicine, South China Agricultural University, Guangzhou, China

Wen Guang Xiong, Yan Lu and Zhen Ling Zeng
National Laboratory of Safety Evaluation of veterinary Drugs, College of Veterinary Medicine, South China Agricultural University, Guangzhou, China
National Laboratory of Safety Evaluation (Environmental Assessment) of Veterinary Drugs, College of Veterinary Medicine, South China Agricultural University, Guangzhou, China

Elena L. Sassu and Isabel Hennig-Pauka
University Clinic for Swine, Department of Farm Animals and Veterinary Public Health, University of Veterinary Medicine Vienna, Vienna, Austria

Janna Frömbling, Tom Grunert, Joachim Spergser and Monika Ehling-Schulz
Department of Pathobiology, Functional Microbiology, Institute of Microbiology, University of Veterinary Medicine Vienna, Vienna, Austria

J. Catharina Duvigneau, Ingrid Miller and Andrea Müllebner
Department of Biomedical Sciences, Institute for Medical Biochemistry, University of Veterinary Medicine Vienna, Vienna, Austria

Ana M. Gutiérrez
Department of Animal Medicine and Surgery, University of Murcia, Murcia, Spain

Martina Patzl and Armin Saalmüller
Department of Pathobiology, Institute of Immunology, University of Veterinary Medicine Vienna, Vienna, Austria

Alexandra von Altrock, Anne Menzel and Martin Ganter
Forensic Medicine and Ambulatory Services, Clinic for Swine and Small Ruminants, University of Veterinary Medicine Hannover, Hannover, Germany

Marion Hewicker-Trautwein
Department of Pathology, University of Veterinary Medicine Hannover, Hannover, Germany

Jutta Verspohl
Institute for Microbiology, University of Veterinary Medicine Hannover, Hannover, Germany

M. M. Bumby, M. C. Williams, J. C. A. Steyl and S. J. Clift
Section Pathology, Department of Paraclinical Sciences, Faculty of Veterinary Science, University of Pretoria, Onderstepoort 0110, South Africa

R. Harrison-White
Wildlife Damage- Research and Management, North West Parks and Tourism Board, Madikwe and SA Lombard Nature Reserves, North West province, South Africa, Sandton, Johannesburg 2146, South Africa

H. Lutermann
Mammal Research Institute, Department of Zoology and Entomology, University of Pretoria, Hatfield, Pretoria 0028, South Africa

G. T. Fosgate
Department of Production Animal Studies, Faculty of Veterinary Science, University of Pretoria, Onderstepoort 0110, South Africa

P. J. de Waal and J. Mitha
Department of Genetics, University of Pretoria, Pretoria 0002, South Africa

Zhenguang Li and Hua Wu
Sinovet (Beijing) Biotechnology Co., Ltd., Kaituo Road 5, Haidian District, Beijing 100085, China
State Key Laboratory of Special Economic Animal Molecular Biology, Institute of Special Economic Animal and Plant Sciences, Chinese Academy of Agricultural Sciences, Juye Street 4899, Changchun, Jilin 130122, China

Yanliang He, Shufen Li and Mingqi Xia
Sinovet (Beijing) Biotechnology Co., Ltd., Kaituo Road 5, Haidian District, Beijing 100085, China

Xiaoqin Xu
Jiangyan Animal Health Inspection Institute, Jiangguan Road 251, Taizhou, Jiangsu 225529, China

Xue Leng, Yongjun Wen, Fengxue Wang and Shipeng Cheng
State Key Laboratory of Special Economic Animal Molecular Biology, Institute of Special Economic Animal and Plant Sciences, Chinese Academy of Agricultural Sciences, Juye Street 4899, Changchun, Jilin 130122, China

Jifei Yang, Zhijie Liu, Qingli Niu, Junlong Liu, Jingying Xie, Qiuyu Chen, Ze Chen, Guiquan Guan, Guangyuan Liu and Jianxun Luo
State Key Laboratory of Veterinary Etiological Biology, Key Laboratory of Veterinary Parasitology of Gansu Province, Lanzhou Veterinary Research Institute, Chinese Academy of Agricultural Science, Xujiaping 1, Lanzhou, Gansu 730046, P. R. China

Hong Yin
State Key Laboratory of Veterinary Etiological Biology, Key Laboratory of Veterinary Parasitology of Gansu Province, Lanzhou Veterinary Research Institute, Chinese Academy of Agricultural Science, Xujiaping 1, Lanzhou, Gansu 730046, P. R. China
Jiangsu Co-innovation Center for Prevention and Control of Important Animal Infectious Diseases and Zoonoses, Yangzhou 225009, P. R. China

Rana Majed Jamous, Mohammed Saleem Ali-Shtayeh and Salam Yousef Abu-Zaitoun
Biodiversity & Environmental Research Center - BERC, Til, Nablus, Palestine

Alex Markovics
Kimron Veterinary Institute, Ministry of Agriculture and Rural Development, Jerusalem, Israel

Hassan Azaizeh
The Institute of Applied Research, The Galilee Society, 20200 Shefa-Amr, Israel
Tel Hai College, Department of Environmental Science, 2208 Upper Galilee, Israel

Jana Sonnenburg
Federal Research Institute for Animal Health, Friedrich-Loeffler-Institut, Institute of Epidemiology, Südufer 10, 17493 Greifswald, Insel Riems, Germany
National Veterinary Institute, Technical University of Denmark, Bülowsvej 27, Building 1-6, 1870 Frederiksberg C, Denmark

Marie-Pierre Ryser-Degiorgis
Centre for Fish and Wildlife Health, Department Infectious Diseases and Pathobiology, Vetsuisse Faculty, University of Bern, Länggass-Str. 122, Postfach 8466, CH-3001 Bern, Switzerland

Thijs Kuiken
Department of Viroscience, Erasmus Medical Centre, 3000, CA, Rotterdam, The Netherlands

Ezio Ferroglio
Dipartimento di Scienze Veterinarie, Università degli Studi di Torino, Largo Paolo Braccini, 2 (già Via L. DaVinci, 44), 10095 Grugliasco, TO, Italy

Rainer G. Ulrich
Federal Research Institute for Animal Health, Institute of Novel and Emerging Infectious Diseases, Friedrich-Loeffler-Institut, Südufer 10, 17493 Greifswald, Insel Riems, Germany

Franz J. Conraths and Christoph Staubach
Federal Research Institute for Animal Health, Friedrich-Loeffler-Institut, Institute of Epidemiology, Südufer 10, 17493 Greifswald, Insel Riems, Germany

Christian Gortázar
SaBio Instituto de Investigaciónen Recursos Cinegéticos IREC Universidad de Castilla—La Mancha & CSIC, Ronda de Toledo s/n, 13071 Ciudad Real, Spain

Hung-Hsun Yen and Helen M. S. Davies
Faculty of Veterinary and Agricultural Sciences, The University of Melbourne, Parkville, Victoria 3010, Australia

Maria Raquel V. Cosate, Tetsu Sakamoto, Tiago Antônio de Oliveira Mendes and José Miguel Ortega
Instituto de Ciências Biológicas, Departamento de Bioquímica e Imunologia, Universidade Federal de Minas Gerais, Belo Horizonte, MG, Brazil

Élvio C. Moreira, Camila S. F. Oliveira, Rômulo C. Leite and João Paulo Haddad
Departamento de Medicina Veterinária Preventiva, Escola de Veterinária, Universidade Federal de Minas Gerais, Belo Horizonte, MG, Brazil

Carlos G. Regis da Silva
Laboratório de Biologia Parasitária, Centro de Pesquisas Gonçalo Moniz- Fiocruz, Salvador, BA, Brazil

Bruno S. A. F. Brasil
Embrapa Agroenergia, Brasília, Brazil

Vasco Ariston de Azevedo
Universidade Federal de Minas Gerais, Departamento de Genética - Instituto de Ciências Biol'ogicas de Minas Gerais, Belo Horizonte, Brazil

Evelyn Walker
Centre for Animal Health Innovation, Faculty of Science, Health, Education & Engineering, University of the Sunshine Coast, Maroochydore, QLD, Australia
Central West Local Land Services, Dubbo & Coonabarabran, NSW, Australia

Cecily Moore
Central West Local Land Services, Dubbo & Coonabarabran, NSW, Australia

Patrick Shearer
State Veterinary Diagnostic Laboratory, Elizabeth Macarthur Agricultural Institute, Menangle, NSW, Australia

Martina Jelocnik, Sankhya Bommana, Peter Timms and Adam Polkinghorne
Centre for Animal Health Innovation, Faculty of Science, Health, Education & Engineering, University of the Sunshine Coast, Maroochydore, QLD, Australia

Zsuzsa Kreizinger, Dénes Grózner, Kinga M. Sulyok, Kristin Nilsson, Veronika Hrivnák and Miklós Gyuranecz
Institute for Veterinary Medical Research, Centre for Agricultural Research, Hungarian Academy of Sciences, Hungária körút 21, Budapest 1143, Hungary

Dušan Benčina
Biotechnical Faculty, University of Ljubljana, Groblje 3, SI-1230 Domžale, Slovenia

Arya Sobhakumari, Robert H. Poppenga and J. Brad Pesavento
California Animal Health and Food Safety Laboratory System, Davis branch, School of Veterinary Medicine, University of California Davis, Davis, USA

Francisco A. Uzal
California Animal Health and Food Safety Laboratory System, San Bernardino branch, School of Veterinary Medicine, University of California Davis, 105 W Central Ave, San Bernardino, CA 92408, USA

Yunjeong Kim, Changin Oh, Vinay Shivanna, Richard A. Hesse and Kyeong-Ok Chang
Diagnostic Medicine and pathobiology, College of Veterinary Medicine, Kansas State University, 1800 Denison Avenue, Manhattan, KS 66506, USA

Pãmella A. Macêdo-Sales
Applied Microbiology e Parasitology Postgraduation Program, Fluminense Federal University (UFF), Niterói, RJ, Brazil

Simone R. L. S. Souto
Veterinary Medicine Postgraduation Program, Fluminense Federal University (UFF), Niterói, RJ, Brazil

Carolina A. Destefani, Ricardo P. Lucena, Ricardo Luiz D. Machado, Marcia R. Pinto, Elisabeth M. S. Rocha and Andréa Regina S. Baptista
Medical and Molecular Mycology Laboratory, Microbiology and Parasitology Department, Biomedical Institute, Fluminense Federal University (UFF), Rua Prof. Hernani Melo, 101 São Domingos, Niterói, RJ CEP: 24210-130, Brazil

Anderson M. Rodrigues
Microbiology, Immunology and Parasitology Department, São Paulo Federal University (UNIFESP), São Paulo, SP, Brazil

Leila M. Lopes-Bezerra
Cellular Mycology and Fungal Proteomics Laboratory, Rio de Janeiro State University (UERJ), Rio de Janeiro, RJ, Brazil

Marianne Kaiser and Stine Jacobsen
Department of Veterinary Clinical Sciences, Faculty of Health and Medical Sciences, Copenhagen University, Højbakkegård Alle 5, 2630 Taastrup, Denmark

Magdalena Jacobson and Pia Haubro Andersen
Department of Clinical Sciences, Faculty of Veterinary Medicine and Animal Science, Swedish University of Agricultural Sciences, SE-750 07 Uppsala, Sweden

Poul Bækbo
SEGES, Danish Pig Research Center, Danish Agriculture & Food Council, Agro Food Park 15, 8200 Aarhus N, Denmark

José Joaquin Cerón and Damián Escribano
Department of Animal Medicine and Surgery, Regional "Campus of Excellence Mare Nostrum", University of Murcia, 30100 Espinardo, Murcia, Spain

Jan Dahl
Danish Agriculture and Food Council, Axelborg, Axeltorv 3, 1709 Copenhagen V, Denmark

Zuoyong Zhou, Hexian Li, Haoyue Yang, Xiaoxia Li, Xinyue Song and Zhiying Wang
College of Animal Science, Rongchang Campus of Southwest University, No. 160 Xueyuan Road, Rongchang District, Chongqing 402460, China
Veterinary Science Engineering Research Center of Chongqing, No. 160 Xueyuan Road, Rongchang District, Chongqing 402460, China

Mengsi Zhang
College of Animal Science, Rongchang Campus of Southwest University, No. 160 Xueyuan Road, Rongchang District, Chongqing 402460, China
Veterinary Science Engineering Research Center of Chongqing, No. 160 Xueyuan Road, Rongchang District, Chongqing 402460, China
College of Veterinary Medicine and State Key Laboratory of Agrobiotechnology, China Agricultural University, No. 2 Yuanmingyuan West Road, Haidian District, Beijing 100193, China

Hua Li, Ting Li, Yujie Guo, Yujun Li, Yan Zhang, Na Teng, Fumiao Zhang and Guiwen Yang
Shandong Provincial Key Laboratory of Animal Resistance Biology, College of Life Sciences, Shandong Normal University, No. 88 East Wenhua Road, Jinan 250014, People's Republic of China

Index